250 Cases in Clinical Medicine

SIXTH EDITION

250 Cases in Clinical Medicine

EIRINI V. KASFIKI
Consultant Physician
Hull University Teaching Hospitals NHS Trust
Hull, United Kingdom

CIARAN W.P. KELLY
General Practitioner
The Old Fire Station Surgery
Beverley, United Kingdom

For additional online content visit eBooks+.com

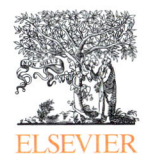

ELSEVIER

© 2024, Elsevier Limited. All rights reserved.

First edition 1997
Second edition 1999
Third edition 2002
Fourth edition 2012
Reprinted 2012 (twice), 2014, 2015
Fifth edition 2019

The right of Eirini V. Kasfiki and Ciaran W.P. Kelly to be identified as authors of this work has been asserted by them in accordance with the Copyright, Designs and Patents Act 1988.

No part of this publication may be reproduced or transmitted in any form or by any means, electronic or mechanical, including photocopying, recording, or any information storage and retrieval system, without permission in writing from the publisher. Details on how to seek permission, further information about the Publisher's permissions policies and our arrangements with organizations such as the Copyright Clearance Center and the Copyright Licensing Agency, can be found at our website: www.elsevier.com/permissions.

This book and the individual contributions contained in it are protected under copyright by the Publisher (other than as may be noted herein).

Notices

Practitioners and researchers must always rely on their own experience and knowledge in evaluating and using any information, methods, compounds or experiments described herein. Because of rapid advances in the medical sciences, in particular, independent verification of diagnoses and drug dosages should be made. To the fullest extent of the law, no responsibility is assumed by Elsevier, authors, editors or contributors for any injury and/or damage to persons or property as a matter of products liability, negligence or otherwise, or from any use or operation of any methods, products, instructions, or ideas contained in the material herein.

ISBN: 978-0-323-93786-3
978-0-323-93812-9

Content Strategist: Alexandra Mortimer
Content Project Manager: Tapajyoti Chaudhuri
Cover Designer: Patrick C. Ferguson
Marketing Manager: Deborah Watkins

Printed in Poland

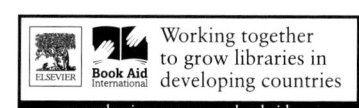

Last digit is the print number: 9 8 7 6 5 4 3 2 1

For Claudia-Maria

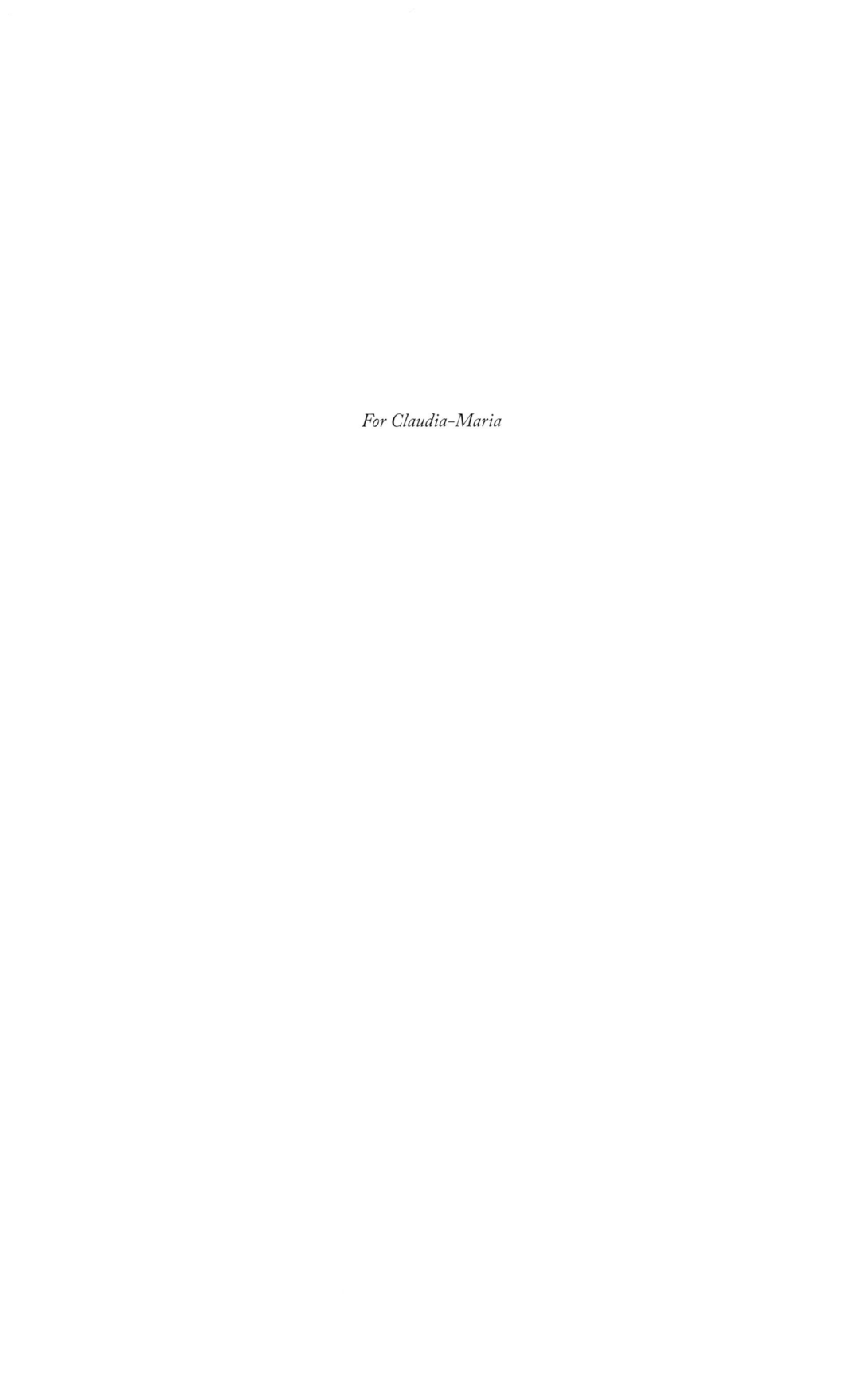

CONTENTS

Preface   xvii

Acknolwedgements   xix

SECTION I   **Respiratory Cases**   **1**

1. Respiratory Case   2
2. Asthma   6
3. Bronchiectasis   10
4. Cystic Fibrosis   15
5. Chronic Obstructive Pulmonary Disease   20
6. Idiopathic Pulmonary Fibrosis   28
7. Cor Pulmonale   33
8. Cough   35
9. Fever   37
10. Collapsed Lung   41
11. Obstructive Sleep Apnoea   43
12. Bronchogenic Carcinoma   46
13. Pulmonary Tuberculosis   50

SECTION II   **Cardiology Cases**   **53**

14. Cardiovascular Case   54
15. Aortic Regurgitation   58
16. Aortic Stenosis   63
17. Mixed Aortic Valve Disease   70
18. Mitral Regurgitation   72
19. Mitral Stenosis   76
20. Mitral Valve Prolapse   83
21. Mixed Mitral Valve Disease   86
22. Mixed Mitral and Aortic Valve Disease   88

23	Prosthetic Heart Valves	90
24	Tricuspid Regurgitation	93
25	Pulmonary Stenosis	96
26	Atrial Septal Defect	100
27	Ventricular Septal Defect	106
28	Patent Ductus Arteriosus	110
29	Ebstein's Anomaly	113
30	Fallot's Tetralogy	116
31	Dextrocardia	121
32	Eisenmenger Syndrome	123
33	Hypertrophic Cardiomyopathy	127
34	Congestive Cardiac Failure	132
35	Constrictive Pericarditis	136
36	Weight Loss	139

SECTION III *Abdominal Cases* 145

37	Abdominal Case	146
38	Swallowing Difficulties	149
39	Diarrhoea	152
40	Crohn's Disease	155
41	Abdominal Mass	159
42	Ascites	161
43	Cirrhosis of the Liver	165
44	Jaundice	170
45	Hepatomegaly	173
46	Splenomegaly	176
47	Haemochromatosis	179
48	Wilson Disease	183
49	Felty Syndrome	186

CONTENTS

SECTION IV *Renal Cases* *189*

50 Unilateral Palpable Kidney 190

51 Polycystic Kidney Disease 192

52 Nephrotic Syndrome 197

53 Transplanted Kidney 200

54 Hypertension 203

SECTION V *Haematology Cases* *209*

55 Anaemia 210

56 Bruising 215

57 Multiple Myeloma 218

58 Myelodysplastic Syndrome 222

59 Chronic Lymphocytic Leukaemia 225

60 Chronic Myeloid Leukaemia 228

61 Acute Leukaemia 231

62 Lymphadenopathy 235

SECTION VI *Rheumatology Cases* *241*

63 Rheumatology Case 242

64 Ankylosing Spondylitis 247

65 Charcot Arthropathy 251

66 Ehlers–Danlos Syndrome 254

67 Gout 258

68 Osteoarthritis 262

69 Psoriatic Arthritis 266

70 Rheumatoid Hands 269

71 Dermatomyositis—Proximal Muscle Weakness 275

72 Scleroderma 279

73 Systemic Lupus Erythematosus 284

74 Small-Vessel ANCA-Associated Vasculitis 290

SECTION VII **Endocrinology Cases** 295

- 75 Acromegaly   296
- 76 Hypopituitarism (Simmonds Disease)   300
- 77 Endocrinology Case   302
- 78 Graves Disease   305
- 79 Orbitopathy   310
- 80 Multinodular Goitre   315
- 81 Hypothyroidism   319
- 82 Hypoparathyroidism   325
- 83 Primary Hyperparathyroidism   328
- 84 Addison Disease   331
- 85 Cushing Syndrome   334
- 86 Carcinoid Syndrome   338
- 87 Gynaecomastia   341
- 88 Falls—Osteoporosis   343
- 89 Obesity   346
- 90 Type 1 Diabetes   351
- 91 Type 2 Diabetes Mellitus   354
- 92 Diabetic Foot   358

SECTION VIII **Eye Cases for Internal Medicine** 363

- 93 The Eye Case   364
- 94 Age-Related Macular Degeneration   366
- 95 Cataracts   371
- 96 Cholesterol Embolus in the Fundus   373
- 97 Diabetic Retinopathy   376
- 98 Hypertensive Retinopathy   383
- 99 Optic Atrophy   387
- 100 Osteogenesis Imperfecta   390
- 101 Papilloedema   392
- 102 Retinal Detachment   396

103 Retinal Vein Occlusion 399

104 Retinitis Pigmentosa 402

105 Subhyaloid Haemorrhage 405

106 Vitreous Opacities 408

SECTION IX **Dermatology Cases for Internal Medicine** *409*

107 Acanthosis Nigricans 411

108 Acne Vulgaris 413

109 Alopecia Areata 416

110 Arterial Leg Ulcer 419

111 Arteriovenous Fistula 422

112 Atopic Dermatitis—Eczema 425

113 Bullous Eruption 428

114 Mycosis Fungoides (Cutaneous T-Cell Lymphoma) 432

115 Dermatitis Herpetiformis 435

116 Eruptive Xanthomata 438

117 Erythema Ab Igne 440

118 Erythema Multiforme 443

119 Erythema Nodosum 446

120 Fungal Nail Disease 448

121 Hairy Leukoplakia 452

122 Henoch–Schönlein Purpura 454

123 Hereditary Haemorrhagic Telangiectasia (Osler–Weber–Rendu Syndrome) 458

124 Herpes Simplex 462

125 Herpes Zoster Syndrome (Shingles) 465

126 Ichthyosis 468

127 Lichen Planus 471

128 Lichen Simplex 474

129 Lipodystrophy 476

130 Lupus Pernio 479

131 Maculopapular Rash 483

132 Malignant Melanoma   485
133 Molluscum Contagiosum   489
134 Nail Changes   491
135 Necrobiosis Lipoidica   494
136 Neurofibromatosis   496
137 Onycholysis   501
138 Palmar Xanthomata   503
139 Peutz–Jeghers Syndrome   505
140 Phlebitis Migrans   508
141 Pretibial Myxoedema   510
142 Pseudoxanthoma Elasticum   513
143 Psoriasis   517
144 Purpura   521
145 Pyoderma Gangrenosum   523
146 Raynaud's Phenomenon   527
147 Rosacea   530
148 Seborrhoeic Dermatitis   532
149 Sturge–Weber Syndrome (Encephalotrigeminal Angiomatosis)   535
150 Tuberous Sclerosis (Bourneville or Pringle Disease)   539
151 Urticaria   544
152 Urticaria Pigmentosa   547
153 Venous Ulcer   549
154 Vitiligo   553
155 Xanthelasma   556
156 Xanthomata   558

SECTION X **Neurology and Elderly Care Medical Cases   561**

157 Neurology Case   563
158 Headache   573
159 Memory Loss   577
160 Lower Urinary Tract Symptoms   581

161	Abnormal Gait	583
162	Argyll Robertson Pupil	586
163	Muscular Dystrophy	588
164	Spastic Paraplegia	592
165	Bitemporal Hemianopia	596
166	Brown-Séquard Syndrome	597
167	Carpal Tunnel Syndrome	599
168	Central Scotoma	603
169	Cerebellar Syndrome	605
170	Cerebellar Dysarthria	608
171	Cerebellopontine Angle Tumour	610
172	Charcot–Marie–Tooth Disease (Peroneal Muscular Atrophy)	613
173	Chorea	617
174	Lateral Popliteal Nerve Palsy, L4, L5 (Common Peroneal Nerve Palsy)	621
175	Expressive Dysphasia	623
176	Facioscapulohumeral Dystrophy (Landouzy–Déjérine Syndrome)	627
177	Friedreich's Ataxia	630
178	Hemiballismus	633
179	Hemiplegia	635
180	Homonymous Hemianopia	642
181	Internuclear Ophthalmoplegia	644
182	Jerky Nystagmus	647
183	Limb-Girdle Dystrophy	649
184	Motor Neurone Disease	652
185	Multiple Sclerosis	657
186	Multiple System Atrophy	664
187	Myasthenia Gravis	668
188	Myotonia Congenita	672
189	Myotonic Dystrophy	674
190	Parkinson Disease	679

191 Peripheral Neuropathy 687
192 Proximal Myopathy 690
193 Pseudobulbar Palsy 692
194 Ptosis and Horner Syndrome 694
195 Radial Nerve Palsy 699
196 Seventh Cranial Nerve Palsy 702
197 Sixth Cranial Nerve Palsy 707
198 Syringomyelia 709
199 Tetraplegia 714
200 Third Cranial Nerve Palsy 717
201 Tremor 720
202 Deformity of a Lower Limb 724
203 Ulnar Nerve Palsy 728
204 Wallenberg Syndrome (Lateral Medullary Syndrome) 732
205 Wasting of the Small Muscles of the Hand 734
206 Long Thoracic Neuropathy 737
207 Anxiety 739
208 Back Pain 741
209 Pruritus 744
210 Speech Disturbance 748
211 Unsteadiness 751

SECTION XI **Acute Internal Medical Cases** 755

212 Absent Radial Pulse 757
213 Confusion 761
214 Acute Kidney Injury 765
215 Acute Pancreatitis 768
216 Anaphylaxis 772
217 Chest Pain—Angina 777
218 Cauda Equina Syndrome 782

219	Cellulitis	784
220	Coarctation of Aorta	787
221	Deep Vein Thrombosis	792
222	Gallop Rhythm	797
223	Guillain–Barré Syndrome	800
224	Hyperkalaemia	804
225	Hypernatraemia	806
226	Hypokalaemia	809
227	Hyponatraemia	812
228	Melaena	816
229	Paracetamol Overdose	821
230	Pericardial Rub	824
231	Pleural Effusion	827
232	Sepsis	834
233	Consolidation	838
234	Pulmonary Embolism	843
235	Jugular Venous Pulse	846
236	Seizures	849
237	Painful Knee Joint	853
238	Slow Pulse Rate	855
239	Spontaneous Pneumothorax	859
240	Subacute Combined Degeneration of the Spinal Cord	864
241	Subarachnoid Haemorrhage	868
242	Syncope	872
243	The Pregnant Patient	879
244	Central Line Insertion	883
245	Chest Drain Insertion for Spontaneous (Nontraumatic) Pneumothorax	886
246	Emergency Synchronized Direct Current Cardioversion	889
247	Knee Arthrocentesis	892
248	Lumbar Puncture	895

249 Therapeutic Abdominal Paracentesis 897

250 Temporary External Pacing 900

Bibliography 903

Index 907

PREFACE

The art of medicine consists in amusing the patient while nature cures the disease.

Voltaire

It is much more important to know what sort of a patient has a disease than what sort of disease a patient has.

William Osler

On the bookshelf of the medical section of my chosen bookshop at medical school, I found a host of learned tomes on the hows, whys and wherefores of recognizing, diagnosing and treating illness, and yet more learned, heavier and more expensive encyclopaedias written on the minutiae of diseases that I had not heard of then and certainly have never seen since. The reason I picked *250 Clinical Cases in Medicine* from this morass of literature is that while imparting sound clinical knowledge and handy examination tips, it also made a good read. Voltaire says that the art of medicine is amusing the patient and I think that the art of medical education is to amuse the doctor (or medical student) while their natural intelligence soaks up the knowledge. This is a book that does that.

Like medicine itself however, books instructing students must also evolve with the times. Baliga's book has evolved from its first iteration describing illnesses and the characteristics of the patients afflicted, together with a shortened history of the medicine surrounding the identification of the disease, into an essential preparation text for candidates for medical examinations.

Medical curricula change to reflect the changing roles of doctors and the changing face of disease. Treatments and advances in technology move at an ever more dizzying pace and it takes a doctor committed to continuing professional development to keep up. This edition has been updated to reflect the changing form of the Royal College of Physicians (RCP) curriculum so that some chapters from the previous edition have been dispensed with entirely to allow new, more clinically relevant topics to be included. A recognition that patients rarely come with a sign or badge declaring their diagnosis has led to the addition of symptom-based chapters and the inclusion of acute medical problems and their management.

Astute clinicians utilize gist-based reasoning to arrive at diagnoses based on pattern recognition; however, it is not sufficient to try and pass an examination simply by seeing patients. There is a pre-requisite level of knowledge that is required in order to manage patients in the real world and pass an examination. This book is best used by seeing representative patients who present with the illnesses described and, crucially, presenting your findings to colleagues, so that by the time it comes to the exam the findings are articulated slickly and confidently to the examiners. Style can matter as much as substance, and this only happens with practice. The sixth edition of this book continues to be useful for MBBS, PLAB, MRCP (UK), MRCPI, MD (New Zealand, Malaysia, Singapore, India, Pakistan, Sri Lanka and Bangladesh), FRACP, FCCP and postgraduate medical examinations in the USA including United States Medical Licensing Examination (USMLE) and American Board of Internal Medicine (ABIM). The structure of each case remains unchanged and is discussed under the following headings: Instruction: This is the information typically given to the candidate at the start of their examination. Salient Features: This is the basic information that the candidate will be expected to elicit and includes aspects of the history, clinical examination and what to tell the examiner in order to satisfy the examiner that the candidate has reached a 'safe' level to be a competent clinician.

Diagnosis: In most cases, candidates will be expected to reach a diagnosis based on their findings. This section is designed to help the candidate to present their diagnosis in a clear and confident manner.

Questions: Common 'viva voce' examination questions and answers are provided in this section. Although not an exhaustive list of questions, these are typical of the questions that would be asked by examiners. Some cases have 'advanced-level questions' which may be asked by examiners when they feel a candidate could demonstrate excellence and deserves the opportunity to demonstrate their clinical acumen.

Some cases have key resources, references and a historical background. This knowledge is certainly not expected from the candidate and has little relevance to patient management, but wider knowledge such as this communicates to the examiner that the candidate is clearly of the right standard to be successful and may give them leeway to soften their questioning for other cases. A happy examiner leads to a happy candidate.

Good luck!

Ciaran W.P. Kelly

ACKNOLWEDGEMENTS

The authors gratefully acknowledge the contributions of Dr Evangelia Florou, Consultant Pulmonologist, and Dr Radhika Raghunath, Consultant Rheumatologist.

The publisher would also like to acknowledge and thank Ragavendra R. Baliga for laying the excellent foundations of this title over earlier editions.

SECTION I

Respiratory Cases

SECTION OUTLINE

1. Respiratory Case
2. Asthma
3. Bronchiectasis
4. Cystic Fibrosis
5. Chronic Obstructive Pulmonary Disease
6. Idiopathic Pulmonary Fibrosis
7. Cor Pulmonale
8. Cough
9. Fever
10. Collapsed Lung
11. Obstructive Sleep Apnoea
12. Bronchogenic Carcinoma
13. Pulmonary Tuberculosis

CHAPTER 1

Respiratory Case

Instruction

Examine this patient's respiratory system.

Salient Features

HISTORY

- Cough
- Sputum
- Haemoptysis (acute infection, including in chronic obstructive pulmonary disease (COPD), pulmonary infarction, bronchogenic carcinoma, bronchiectasis, tuberculosis, Goodpasture syndrome, pulmonary haemosiderosis, mitral stenosis)
- Degree of dyspnoea: what the patient can do without becoming breathless:
    - Normal
    - Walk normally on the level but not on stairs or hills
    - Walk on the level for 1.5 km (1 mile) but cannot keep up with people of a similar age
    - Walk about 1.5 km (1 mile) on the level
    - Breathless at rest or on minimal effort
- Onset of dyspnoea:
    - Intermittent: asthma, recurrent pulmonary oedema, exacerbations of COPD
    - Over days: pleural fluid, carcinoma of bronchus, heart failure
    - Over months to years: COPD, fibrosing alveolitis, anaemia, fibrotic lung disease
    - Over a few hours: pulmonary oedema, bronchial asthma, pneumonia
    - Acute or sudden: pneumothorax, pulmonary oedema, inhaled foreign body
- Wheezing: airways limitation including asthma, COPD
- Chest pain: pleurisy, tracheitis
- Smoking
- Family history.

EXAMINATION

- Place the patient in a sitting position and ask whether he or she is comfortable.
- Examine the sputum cup and comment on the sputum.
- Examine the patient from the foot end of the bed and comment as follows:
    - Whether the patient is breathless at rest
    - On wasting, if any, in the infraclavicular region
    - On diminished movement on the right or left side
    - Count the respiratory rate
    - Comment on pattern of breathing (Fig. 1.1).
- Examine the hands:
    - Clubbing

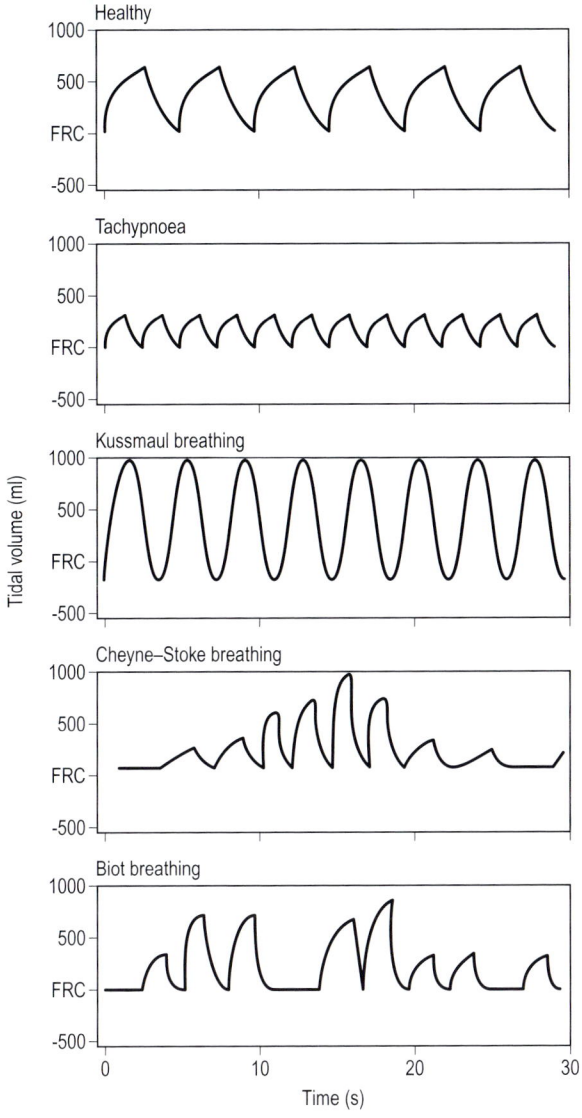

Fig. 1.1 Different patterns of breathing. *FRC*, functional residual capacity. (Mettler, F.A., 2004. *Essentials of Radiology*, second edn. Saunders-Elsevier, Philadelphia, PA.)

- Cyanosis
- Tar staining (The yellow 'nicotine' staining is actually tar.)
- Examine the pulse for bounding pulse and asterixis: signs of carbon monoxide narcosis.
- Examine the face:
    - Comment on the tongue, looking for central cyanosis.
    - Comment on the eyes, looking for pallor and evidence of Horner syndrome.
- Examine the neck:
    - Comment on neck veins.
    - Check for cervical lymphadenopathy.

- Comment on the trachea: any deviation, distance between the cricoid cartilage and suprasternal notch.
- Palpate:
  - Apex beat
  - Movements on both sides with the fingers symmetrically placed in the intercostal spaces on both sides
  - Vocal fremitus (Tell the examiner that you would prefer to do vocal resonance because it gives the same information and is more reliable.)
- Percussion: percuss over supraclavicular areas, clavicles, upper, middle, and lower chest on both sides.
- Auscultation:
  - Over the supraclavicular areas, upper, middle, and lower chest on both sides: comment on breath sounds (whether vesicular or bronchial) and on adventitious sounds (wheeze, crackles, or pleural rub).
  - If crackles are heard, ask the patient to cough and then repeat auscultation. It is important to time the crackles to ascertain whether they occur in early, mid, or late inspiration.
  - While auscultating the front of the chest, seize the opportunity to listen to the second pulmonary sound.
  - Check for vocal resonance by asking the patient to repeat 'one, one, one'.
  - Check for forced expiratory time (FET) if your diagnosis is COPD by asking the patient to exhale forcefully after full inspiration while you are listening over the trachea: if the patient takes more than 6 s, airway disease is indicated (be prepared to discuss spirometry findings; Fig. 1.2).
- Ask the patient to sit forward:
  - Palpate: assess expansion posteriorly
  - Percuss: on both sides including axillae
  - Auscultate: posteriorly including the axillae.
- Remember to look for signs of middle lobe disease in the right axilla and correlate your findings with common clinical conditions.

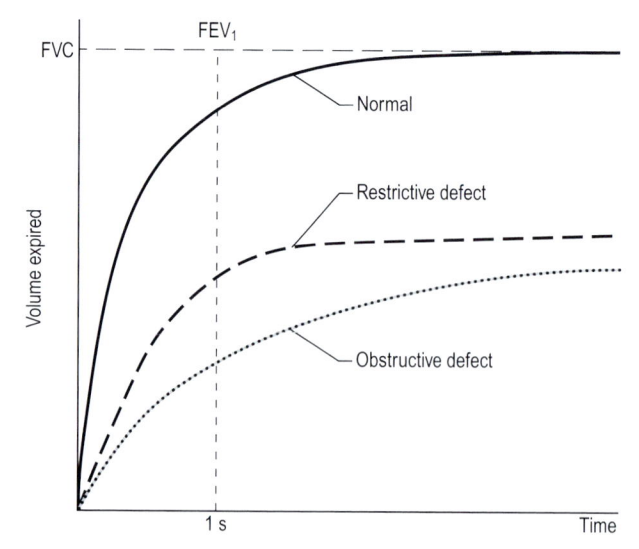

Fig. 1.2 Typical spirometry. *FEV1*, forced expiratory volume in 1 s; *FVC*, forced vital capacity.

1—RESPIRATORY CASE

Tell the examiner you would like to do a chest X-ray or chest computed tomography (and be prepared to comment on the findings):
- Normal: airways disease, neuromuscular disease, pulmonary emboli, anaemia
- Abnormal lung fields: pleural thickening, effusion, tumour, lobar collapse, diffuse infiltration
- Abnormal mediastinum: lymphadenopathy, large pulmonary vessels
- Cardiomegaly with upper lobe blood diversion: pericardial effusion, left ventricular failure.

Questions

Name some respiratory diseases that produce an obstructive picture on spirometry and diseases that produce a restrictive pattern.
Emphysema, asthma, bronchiectasis, and bronchitis can give an obstructive picture on spirometry, whereas interstitial lung disease, pulmonary oedema, pulmonary haemorrhages, and skeletal defects can give a restrictive pattern.

Name some causes of increased and decreased diffuse capacity of carbon monoxide (KCO).
KCO is decreased in all cases with restrictive patterns with the exception of pulmonary haemorrhage, where it is increased, and skeletal deformities where it can be normal or decreased. KCO is also decreased with all obstructive patterns with the exception of acute asthma attacks when it can be decreased, normal, or increased. Increased KCO is seen in polycythaemia and in left to right shunt.

How do respiratory flow loops look in obstructive and restrictive disease?
The normal flow loop is shown (Fig. 1.3). Here the inspiratory flow limb is semicircular and the expiratory flow limb is triangular. In obstructive airway disease, the initial peak of expiration is not as high as in normal spirometry, and the peak is followed by a flatter curve than normal. In restrictive disease the flow loop looks like the normal loop with the difference that the total lung volume is much smaller than expected.

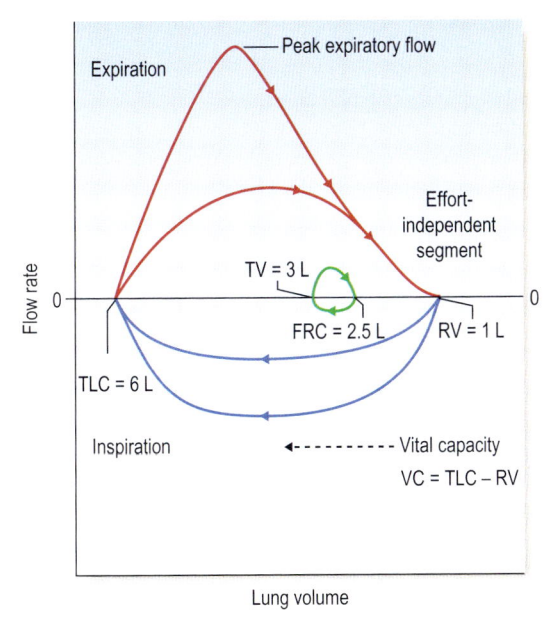

Fig. 1.3 Normal flow–volume loop for increasing inspirations. Both meet in a common effort-independent segment. A normal tidal volume (TV) breath is shown. *FRC*, Functional respiratory capacity; *RV*, residual volume; *TLC*, total lung capacity. (With permission from Donaldson, G., Naish, J., Syndercombe Court, D., 2019. Medical Sciences, third edn, Elsevier.)

CHAPTER 2

Asthma

Instruction

Examine this patient's chest.

Salient Features

HISTORY

- History of reversible airway obstruction: wheezing and breathlessness
- Daily or seasonal variation of the symptoms
- Chest tightness
- Recurrent cough
- Exacerbation of cough or wheeze at night or after exercise
- Improvement of the cough or wheeze with bronchodilator therapy
- Fever, yellowish sputum
- History of atopy (eczema, hay fever)
- History of rhinitis, nasal polyps
- History of trigger factors such as cold air, emotion, vapours, dust, drugs (e.g. beta-blockers), pollution, viral infections, pets, pollen.

EXAMINATION

- Bilateral scattered expiratory polyphonic wheeze
- Examine the sputum cup.

Comment on accessory muscles of respiration, tachycardia, pulsus paradoxus, and if the patient can speak in sentences without stopping to take a breath.

Diagnosis

This patient has a history of hay fever and bilateral scattered wheeze (lesion) caused by bronchial asthma (aetiology) and is breathless at rest (functional status).

Questions

Mention a few trigger factors known to aggravate asthma.
- Infection
- Emotion
- Exercise
- Drugs, e.g. beta-blockers
- External allergens.

2—ASTHMA

What do you understand by the term asthma?
Asthma is an inflammatory disorder characterized by hyperresponsiveness of the airway to various stimuli, resulting in widespread narrowing of the airways. The changes are reversible, either spontaneously or with therapy. The inflammatory response includes T-lymphocytes, mast cells, and eosinophils and is associated with exudation of plasma, oedema, smooth muscle hypertrophy, deposition of matrix, mucus plugging, and epithelial damage.

What are some objective tests for diagnosing asthma and when are they considered to be positive?
- Fractional exhaled nitric oxide (FeNO)—a positive test is >40 ppb.
- Formal spirometry with bronchodilator reversibility test—asthma has an obstructive picture with a ratio of forced expiratory volume in 1 second/forced vital capacity (FEV1/FVC) <70% with 12% improvement in FEV1 postbronchodilator.
- Peak flow variability—a variability in peak expiratory flow (PEF) of more than 20% is considered consistent with a diagnosis of asthma.
- Direct bronchial challenge with histamine or methacholine—when provocative concentration of methacholine causes FEV1 to fall more than 20%, the test is considered positive.

What do you understand by intrinsic asthma?
Intrinsic asthma is of nonallergic aetiology and usually begins after the age of 30 years. It tends to be more continuous and more severe; status asthmaticus is common in this group.

What do you understand by extrinsic asthma?
Extrinsic asthma has a clearly defined history of allergy to a variety of inhaled factors and is characterized by a childhood onset and seasonal variation.

What are the indications for steroids in chronic asthma?
- Sleep is disturbed by wheeze.
- Morning tightness persists until midday.
- Symptoms and PEFs progressively deteriorate each day.
- Maximum treatment with bronchodilators not controlling symptoms.
- Emergency nebulizers are needed.

What is the effect of reducing or discontinuing inhaled budesonide in patients with mild asthma?
Early treatment with inhaled budesonide results in long-lasting control of mild asthma (i.e. the forced expiratory volume is >85% of predicted value). Maintenance therapy can usually be given at a reduced dose, but discontinuation of treatment is often accompanied by exacerbation of the disease.

How would you manage a patient with acute asthma?
- Nebulized beta-agonists, e.g. terbutaline or salbutamol
- Oxygen as needed to maintain normal oxygen saturations (94%–98%)
- High-dose steroids: intravenous hydrocortisone or oral prednisolone
- Blood gases monitoring
- Chest radiography to rule out pneumothorax.

When life-threatening features are present:
- Add ipratropium to nebulized beta-agonist.
- Intravenous magnesium sulphate, aminophylline or salbutamol or terbutaline.

What do you know about the British Thoracic Society step care regimen for the management of chronic asthma in adults?

Patients should be started on treatment at the step most appropriate to the initial severity. A rescue course of prednisolone may be needed at any time and at any step. Stepwise reduction in treatment should be undertaken after the asthma has been stable over a period of 3–6 months.

- Step 1: inhaled short-acting beta2-agonist (LABA) used as required for symptom relief
- Step 2: step 1 plus inhaled steroid therapy—inhaled corticosteroids (ICS) (equivalent to budesonide 400 µg/day)
- Step 3: step 2 plus a long-acting beta-2 agonist (LAMA) daily or increase the inhaled steroid
- In adults who still suffer from asthma exacerbations on step 3, consider combination inhaler (ICS-LAMA) daily or alternatively choose the maintenance and reliever therapy (MART), where a combination ICS-LABA inhaler is used both regularly and as needed.
- Consider adding a fourth drug such as leukotriene receptor antagonist (e.g. montelukast), sustained-release theophylline, long-acting muscarinic antagonist (tiotropium), and at the same time, patients who have reached this step of therapy would need a referral to a respiratory physician for further tests and escalation of treatment, such as:
  - Continuous use of oral or frequent steroids (low-dose oral steroids or maintain inhaled steroid at 2000 µg/day)
  - Monoclonal antibodies to minimize steroid therapy (omalizumab, mepolizumab, benralizumab, reslizumab)—newer agents are undergoing trials (astegolimab, tezepelumab)
  - If available, referral for bronchial thermoplasty.

What are the features of acute severe asthma?

- Inability to complete a sentence in one breath
- Respiration rate >25 breaths/min
- Pulse rate >110 beats/min
- PEF rate <50% of predicted or best.

What are the life-threatening indicators in acute asthma?

- PEF rate <33% of predicted or best
- Exhaustion, confusion, coma
- Silent chest, cyanosis, or feeble respiratory effort
- Bradycardia or hypotension.

Note: Arterial blood gases should be measured if *any* of these features are present or if oxygen saturation is <92%.

What are the indicators of a very severe, life-threatening attack?

- Normal (5–6 kPa, 36–45 mm Hg) or increased (>6 kPa or 45 mm Hg) carbon dioxide tension
- Severe hypoxia of <8 kPa (60 mm Hg)
- Low or falling arterial pH.

What is the value of assessing pulsus paradoxus in a patient with acute severe asthma?

It is a poor guide to the severity of acute asthma as it compares poorly with the measurement of peak flow.

In which other conditions is wheeze a prominent sign?
Chronic obstructive pulmonary disease (COPD), left ventricular failure (cardiac asthma), polyarteritis nodosa, eosinophilic lung disease, recurrent thromboembolism, tumour causing localized wheeze.

What are the indications for mechanical ventilation with intermittent positive pressure ventilation?
- Worsening hypoxia (arterial partial pressure of oxygen (PaO_2) <8 kPa) despite 60% inspired oxygen
- Hypercapnia ($PaCO_2$ >6 kPa)
- Drowsiness
- Unconsciousness.

What do you understand by the term severe brittle asthma?
This condition is characterized by life-threatening attacks, which can develop within hours or sometimes even within minutes and can lead to sudden death.

What do you know about beta-receptor polymorphisms in asthma?
- Glycine homozygous patients do well on regular beta2-agonists, whether short or long acting.
- Long- and short-acting beta2-agonists produce disparate responses: for example, a lack of increased bronchial hyper-responsiveness associated with LABAs but is commonly seen with short-acting beta2-agonists.
- All genotypes and beta2-agonists are associated with receptor desensitization but not associated with worsening asthma.

Can you describe some limitations when using LABA inhalers in asthma?
- The use of LABAs for asthma in patients of all ages is contraindicated without concomitant use of an asthma-controller medication such as an inhaled corticosteroid.
- Stop use of the LABA, if possible, once asthma control is achieved and maintain the use of an asthma-controller medication, such as an inhaled corticosteroid.
- Recommend against LABA use in patients whose asthma is adequately controlled with a low- or medium-dose inhaled corticosteroid.
- Recommend that a fixed-dose combination product containing a LABA and an inhaled corticosteroid be used to ensure compliance with concomitant therapy in paediatric and adolescent patients who require the addition of a LABA to an inhaled corticosteroid.

CHAPTER 3

Bronchiectasis

Instruction

This patient presented with productive cough and shortness of breath. Please examine.

Salient Features

HISTORY

- Cough with copious purulent sputum, recurrent haemoptysis
- Intermittent fever and night sweats
- History of recurrent chest infections
- Weight loss.

EXAMINATION

- Inspection of the room for oxygen, inhalers, sputum pots, nebulizer
- Copious purulent expectoration (remember to check the sputum cup in a chest case)
- Finger clubbing
- Scars from previous lung resection for localized bronchiectasis
- Mixed inspiratory and expiratory coarse crackles that alter with coughing.

Proceed as follows:
Comment on any signs of pulmonary hypertension (raised jugular venous pressure, parasternal heave, loud P2 component of second heart sound, and peripheral oedema).

Diagnosis

This patient has bilateral, coarse, late inspiratory crackles with purulent sputum (lesion) caused by bronchiectasis (aetiology) and is cyanosed at rest (functional status).

Questions

What do you understand by bronchiectasis?
Bronchiectasis is a respiratory condition characterized by persistent or recurrent bronchial inflammation related to irreversibly damaged and dilated bronchi.

Mention the causes of bronchiectasis.
- History of previous severe lower respiratory tract infections due to bacterial or viral pneumonia, pertussis, tuberculosis (TB), opportunistic mycobacteria
- Mechanical bronchial obstruction as in TB, malignancy, nodal compression, foreign body aspiration
- Allergic bronchopulmonary aspergillosis (ABPA)
- Underlying immune deficiency, particularly antibody deficiency

- Gastric aspiration
- Disorders of ciliary function (primary ciliary dyskinesia, Kartagener syndrome, Young syndrome)
- Cystic fibrosis
- Congenital defects of large airways such as Williams–Campbell syndrome (bronchial cartilage deficiency), tracheobronchomegaly (Mounier–Kuhn syndrome), Marfan syndrome, H-type tracheobronchial and oesophagobronchial fistula or sequestration
- Neuropathic disorders (Riley–Day syndrome, Chagas disease)
- Connective tissue disorders, e.g. rheumatoid arthritis
- Inflammatory bowel disease
- Primary bronchiolar disorders
- α1-antitrypsin deficiency
- Yellow nail syndrome.

What investigations would you do in such a patient?
- Full blood count
- Sputum culture
- Chest radiography
- High-resolution computed tomography (HRCT) of the chest to confirm the diagnosis
- Full lung function tests (usually obstructive pattern, but may be mixed)
- Immunoglobulin levels and serum electrophoresis, especially with a history of recurrent infections in younger patients
- Mutation analysis for the cystic fibrosis transmembrane conductance regulator gene (CFTR)
- Serum immunoglobulin E (IgE), serum IgE testing to *Aspergillus fumigatus* and *Aspergillus precipitins*
- Autoimmune screen, rheumatoid factor
- Bronchoscopy (suspicion of proximal obstruction).

How can computed tomography assess bronchiectasis?
HRCT is the radiological investigation of choice to establish the diagnosis of bronchiectasis (Fig. 3.1).

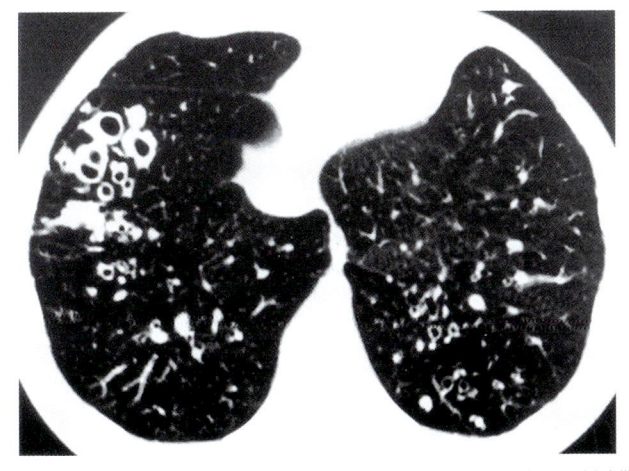

Fig. 3.1 Severe bronchiectasis in the right lower lobe with plugging of the dilated bronchi. Mild, cylindric bronchiectasis in the left lower lobe showing the signet ring sign. (With permission from Albert, R.K., Spiro, S.G., Jett, J.R., 2008. Clinical Respiratory Medicine, third edn. Mosby, Philadelphia, PA.)

Bronchial wall dilation in HRCT is defined by the internal lumen diameter being greater than the accompanying pulmonary artery or by lack of tapering. When the bronchiectatic bronchus with the accompanying vessel are seen in cross-section images, they may create the 'signet ring sign'. Bronchial wall thickening is often also present although is harder to define. Other nonspecific abnormalities found with HRCT are mucus plugging of the smaller peripheral and centrilobular airways producing V- and Y-shaped opacities, the so-called 'tree-in-bud' pattern. Furthermore, the larger plugged bronchi will be visible as lobulated or branching opacities and the mosaic attenuation pattern reflects coexisting constrictive obliterative bronchiolitis.

Is high-resolution computed tomography only helpful for diagnosing bronchiectasis?
Apart from being the gold standard for diagnosing bronchiectasis, it also gives information about the distribution of the disease, which can be helpful in identifying the underlying cause. The pattern of bronchiectasis and associated computed tomography (CT) features may be sufficiently characteristic for a specific underlying cause. Here are a few examples:
- Cystic fibrosis involves an upper-lobe distribution.
- ABPA changes are typically upper zone and central in distribution.
- Hypogammaglobulinaemia-related disease demonstrates a lower and middle lobe distribution of cylindrical bronchiectasis with marked bronchial wall thickening.
- Tracheobronchomegaly (Mounier-Kuhn syndrome) may be identified because of the marked dilation of the major airways and grape-like bronchiectasis.
- In opportunist mycobacterial infection, notably *Mycobacterium avium intracellulare* complex is characterized by a triad of mild bronchiectasis concentrated in the right middle lobe and lingula, a 'tree-in-bud' pattern, and randomly scattered (+/− cavitated) nodules 1 to 2 cm in diameter.

What is the difference between standard and high-resolution computed tomography?
In standard CT, the resolution is 10 mm thick, whereas with HRCT, the slices are 1 to 1.5 mm thick and high-spatial-resolution algorithms are used to reconstruct images.

What are the complications of bronchiectasis?
- Pneumonia, pleurisy, pleural effusion, pneumothorax
- Sinusitis
- Haemoptysis (life-threatening haemoptysis is >600 mL/day)
- Brain abscess
- Amyloidosis.

What are the major respiratory pathogens in bronchiectasis?
Staphylococcus aureus, *Haemophilus influenzae*, and *Pseudomonas aeruginosa*. *H. influenzae* is the most frequently isolated pathogen, followed by *P. aeruginosa*, *Streptococcus pneumoniae*, *S. aureus*, and *Moraxella catarrhalis*, and atypical mycobacteria are also seen. Aspergillus species are reported in a small number of patients.

Interestingly, during the COVID-19 pandemic (2020–2021) there was a major reduction (about 60%) in hospitalizations from bronchiectasis exacerbations. This is believed to have occurred from the reduced exposure to respiratory viruses and pathogens due to global infection transmission measures.

How would you treat such patients?
- Identification of acute exacerbations and administration of antibiotics
- Sputum cultures
- Treatment of underlying conditions
- Promotion of airway clearance techniques

3 — BRONCHIECTASIS

- Identification and treatment of underlying cause to prevent disease
- Maintenance or improvement of pulmonary function
- Improvement of quality of life by reducing daily symptoms and exacerbations
- Pulmonary rehabilitation (regular physiotherapy-led techniques for airway clearance is the single most important long-term intervention and the cornerstone of treatment for bronchiectasis)
- Bronchodilators (check airflow obstruction for reversibility to bronchodilators and provide therapy where lung function or symptoms improve with therapy)
- Control of bronchial haemorrhage (bronchial artery embolization and/or surgery)
- Surgery in selected cases: surgical removal of extremely damaged segments or lobes that may be a nidus for infection or bleeding
- Oxygen therapy/noninvasive ventilation in cases of respiratory failure.

What abnormalities may be associated with bronchiectasis?
- Congenital absence of bronchial cartilage (Williams–Campbell syndrome)
- Tracheobronchomegaly (Mounier–Kuhn syndrome)
- Obstructive azoospermia and chronic sinopulmonary infection (Young syndrome), said to be caused by mercury intoxication. First described in the north of England by Young in 1970
- Congenital kyphoscoliosis
- Situs inversus and paranasal sinusitis (Kartagener syndrome)
- Unilateral absence of pulmonary artery.

What are the indications for surgery in bronchiectasis?
Lung resection surgery may be considered in patients with localized disease in whom symptoms are uncontrolled by medical treatment and in massive haemoptysis.

What are the most common sites for localized disease?
Left lower lobe and lingula.

What do you understand by the term bronchiectasis sicca?
Bronchiectasis or 'dry' bronchiectasis is that which presents with recurrent dry cough associated with intermittent episodes (months or years apart) of haemoptysis. The haemoptysis can be life-threatening as bleeding is from bronchial vessels with systemic pressures. There is usually a history of granulomatous infection, particularly TB. The upper lobes are often primarily affected, allowing good drainage.

What is yellow nail syndrome?
A rare medical condition characterized by the combination of lymphoedema, yellow dystrophic nails, bronchiectasis, and pleural effusions.

What do you know about Reid's classification of bronchiectasis?
In 1950, Reid correlated pathological changes with bronchography and described three different appearances:
- Cylindrical bronchiectasis: bronchi that are uniformly dilated (to >2 mm but can be so large as to admit a finger) and do not taper but rather end abruptly; this is caused by plugging of smaller bronchi by thick mucus and casts
- Varicose bronchiectasis: dilated bronchi with irregular bulging contours similar to a varicose vein and no tapering; terminations are bulbous and bronchial subdivisions are reduced

- Cystic or saccular bronchiectasis is the most severe form and is characterized by sharply reduced bronchial subdivisions and dilated bronchi ending in cystic pus-filled cavities. It usually runs a more severe course.

All three types can be present in the same patient.

What are the modes of presentation of bronchiectasis?

Bronchiectasis may be diffuse or focal disease. There are three types of focal airway obstruction that may lead to bronchiectasis:
- Luminal blockage by a foreign body, broncholith, or slowly growing benign tumour
- Extrinsic narrowing caused by enlarged lymph nodes (e.g. in middle lobe syndrome, which involves a small angulated orifice surrounded by a collar of lymph nodes that may enlarge and encroach on the main airway after granulomatous disease caused by infection with mycobacteria or fungi)
- Twisting or displacement of the airways after a lobar resection (e.g. the occasional cephalad displacement of a lower lobe after surgery for the resection of the upper lobe).

Recurrent or persistent lobar pneumonia is a key distinguishing feature of the first two types of focal bronchiectasis. It is important to recognize as interventional bronchoscopy or surgery may result in symptom control and sometimes cure.

Further Information

Laennec was the first to describe bronchiectasis in 1819.

M. Kartagener (1897–1975), a Swiss physician.

C.M. Riley and R.L. Day, both US paediatricians. Riley–Day syndrome consists of dysautonomia and lack of coordination in swallowing.

C.J.R. Chagas (1879–1934), a Brazilian physician.

CHAPTER 4

Cystic Fibrosis

Instruction

This 24-year-old male patient presents with weight loss and foul-smelling fatty stools despite a normal appetite. Please examine his chest.

Salient Features
HISTORY

- Cough with purulent and viscous expectoration
- Diabetes mellitus
- Gastrointestinal (GI) symptoms (steatorrhoea, failure to thrive in childhood, rectal prolapse, meconium ileus, or distal intestinal obstruction)
- Heat stroke, salt depletion
- Sterility in men and decreased fertility in women.

EXAMINATION

- Purulent sputum
- Patient is short of breath
- Central cyanosis
- Finger clubbing
- Bilateral coarse crackles that alter with coughing
- Sinonasal symptoms.

Proceed as follows:
- Tell the examiner that you would like to check the following:
- Glucose
- Faecal fat
- Sweat chloride.

Note: Cystic fibrosis (CF) is defined as the presence of a coherent clinical syndrome, plus either evidence of CF transmembrane conductor regulator (CFTR) dysfunction (an abnormal value for sweat chloride or nasal potential difference) or confirmation of CF-causing mutations on both alleles.

Diagnosis

This patient has clubbing with bilateral coarse crackles that alter with coughing, weakness, and foul fatty stool (lesion) caused by CF (aetiology) and requires continuous oxygen indicating respiratory failure (functional status).

15

Questions

What are the chances of this male patient having a child?
Males are infertile because of abnormalities of development of the vas deferens and epididymis.

What are the clinical manifestations of this condition?
- Neonates: recurrent chest infections, failure to thrive, meconium ileus, and rectal prolapse
- In childhood and young adults:
    - Respiratory: infection, bronchiectasis (Fig. 4.1), pneumothorax, haemoptysis, nasal polyps, recurrent sinusitis, allergic bronchopulmonary aspergillosis, cor pulmonale
    - GI: rectal prolapse, distal ileal obstruction (meconium ileus equivalent), cirrhosis, gallstones, intussusception, pancreatic insufficiency of the exocrine pancreas with malabsorption
    - Miscellaneous: male infertility, CF-related diabetes mellitus, hypertrophic pulmonary osteoarthropathy, osteoporosis, anaemia, nephrolithiasis.

How would you treat steatorrhoea?
- Low-fat diet
- Oral supplementation with vitamins and minerals
- Pancreatic enzyme replacement therapy
- Proton pump inhibitor or H2 receptor antagonists.

How would you treat chest complications?
- Postural drainage
- Antibiotics

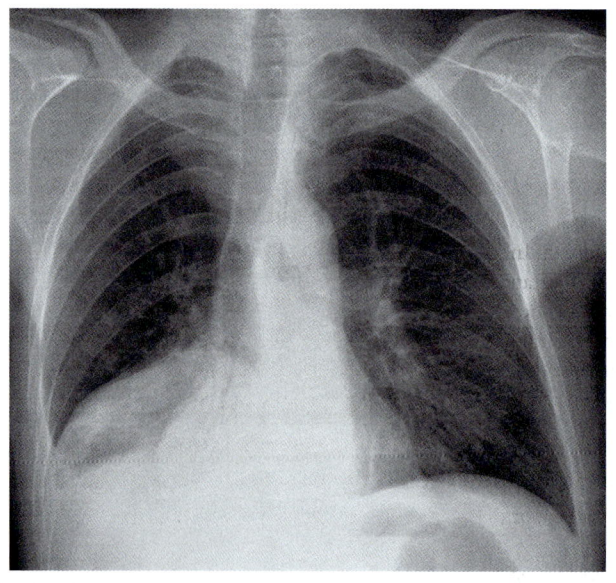

Fig. 4.1 Cystic fibrosis. There is slight overinflation and multiple thin-walled ring shadows in the right lung and the upper part of the left lung, reflecting cystic bronchiectasis. Some ring shadows contain air–fluid levels. (With permission from Adam, A., Dixon, A.K., Grainger, R.G., Allison, D.J., 2008. Grainger and Allison's Diagnostic Radiology, fifth edn. Churchill Livingstone, Edinburgh.)

- Aerosolized medication for pseudomonas colonization: tobramycin
- Bronchodilators
- Heart–lung transplantation.

What is the role of physiotherapy?
Specialist CF physiotherapy is very important, but there is considerable debate regarding the effectiveness of different techniques for airway clearance, including active cycle of breathing technique, autogenic drainage, positive expiratory pressure technique, oscillatory devices, and traditional postural drainage. There is good evidence that physical exercise improves both cardiorespiratory and muscular function in patients with CF.

What is the inheritance pattern for cystic fibrosis?
Autosomal recessive. On the long arm of chromosome 7 resides the gene encoding CFTR, a protein of 1480 residues that acts as a cyclic adenosine monophosphate (AMP)-regulated chloride channel. This gene is carried by 1 in 20 White, with an incidence of 1 in 2500 live births in the UK, rising to 1 in 1500 in Ireland. There is a mutation on the long arm of chromosome 7 in 70% of patients. There is a deletion of the codon for phenylalanine at position 508 (Δ508). This defect leads to a failure of the chloride channel to open in response to cyclic AMP. More than 175 other lesions in the CF gene are responsible for the disease in the remaining 30% of patients.

How is this condition diagnosed in infancy?
Immunoreactive trypsinogen (IRT) assay in dried blood in neonates as part of the newborn blood spot screening test. A very high IRT concentration suggests pancreatic injury consistent with (but not specific for) CF. This assay is useful for screening rather than diagnosis. Infants who have a high IRT concentration on initial testing undergo further assessment via a repeat IRT 1 to 3 weeks later (IRT/IRT) or by analysis of the initial blood spot for a specified group of CFTR mutations (IRT/DNA).

What do you know about sweat testing?
A sweat sodium concentration >60 mmol/L is indicative of CF. It identifies over 75% of cases by the age of 2 years and about 95% by the age of 12 years. It is more difficult to interpret in older children and adults.

What is the basic defect in the airways of these patients?
The opening of chloride channels at the luminal surface of the airway epithelial cells in normal individuals allows the passive transport of chloride along an electrochemical gradient from the cytoplasm to the lumen. In patients with CF, there is a defect in these channels that prevents this normal secretion. Simultaneously, there is a threefold increase in the reabsorption of sodium from the airway lumen into the cytoplasm of the epithelial cell. As the movement of water into airway secretions follows the movement of salt, it is believed that a decreased secretion of chloride into the airway lumen and the increased reabsorption of sodium from the airway lumen combine to reduce water content and increase the viscosity and tenacity of the airway secretions.

If the patient has persistent purulent cough, which organisms are usually responsible?
Staphylococcus aureus, Haemophilus influenzae, Burkholderia cepacia, and *Pseudomonas aeruginosa*. The last is associated with poor prognosis as this organism is almost impossible to eradicate.

What is the risk of cancer in patients with cystic fibrosis?
The overall risk of cancer is similar to that of the general population, but there is an increased risk of digestive tract cancers. Persistent or unexplained GI symptoms in these patients should be investigated carefully.

What is the lifespan in such patients?
The median age of survival is currently in the late 40 s. It is possible that a child born today will have a longer median survival as the current studies do not consider the impact of the modulator therapy for CF.

What is the cause of death in cystic fibrosis?
Death occurs from pulmonary complications, such as pneumonia, pneumothorax, massive haemoptysis, or from terminal chronic respiratory failure.

What parameters can predict death in cystic fibrosis?
Prediction of death within 2 years can be made for 50% of the patients whose forced expiratory volume in 1 s (FEV1) is <30%. Thus, the necessity for referral for transplantation can be anticipated about 1 year in advance of death.

How would you manage a patient who has been accepted for transplantation?
The aim is to sustain life by aggressive therapy with nocturnal oxygen, continuous intravenous antibiotics, enteral feeding, respiratory stimulants, and nasal intermittent positive pressure ventilation.

If this patient requires lung transplantation, which type of transplantation is the treatment of choice?
Bilateral lung transplantation is necessary for patients with chronic bronchial disease such as CF (or bronchiectasis) to avoid contamination of the donor lung by spillover of infected material from the recipient's remaining lung.

What are the complications of lung transplantation?
Early posttransplantation lung oedema, infection, and rejection (including obliterative bronchiolitis).

What are the indications for a combined heart–lung transplantation?
The combined heart–lung transplantation has relatively few indications, the primary one being congenital heart disease with Eisenmenger syndrome.

What are the new methods of treatment available for cystic fibrosis?
- High-dose ibuprofen in young patients with mild disease (FEV1 of at least 60% of the predicted value), taken consistently for long periods, has shown to slow the progression of lung disease without serious adverse effects, but this is not a treatment option for adult patients with CF, as the effects on more severe than mild disease and adult patients are not proven.
- CFTR modulator therapies are designed to alter the function of the protein coded for by the defective CFTR gene. These are effective in patients with specific gene mutations.
- Gene therapy: the gene is transferred in a 'carrier' (a cationic lipid envelope known as a liposome). On transferring the gene for CF to the nasal epithelium using these liposomes, the deficit is partly removed without provoking a local inflammatory response. Some modestly significant results have been obtained but it is not the magic wand that had been hoped for so far.
- Inhalation of hypertonic saline produces a sustained acceleration of mucus clearance and improved lung function. This treatment may protect the lung from insults that reduce mucus clearance and produce lung disease. Inhaled mannitol is currently in phase 3 trials.
- Immunization against various components of *Pseudomonas* has remained an elusive goal.

What advice would you give a patient with cystic fibrosis who wishes to become pregnant?
- The couple will be offered genetic counselling and the man will be offered testing to determine his genetic status. If he is a carrier, chorionic villous sampling will be considered, as the risk of the couple conceiving an infant with CF is one in two and they may wish to consider selective termination in the first trimester. The hazards of general anaesthesia (as lung function is impaired) for termination of pregnancy will be brought to their attention. Termination of pregnancy either with spinal anaesthesia or medications is an alternative.
- Women with severe disease will be informed that they may be unable to complete pregnancy and that their premature demise may leave a motherless child.
- In women with an FEV_1 <60% of the predicted value, there is an increased risk of premature delivery, an increased rate of caesarean section, some loss of lung function, and risk of respiratory complications and early death of the mother.
- Pregnancy after heart–lung transplantation offers better health and increased longevity in the mother, but the risk of organ rejection and exposure of the fetus to potentially teratogenic immunosuppressants means that pregnancy should not be attempted by women with transplants.

What is the *forme fruste* of cystic fibrosis?
Increasingly, with the availability of neonatal screening with IRT and thorough diagnosis by genetic studies, milder forms of disease have been recognized without the increase in sweat sodium. It is predicted that a considerable number will present with a pattern of disease in adult life that has not been recognized in the past as being caused by CF.

Further Information

Quinton established that sweat ducts are impermeable to chloride in 1986.
Christiaan Barnard performed the first heart transplant in 1967. Sir Magdi H. Yacoub, contemporary Egyptian-born cardiothoracic surgeon, popularized cardiac transplantation in the UK at Harefield Hospital, London.
The first successful pregnancy in a woman with CF was reported in 1960.

CHAPTER 5

Chronic Obstructive Pulmonary Disease

Instruction
This patient presents with productive cough and shortness of breath. Please examine his respiratory system.

Salient Features

HISTORY
- Productive cough
- Increasing dyspnoea
- Weight loss
- History of smoking or exposure to outdoor, occupational, and indoor air pollution (e.g. burning of biomass)
- History of α_1-antitrypsin deficiency or poor lung growth during childhood.

EXAMINATION
- Begin with examination of the *sputum pot*.
- Observe from the end of the bed for obvious breathlessness, pursed lip breathing, and symmetrical chest movement. Count the respiratory rate.
- Look for finger staining from tar and smell for tobacco foetor.
- Feel the palms for warmth and the pulse for a rapid bounding pulse (signs of carbon dioxide retention).
- Look at the lips and tongue for central cyanosis.
- Comment on the active contractions of the accessory muscles of respiration such as sternomastoids, scalenes, and trapezii.
- Palpate for tracheal deviation and measure the distance between the cricoid cartilage and suprasternal notch (less than three fingers' breadth in emphysema).
- Comment on the raised jugular venous pressure.
- Comment on barrel-shaped chest (Fig. 5.1).
- Look for inspiratory retraction of the lower ribs (Hoover's sign).
- Comment on use of accessory muscles of respiration.
- Palpate for:
  - apex beat
  - chest expansion
  - vocal fremitus
- Percuss looking for:
  - hyperresonance and obliteration of cardiac and liver dullness

5—CHRONIC OBSTRUCTIVE PULMONARY DISEASE

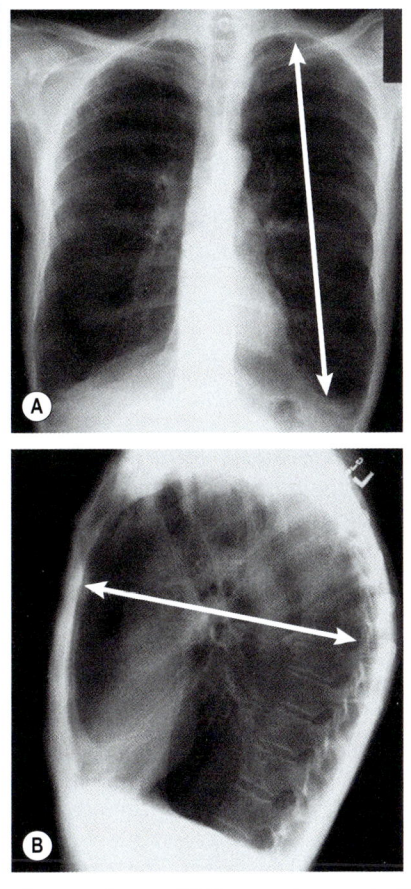

Fig. 5.1 Chronic obstructive pulmonary disease. **(A)** The superior aspect of the hemidiaphragms is at the same level as the posterior aspect of the twelfth ribs. **(B)** Hyperinflation. (Mettler, F.A., 2004. Essentials of radiology, second edn. Saunders-Elsevier, Philadelphia, PA.)

- Auscultate for:
  - breath sounds (diminished breath sounds)
  - vocal resonance
  - forced expiratory time (the end-point is detected by auscultating over the trachea in the suprasternal notch; normal individuals can empty their chest from full inspiration in ≤4 s and prolongation to >6 s indicates airflow obstruction)
  - loud pulmonary second heart sound
- Palpable liver to look for hepatic displacement (comment on upper border of liver by percussion).

Proceed as follows:
Tell the examiner that this patient is at increased risk for cardiovascular disease, osteoporosis, lung cancer, and depression.

Remember: Airflow obstruction as measured by spirometry is defined as a ratio of the post-bronchodilator forced expiratory volume in 1 s (FEV1) to forced vital capacity (FVC) of <0.70.

Diagnosis

This patient has features of chronic obstructive pulmonary disease (COPD) (lesion) caused by tobacco smoking (aetiology) and is breathless at rest (functional status).

Questions

What do you understand by the term chronic bronchitis?
Chronic bronchitis is cough with sputum production for at least 3 months in a year for 2 successive years.

What is the definition of emphysema?
Emphysema is the destruction of lung parenchyma, leading to loss of alveolar attachments to small airways.

What do you understand by the term chronic obstructive pulmonary disease?
COPD denotes persistent respiratory symptoms and airflow limitation caused by airway and/or alveolar abnormalities due to significant exposure to noxious particles or gases. The chronic airflow limitation that is characteristic of COPD is caused by a mixture of small airways disease and parenchymal destruction.

What is the mechanism of reduction in expiratory capacity in chronic COPD?
Dynamic hyperinflation is considered an important factor in the reduction of exercise capacity and the development of dyspnoea.

COPD is caused by a variable mixture of three pathological processes: loss of alveolar attachments, inflammatory obstruction of the airway, and luminal obstruction with mucus. Alveolar attachments ensure a radial tethering effect, which is important for keeping small airways patent in the normal lung. At smaller lung volumes, airways narrow because of decreased lung elasticity and weaker tethering effects. As a result, maximal expiratory airflow decreases as the lung empties and ceases at 25% to 35% of total lung capacity. The remaining air (or residual volume) may account for as much as 60% to 70% of predicted total lung capacity. Patients with COPD must breathe at larger lung volumes to optimize expiratory airflow, but this requires greater respiratory work because the lungs and chest wall become stiffer at larger volumes. These effects are worse with exercise. A normal lung meets the increased ventilatory demands of exercise by increasing both tidal volume and respiratory rate, with little change in the final end-expiratory lung volume. Whereas in COPD, the respiratory rate does increase in response to exercise, but with insufficient expiratory time, breaths become increasingly shallow and end-expiratory lung volume progressively enlarges, a phenomenon called dynamic hyperinflation.

What is the role of inflammatory mechanisms in COPD?
In COPD, reactive oxygen species, pathogen-associated molecular patterns, and damage-associated molecular patterns activate families of pattern recognition receptors that include the toll-like receptors. This understanding has led to the hypothesis that COPD is also a disease of innate immunity. COPD is characterized by abnormal response to injury, with altered barrier function of the respiratory tract, an acute phase reaction, and excessive activation of macrophages, neutrophils, and fibroblasts in the lung. Macrophages and epithelial cells in airways are activated by cigarette smoke and other irritants (in developing countries, the inhalation of smoke from biomass fuels is an important cause of COPD, particularly among women who cook in poorly ventilated homes) and these release neutrophil chemotactic factors, including interleukin-8 and leukotriene B_4. Neutrophils and macrophages then release proteases that

5 — CHRONIC OBSTRUCTIVE PULMONARY DISEASE

break down connective tissue in the lung parenchyma, resulting in emphysema and stimulating hypersecretion of bronchial mucus. The chronic inflammatory process in COPD differs markedly from that seen in bronchial asthma, with different inflammatory cells, mediators, inflammatory effects, and responses to treatment.

What is the role of proteolysis in COPD?

In COPD, the protease-antiprotease balance is tipped in favour of proteolysis because of either an increase in proteases (including neutrophil elastase, proteinase 3, cathepsins, matrix metalloproteases 1, 2, 9, and 12) or a deficiency of antiproteases (including α_1-antitrypsin, elafin, secretory leukoprotease inhibitor, and tissue inhibitors of matrix metalloproteases).

What is the main cause of death and disability in COPD?

Mortality and disability from COPD are related to an accelerated decline in lung function over time, with a loss of >50–60 mL/year in FEV1, compared with a normal loss of 20–30 mL/year. The progressive reduction in FEV1 and increasing severity of disease over time result in increasing dyspnoea on exertion, which slowly advances to respiratory failure.

What is the role of high-resolution computed tomography in the diagnosis of emphysema?

This is the most sensitive technique for the diagnosis of emphysema. It is useful in evaluating symptomatic patients with almost normal pulmonary function except for a low carbon monoxide diffusing capacity – a combination of findings that occurs in emphysema, interstitial lung disease, and pulmonary vascular disease.

What is the differential diagnosis in a patient with suspected COPD?

Any process presenting with chronic dyspnoea and cough poses the differential of COPD. One of the main differentials, especially in the younger population, is asthma. Asthma patients, as opposed to COPD patients, tend to have diurnal and seasonal variation of their symptoms (also demonstrated by wide variation of peak expiratory flow diary), they are younger at diagnosis, and they may have other atopic features in their history. Sometimes, differentiating between the two conditions is difficult, and there is a group of people that have a combination of the two pathologies (asthma–COPD overlap syndrome). Other possible differentials are left ventricular failure, bronchiectasis, bronchiolitis, and tuberculosis.

How would you classify the severity of airflow obstruction in COPD patients?

The presence of airway obstruction is defined by a ratio of FEV1/FVC less than 70%. Once airflow obstruction is demonstrated on spirometry, the reduction in FEV1 determines the severity of the obstruction, ranging from mild to very severe.

Are you aware of any tools to assess patients' symptoms?

A simple measure of breathlessness is the Modified British Medical Research Council questionnaire on respiratory symptoms, which correlates well with other measures of health status and predicts future mortality risk.

Another tool used is the COPD Assessment Test. Both tools take into account patients' symptoms and functional status.

What medications are commonly used in outpatient treatment of COPD?

- Short-acting bronchodilators:
  - Beta2-adrenergic agonist: albuterol
  - Anticholinergic agent: ipratropium, oxitropium
  - Combination: albuterol–ipratropium

- Long-acting bronchodilators:
  - Beta2-adrenergic agonists: salmeterol, formoterol, arformoterol, indacaterol, oladaterol vilanterol
  - Anticholinergic agent: tiotropium, aclidinium, glycopyrronium bromide, umeclidinium.
- Combination long-acting beta2-adrenergic agonist bronchodilator (LABA) with long-acting antimuscarinic antagonist (LAMA): formoterol/aclidinium, formoterol/glycopyrronium, indacaterol/glycopyrronium.

Combination therapy with LABA/LAMA increases FEV1 and reduces symptoms compared to monotherapy. Additionally, it reduces exacerbation compared to monotherapy

- Combination beta2-adrenergic agonist bronchodilator with inhaled corticosteroid (ICS):
  - Fluticasone–salmeterol
  - Budesonide–formoterol
  - Triple inhaled therapy combination of ICS/LAMA/LABA, which improves lung function, symptoms, and health status and reduces exacerbations compared to ICS/LABA or LAMA alone
- Phosphodiesterase-4 inhibitors:
  - Roflumilast reduces moderate and severe exacerbations treated with systemic corticosteroids in patients with chronic bronchitis, severe to very severe COPD, and a history of exacerbations
- Methylxanthine: theophylline
- Alpha 1 antitrypsin augmentation therapy may slow emphysema progression

Note: Smoking cessation, influenza and pneumococcal vaccinations, and pulmonary rehabilitation (including education, exercise, behaviour modification, and interventions to improve social and psychological functioning), ventilatory support in COPD–sleep apnoea overlap syndrome, and lung volume reduction are important therapeutic measures in COPD.

How would you treat an acute exacerbation?
- Assess severity of symptoms
- Use supplemental oxygen therapy (obtain blood gas, monitoring pulse oximetry)
- Use bronchodilators:
  - Increase doses and/or frequency of short-acting beta2 bronchodilators/combine short-acting beta2-agonists and anticholinergics
  - Consider LABAs when patient becomes stable
  - Use spacers and air-driven nebulizers where appropriate
- Consider systemic corticosteroids
- Consider antibiotics in case of signs of bacterial infection
- Use noninvasive mechanical ventilation
- Identify and treat comorbidities or associated conditions (e.g. heart failure, arrhythmias, pulmonary embolism, low molecular weight heparin for thromboembolism prophylaxis etc.).

What is the role of inhaled steroids in COPD?
An ICS/LABA combination is more effective than the individual components in improving lung function and health status and contributes in exacerbation reduction in patients suffering from moderate to very severe COPD. Moreover, the triple inhaled therapy is superior in terms of lung function, symptoms, and health status compared with ICS/LABA and LAMA monotherapy. Regular treatment with ICS alone does not does not modify the long-term FEV1 decline nor the mortality and increases the risk of pneumonia.

What are the organisms commonly associated with exacerbations of COPD?

The infectious agents in COPD can be viral or bacterial. *Haemophilus influenzae* and *Streptococcus pneumoniae* are the commonest organisms identified in the sputum during exacerbations of COPD, accounting for 43% and 25%, respectively, of positive cultures in one study. *Moraxella catarrhalis* is also frequently isolated from sputum during exacerbations and, less commonly, *Chlamydia pneumoniae*. *Klebsiella* and other Gram-negative organisms such as *Pseudomonas aeruginosa* have been associated with severe disease and other risk factors such as cardiac disease, home oxygen use, chronic oral steroid use, or recent antibiotic use.

What clinical features would suggest that this patient is suitable for long-term domiciliary oxygen therapy?

The long-term administration of oxygen (>15 h per day) to patients with chronic respiratory failure has been shown to increase survival in patients with severe resting hypoxaemia
- Arterial PaO_2 ≤55 mm Hg (≤7.3 kPa) or SpO_2 ≤88% with or without hypercapnia
- 55 mm Hg (≤7.3 kPa), PaO_2 ≤60 mm Hg (≤8 kPa), or SpO_2 ≥88% with evidence of pulmonary hypertension, congestive heart failure, or polycythemia (haematocrit >55%).

How can the sensation of breathlessness be reduced?

Opiates, neuromuscular electrical stimulation, and oxygen therapy can relieve breathlessness.

How would you treat acute respiratory failure?

- Administer titrated oxygen to improve hypoxaemia (target saturation should be individualized to patients, with a target of 88%–92% in patients with CO_2 retention/oxygen sensitivity)
- Arterial blood gases should be monitored frequently to ensure adequate oxygenation and exclude carbon dioxide retention or worsening acidosis
- Noninvasive ventilation is preferred to treat acute type 2 respiratory failure in patients with acute exacerbations of COPD. Any COPD patient who presents with an acute exacerbation with respiratory acidosis that has failed to improve after an hour of optimal medical treatment needs noninvasive ventilation. Mortality, intubation rates, and related complications (such as ventilator-associated pneumonia or length of hospitalization) are reduced compared to invasive ventilation. A clear escalation plan should be discussed with the patient and family prior to commencing noninvasive ventilation. Its use requires a high-dependency/close-monitoring environment, trained staff, and regular arterial blood gas monitoring.

What do you know about noninvasive ventilation?

Noninvasive ventilation is an alternative approach to endotracheal intubation to treat hypercapnic ventilatory failure, which occurs in COPD. It reduces the complications of endotracheal intubation such as infection and injury to the trachea. Noninvasive ventilation is pressure-support ventilation delivered with a face mask. Noninvasive ventilation has been shown to reduce the need for endotracheal intubation, length of hospital stay, and in-hospital mortality rate in selected patients with acute exacerbations of COPD.

What do you know about the BODE index?

The BODE index combines information about several predictors in a score ranging from 0 to 10, including:
- **B**ody mass index
- Airflow **O**bstruction (FEV1)
- **D**yspnoea (Medical Research Council dyspnoea scale)
- **E**xercise capacity (6 min walk distance) in a score ranging from 0 to 10

This prognostic index predicts mortality significantly better than FEV (the traditional prognostic COPD indicator) alone.

What do you know about molecular genetics of COPD?
Deficiency of α_1-antitrypsin:
- First described in Sweden, the patient is deficient in α_1-antitrypsin with activity approximately 15% of normal values; concentrations of 40% or more are required for health. The patient is homozygous for the gene (*Z*) encoding a protease inhibitor (Pi). Other genetic combinations and their percentage of normal activity are *MS* (80%), *MZ* (60%), *SS* (60%), and *SZ* (40%). Six percent of the population is heterozygous for S(PiMS) and 4% for Z(PiMZ), making an overall frequency of 1 in 10 for the carriage of the defective gene. Liver transplantation results in conversion to the genotype of the donor.
- In the lung, α_1-antitrypsin inhibits the excessive actions of neutrophil and macrophage elastase, which cigarette smoke promotes. When the lung is heavily exposed to cigarette smoke, the protective effect of α_1-antitrypsin may be overwhelmed by the amount of elastase released or by a direct oxidative action of cigarette smoke on the α_1-antitrypsin molecule. The emphysema is panacinar and is seen in the lower lobes of the lungs. Smoking increases the severity, and lowers the age of onset, of emphysema. Liver disease is a much less common complication. Human α_1-antitrypsin is prepared from pooled plasma from normal donors. Never- or ex-smokers with an FEV1 of 35%–60% are suggested to be the most suitable for α1-antitrypsin deficiency augmentation therapy.
- The siblings of an index case should be screened for this disorder. Their identification should be followed by counselling to avoid smoking and occupations with atmospheric pollution. Children of homozygotes will inherit at least one Z gene and hence will be heterozygotes. They should avoid pairing with another heterozygote if they wish to avoid the risk of producing an affected homozygote.

Tumour necrosis factor-alpha (TNF-α):
- COPD is 10 times more common in the Taiwanese population with a polymorphism in the promoter region of the gene for TNF-α, resulting in its increased production. However, the same polymorphism in the UK population is not associated with increased risk of COPD.

Microsomal epoxide hydrolase:
- A polymorphism variant of microsomal epoxide hydrolase, an enzyme involved in the metabolism of the epoxides that may be generated in tobacco smoke, has been associated with a quintupling of the risk of COPD.

What is the role of surgery in COPD?
- Bullectomy is the removal of a large bulla that does not contribute to gas exchange and may be responsible for complications and lung parenchyma compression. In selected patients, this surgical procedure is associated with improved gas exchange, lung function, exercise tolerance, and decreased dyspnoea. Lung-volume reduction surgery results in functional improvements including increased FEV1, reduced total lung capacity, improved function of respiratory muscles, improved exercise capacity, and improved quality of life. The National Emphysema Treatment Trial Group found that lung-volume reduction surgery increased the chance of improved exercise capacity but did not confer a survival advantage over medical therapy. It did yield a survival advantage for patients with both predominantly upper-lobe emphysema and low baseline exercise capacity. Patients previously reported to be at high risk and those with non-upper-lobe emphysema and high baseline exercise capacity are poor candidates for lung-volume reduction surgery because of increased mortality and negligible functional gain.

- Single lung transplantation has been successful for at least 3–4 years in patients with COPD. The criteria for selecting patients for transplantation have not been established. It does not improve survival but improves quality of life.

What is the best method for communicating spirometry findings to patients?

Results from studies suggest that providing feedback on lung age with graphic displays may be the best option so far for communicating the results of spirometry. More patients are likely to stop smoking when spirometry results, as communicated using Fletcher and Peto's diagram (a pictorial representation of how smoking ages the lungs), are shared with the patient.

What are the general indications for lung transplantation?

The general indication is end-stage lung disease without alternative forms of therapy. Patients should be <60 years of age and should have a life expectancy of <12–18 months; they should not have an underlying cancer or other serious systemic illness. The most common lung diseases are pulmonary fibrosis, emphysema (particularly α_1-antitrypsin deficiency), bronchiectasis, cystic fibrosis, and primary pulmonary hypertension.

What is the role of nutrition in COPD?

Malnutrition is associated with reduced respiratory muscle function and increased mortality rate. A high dietary intake of *n*-3 fatty acids may protect cigarette smokers against COPD.

Mention some newer treatments for COPD.

- Antagonists of inflammatory mediators: 5-lipoxygenase inhibitors, leukotriene B_4 antagonists, interleukin-8 antagonists, tumour-necrosis factor inhibitors and antioxidants
- Protease inhibitors: neutrophil elastase inhibitors, cathepsin inhibitors, nonselective matrix metalloprotease inhibitors, elafin, secretory leukoprotease inhibitor, α_1-antitrypsin
- New antiinflammatory agents: phosphodieasterase-4 inhibitors, nuclear factor-κB inhibitors, adhesion molecule inhibitors, and p38 mitogen-activated protein kinase inhibitors.

Further Information

The first association between tobacco smoking and chronic respiratory disease was made in 1953 by Dr George Waldbott in a disease he called smoker's respiratory syndrome.

The term emphysema was first used by Rene Laennec in 1837 in his treatise on chest diseases. He had by that stage already invented the stethoscope in 1816.

CHAPTER 6

Idiopathic Pulmonary Fibrosis

Instruction

Examine this patient's chest.
Examine the respiratory system from the back.

Salient Features

HISTORY

- Progressive exertional dyspnoea
- Chronic cough
- Arthralgia/arthritis
- Constitutional symptoms (fevers, chills, weight loss, fatigue suggest collagen disorders)
- Smoking history
- Occupational history
- Family history
- Drug history (amiodarone, nitrofurantoin, methotrexate, bleomycin, busulfan).

EXAMINATION

- Clubbing (Fig. 6.1)
- Central cyanosis
- Bilateral, basal, fine, end-inspiratory crackles that disappear or become quieter on leaning forwards and, furthermore, do not disappear on coughing (unlike those of pulmonary oedema), which have been called 'velcro' or 'cellophane' crackles
- Tachypnoea (in advanced disease).

Proceed as follows:
- Examine the following:
  - Hands (for rheumatoid arthritis, systemic sclerosis)
  - Face (for typical rash of systemic lupus erythematosus (SLE), heliotropic rash of dermatomyositis, typical facies of systemic sclerosis, lupus pernio of sarcoid)
  - Mouth (for aphthous ulcers of Crohn's disease, dry mouth of Sjögren syndrome)
- Look for signs of pulmonary hypertension: 'a' wave in the jugular venous pressure, left parasternal heave, and P_2.

Diagnosis

This patient has bilateral, basal, fine end-inspiratory crackles (lesion) caused by idiopathic pulmonary fibrosis (IPF) (aetiology) and is tachypnoeic at rest (functional status).

6 — IDIOPATHIC PULMONARY FIBROSIS

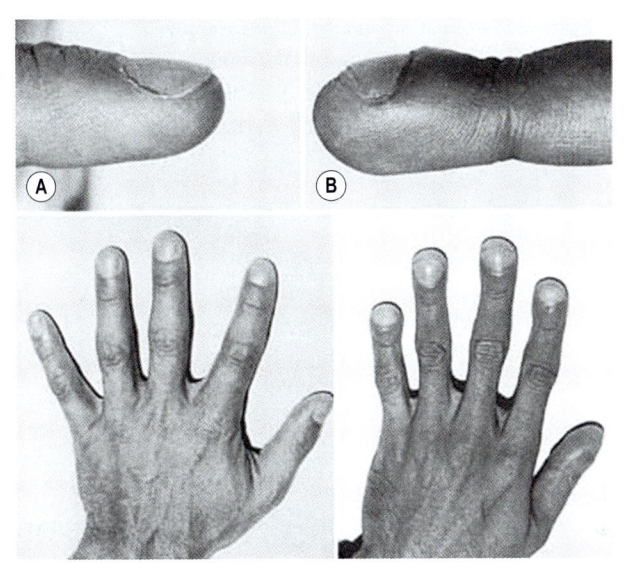

Fig. 6.1 Hands and index fingers of a normal person (A) and a person with clubbing of the digits (B) secondary to severe diffuse pulmonary interstitial fibrosis. (With permission from Mason, R.J., Broaddus, V.C., Murray, J.F., Nadel, J.A., 2005. Murray & Nadel's Textbook of Respiratory Medicine, fourth edn. Saunders, Philadelphia, PA.)

Questions

In which other conditions is clubbing associated with crackles?
- Bronchogenic carcinoma (crackles are localized)
- Bronchiectasis (coarse crackles)
- Asbestosis (history of exposure to asbestos)
- Sarcoidosis (fibrosing stage)
- Collagen vascular diseases (rheumatoid arthritis, SLE, systemic sclerosis, mixed connective tissue diseases)
- Idiopathic interstitial pneumonias.

Mention some conditions which can cause fibrosis in the lungs.
- Rheumatoid arthritis, SLE, dermatomyositis, ulcerative colitis, systemic sclerosis
- Pneumoconiosis
- Granulomatous disease: sarcoid, tuberculosis (TB)
- Chronic pulmonary oedema
- Radiotherapy
- Lymphangitis carcinomatosa
- Extrinsic allergic alveolitis: farmer's lung, bird fancier's lung.

What is the pathology in idiopathic pulmonary fibrosis?
The histopathological pattern is usual interstitial pneumonia (UIP). It is defined by alveolar septal thickening with predominately subpleural distribution, accompanied by fibroblastic foci.

What is the classification of idiopathic interstitial pneumonias?
According to the official American Thoracic Society/European Respiratory Society Statement: Update of the International Multidisciplinary Classification of the Idiopathic Interstitial Pneumonias, they are classified as follows:
- Major idiopathic interstitial pneumonias:
  - IPF
  - Idiopathic nonspecific interstitial pneumonia
  - Respiratory bronchiolitis–interstitial lung disease
  - Desquamative interstitial pneumonia
  - Cryptogenic organizing pneumonia
  - Acute interstitial pneumonia
- Rare idiopathic interstitial pneumonias:
  - Idiopathic lymphoid interstitial pneumonia
  - Idiopathic pleuroparenchymal fibroelastosis
- Unclassifiable idiopathic interstitial pneumonias.

How would you investigate this patient?
- Chest radiography: typically shows small lung volumes and bilateral basal reticulonodular shadows, which progress upwards as the disease progresses. In advanced disease, there is marked destruction of the parenchyma, causing 'honeycombing' (caused by groups of closely set ring shadows), and nodular shadows are not conspicuous. The mediastinum may appear broad as a result of a decrease in lung volume.
- Blood gases: arterial desaturation worsens while upright and improves on recumbency. There is arterial hypoxaemia and hypocapnia.
- Pulmonary function tests: in the early stages, lung volumes may be normal, but there is arterial desaturation following exercise. Typically, there is a restrictive defect with reduction in both gas transfer factor and gas transfer coefficient.
- Blood tests: full blood count, C-reactive protein, raised immunoglobulins, anti-nuclear factor, rheumatoid factor, angiotensin-converting enzyme, c-anti-neutrophil cytoplasmic antibody (ANCA), p-ANCA, SCL-70, ds-DNA, anti-Jo1, anti-RNP, anti-Ro, anti-La antibodies to exclude connective tissue disease.
- High-resolution computed tomography (HRCT) is considered the gold standard for imaging patients with suspected interstitial lung diseases.
- Bronchial lavage: bronchoalveolar lavage (BAL) is helpful in order to exclude infection, malignancy, or other specific diseases (histiocytosis Langerhans/CD-1a, pulmonary alveolar proteinosis, eosinophilic pneumonias, diffuse alveolar haemorrhage). It is not diagnostic for IPF, but an increased percentage of BAL neutrophils appears to correlate with a poor prognosis.
- Lung biopsy: surgical lung biopsy is not necessary in the diagnostic algorithm for IPF if there is UIP pattern on HRCT (reticular abnormalities with subpleural and basal predominance accompanied by honeycombing ± traction bronchiectasis).

Mention factors associated with increased mortality in IPF.
- Dyspnoea and hypoxaemia
- Pulmonary functional status (diffusing capacity of the lung for carbon monoxide (DLCO), 40% predicted, decrease in forced vital capacity by >10% absolute value)
- Desaturation <88% during 6-min walk test
- Extent of honeycombing or worsening of fibrosis on HRCT
- Pulmonary hypertension.

How would you manage a patient with IPF?
- Nintedanib (tyrosine kinase inhibitor)
- Pirfenidone (regulator of important profibrotic and proinflammatory pathways)
- Current data against the use of combination therapy of *N*-acetylcysteine, azathioprine, and prednisolone
- Consideration of antacid treatment because abnormal gastroesophageal reflux (GER), including clinically silent acid (or at least untreated acid), has been observed in up to 90% of patients with IPF
- Long-term oxygen therapy (in patients with hypoxaemia)
- Lung transplantation.

What is the prognosis?
The median survival of patients with the disease ranges from 2 to 3 years from the time of diagnosis.

What are the causes of death in such patients?
- Respiratory failure or cor pulmonale precipitated by chest infection
- Bronchogenic carcinoma, 10-fold increase compared with normal controls.

What is the role for lung transplantation?
Single lung transplantation is now an established and effective form of treatment for certain individuals. Survival rate at 5 years is estimated at approximately 50% to 55%.

What do you know about the Hamman–Rich syndrome?
The Hamman–Rich syndrome is a rapidly progressive and fatal variant of interstitial lung disease.

Mention indications for transbronchial and open lung biopsy in interstitial lung diseases.
- Transbronchial biopsy: sarcoidosis, TB, berylliosis, lymphangitis carcinomatosa, extrinsic allergic alveolitis
- Open lung biopsy: idiopathic interstitial lung diseases, IPF, connective tissue diseases, pulmonary vasculitis, lymphangioleiomyomatosis, Langerhan's cell histiocytosis.

Mention some genetic disorders with pulmonary fibrosis.
- Dyskeratosis congenita: pulmonary fibrosis is present in 20% of patients. Dyskeratosis congenita is also typically associated with a triad of mucocutaneous manifestations: skin hyperpigmentation, oral leukoplakia, and nail dystrophy.
- Hermansky–Pudlak syndrome: oculocutaneous albinism, a bleeding diathesis, and pulmonary fibrosis.

What is the role of caveolin in pulmonary fibrosis?
Caveolin-1 (the most abundant protein found within caveolae, which are flask-shaped invaginations of the plasma membrane abundantly present in many terminally differentiated cells) is a protective regulator of pulmonary fibrosis and it limits transforming growth factor-β_1-induced production of extracellular matrix and restores alveolar epithelial repair processes. It attenuates the development of pulmonary fibrosis in a mouse model of the disease. Therapeutic approaches that augment caveolin-1 bioavailability may help to restore normal alveolar epithelial repair and regeneration and may help patients with IPF to breathe more easily and live longer.

Further Information

L.V. Hamman (1877–1946), physician, and A.R. Rich (1893–1968), pathologist, worked at the Johns Hopkins Hospitals, Baltimore.

Dame Margaret Turner-Warwick (1924–2017) was the first woman president of the Royal College of Physicians, London; her chief interest was fibrotic lung disease.

CHAPTER 7

Cor Pulmonale

Instruction
This patient presents with worsening dyspnoea on exertion. Please examine this patient's chest.

Salient Features
HISTORY
- Symptoms of chronic obstructive pulmonary disease (COPD) or other respiratory condition, with rapidly progressive dyspnoea
- Easy fatigability, shortness of breath on exertion, weakness, syncope, or presyncope
- Leg oedema and right upper quadrant pain.

EXAMINATION
- The patient is short of breath at rest and is centrally cyanosed.
- There is tar staining of the fingers.
- Jugular venous pressure is raised: both 'a' and 'v' waves are seen, with 'v' waves being prominent if there is associated tricuspid regurgitation.
- There are bilateral wheeze/bilateral fine end inspiratory crepitations (auscultation signs depend entirely on the underlying respiratory pathology that has led to pulmonary hypertension).

Proceed as follows:
- Examination of the cardiovascular system for signs of pulmonary hypertension
    - Left parasternal heave (often absent when the chest is barrel shaped)
    - Right ventricular gallop rhythm
- Loud and narrow split second heart sound, loud ejection click
- Pansystolic murmur of tricuspid regurgitation
- Early diastolic Graham Steell murmur in the pulmonary area
- Look for signs of:
    - hepatomegaly
    - pedal oedema.

Diagnosis
This patient has chronic cor pulmonale (lesion) caused by long-standing COPD (aetiology) and is in congestive cardiac failure (functional status).

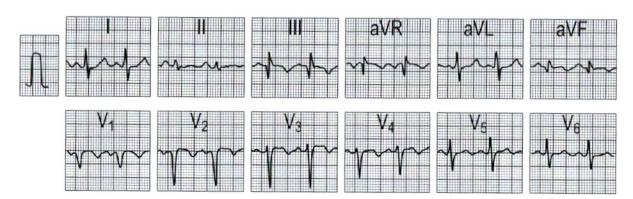

Fig. 7.1 Acute cor pulmonale secondary to pulmonary embolism simulating inferior and anterior infarction. An S1Q3T3, a QR in V_1 with poor R wave progression in the right precordial leads ('clockwise rotation'), and right precordial to midprecordial T-wave inversion (V_1 to V_4). The S1Q3 pattern is usually associated with a QR or QS complex, but not an RS, in aVR. Furthermore, acute cor pulmonale per se does not cause prominent Q waves in II (only in III and aVF).

Questions

What do you understand by the term cor pulmonale?
Pulmonary hypertension is classified by the World Health Organization into five groups, depending on the leading cause of pulmonary hypertension; Group 3 pulmonary hypertension or cor pulmonale refers to pulmonary hypertension caused by underlying chronic respiratory disease, COPD, interstitial lung disease, or mixed pathologies (Fig. 7.1).

Mention respiratory diseases that can be complicated by cor pulmonale.
- COPD
- Interstitial lung disease
- Overlap syndromes
- Sleep-disordered breathing
- Alveolar hypoventilation disorders
- High-altitude lung disease
- Developmental lung disease.

How would you manage a patient with cor pulmonale?
- Treatment of the underlying cause
- General measures (smoking cessation, vaccinations, pulmonary rehabilitation programmes)
- Oxygen (long-term oxygen therapy has shown survival benefit in specific conditions such as COPD-related cor pulmonale with documented hypoxaemia)
- Treatment of cardiac failure with furosemide
- Consideration of heart–lung transplantation in young patients.

What is the prognosis in cor pulmonale?
Once cor pulmonale develops, mortality from the underlying respiratory disease increases, regardless of the underlying cause. Approximately 50% of patients succumb within 5 years.

What is the relationship between chronic obstructive pulmonary disease and left ventricular function?
Even early-stage COPD influences stroke volume and left ventricular size. Left ventricular volume and stroke volume are decreased in COPD without changes in the left ventricular ejection fraction. This decrease is related to the percentage of emphysema and to the degree of airway obstruction. This impairment in left ventricular filling is probably caused by endothelial dysfunction (and not just loss) of the pulmonary microvasculature as a result of smoking.

CHAPTER 8

Cough

Instruction

This patient has a cough. Please assess him.

Salient Features

This chapter focuses on subacute and chronic cough. The causes of acute cough are dealt with in separate chapters of this book.

HISTORY

- How long has the cough been there? Acute cough, <3 weeks duration; subacute cough, 3 to 8 weeks; and chronic cough, >8 weeks
- Productive or dry?
- Haemoptysis
- Medication: angiotensin-converting enzyme inhibitors
- Smoking history
- 'The three Rs' (reversible airways disease (i.e. asthma), reflux, and rhinosinusitis)
- Recent respiratory tract infection
    - Patients can present weeks after the acute infection with a persistent cough (the cough lingers long after the patient has recovered from the initial illness)
- Atypical infections—mycoplasma, pertussis, tuberculosis
- 'Red flag' symptoms—unexplained weight loss, recurrent haemoptysis, finger clubbing, and lymphadenopathy (cervical and supraclavicular—needs urgent assessment to exclude cancer, either a primary lung tumour or a metastasis)
- Does the patient need emergency admission to hospital? Signs of pulmonary embolism, pneumothorax, foreign body aspiration, severe exacerbation of preexisting lung disease (asthma, chronic obstructive pulmonary disease, bronchiectasis), and respiratory sepsis require prompt treatment.

EXAMINATION

- Observations—oxygen saturations, vital signs
- Chest exam (breath sounds, added sounds, muscles of respiration)
- Brief eyes, nose, and throat examination—pharynx, nose, neck
- Sputum pot, inhalers, nebulizer, long-term oxygen therapy
- Consider arterial blood gas analysis, chest radiography, and peak expiratory flow rate (PEFR)/spirometry.

Diagnosis

This patient with underlying asthma has a subacute cough (lesion), caused by a respiratory tract infection (aetiology). After using his bronchodilator inhaler, he is comfortable at rest (functional status).

Questions

How do antitussive cough medicines work?
Antitussives either work centrally on the cough centre in the brain or peripherally.

Centrally acting drugs are by far the most commonly used medication for symptomatic relief of the cough symptom. Synthetic opiates such as dextromethorphan and pholcodine, and natural opiates codeine and morphine are used widely around the world and may be effective in some patient groups. Care must be taken to counsel patients of the addictive nature of natural opiate compounds.

γ-Aminobutyric acid analogues (pregabalin and gabapentin) have been successfully used in chronic cough though are not licensed for this use.

Peripherally acting drugs are used very rarely. Thalidomide can be used in idiopathic pulmonary fibrosis. Benzonatate and butamirate are marketed in the USA. Nebulized lidocaine is effective in reducing cough but has unpleasant side effects, including taste disturbance and choking on food or fluids.

How would you treat a chronic persistent cough refractory to conventional treatment?
Once empiric treatment of respiratory disease, suspected nasal conditions, and a trial of reflux treatment have failed, these patients probably have a form of cough hypersensitivity syndrome, whereby there is a complex dysfunction of sensory neurons leading to hypersensitivity of the upper airway. This is influenced by a variety of factors, both local and systemic. Inflammation and damage to the epithelium of the aerodigestive and respiratory tract, together with afferent sensory neural dysfunction, are thought to be involved in the pathogenesis of this condition.

Women are known to consult doctors more often than men do for cough, have a more prominent cough reflex, and are more likely to experience chronic cough, suggesting a genetic influence on the neurophysiology of the upper respiratory tract.

Treatment is directed at the potentially modifiable factors such as environment, occupation, smoking, acid and non-acid reflux disease, sinonasal disease, and asthma/airway allergy.

What is the cough reflex arc?
Cough receptors are located in the upper and lower respiratory tract epithelium, as well as the pericardium, oesophagus, stomach, and diaphragm. They may be sensitive to chemical stimuli such as acid, capsaicin (chilli), and temperature extremes, as well as mechanical stretch.

These receptors, when stimulated, induce ion-channel activation of transient receptor potential vanilloid type 1 and transient receptor potential ankyrin type 1 classes. These signals travel via the vagus nerve to the cough centre, located in the medulla. The cough centre also receives input from higher cortical centres. This cough centre generates a signal transmitted via vagus, phrenic, and spinal motor nerves to expiratory muscles which contract forcefully to produce a cough.

Do you know of any pathways that may be targeted to reduce cough hypersensitivity syndrome?
Recent attention on the P2X3 receptor and the role of adenosine triphosphate (ATP) gives the exciting prospect of drugs that may target the central cough reflex and help those patients where treatment of common conditions thought to underpin the majority of chronic cough has failed. Gefapixant is being trialled in those with a persistent cough in the context of idiopathic pulmonary fibrosis and, although not used out of a research environment as yet, may yet offer a panacea to those patients whose lives are ruled by an unrelenting cough.

CHAPTER 9

Fever

Instruction

This patient presents to the ambulatory care unit with intermittent fever for the last 2 weeks. Please take a focused history, assess the patient, and advise on further management.

Salient Features

HISTORY

- History of pyrexia, degree of fever, spike frequency, response to antipyretics, diurnal variation, and relationship of fever to any other symptoms
- Associated symptoms (systemic enquiry) to include weight loss, night sweats, and 'B' symptoms
- Travel history (detailed geography and dates) and tuberculosis exposure history
- Occupational history and pet exposure
- Outdoor activities and frequency (e.g. camping)
- Immunosuppression and full medical history, including immunization history
- Gynaecological history if relevant
- Full drug history.

EXAMINATION

- Cardiovascular examination: peripheral stigmata of infective endocarditis, fundoscopy for Roth spots, auscultation for murmurs, urine dip for protein and blood
- Respiratory examination: presence of clubbing or onychodystrophy; chest examination, looking for signs of infection, bronchiectasis, and interstitial lung disease; and palpate for lymph nodes
- Neurological: signs of meningism, examination of peripheral and central nervous systems and assessment of cognition, palpation of temporal regions for signs of temporal arteritis, palpation over muscle groups for signs of myositis
- Abdominal examination: palpation for masses and organomegaly, localized tenderness, testicular examination if relevant and lymph node palpation of all major groups
- Musculoskeletal and skin examination: inspection for rashes; vasculitic, cellulitic rashes, joint problems, and examination of all joints for arthritis/synovitis, palpation of whole spine to reveal areas of localized tenderness.

Diagnosis

This young man has fever, cough, and breathlessness (lesions) caused by infection with SARS-CoV-2 (aetiology). He is hypoxic and requires supplemental oxygen to maintain normal saturations (functional status).

Questions

Name some differential diagnoses of pyrexia of unknown origin.
The most common causes of pyrexia of unknown origin are categorized into infections, connective tissue disorders, malignancy, and drug-induced pyrexia:
- Infections:
  - Tuberculosis, brucellosis, malaria, typhoid, paratyphoid fever, mononucleosis, parasitic infection, dengue fever, leishmaniasis, Lyme disease, amoebiasis, echinococcus, culture-negative infective endocarditis, intraabdominal and retroperitoneal abscess, dental abscess, viral illness
- Connective tissue disorders:
  - Adult-onset Still disease, vasculitis, systemic lupus erythematosus
- Malignancy:
  - Haematological malignancy (lymphoma and leukaemia), occult malignancy, especially renal cell carcinoma, and hepatocellular carcinoma
- Other causes:
  - Veno-occlusive disease, endocrine abnormalities (e.g. thyroid disease), hypothalamic disorders (e.g. stroke, anoxic brain insult), hereditary conditions (e.g. familial Mediterranean fever)
- Drug-induced pyrexia:
  - Multiple medications can induce fever, either because of an allergic reaction or due to an idiosyncratic reaction of thermoregulation. The fever can be caused on initiation of the medication or much later. Once other more sinister causes have been excluded, a trial of stopping medications should be initiated. The list of medications causing fever is long, including even medications that can treat fever (e.g. nonsteroidal antiinflammatory drugs), antimicrobials (e.g. penicillins), and medications that are used in everyday practice in hospitalized patients (low-molecular-weight heparin).

What investigations would you request for this patient?
- Routine blood tests: full blood count, urea and electrolytes, liver function test, coagulation screen, C-reactive protein, erythrocyte sedimentation rate, thyroid function tests, lactate dehydrogenase
- Blood film, including thick and thin films for malaria
- Respiratory viral screen
- Repeated blood cultures
- Full autoimmune screen, including rheumatoid factor
- Serum protein electrophoresis and immunoglobulins
- HIV assay, hepatitis serology (hepatitis A, B, C, E), and hepatomimetic virus serology (cytomegalovirus, Epstein–Barr virus)
- Imaging (computed tomography scan of chest–abdomen–pelvis)
- Echocardiogram (transthoracic echocardiography or transoesophageal echocardiography depending on clinical suspicion of infective endocarditis)
- Bone marrow biopsy.

What are the main mechanisms by which a medication can induce fever?
- Hypersensitivity reaction to the medication
- Idiosyncratic reaction to the medication
- Due to the pharmacological properties and actions of the medication
- Due to altering the thermoregulatory mechanisms in the hypothalamus.

What other complications can follow drug-induced fever?
Although fever can be in isolation, a clinical sign of a drug hypersensitivity reaction, some patients may develop other systemic symptoms or even life-threatening organ failure.

Are you aware of any life-threatening syndromes associated with drug-induced hypersensitivity reactions?
Drug reaction with eosinophilia and systemic symptoms (DRESS) syndrome: it is caused by a number of drugs, but most commonly seen after the use of allopurinol. It presents with fever, malaise, lymphadenopathy, and a generalized rash and can lead to multiple organ failure, particularly liver and kidney failure. It is also reported to cause reactivation of herpesviruses. Patients with DRESS syndrome are treated with cessation of the offensive drug and supportive measures.

What is neuroleptic malignant syndrome?
Neuroleptic malignant syndrome is a life-threatening condition associated with neuroleptic drugs, characterized by high fever, reduced consciousness level, rigidity, and autonomic dysfunction.

It is mostly caused by potent agents like haloperidol, but atypical antipsychotics and withdrawal of antiparkinsonian medication have also been associated with the syndrome. The pathophysiology is poorly understood, but it is thought that dopamine receptor blockade in the hypothalamus results in the clinical features of the syndrome.

The diagnosis is mainly clinical and the treatment is supportive. Cessation of the causative medication is essential, and if supportive measures fail to treat the hyperthermia, then medications such as dantrolene can be used.

What are the clinical features of SARS-CoV-2 infection, the coronavirus that gave rise to the COVID-19 pandemic?
Around one-third of the population affected and testing positive for the virus on polymerase chain reaction (PCR) test will be asymptomatic. Most people infected will have upper respiratory symptoms (fever, dry cough, headache, fatigue, myalgias, sore throat) or mild lower respiratory tract symptoms (mild dyspnoea, cough). Around 20% of the population will have severe disease (dyspnoea with hypoxaemia), of which one-fourth will develop critical illness (acute respiratory distress syndrome, severe hypoxia, hypotension) requiring organ support in intensive care mainly due to respiratory failure. Risk factors for developing critical disease are identified as increasing age, coexistent malignancy, cardiovascular risk factors, coexistent respiratory, liver, or kidney disease, obesity, and smoking. Once hospitalized the overall mortality is estimated around 10%. Vaccinations have changed the previous statistics and will continue changing as time progresses as they have proven very effective in preventing severe disease. Protection against infection has probably varied amongst different emerging variants but protection against critical illness has remained high regardless of the variant.

Name some complications of COVID-19 infection in adults.
- Long COVID—symptoms persisting for months after the initial infection. Those symptoms include general symptoms like fatigue and low energy levels, headaches, myalgias, mild respiratory symptoms such as dry cough, cognitive symptoms like memory loss, poor concentration ability, anxiety and depression, and persisting lung pathology with dyspnoea.
- Thrombosis—severe and critical illnesses are associated with increased risk of thrombotic episodes.
- Anosmia—or dysosmia that can persist for months after the initial infection.
- Cardiac complications—myocarditis and cardiomyopathy.

Are there any pharmacological treatment options for mild COVID-19 disease?
This is a new disease so guidelines, treatment options, and hospitalization indications have evolved and will continue to evolve for the next few years as we understand more about the effects of this novel virus. So far, those needing admission to hospital have been given antivirals (remdesivir) and steroids (dexamethasone). Patients treated at home would be advised about simple measures (isolation, hydration, analgesia). Newer antiviral agents are now available to patients with known risk factors for developing severe disease to be taken at the start of the illness while symptoms are still mild. One example of these agents is molnupiravir, a nucleoside analogue that inhibits viral replication. Monoclonal antibodies are also used with success in mild disease but they are not widely available. One example is sotrovimab, which is given as a single infusion in patients infected with the omicron variant.

CHAPTER 10

Collapsed Lung

Instruction
This patient presented with shortness of breath. Please examine this patient's chest.

Salient Features
HISTORY
- Sudden onset of breathlessness
- History of cough
- History of asthma, tuberculosis (TB), lung cancer.

EXAMINATION
- Trachea deviated to the affected side
- Movements decreased on the affected side
- Percussion note dull on the affected side
- Breath sounds diminished on the affected side.

Proceed as follows:
- Tell the examiner that you would like to look for tar staining (tobacco smoking), clubbing, and cachexia (bronchogenic carcinoma).
- Be prepared to discuss the patient's chest radiography (Fig. 10.1).

Diagnosis
This patient has a collapsed lung (lesion); he is breathless at rest (functional status). I would like to exclude malignancy (aetiology).

Questions
What are the causes of lung collapse?
- Bronchogenic carcinoma
- Mucus plugs (asthma, allergic bronchopulmonary aspergillosis)
- Extrinsic compression from hilar adenopathy (e.g. primary TB, sarcoidosis)
- TB (Brock syndrome)
- Other intrabronchial lesions (carcinoid tumour, inflammatory strictures, obstructive granulation tissue, amyloidosis, and benign tumours)
- Foreign body aspiration
- Ventilation-induced lung injury.

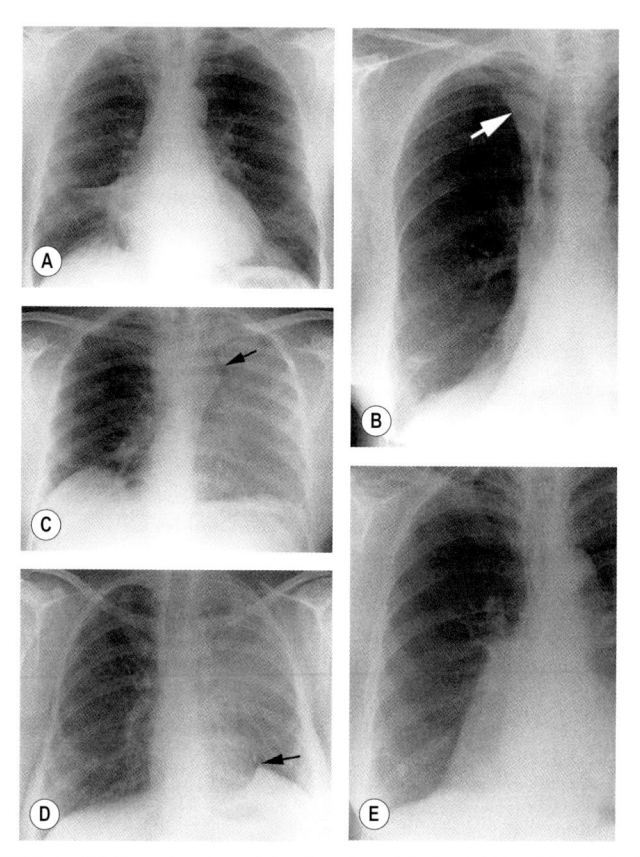

Fig. 10.1 Collapsed lung. **(A)** Triangular-shaped density adjacent to the right heart border in right middle lobe collapse. **(B)** Superior triangle sign in right upper lobe collapse *(arrow)*. **(C)** Paramediastinal lucency (Luftsichel sign; *arrow*) in left upper lobe collapse. **(D)** A small triangular density (juxtaphrenic peak sign/Kattan sign; *arrow*) in left upper lobe collapse (indicates reorientation of an inferior accessory fissure). **(E)** Shifting granuloma sign in right lower lobe collapse. (With permission from Adam, A., Dixon, A.K., Grainger, R.G., Allison, D.J., 2008. Grainger and Allison's Diagnostic Radiology, fifth edn. Churchill Livingstone, Edinburgh.)

What are the chest radiograph findings of collapse of the right middle lobe?
The loss of definition of the right heart border (Fig. 10.1A) reflects collapse (or consolidation) affecting the right middle lobe.

What is Brock syndrome?
It is collapse caused by compression of the right middle lobe bronchus by an enlarged lymph node.

Further Information
Sir Russell C. Brock (1903–1980) graduated from Guy's Hospital and was surgeon at Guy's and Brompton Hospitals. His interests included both thoracic and cardiac surgery. He was the President of the Royal College of Surgeons, 1963–1966.

CHAPTER 11

Obstructive Sleep Apnoea

Instruction
Look at this patient.

Salient Features

HISTORY
- Daytime somnolence
- Unrefreshing sleep
- Daytime fatigue
- Snoring with witnessed apnoeas
- Episodes of gasping during sleeping
- Shortness of breath
- Headache particularly in the morning
- Decreased libido
- Memory impairment
- Irritability/change in personality
- Poor concentration
- Nocturia
- Weight gain
- Gastroesophageal reflux
- Rarely insomnia (usually in women)
- Poor quality of life
- History of hypertension (especially refractory hypertension) and/or arrhythmias
- History of stroke (Obstructive sleep apnoea significantly increases the risk of stroke or mortality from any cause, and the increase is independent of other risk factors, including hypertension.)
- History of sleep-related car accident
- Medication (sedative or hypnotic drugs)
- Alcohol.

EXAMINATION
- Obese patient
- Upper airway anatomy evaluation (e.g. acroglossia, tonsillar hypertrophy, nasal septal deviation, retrognathia, micrognathia, maxillary or mandibular hypoplasia)
    - May be nodding off to sleep
    - Inherited diseases (e.g. Down syndrome, Treacher Collins syndrome).
- Neck circumference
- Systemic hypertension

43

- Disorders of endocrine glands (hypothyroidism, acromegaly)
- Signs of pulmonary hypertension and right heart failure.

Remember: Nearly 50% of patients with sleep apnoea syndrome are *not* obese.

Diagnosis

This patient has marked obesity and hypersomnolence with signs of pulmonary hypertension (lesion), which indicates that she has hypoventilation syndrome secondary to morbid obesity (aetiology). The patient is in cardiac failure (functional status).

Questions

What is obstructive sleep apnoea?
It consists of repetitive episodes of partial (hypopnoeas) or total (apnoeas) upper airway cessations, usually followed by oxygen desaturations of >3%. Fifteen events per hour or five or more events per hour together with one or more clinical symptoms of obstructive sleep apnoea are required for diagnosis.

Severity classification is according to the apnoea–hypopnoea index (AHI):
AHI 5 to 14: mild
AHI 15 to 29: moderate
AHI >30: severe.

What are the diagnostic criteria for obesity hypoventilation syndrome?
1. Body mass index >30 kg/m²
2. Awake arterial daytime hypercapnia ($PaCO_2$ >45 mm Hg)
3. Other causes of hypoventilation ruled out
4. Obstructive sleep apnoea (AHI ≥5 events/hour) or nonobstructive sleep hypoventilation (AHI <5 events/hour, O_2 saturation ≤88% for at least 5 min in the absence of any obstructive event).

What is the cause of cyanosis in such a patient?
A mixture of obstructive apnoea and sleep-induced hypoventilation (Fig. 11.1). The blood gas picture is hypoxia and carbon dioxide retention.

Where is the obstruction?
The obstruction, which may have both anatomical and neuromuscular origins, usually occurs in the retropalatal and retroglossal parts of the pharyngeal wall.

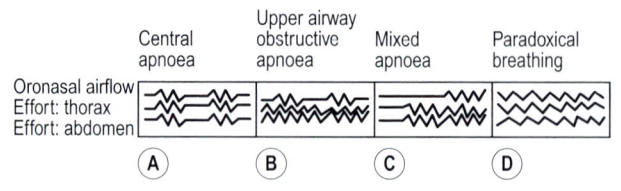

Fig. 11.1 Patterns of sleep-disordered breathing.

What is the significance of neck circumference?

A prediction rule based on neck circumference is used to estimate a patient's probability of having a sleep test result that is diagnostic of sleep apnoea. Calculating the neck circumference/height ratio (NHR) is a sensitive screening tool in obese individuals and may prompt early sleep study to formally diagnose obstructive sleep apnoea.

How would you treat such a patient?

- Reduce weight.
- Avoid smoking and alcohol, sedatives, or hypnotic drugs.
- Apply position therapy (avoid the supine position if polysomnography indicates elevated AHI in the supine position compared to left or right position).
- Use continuous nasal positive airway pressure (CPAP) delivered by a nasal mask. CPAP is recommended even if the AHI is in the mild range (5–14) in patients with cardiovascular diseases and symptoms of daytime somnolence or cognitive impairment. CPAP acts like a pneumatic splint, resulting in patency of the upper airway during inspiration and expiration. The resultant reductions in gas-exchange perturbations, respiratory effort, abrupt arousals, and blood pressure surges all probably ameliorate symptoms.
- Use oral appliances (a treatment option in patients with mild obstructive sleep apnoea or in those who cannot tolerate CPAP).
- Perform surgery in selected patients:
  - Single-level surgery, e.g. nasal surgery, adenotonsillectomy, uvulopalatopharyngoplasty
  - Multilevel surgery tailored to the patient that may include linguoplasty, genioglossus and hyoid advancement, mandibular advancement
  - Upper airway stimulation (UAS) is emerging as an effective treatment modality in selected patients.
  - Bariatric surgery.

Further Information

William Howard Taft, US President from 1909 to 1913, had a minimum body mass index of $42\,kg/m^2$, wore size 54 pyjamas, had a neck size of 19 in (47.5 cm), snored, and had hypersomnolence. He appears to have become symptomatic at approximately 300 lb (140 kg). Within 12 months of leaving office, Taft permanently lost over 60 lb (27 kg). His somnolence resolved. As Chief Justice of the United States from 1921 to 1930, he was not somnolent.

Mr. Pickwick is a character in the novel *Pickwick Papers*, written by Charles Dickens, and this term was applied by Sir William Osler. In Charles Dickens' *The Posthumous Papers of the Pickwick Club*, Dickens describes the first meeting of Mr. Wardle with his servant:

> *Damn that boy, said the old gentleman, he's gone to sleep again.*
>
> *Very extraordinary boy, that, said Mr. Pickwick, does he always sleep in this way?*
>
> *Sleep! said the old gentleman, he's always asleep. Goes on errands fast asleep, and snores as he waits at the table.*
>
> *How very odd! said Mr. Pickwick.*
>
> *Ah! Odd indeed, returned the old gentleman; I'm proud of that boy—wouldn't part with him on any account—damn, he's a natural curiosity!*

CHAPTER 12

Bronchogenic Carcinoma

Instruction
Examine this patient's chest.

Salient Features

HISTORY
- Symptoms related to primary tumour: cough, dyspnoea, haemoptysis, postobstructive pneumonia, atelectasis, pneumothorax
- Symptoms related to mediastinal spread:
  - Hoarseness with left-sided lesions (caused by recurrent laryngeal nerve palsy)
  - Obstruction of the superior vena cava with right-sided tumours or associated lymphadenopathy
  - Elevation of the hemidiaphragm from phrenic nerve paralysis
  - Dysphagia from oesophageal obstruction
  - Pericardial tamponade.
- Symptoms related to metastases:
  - Sites include liver, brain, pleural cavity, bone, adrenal glands, contralateral lung, and skin
  - Initial presentation with symptoms from a metastatic focus is particularly common with adenocarcinoma.
- Paraneoplastic syndrome (10%–20% in patients with bronchogenic carcinoma):
  - Pain or arm in legs caused by hypertrophic osteoarthropathy
  - Symptoms of hypercalcaemia usually caused by squamous cell carcinoma or bone metastasis
  - Endocrine syndromes (Cushing syndrome, syndrome of inappropriate antidiuretic hormone (SIADH), carcinoid syndrome, hyperglycaemia/hypoglycaemia)
  - Neurological syndromes (e.g. Lambert–Eaton, peripheral neuropathy, encephalopathy).
- Systemic effects: anorexia, weight loss, weakness, and profound fatigue
- History of smoking.

EXAMINATION
Patient 1
- Clubbing and tar staining of the fingers
- Dull percussion notes at the apex with absent breath sounds

Look for Horner syndrome and wasting of the small muscles of the hand.

Patient 2
- Signs of pleural effusion on one side.

Patient 3

- Signs of unilateral collapse or consolidation of the upper lobe on one side

Note: If you suspect bronchogenic carcinoma, always look for clubbing, tar staining, cervical lymph nodes, radiation marks, and comment on cachexia.

Diagnosis

This patient with marked clubbing and large pleural effusion (lesion) probably has bronchogenic carcinoma (aetiology) and is very short of breath because of the large effusion (functional status).

Questions

How may patients with bronchogenic carcinoma present?

- Cough (50%–75%), haemoptysis (25%–50%), chest pain (25%), dyspnoea (25%), loss of weight, anorexia
- Skeletal manifestations: clubbing (in 30%)
- Local pressure effects: recurrent laryngeal palsy, superior vena cava obstruction, Horner syndrome
- Endocrine manifestations (12% of tumours), particularly with small cell tumours, present with a SIADH, hypercalcaemia, adrenocorticotrophic hormone (ACTH) secretion, or gynaecomastia. SIADH does not usually cause symptoms. When Cushing syndrome occurs, the manifestations are primarily metabolic (hypokalaemic alkalosis).
- Neurological manifestations: Eaton–Lambert syndrome, cerebellar degeneration, polyneuropathy, dementia, proximal myopathy, encephalomyelitis, subacute sensory neuropathy, limbic encephalitis, opsoclonus, myoclonus
- Cardiovascular: thrombophlebitis migrans, atrial fibrillation, pericarditis, nonbacterial thrombotic endocarditis
- Cutaneous manifestations: dermatomyositis, acanthosis nigricans, herpes zoster
- Haematologic manifestations: anaemia, disseminated intravascular coagulation, thrombotic thrombocytopenic purpura, thrombocytosis, hypercoagulopathy, eosinophilia
- Membranous glomerulonephritis.

How would you investigate this patient?

- Sputum cytology: higher yield for central endobronchial tumours. Usually is reserved for patients who have centrally placed lesions and are unable to tolerate, or unwilling to undergo, bronchoscopy, or other invasive diagnostic methods
- Chest radiography (Fig. 12.1)
- Bronchoscopy: the diagnostic yield depends on factors such as lesion size, distance of the lesion from the hilum, and presence of the bronchus sign on computed tomography (CT) (bronchus leading to a lung lesion). The efficacy of bronchoscopy is highest in central tumours because of the combination of methods used (endobronchial washes, bronchoalveolar lavage, protected brushing, and biopsies).
- Chest CT (contrast enhanced) offers better diagnostic spectrum and disease staging. The scan should also include the liver and adrenals to exclude metastasis.
- CT or ultrasound-guided transthoracic needle biopsy with peripheral lung lesions
- Positron emission tomography (PET)-CT in patients who may be suitable for treatment with curative intent. PET findings that alter treatment should be followed by pathological confirmation.

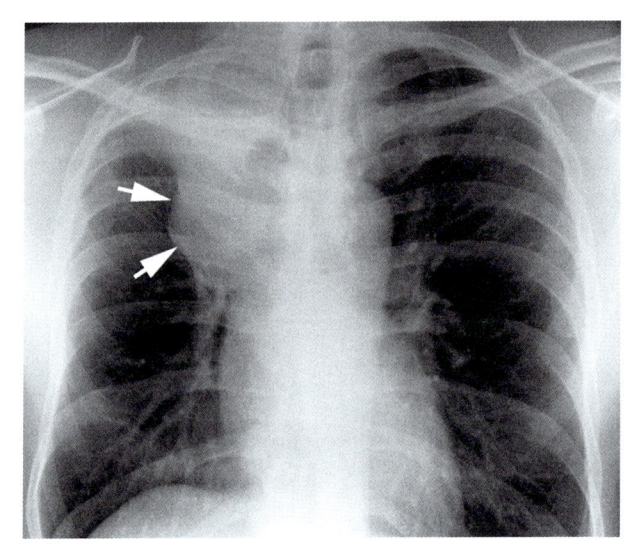

Fig. 12.1 Right upper lobe collapse with peripheral concavity and central convexity (*arrows*) caused by an underlying bronchogenic carcinoma resulting in a reverse S shape (Golden's 'S' sign). (With permission from Adam, A., Dixon, A.K., Grainger, R.G., Allison, D.J. 2008. Grainger and Allison's Diagnostic Radiology, fifth edn. Churchill Livingstone, Edinburgh.)

- Consider endobronchial ultrasound (EBUS)-guided transbronchial needle aspirate (TBNA) for biopsy of paratracheal, peribronchial, or intraparenchymal lung lesions.
- If symptoms and clinical examination indicate another organ involvement, proceed to CT or magnetic resonance imaging (MRI) of the brain, bone scintigraphy, bone marrow aspiration.
- Pleural fluid cytology.

What is the aim of staging?
The main aim of staging is to identify candidates for surgical resection, since this approach offers the highest potential cure for lung cancer. The staging assessment covers three major issues: distant metastases, the state of chest and mediastinum, and the condition of the patient.

What is the role of surgery in lung carcinoma?
Surgery is beneficial in early stages of non-small cell lung cancer (NSCLC). Surgery should include anatomical resection and mediastinal node mapping. Complete lymph node dissection should be performed if the tumour is resectable and mediastinal nodes are involved. The role of surgery in small cell lung cancer (SCLC) is limited because only one-third of the patients are diagnosed with localized disease and should also receive adjuvant chemotherapy and radiotherapy.

Which tumours respond well to chemotherapy?
SCLC: cisplatin or carboplatin and etoposide are first-line agents. If etoposide is contraindicated, it can be replaced by irinotecan or gemcitabine.

What are the drugs used in non-small cell lung cancer?
- Old agents: cisplatin, carboplatin, etoposide, vinblastine, vindesine
- Newer agents: docetaxel, paclitaxel, irinotecan, vinorelbine, gemcitabine
- Vascular endothelial growth factor inhibitors: bevacizumab

- Epidermal growth factor receptor (EGFR) tyrosine kinase inhibitors (e.g. gefitinib, erlotinib, cetuximab, afatinib): most effective in women, patients who have never smoked, patients with pulmonary adenocarcinomas, and patients of Asian origin
- Anaplastic lymphoma kinase inhibitors: crizotinib
- BRAF, HER2 mutations or ROS1, RET translocations: crizotinib, vandetanib, dabrafenib, trastuzumab (limited evidence).

The EGFR family of surface-receptor tyrosine kinases contains four members, which can form homodimers or heterodimers after ligand binding. Dimerization results in the activation of tyrosine kinases, which is followed by stimulation of three major signalling pathways, eventually leading to the activation of five of the six hallmarks of cancer: angiogenesis, resistance to antigrowth signals, invasion and metastasis, self-sufficiency in growth signals, and evasion of apoptosis (the sixth hallmark being limitless replication). The vast majority of *EGFR* mutations are either a deletion of a conserved sequence in exon 19 or a single point mutation in exon 21 (L858R).

What are the indications for radiotherapy?
Radiotherapy is administered for palliation in the following circumstances:
- Pain: either local or metastatic
- Breathlessness caused by bronchial obstruction
- Dysphagia
- Haemoptysis
- Superior venal caval obstruction
- Pancoast tumour
- Before and after operation in selected patients
- Cerebral metastases.

What are the contraindications for surgery?
Consider using a global risk score (e.g. Thoracoscore) to estimate the mortality risk:
- Metastatic carcinoma
- Forced expiratory volume in 1 s (FEV1) <40%
- Estimated postoperative FEV1 or transfer factor of the lung for carbon monoxide (TLCO) ≤30%, which is the recommended limit
- Uncontrolled major cardiac arrhythmias
- Patients with moderate to high risk of postoperative dyspnoea and VO_2 max ≤15 mL/kg/min in cardiopulmonary exercise test
- Myocardial infarction in the past month.

Is the progression of cancer associated with genetic change?
In early-stage NSCLC the increased activation of Src, tumour necrosis factor (TNF), and signal transducer and activator of transcription 3 (STAT3) pathways may be factors of prognostic value. Single-nucleotide polymorphisms (e.g. in the promoter region of Yes-associated protein 1 (YAP1) on chromosome 11q22, 5p15.33, 15q25.1, 6p22.1, 6q27, 7p15.3) may affect survival in SCLC patients.

What is the prognosis?
For limited-stage SCLC disease treated with chemotherapy plus chest radiation, a 17-month survival is reported.

A 5-year survival rate of 70% was reported for 65-year-old patients with early-stage NSCLC.

Further Information
Henry K. Pancoast (1875–1939), an American radiologist, pioneered the use of contrast media in X-ray images.

CHAPTER 13

Pulmonary Tuberculosis

Instruction

This patient presented with cough and malaise for 2 months. Please assess them.

Salient Features

HISTORY

- Fever, night sweats
- Malaise, fatigue, anorexia
- Weight loss
- Cough productive of sputum
- Chest pain
- Haemoptysis
- History of tuberculosis (TB) exposure or previous TB treatment
- Travel to endemic area and known contacts
- Social history and living conditions
- Immunosuppression (HIV infection).

Tell the examiner that with a suspicion of pulmonary TB, all body systems must to explored to exclude systemic involvement such as:

Tuberculous meningitis: headache, confusion, and low-grade fever
Urinary TB: dysuria, haematuria, frequency, urgency, flank pain, palpable inguinal lymph nodes
Bony TB (Pott disease): back pain and paraplegia
Gastrointestinal TB: abdominal pain, abdominal distention, dysphagia, diarrhoea, and malabsorption.

EXAMINATION

- Respiratory signs common to many chest diseases (crackles in the case of consolidation, dullness in the case of pleural thickening or effusion, signs of previous pneumonectomy, etc.)
- Lymphadenopathy
- Weight loss.

Diagnosis

This young man who is an intravenous drug user has a productive cough, weight loss, and intermittent fevers (lesion). His sputum is positive for acid-fast bacilli in keeping with pulmonary TB (aetiology).

Questions

List some risk factors for developing tuberculosis.
- Patient born in an endemic country

13 — PULMONARY TUBERCULOSIS

- Older age
- Previous TB infection
- Immunocompromised
- Preexisting condition (diabetes, renal failure, alcohol excess, intravenous drug use, haematological malignancy)
- Contact with people with pulmonary or laryngeal TB
- Occupational risk (doctors, nurses, chest physiotherapists, prison staff, residential healthcare workers, staff working in homeless or refugee shelters, people who are sent to work in an endemic country for more than 3 months).

Would you isolate this patient with newly diagnosed, sputum-positive pulmonary tuberculosis?
In the hospital setting, any patient with clinical suspicion of TB should be isolated and once TB is confirmed needs to be screened for multidrug-resistant TB. Those at low risk should be treated in isolation in a single room, whereas high-risk patients should be provided with a negative pressure room. Healthcare workers entering the room to provide care for these patients should follow all necessary airborne precautions. The risk of having TB is determined by the history and the patient's risk factors. In the outpatient setting, patients suspected to have TB should be advised to stay at home in relative isolation.

Does the bacille Calmette–Guérin vaccine protect against tuberculosis infection?
Depending on disease prevalence, immunization programmes differ by country. Countries where TB is endemic mostly have bacille Calmette–Guérin (BCG) vaccine as part of their infant immunization programme. In some countries where TB risk is low, BCG is still a recommended vaccination for older children, and other countries like the United Kingdom have removed BCG vaccination from their routine vaccination programme but offer it to some children at high risk. Primary immunization in infants and newborns is very effective in preventing TB, as well as preventing severe complications like disseminated disease, tuberculous meningitis, and death. Primary immunization of older children has shown to offer partial protection against TB but immunity wanes quickly.

How are contacts investigated?
Screening of contacts should take place as soon as a case of TB is confirmed. Patients who have symptoms of TB with sputum positive for acid-fast bacilli test are considered to have been infectious for the last 3 months prior to the diagnostic confirmation, so all contacts during that period should be investigated by a tuberculin skin test (Mantoux) or an interferon-γ release assay (IGRA).

How is latent tuberculosis infection diagnosed?
Latent TB infection is a clinical diagnosis. It consists of a combination of a positive tuberculin test or IGRA with no symptoms of active TB. If untreated, 1 in 10 people with latent TB will progress to active disease during their lifetime. As such it is important, once latent TB is diagnosed, for chemoprophylaxis to be given as appropriate.

Which rapid test allows early diagnosis of tuberculosis?
Microbiological and molecular testing. Detecting acid-fast bacilli in stained sputum samples under the microscope is the traditional initial test for all patients. Molecular testing is performed at the same time in most centres: The Xpert MTB/RIF test can establish a diagnosis of TB and assess resistance to rifampicin within 2 hours.

Name one regimen for treating susceptible tuberculosis.
Isoniazid and rifampicin for the intensive and the continuous phase, with the addition of pyrazinamide and ethambutol for the intensive phase.

List a few side effects of antituberculous treatment.
- Hepatotoxicity
- Optic nerve dysfunction with ethambutol
- Photosensitivity with pyrazinamide and other dermatological reactions with most of the antituberculous drugs
- Drug reaction with eosinophilia and systemic symptoms (DRESS) syndrome with isoniazid
- Peripheral neuropathy and seizures with isoniazid.

When should antiretroviral therapy be started in patients with tuberculosis and HIV infection?
Initiation of antiretroviral treatment early (<1 month after initiation of TB treatment in patients with confirmed TB and HIV infection) may reduce progression to AIDS and death. In patients with higher CD-4 T-cell counts, antiretroviral therapy could be postponed until the continuation phase of TB therapy. Rifampicin should be avoided in patients who receive protease inhibitors. Be aware of immune reconstitution inflammatory syndrome in such patients.

Further Information

Robert Koch (1843–1910), a German physician and microbiologist, first described Koch's postulates which are still the basis of infectious disease science and microbiology. His work on TB led him to isolate the mycobacterium responsible, work which earned him the Nobel Prize in Medicine in 1905.

SECTION II

Cardiology Cases

SECTION OUTLINE

14 Cardiovascular Case
15 Aortic Regurgitation
16 Aortic Stenosis
17 Mixed Aortic Valve Disease
18 Mitral Regurgitation
19 Mitral Stenosis
20 Mitral Valve Prolapse
21 Mixed Mitral Valve Disease
22 Mixed Mitral and Aortic Valve Disease
23 Prosthetic Heart Valves
24 Tricuspid Regurgitation
25 Pulmonary Stenosis
26 Atrial Septal Defect
27 Ventricular Septal Defect
28 Patent Ductus Arteriosus
29 Ebstein's Anomaly
30 Fallot's Tetralogy
31 Dextrocardia
32 Eisenmenger Syndrome
33 Hypertrophic Cardiomyopathy
34 Congestive Cardiac Failure
35 Constrictive Pericarditis
36 Weight Loss

CHAPTER 14

Cardiovascular Case

Instruction
Examine this patient's cardiovascular system.

Salient Features

HISTORY
- Chest pain: exertional, at rest (when angina present, comment on the Canadian Cardiovascular Angina class)
- Shortness of breath: exertional, at rest (when dyspnoea is present, comment on the New York Heart Association (NYHA) class), paroxysmal nocturnal dyspnoea
- Palpitations
- Dizziness, presyncope, syncope
- Swelling of feet.

EXAMINATION
1. Introduce yourself: 'I am Dr/Mr/Ms [etc.]. May I examine your heart?'
2. Ensure adequate exposure of the precordium: 'Would you take your top off, please?' However, be sensitive of the feelings of female patients.
3. Get the patient to sit at 45 degrees: use pillows to support the neck.
4. Inspection: comment on the patient's decubitus (whether they are comfortable at rest or obviously short of breath); comment on malar flush (seen in mitral stenosis).
5. Examine the pulse: rate (count for 15 s), rhythm, character, volume; lift the arm to feel for a collapsing pulse. Feel the other radial pulse simultaneously.
6. Comment on scars at the antecubital fossa (cardiac catheterization scars).
7. Look at the tongue for pallor, central cyanosis.
8. Look at the eye for pallor, Argyll Robertson pupil.
9. Examine the jugular venous pulse: comment on the waveform and height from the sternal angle. Check the abdominojugular reflux.
10. Comment on any carotid pulsations (Corrigan's sign of aortic regurgitation).
11. Examine the precordium: comment on surgical scars (midline sternotomy scars; thoracotomy scars for mitral valvotomy may be missed under the female breast).
12. Feel the apex beat: position and character.
13. Feel for left parasternal heave and thrills at the apex and on either side of the sternum.
14. Listen to the heart, beginning from the apex: take care to palpate the right carotid pulse simultaneously so that the examiner notices that you are timing the various cardiac events:
    - Always comment on the first and second heart sounds; mention any additional heart sounds (Fig. 14.1); listen to the heart murmurs and *be prepared to draw what you hear*.
    - If you do not hear the middiastolic murmur of mitral stenosis, make sure you listen to the apex in the left lateral position with the bell of the stethoscope.

14 — CARDIOVASCULAR CASE

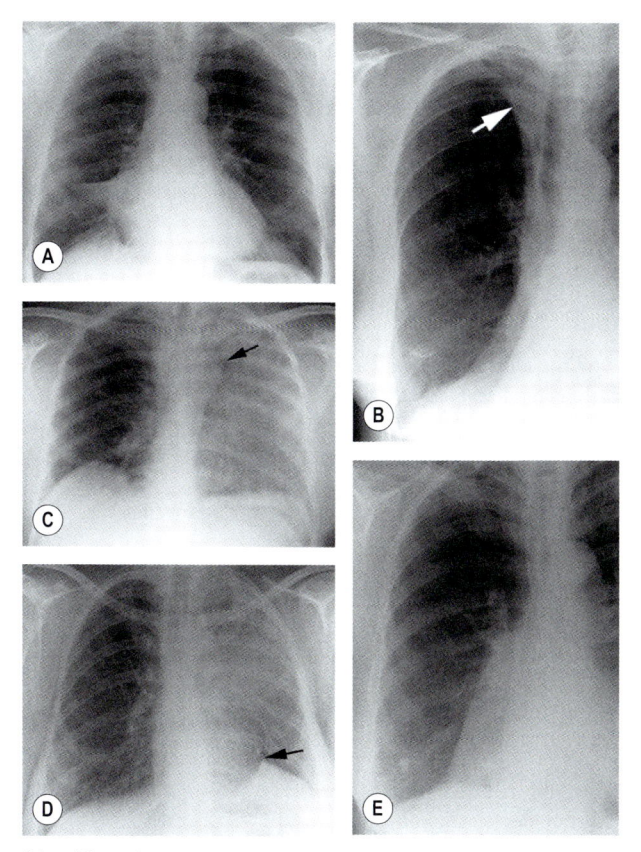

Fig. 14.1 Timing of the different heart sounds and added sounds.

- If you hear a murmur at the apex, ensure that you get the patient to breathe in and out: the examiner will be observing whether or not you are listening for the variation in intensity with respiration.
- If you hear a pansystolic murmur, listen at the axilla (mitral regurgitant murmurs are conducted to the axilla).

Note: Be prepared to discuss the approach of systolic and diastolic murmurs (see later).

15. Using the diaphragm of your stethoscope, listen at the apex, below the sternum, along the left sternal edge, the second right intercostal space, and the neck (for ejection systolic murmur of aortic stenosis, aortic sclerosis).
16. Request the patient to sit forward and listen with the diaphragm along the left sternal edge in the third intercostal area with the patient's breath held in expiration for early diastolic murmur of aortic regurgitation.
17. Tell the examiner that you would like to do the following:
    - Listen to lung bases for signs of cardiac failure
    - Check for sacral and leg oedema
    - Examine the liver (tender liver of cardiac failure), splenomegaly (endocarditis)
    - Check blood pressure
    - Check the peripheral pulses and also check for radiofemoral delay.

Systolic Murmur

What is the effect on the murmur of inspiration?
- (a) Increases with inspiration (right sided):
  - Ejection or regurgitant?
  - If ejection, is there an ejection sound?
  - If no ejection sound, is S_2 fixed or not fixed?
- (b) No increase with inspiration (left sided):
  - Is it ejection, regurgitant or uncertain?
  - For each, what is the effect of the Valsalva manoeuvre or squatting?

Diastolic Murmur

What is the effect on the murmur of inspiration?
- (a) Increases with inspiration (right sided):
  - Assess the quality of murmur and location.
  - Is there pulmonary regurgitation?
- (b) No increase with inspiration (left sided):
  - Assess quality of murmur (high or low pitched) and location.

Questions

How do you classify the severity of heart failure?
The severity of heart failure is classified by the NYHA classification, which grades symptoms and gives estimated mortality.

NYHA Class	Symptoms	Estimated 1-Year Mortality (%)
I	Mild: no limitation of physical activity	5–10
II	Mild to moderate: slight limitation of physical activity, comfortable at rest but dyspnoea and fatigue on ordinary physical activity	15–30
III	Moderate: marked limitation of physical activity, comfortable at rest but dyspnoea and fatigue on less than ordinary physical activity	15–30
IV	Severe: symptoms at rest	50–60

Name the causes of bilateral leg oedema.
- Heart failure
- Chronic venous insufficiency
- Hypoalbuminaemia
- Immobility
- Lymphoedema
- Thiamine deficiency
- Iatrogenic (amlodipine, steroids).

Further Information

British physician Sir John Forbes (1787–1861) is best remembered for popularizing the stethoscope among English-speaking doctors. Forbes was born in Banff in the north-east of Scotland. He studied at Marischal College, Aberdeen, before he went to Edinburgh, where he received his medical education. Forbes translated Laennec's monograph into English in 1821 and published his own book on the subject in 1824 (Forbes, 1824). The latter included a brief biographical sketch of the Austrian physician Leopold Auenbrugger and the first English translation of his essay (which was in Latin) on percussion. It also contained a summary of Parisian physician Victor Collin's recent manual on cardiac physical diagnosis.

CHAPTER 15

Aortic Regurgitation

Instruction

This patient presented with progressive dyspnoea and tiredness. Please examine this patient's cardiovascular system.

Salient Features

HISTORY

- Asymptomatic (but may have normal or depressed left ventricular (LV) function)
- Dyspnoea and fatigue (from LV impairment and low cardiac output, initially on exertion)
- Symptoms of LV failure in later stages
- Angina pectoris is less common than in aortic stenosis; usually indicates coronary artery disease.

EXAMINATION

Pulse

- Collapsing pulse (large volume, rapid fall with low diastolic pressure)
- Visible carotid pulsation in the neck (dancing carotids or Corrigan's sign)
- Capillary pulsation in the fingernails (Quincke's sign)
- A booming sound heard over the femorals ('pistol-shot' femorals or Traube's sign)
- To and fro systolic and diastolic murmur produced by compression of femorals by stethoscope (Duroziez's sign or murmur).

Heart

- Heart sounds are usually normal.
- Apex beat will be displaced outwards and forceful; may be seen and/or felt.
- Third heart sound is heard (in early systole with bicuspid aortic valve).
- Early diastolic, high-pitched, decrescendo murmur is heard at the left sternal edge with the diaphragm; if not readily apparent, it is important to sit the patient forward and auscultate with the patient's breath held at the end of expiration (Fig. 15.1). When the ascending aorta is dilated and displaced to the right, the murmur may be heard along the right sternal border.
- An ejection systolic murmur may be heard at the base of the heart in severe aortic regurgitation (without aortic stenosis). This murmur may be as loud as grade 5 or 6, and underlying organic stenosis can be ruled out only by investigations.
- Ejection click suggests underlying bicuspid aortic valve.
- Middiastolic murmur of Austin Flint may be heard at the apex. It is typically low pitched, similar to the murmur of mitral stenosis but without preceding opening snap.
- There is a loud pulmonary component of the second sound (suggests pulmonary hypertension).

15—AORTIC REGURGITATION

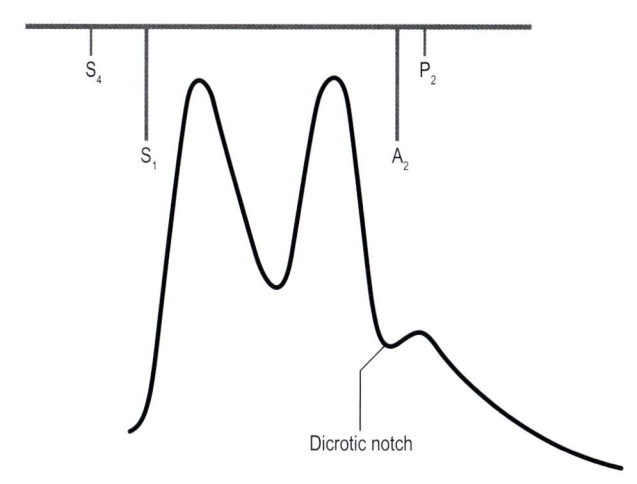

Fig. 15.1 Carotid pulse waveform and heart sound in severe aortic regurgitation; bifid pulse with two systolic peaks.

General Examination
- Head nodding in time with the heart beat (de Musset's sign) may be present.
- Visible carotid pulsation may be obvious in the neck: dancing carotids or Corrigan's sign.
- Blood pressure indicates wide pulse pressure.
- Look for systolic pulsations of the uvula (Muller's sign).
- Check the pupils for Argyll Robertson pupil of syphilis.
- Look for stigmata of Marfan syndrome: high-arched palate, arm span greater than height.
- Check joints for ankylosing spondylitis and rheumatoid arthritis.

Diagnosis

This patient has pure aortic regurgitation (lesion), which is caused by associated ankylosing spondylitis (aetiology), and is in cardiac failure (functional status).

Questions

Mention a few causes of chronic aortic regurgitation.
- Rheumatic fever
- Hypertension (accentuated tambour quality of second sound)
- Atherosclerosis
- Bacterial endocarditis
- Idiopathic dilatation of the aortic root and annulus
- Syphilis
- Marfan syndrome
- Rheumatoid arthritis
- Cystic medial necrosis of the aorta
- Seronegative arthritis (ankylosing spondylitis, Reiter syndrome)
- Bicuspid aortic valve.

How would you investigate a patient with aortic regurgitation?
- *Chest radiograph* is usually normal in mild aortic regurgitation, possibly valvular calcification, cardiomegaly.
- *Electrocardiogram* (Fig. 15.2) typically shows features of LV hypertrophy and strain (increased QRS amplitude and ST/T wave changes in precordial leads) and left atrial hypertrophy (wide P wave in lead II and biphasic P in lead V_1).
- *Echocardiogram* is indicated to confirm the diagnosis of aortic regurgitation; determine aetiology; assess valve morphology; acquire a semiquantitative estimate of the severity of regurgitation; assess LV dimension, mass, and systolic function; assess aortic size; estimate the degree of pulmonary hypertension (when tricuspid regurgitation is present); and determine whether there is rapid equilibration of aortic and LV diastolic pressure. Doppler is the most sensitive method for detecting an aortic regurgitation jet.
- *Exercise testing* in severe aortic regurgitation, when sedentary or where there are equivocal symptoms, is useful to assess functional capacity, symptomatic responses, and haemodynamic effects of exercise.
- *Cardiac catheterization* and angiography are necessary when coronary artery disease is suspected (e.g. in patients >40 years) and when the severity of aortic regurgitation is doubted; injection of contrast into the aortic root gives information on the degree of regurgitation and state of aortic root (presence of dilatation, dissection, root abscesses).
- Computed tomography and cardiac magnetic resonance can be used to assess aortic regurgitation if echocardiogram is insufficient.

How can you explain the wide pulse pressure in aortic regurgitation?
Regardless of the aetiology, in aortic regurgitation the leaflets of the aortic valve cannot fully close during diastole. A percentage of the stroke volume leaks back into the left ventricle. The left ventricle responds with concentric hypertrophy in pressure overload and eccentric hypertrophy in volume overload. In this scenario the added volume of blood that regurgitates back to the left ventricle causes compensatory eccentric hypertrophy. As the left ventricle enlarges, the stroke volume increases which causes an increase in systolic blood pressure. With each diastole the regurgitant stroke volume causes an immediate fall in the arterial wall pressure and collapse of the arteries, which translates into a diminished diastolic blood pressure. Overall, the pulse pressure is larger than in a normally functioning aortic valve.

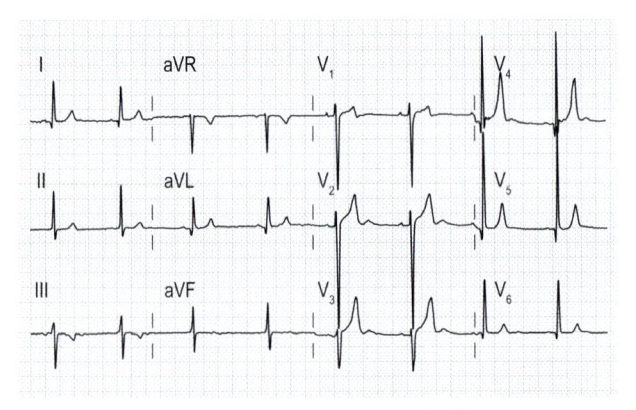

Fig. 15.2 Left ventricular hypertrophy with prominent positive anterior T waves.

15 — AORTIC REGURGITATION

What is the natural history of chronic aortic regurgitation?
- Asymptomatic patients with normal LV systolic function:
  - Progression to symptoms and/or LV dysfunction <6%/year
  - Progression to asymptomatic LV dysfunction <3.5%/year
  - Sudden death <0.2%/year.
- Asymptomatic patients with LV systolic dysfunction:
  - Progression to symptoms >25%/year.
- Symptomatic patients:
  - Mortality rate >10%/year.

What are the clinical signs of severity?
- Wide pulse pressure
- Soft second heart sound
- The duration of the decrescendo diastolic murmur
- Presence of the LV third heart sound
- Austin Flint murmur
- Signs of LV failure.

What do you know of Hill's sign?
Hill's sign is the presence of higher systolic pressure in the leg than in the arm and is said to be an indicator of the severity of aortic regurgitation. In mild aortic regurgitation the difference is <20 mm Hg; in moderate regurgitation, 20 to 40 mm Hg; and in severe regurgitation, it is >60 mm Hg.

Do the characteristics of early diastolic murmur correlate with severity?
Yes. In mild aortic regurgitation the murmur is short, but as the severity of the regurgitation increases the murmur becomes longer and louder and it may extend throughout diastole. It is not uncommon for the murmur to disappear in severe regurgitation with ventricular decompensation, as the aortic and LV diastolic pressures equalize.

What is an Austin Flint murmur?
It is an apical, low-pitched, diastolic murmur caused by vibration of the anterior mitral cusp in the regurgitant jet; it is heard at the apex.

Mention a few causes of acute aortic regurgitation.
- Infective endocarditis
- Aortic dissection
- Trauma
- Failure of prosthetic valve
- Rupture of sinus of Valsalva.

What do you understand by the term cor bovinum?
In chronic aortic regurgitation, there is slow and progressive LV dilatation and hypertrophy in an attempt to normalize wall stress. The heart may therefore become larger and heavier than in any other form of chronic heart disease, which is cor bovinum (bovine or ox heart).

What is the role of vasodilators in aortic regurgitation?
Multiple studies have been carried out over the last two decades investigating the role of vasodilators in aortic regurgitation, and although different outcomes have come out of different groups, it is generally accepted that vasodilators should be used in patients with severe aortic regurgitation

with LV dilation. Groups of patients with severe aortic regurgitation that would benefit from the use of vasodilators are patients who:
- Have symptoms of heart failure, but surgery is contraindicated
- Are awaiting corrective surgery but suffer from symptomatic heart failure
- Have undergone valve replacement but continue to suffer from heart failure.

What are the indications for surgical intervention?
Severe aortic regurgitation is usually treated surgically. The timing of surgery is important and depends on the severity of symptoms and extent of LV dysfunction. Valve replacement should be performed as soon as possible after the onset of ventricular dysfunction. Indications for surgery include:
- Symptoms of heart failure and diminished LV function
- Concomitant coronary artery disease that requires coronary artery bypass grafting
- Existence of another indication for cardiac surgery.

How would you follow up a patient with aortic regurgitation?
Asymptomatic patients with aortic regurgitation should be followed up with clinical assessment annually and have regular echocardiograms, the frequency of which will depend on the severity of the underlying valve lesion (6-monthly to 5-yearly).

Further Information

Alfred de Musset was a French poet whose nodding movements were described by his brother in a biography. When told of this, Alfred put his thumb and forefinger on his neck and the head stopped bobbing.

Austin Flint (1812–1886) was one of the founders of Buffalo Medical College, New York, and reported the murmur in two patients with aortic regurgitation, confirmed by postmortem. He also held chairs at New Orleans, Chicago, and Louisville.

H.I. Quincke (1842–1922) was a German physician who described angioneurotic oedema and benign intracranial hypertension.

P.I. Duroziez (1826–1897), a French physician, was widely acclaimed for his articles on mitral stenosis.

L. Traube (1818–1876), a German physician, was the first to describe pulsus bigeminus.

Antonio Maria Valsalva (1666–1723) was an Italian anatomist and surgeon who discovered the labyrinth and developed the Valsalva manoeuvre to remove foreign bodies from the ear.

CHAPTER 16

Aortic Stenosis

Instruction
This patient presents with several presyncopal episodes while playing football. Please examine this patient's cardiovascular system.

Salient Features
HISTORY
- Asymptomatic (many patients do not have symptoms)
- Fatigue
- Dyspnoea on exertion (the commonest presenting symptom of aortic stenosis)
- Angina (in ~70% of adults; average survival after onset of angina is 5 years)
- Syncope on exertion (in 25% of patients, during or immediately after exercise; average survival after onset of syncope is 3 years).

EXAMINATION
Pulse
- Low volume pulse, with a delayed upstroke (pulsus parvus et tardus). This is caused by a reduction in systolic pressure and a gradual decline in diastolic pressure.
  - Normal pulse in mild aortic stenosis when the gradient is <50 mm Hg
  - Slow rise with diminished 'volume', sometimes with notch on the upstroke ('anacrotic'): indicating severe aortic stenosis with associated aortic regurgitation, double pulse may be felt ('bisferiens') (Fig. 16.1).

Heart
- Apex beat is heaving in nature but is not displaced. (A displaced apex beat indicates left ventricular (LV) dilatation and severe disease.)
- Palpable systolic vibrations over the primary aortic area with the patient in the sitting position during full expiration (often correlates with a gradient of >40 mm Hg).
- Systolic thrill over the aortic area and the carotids.
- Soft second heart sound.
- Ejection click heard 0.1 s after the first heart sound along the left sternal border (indicates valvular stenosis). An ejection sound that moves with respiration is not aortic in origin (Fig. 16.2).
- An atrial (S4) sound may be heard.
- Ejection systolic murmur at the base of the heart conducted to the carotids and the right clavicle (Fig. 16.2). (Listen carefully for an early diastolic murmur as mild aortic regurgitation often accompanies aortic stenosis.)

63

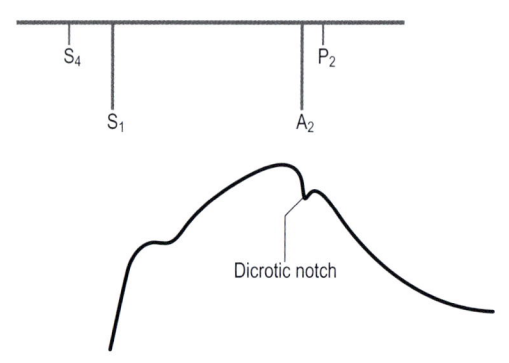

Fig. 16.1 Carotid pulse waveforms and heart sounds in aortic stenosis. Anacrotic pulse with slow upstroke and peak near S_2.

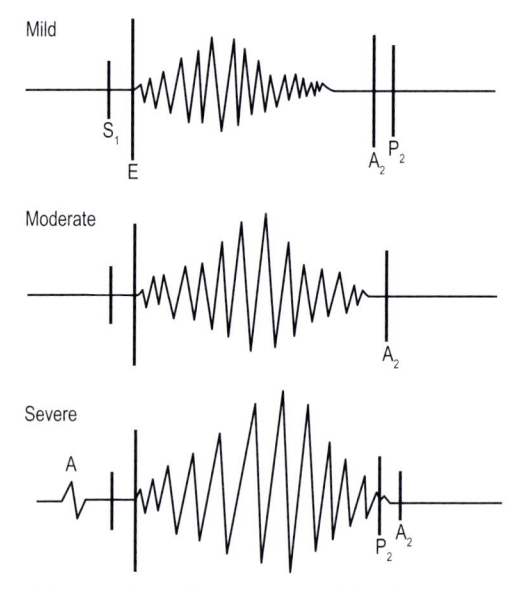

Fig. 16.2 Auscultatory and phonocardiographic signs in bicuspid aortic stenosis.

- Third heart sound: in patients with aortic stenosis, third heart sounds are uncommon but usually indicate the presence of systolic dysfunction and raised filling pressures.

General Examination

- Check blood pressure, keeping in mind that pulse pressure is low in moderate to severe stenosis.

Diagnosis

This patient has pure aortic stenosis (lesion), which may have a rheumatic aetiology or be from a bicuspid aortic valve (aetiology). He has severe aortic stenosis as he gives a history of recurrent syncope (functional status).

Questions

How would you differentiate aortic stenosis from aortic sclerosis?
Aortic sclerosis is seen in the elderly; the pulse is normal volume, the apex beat is not shifted, and the murmur is localized with no radiation.

Mention some causes of aortic stenosis.
- Rheumatic, congenital
- Calcified bicuspid aortic valve
- Degenerative calcification.

What does the second heart sound tell us in this condition?
- A soft second heart sound indicates valvular stenosis (except in calcific stenosis of the elderly, where the margins of the leaflets usually maintain their mobility).
- A single second heart sound may be seen when there is fibrosis and fusion of the valve leaflets.
- Reversed splitting of the second sound indicates mechanical or electrical prolongation of ventricular systole.
- A perfectly normal second heart sound (i.e. normal splitting with A_2 of normal intensity) is strong evidence against the presence of critical aortic stenosis.

What do you understand by the term ejection systolic murmur?
It is a crescendo–decrescendo murmur that begins after the first heart sound (or after the ejection click when present), peaks in mid or late systole, and ends before the second heart sound. This peak is delayed with increasing severity of aortic stenosis.

Does the loudness of the murmur reflect the severity of the aortic stenosis?
No, the loudness of the murmur is related more to the cardiac output and the systolic turbulence surrounding the valve than to the severity of the stenosis. Thus, a loud murmur may be associated with trivial stenosis, and in severe heart failure it may be soft because of decreased flow across the valve from the diminished cardiac output.

What are other causes of ejection systolic murmur at the base of the heart?
- Pulmonary stenosis
- Hypertrophic obstructive cardiomyopathy (HOCM)
- Supravalvular aortic stenosis.

How would you clinically differentiate aortic stenosis from hypertrophic obstructive cardiomyopathy?
- The systolic murmur in aortic stenosis will decrease in intensity when the patient goes from a squatting to a standing position. The opposite will happen in HOCM; the murmur will increase in intensity when the patient goes from a squatting to a standing position.
- Similarly, Valsalva manoeuvre decreases the intensity of the systolic murmur in aortic stenosis, but increases it in HOCM.
- Pulse character is jerky with double impulse in HOCM.
- Aortic stenosis can be associated with an opening click.
- Systolic murmur in aortic stenosis radiates to the carotids whereas the systolic murmur in HOCM radiates to the apex but not the neck.

What is the prevalence of aortic stenosis in the elderly?
According to the Helsinki Ageing Study, almost 3% of individuals aged between 75 and 86 years have critical aortic stenosis.

What is the mechanism of syncope in aortic stenosis?
The LV is suddenly unable to contract (transient electromechanical dissociation) against the stenosed valve. Aortic stenosis is associated with cardiac arrhythmias (bradycardia, ventricular tachycardia, or fibrillation). Marked peripheral vasodilatation without a concomitant increase in cardiac output, particularly after exercise.

What is the mechanism of angina in aortic stenosis?
- Increased oxygen demand by the hypertrophic LV
- Reduced time of diastolic coronary perfusion
- Compression of the small coronary arteries by the hypertrophied myocardial cells
- Concomitant coronary artery disease.

How is the degree of aortic stenosis graded depending on the valve area?
The degree of aortic stenosis is graded as mild (valve area >1.5 cm^2), moderate (>1.0–1.5 cm^2), or severe (≥1.0 cm^2).

What investigations would you do?
- *Electrocardiogram* may show LV hypertrophy, ST-T changes, possibly left axis deviation, later left atrial hypertrophy (negative P waves in V_1), conduction abnormalities from calcification of conducting tissues (first-degree heart block, left bundle branch block).
- *Chest radiograph* may show cardiac enlargement, poststenotic dilatation of aorta (a bicuspid valve should be suspected if the proximal aorta is greatly enlarged), calcification of aortic valve (particularly in older patients) (Fig. 16.3).
- *Echocardiography* is useful in:
    - the diagnosis and assessment of severity of aortic stenosis as it can estimate valve gradient; a normal valve appearance excludes significant aortic stenosis in adults
    - helping to define the level of obstruction (i.e. valvular, supravalvular, subvalvular)
    - identifying calcified valves
    - assessing LV size, function, and/or haemodynamics
    - reevaluating patients with known aortic stenosis with changing symptoms and signs
    - reevaluating asymptomatic patients with severe aortic stenosis
    - assessing patients with known aortic stenosis during pregnancy.
- *Exercise testing* in adults with aortic stenosis has been discouraged largely because of safety; it should not be performed in symptomatic patients as it may be fatal. In asymptomatic patients, an abnormal haemodynamic response (e.g. hypotension) is sufficient to consider aortic valve replacement (AVR). In selected patients, it may be useful to provide a basis for advice about physical activity.
- *Cardiac catheterization* is done to assess the coronary circulation and to confirm or clarify the diagnosis. When the echocardiogram is inadequate, cardiac haemodynamics using both left and right heart catheterization is indicated to establish diagnosis. It is also used to rule out coronary artery disease in patients with angina not explained by the aortic stenosis and in patients with coronary artery disease who are going to undergo AVR, as they may need to have bypass grafting at the same time.
- Cardiac magnetic resonance is used to study the anatomy of the valve, especially when the stenosis is caused by a bicuspid valve.

What are the complications of aortic stenosis?
- LV failure
- Sudden death occurs in 10% to 20% of adults with symptomatic disease. In severe asymptomatic disease, the annual incidence is around 1%, whereas in symptomatic disease, it is much more common.

16—AORTIC STENOSIS

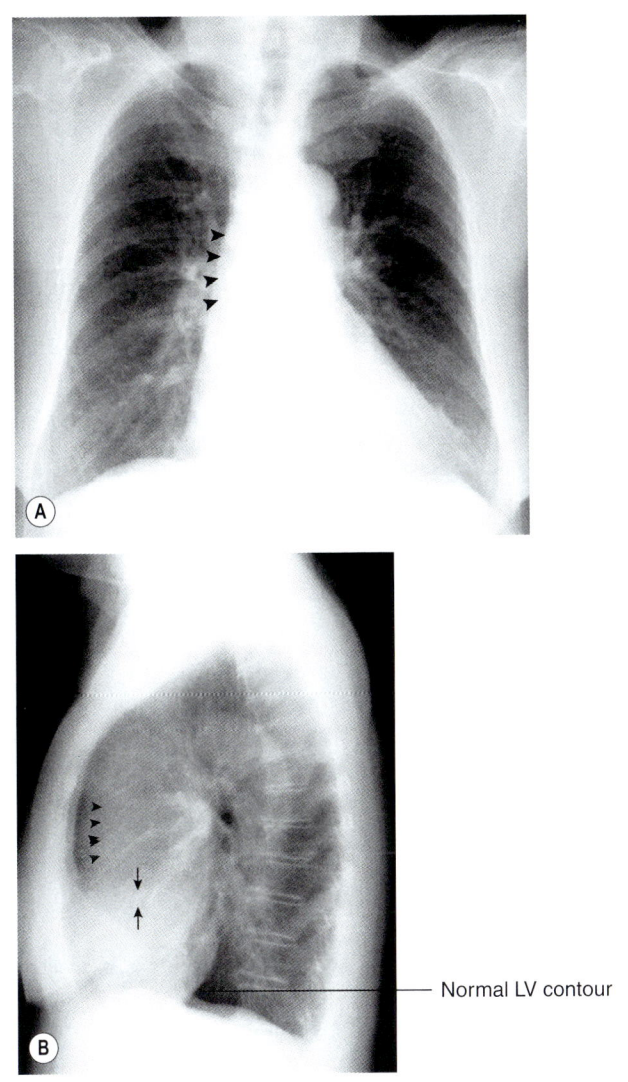

Fig. 16.3 Chest radiographs in severe aortic stenosis. **(A)** Frontal view shows prominent aortic root to the right of the midline *(arrowheads)*. **(B)** Lateral view demonstrates calcification of the aortic valve leaflets *(arrows)*, suggestive of a bicuspid valve. There is a prominent, mildly dilated aortic root *(arrowheads)*. (With permission from Zipes, D.P., Libby, P., Bonow, R.O., Braunwald, E., 2007. Braunwald's Heart Disease. Saunders, Philadelphia, PA.)

- Arrhythmias and conduction abnormalities include ventricular arrhythmias (more common than supraventricular arrhythmias) and heart block (may occur because of calcification of conducting tissues).
- Systemic embolization is caused by disintegration of the aortic valve apparatus or by concomitant aortic atheroma.
- Infective endocarditis (in 10% of cases) should be considered when these patients present with unexplained illness.
- Haemolytic anaemia.

What are the clinical signs of severity of aortic stenosis?
- Narrow pulse pressure
- Soft second sound
- Narrow or reverse split second sound
- Systolic thrill and heaving apex beat
- Fourth heart sound
- Cardiac failure.

What is the treatment for asymptomatic aortic stenosis?
- Asymptomatic patients with mild or moderate disease echocardiographically should be monitored clinically and with frequent echocardiograms.
- Asymptomatic patients but with severe aortic stenosis should undergo intervention.

What is the treatment for symptomatic aortic stenosis?
Symptomatic patients should undergo surgical intervention. AVR and transcatheter aortic valve implantation (TAVI) are the treatment options for symptomatic or severe aortic stenosis. The exception to this rule is in patients who have a predicted survival of less than 1 year and patients whose severe comorbid state makes intervention risky and unlikely to extend life. AVR is the treatment of choice in symptomatic patients who are low-risk surgical candidates. If surgical intervention is otherwise indicated but the patient has a high surgical risk profile, then TAVI is the preferred procedure.

What is the role of medical management in aortic stenosis?
No medical intervention or medication has proven to alter the prognosis of aortic stenosis. Concomitant cardiac conditions like hypertension or coronary artery disease should be treated appropriately.

If a young person presents with signs and symptoms of aortic stenosis but the aortic valve is normal on echocardiography, which condition would you suspect?
Supravalvular or subvalvular aortic stenosis.

What are the genetics of supravalvular stenosis?
- Studies suggest that mutation in the gene for elastin causes supravalvular stenosis.
- In Williams syndrome (also known as Williams–Beurens syndrome), there is a microdeletion in chromosome 7.

If this patient had bleeding per rectum, what unusual cause would come to mind?
Angiodysplasia of the colon.

If the patient was icteric and had haemolytic anaemia, what would the mechanism be?
Microangiopathic haemolysis has been described in severe calcified aortic stenosis, manifesting with anaemia and icterus.

What is the relationship between skin and gastrointestinal tract bleeding and aortic stenosis?
Skin and gastrointestinal tract bleeding is caused by an acquired defect in von Willebrand factor; AVR restores the normal structure of von Willebrand factor and thus restores normal haemostasis. Von Willebrand factor abnormalities are directly related to the severity of aortic stenosis and are improved by valve replacement in the absence of mismatch between patient and prosthesis. The von Willebrand factor normally circulates as very large, homologous multimers composed of 250 kDa subunits. In aortic stenosis, the von Willebrand factor is subjected to high fluid shear

stress as it passes through the stenotic valve, which renders the multimers susceptible to cleavage by ADAMTS 13 (a plasma metalloprotease that acts on von Willebrand factor preferentially under conditions of high fluid shear stress). A deficit in large, haemostatically effective multimers is the result.

What do you understand by 'Gallavardin phenomenon'?
The high-frequency components of the ejection systolic murmur may radiate to the apex. This can then falsely suggest mitral regurgitation. This is known as the Gallavardin phenomenon.

Further Information

Williams syndrome is characterized by elfin facies, supravalvular aortic stenosis, and hypercalcaemia (J.C.P. Williams, New Zealand physician).

CHAPTER 17

Mixed Aortic Valve Disease

Instruction
This patient presents with shortness of breath. Please examine this patient's cardiovascular system.

Salient Features
- Pulse may be biphasic, small volume, or large volume depending on the dominant lesion.
- There is a displaced apex beat (remember a small left ventricle (LV) is inconsistent with chronic severe aortic regurgitation).
- Early diastolic murmur of aortic regurgitation (Fig. 17.1).
- Ejection systolic murmur of aortic stenosis.
- Proceed by telling the examiner that you would like to check the blood pressure (BP), in particular to determine the pulse pressure (systolic minus diastolic pressure).

Diagnosis
This patient has mixed aortic stenosis with aortic regurgitation (lesion) caused by rheumatic heart disease (aetiology). He has a dominant stenosis and is in cardiac failure (functional status).

> **Note:**
> In dominant aortic stenosis:
> - Pulse volume is small.
> - BP is normal and pulse pressure is narrow.
>
> In dominant aortic regurgitation:
> - Pulse is collapsing.
> - Pulse pressure is wide.

Questions

What are common causes of mixed aortic lesions?
- Rheumatic heart disease
- Bicuspid aortic valve
- Degenerative disease.

What is the pathophysiology of mixed aortic valve disease?
- In mixed aortic valve disease, one lesion usually predominates over the other and the pathophysiology resembles that of the pure dominant lesion. When aortic stenosis predominates, the pathophysiology and, therefore, the management resemble that of pure aortic stenosis. The LV in these patients develops concentric hypertrophy rather than dilatation. The timing of aortic valve replacement (like pure aortic stenosis) depends on symptoms.

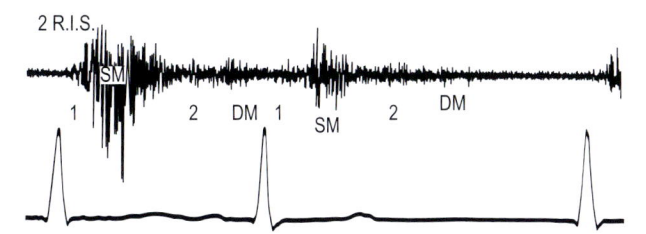

Fig. 17.1 Phonocardiogram of the murmurs present in a patient with valvar aortic stenosis and regurgitation. Note the diamond-shaped systolic murmur peaking in early to midsystole and the high-frequency, lower-intensity murmur throughout diastole. *DM*, Diastolic murmur; *SM*, systolic murmur; *1*, first heart sound; *2*, second heart sound; *2R.I.S.*, second right intercostal space.

- When aortic regurgitation is more than mild and the aortic stenosis is predominant, the concentrically hypertrophied and noncompliant LV is on the steeper portion of the diastolic pressure–volume curve, resulting in pulmonary congestion. Therefore, although neither lesion by itself is severe enough to merit surgery, both together produce substantial haemodynamic compromise requiring surgery.
- When the aortic regurgitation is severe and the aortic stenosis is mild, the high total stroke volume caused by extensive regurgitation may produce a substantial transvalvular gradient. Because the transvalvular gradient varies with the square of the transvalvular flow, a high gradient in predominant regurgitation may be predicted primarily on excess transvalvular flow rather than on a severely compromised orifice area.

In mixed aortic valve disease, is cardiac catheterization more accurate than Doppler echocardiography to measure valve area?
Aortic valve area would be measured inaccurately at the time of cardiac catheterization in mixed aortic valve lesions if the cardiac output is measured by either the Fick or the thermodilution method as both these methods usually underestimate total valve flow. The valve area can be measured more accurately using Doppler echocardiography (by continuity equation) in mixed aortic stenosis and aortic regurgitation. However, the confusing nature of mixed valve disease makes cardiac catheterization necessary to obtain additional haemodynamic information in most patients (including coronary anatomy).

How would you manage such a patient?
- Surgical correction of disease that produces more than mild symptoms
- When the aortic stenosis is dominant, surgery in the presence of even mild symptoms
- When the aortic regurgitation is dominant, surgery can be delayed until symptoms develop or asymptomatic LV dysfunction becomes apparent on echocardiography.

CHAPTER 18

Mitral Regurgitation

Instruction
Examine this patient's heart.

Salient Features
HISTORY
- Asymptomatic or mild symptoms: often
- Shortness of breath (from pulmonary congestion)
- Fatigue (from low cardiac output)
- Palpitation (from atrial fibrillation or left ventricular (LV) dysfunction)
- Fluid retention (in late-stage disease)
- Obtain a history of myocardial infarction, rheumatic fever, connective tissue disorder, infective endocarditis.

EXAMINATION
- Peripheral pulse may be normal or jerky (i.e. rapid upstroke with a short duration).
- Apex beat will be displaced downwards and outwards and will be forceful in character.
- First heart sound will be soft.
- Third heart sound is common (LV gallop sound).
- Pansystolic murmur (Hope murmur) conducted to the axilla is best detected with the diaphragm and on expiration. (Note: It is important to be sure that there is no associated tricuspid regurgitation.)
- Loud pulmonary second sound and left parasternal heave when there is associated pulmonary hypertension.

When mitral regurgitation is caused by LV dilatation and diminished cardiac contractility, the systolic murmur may be mid, late, or pansystolic. Other causes of short systolic murmurs at the apex include mitral valve prolapse, papillary muscle dysfunction, and aortic stenosis. In calcific aortic stenosis of the elderly, the murmur may be more prominent in the apex and may be confused with mitral regurgitation. In such instances, try to listen to the murmur after a pause with premature beat or listen to the beat after a pause with atrial fibrillation. The murmur of aortic stenosis becomes louder, whereas that of mitral regurgitation shows little change.

Diagnosis
This patient has mitral regurgitation (lesion) as evidenced by grade III/VI pansystolic murmur, which is probably caused by ischaemic or rheumatic heart disease (aetiology), and is in cardiac failure as evidenced by bibasal crackles (functional status). The patient is in New York Heart Association class III heart failure.

18 — MITRAL REGURGITATION

Questions

What are causes of chronic mitral regurgitation?
Mitral regurgitation can be classified into primary or secondary, depending on whether the incompetence of the valve is caused by a faulty component of its apparatus or by dilation of the LV causing incompetence of the valve. Some of the causes of mitral regurgitation are the following:
- Infective endocarditis
- Mitral valve prolapse
- Rheumatic heart disease
- LV dilatation
- Coronary artery disease
- Annular calcification
- Papillary muscle dysfunction
- Cardiomyopathy
- Connective tissue disorders.

What are causes of acute mitral regurgitation?
- Acute myocardial infarction (rupture of the papillary muscle)
- Endocarditis (from perforation of the mitral valve leaflet or the chordae)
- Trauma
- Myxomatous degeneration of the valve.

How would you investigate this patient?
- *Electrocardiogram*: look for broad bifid P waves (P mitrale), LV hypertrophy, atrial fibrillation. When coronary artery disease is the cause, there is often evidence of inferior or posterior wall myocardial infarction.
- *Radiography* can assess pulmonary congestion, large heart, left atrial enlargement, and pulmonary artery enlargement (if severe and long-standing).
- *Echocardiography* determines the anatomy of the mitral valve apparatus and left atrial and LV size and function (typical features include large left atrium, large LV, increased fractional shortening, regurgitant jet on colour Doppler, leaflet prolapse, floppy valve, or flail leaflet). The echocardiogram provides baselines estimation of LV and left atrial volume, an estimation of LV ejection fraction, and approximation of the severity of regurgitation. It can be helpful to determine the anatomic cause of mitral regurgitation. In the presence of even mild tricuspid regurgitation, an estimate of pulmonary artery pressure can be obtained.
- *Transoesophageal echocardiogram* is useful when transthoracic echocardiography provides nondiagnostic images. It may give better visualization of mitral valve prolapse. It is utilized to determine the cause of the valve incompetence, as establishing the cause will determine further treatment options. It is also used intraoperatively to establish the anatomic basis for mitral regurgitation and to guide repair.
- *Magnetic resonance imaging* (MRI) of the heart (cardiac MRI) can be used if the severity measures obtained by echocardiography are insufficient to appropriately assess severity.
- *Cardiac catheterization* is useful to determine coexistent coronary artery or aortic valve disease. Large 'v' waves are seen in the wedge tracing. Left ventriculogram and haemodynamic measurements are indicated when noninvasive tests are inconclusive regarding the severity of mitral regurgitation, LV function, or the need for surgery.

How would you differentiate between mitral regurgitation and tricuspid regurgitation?

	Mitral Regurgitation	*Tricuspid Regurgitation*
Pulse	Jerky or normal	Normal
Jugular venous pressure		Prominent 'v' wave
Palpation	LV heave	Left parasternal heave
Auscultation	Pansystolic murmur	Pansystolic murmur
	Intensity increases with expiration	Intensity increases with inspiration
	Radiates to the axilla	
Other signs		Hepatic pulsations

Why may these patients have a jerky pulse?
Because of reduced systolic ejection time, secondary to a large volume of blood regurgitating into the left atrium.

When does the murmur of mitral regurgitation radiate to the neck (i.e. base of the heart)?
Rarely, in involvement of the posterior mitral leaflet or from ruptured chordae tendinae, the regurgitant jet strikes the left atrial wall adjacent to the aortic root and the murmur radiates to the base of the heart; therefore, it may be confused with the murmur of aortic stenosis.

How do you grade systolic murmurs?
Levine's grading of systolic murmurs:
1. Murmur is so faint that it is heard only with special effort.
2. Murmur is faint but readily detected.
3. Murmur is prominent but not loud.
4. Murmur is loud.
5. Murmur is very loud.
6. Murmur is loud enough to be heard with the stethoscope just removed from contact with the chest wall.

What are the causes of pansystolic murmur over the precordium?
- Mitral regurgitation
- Tricuspid regurgitation
- Ventricular septal defect (this generally radiates to the right of the sternum).

Which congenital cardiac conditions can be associated with mitral valve regurgitation?
- Ostium primum atrial septal defect (as a result of cleft mitral valve)
- Partial atrioventricular canal
- Corrected transposition of the great arteries.

What are the mechanisms of mitral regurgitation?
Mechanisms are grossly classified as:
- *functional* (mitral valve is structurally normal and disease results from valve deformation caused by ventricular remodelling), e.g. cardiomyopathy, myocarditis
- *organic* (intrinsic valve lesions), e.g. endocarditis, annular calcification, rheumatic heart disease, ruptured papillary muscle.

They can be subclassified by leaflet movement (Carpentier's classification):
- Type I (normal valve movement, such as annular dilatation or leaflet perforation), e.g. endocarditis
- Type II (excessive movement), e.g. ruptured papillary muscle

- Type III (restrictive movement):
  - IIIa: diastolic restriction, e.g. in rheumatic disease
  - IIIb: systolic restriction, e.g. in functional disease such as cardiomyopathy.

Name some echocardiographic parameters used to determine the severity in primary mitral regurgitation.
A number of clinical and echocardiographic parameters have to be taken into account in order to determine the severity of mitral regurgitation:
- LV size (LV dilation signifies severe incompetence.)
- Left atrial size (Left atrium remains normal in mild incompetence, but in moderate, it is already increased.)
- Mitral apparatus characteristics (coaptation defect, ruptured papillary muscle, flail leaflet)
- Transmitral flow regurgitant jet characteristics in the colour Doppler (large central jet or eccentric jet reaching the posterior left atrial wall)
- Regurgitant volume
- Semiquantitative data (E wave dominant, systolic pulmonary vein flow reversal, wide vena contracta).

What is the significance of third heart sounds in mitral regurgitation?
The prevalence of third heart sounds increases with the severity of mitral regurgitation. However, in patients with mitral regurgitation, the third heart sound is caused by rapid ventricular filling and does not necessarily reflect LV systolic dysfunction or increased filling pressure, since in this situation the third heart sound is caused by rapid filling of the LV by the large volume of blood stored in the left atrium in diastole.

How would you follow a patient with chronic mitral regurgitation?
As a general rule, asymptomatic patients are followed up clinically and echocardiographically or undergo surgical mitral valve repair. Symptomatic patients should be treated medically in the first instance and, depending on their comorbid state, can undergo surgical repair or percutaneous edge-to-edge repair.
  Monitoring: all asymptomatic patients should have annual follow-up with clinical examination and regular echocardiograms, the frequency of which will be determined by the severity of the mitral regurgitation, varying from 6-monthly to 5-yearly.
  Medical therapy: prompt treatment of hypertension and heart failure.
  Intervention: indicated in symptomatic patients with LV ejection fraction more than 30%, asymptomatic patients with LV dysfunction (LV ejection fraction less than 60%), and asymptomatic patients with preserved ejection fraction with atrial fibrillation secondary to the valvular problem, or pulmonary hypertension.

What is the natural history of chronic mitral regurgitation?
Progression of the mitral regurgitation is variable and is determined by progression of lesions or mitral annulus size.

Further Information

Samuel A. Levine was Professor of Cardiology at Harvard Medical School and Peter Bent Brigham Hospital in Boston.

James Hope (1801–1841) was an English physician who worked at St George's Hospital, London, and wrote a book in 1831 entitled *Diseases of the Heart and Great Vessels*.

CHAPTER 19

Mitral Stenosis

Instruction

This patient complains of shortness of breath on exertion of recent onset. Please examine their cardiovascular system.

Salient Features

HISTORY

- Dyspnoea on exertion along with reduced exercise tolerance as the presenting complaint may be the only symptom of mitral stenosis. A detailed history of the onset and progression of this symptom should be obtained. It is not a sign of left-sided heart failure, especially in the early stages of mitral stenosis, rather of increased left atrial and consequent pulmonary pressure.
- Symptoms of left-sided heart failure: exertional dyspnoea, orthopnoea, paroxysmal dyspnoea, fatigue, and dizziness from low output
- Symptoms of right-sided failure (These symptoms are somewhat more specific for mitral stenosis.)
- Complications related to mitral stenosis (palpitations if atrial fibrillation has developed, embolic events, voice hoarseness from left atrial enlargement, symptoms of pulmonary hypertension including haemoptysis)
- Obtain a history of rheumatic fever in childhood.

EXAMINATION

- Pulse is regular or irregularly irregular (from atrial fibrillation).
- Jugular venous pressure (JVP) may be raised.
- Malar flush
- Tapping apex beat in the fifth intercostal space just medial to the midclavicular line
- Left parasternal heave (indicating right ventricular enlargement)
- Loud first heart sound
- Opening snap (OS; often difficult to hear; a high-pitched sound that can vary from 0.04 to 0.10 s after the second sound (S) and is heard best at the apex with the patient in the lateral decubitus position)
- Rumbling, low-pitched, middiastolic murmur, best heard in the left lateral position on expiration. In sinus rhythm, there may be presystolic accentuation of the murmur.
- Increasing the flow across the mitral valve will make the murmur heard better; ask the patient to perform sit-ups or to hop to increase the heart rate. However, increasing the flow across a stenotic valve can precipitate symptoms, so perhaps it is not appropriate for a candidate to ask the patient in an examination setting.
- Pulmonary component of second sound (P) is loud.

> **Notes:**
> The signs of pulmonary hypertension include loud P_2, right ventricular lift, elevated neck veins, ascites, and oedema. This is an ominous sign of disease progression because pulmonary hypertension increases the risk associated with surgery.
>   In patients with valvular lesions, a candidate would be expected to comment on rhythm, the presence of heart failure, and signs of pulmonary hypertension.
>   In atrial septal defect, large flow murmurs across the tricuspid valve can cause middiastolic murmurs. The presence of wide, fixed splitting of second sound, absence of loud first heart sound, and an OS and incomplete right bundle branch block should indicate the correct diagnosis. However, about 4% of patients with atrial septal defect have mitral stenosis, a combination called Lutembacher syndrome.

Diagnosis

This patient has mitral stenosis (lesion), which may be caused by rheumatic heart disease (aetiology), and has atrial fibrillation, pulmonary hypertension, and congestive cardiac failure (functional status).

Questions

What is the commonest cause of mitral stenosis?
Rheumatic heart disease.

What is the pathology of mitral stenosis?
The main features are leaflet thickening, nodularity, and commissural fusion, all of which result in narrowing of the valve to the shape of a fish mouth.

What is the natural history of mitral stenosis?
- From the occurrence of rheumatic fever to the onset of symptoms, there is a long latent period of 20 years, with wide variability among countries.
- Moreover, there is a further period of about 10 years before symptoms become disabling.
- The prognosis worsens once symptoms develop.
- The 10-year survival of untreated patients is 50% to 60%, depending on symptoms at presentation:
    - When the patient is asymptomatic or minimally symptomatic, the survival is >80% at 10 years, with 60% of patients having no progression of symptoms.
    - Once significant limiting symptoms occur, the 10-year survival rate is poor (0%–15%).
    - When there is severe pulmonary hypertension, mean survival drops to <3 years.
- Mortality of untreated patients is caused by:
    - progressive heart failure in 60% to 70%
    - systemic embolism in 20% to 30%
    - pulmonary embolism in 10%
    - infection in 1% to 5%.

What is the mechanism of tapping apex beat?
It is from an accentuated first heart sound.

What does the opening snap indicate?
The OS is caused by the opening of the stenosed mitral valve and indicates that the leaflets are pliable. The OS is usually accompanied by a loud first heart sound. It is absent when the valve is diffusely calcified. When only the tips of the leaflets are calcified, the OS persists.

What is the mechanism of a loud first heart sound?
The loud first heart sound occurs when the valve leaflets are mobile. The valve is open during diastole and is suddenly slammed shut by ventricular contraction in systole.

What is the mechanism of presystolic accentuation of the murmur?
In sinus rhythm, it is caused by the atrial systole, which increases flow across the stenotic valve from the left atrium to the left ventricle (LV); this causes accentuation of the loudness of the murmur. This may also be seen in atrial fibrillation and is explained by the turbulent flow caused by the mitral valve starting to close with the onset of ventricular systole. This occurs before the first heart sound and gives the impression of falling in late diastole. It is, however, caused by the start of ventricular systole.

What are the complications?
- Left atrial enlargement and atrial fibrillation
- Systemic embolization, usually cerebral hemispheres
- Pulmonary hypertension
- Tricuspid regurgitation
- Right heart failure

How does one determine clinically the severity of the stenosis?
- The narrower the distance between the second sound and the OS, the greater the severity. The converse is not true. (Note: This time interval between the second sound and OS is said to be inversely related to the left atrial pressure.)
- The longer the duration of the diastolic murmur, the greater the severity. Note that in tight mitral stenosis, the murmur may be less prominent or inaudible and the findings may be primarily those of pulmonary hypertension.

What are the investigations you would do?
- *Electrocardiogram* shows broad bifid P wave (P mitrale); atrial fibrillation in advanced disease, left atrial enlargement, right ventricular hypertrophy (Fig. 19.1).
- *Chest radiography* (Fig. 19.2) shows:
    - congested upper lobe veins
    - double silhouette from enlarged left atrium
    - straightening of the left border of the heart caused by prominent pulmonary conus and filling of the pulmonary bay by the enlarged left atrium

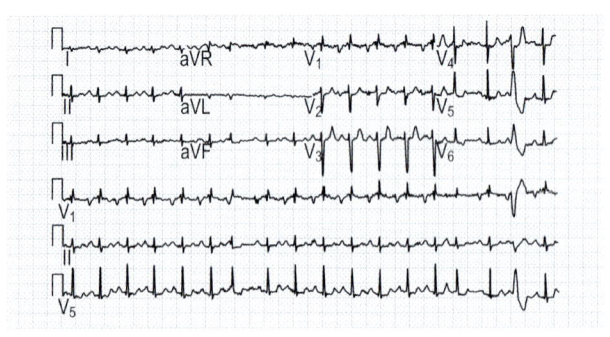

Fig. 19.1 Electrocardiography in severe mitral stenosis, showing right ventricular hypertrophy and left atrial enlargement.

19 — MITRAL STENOSIS

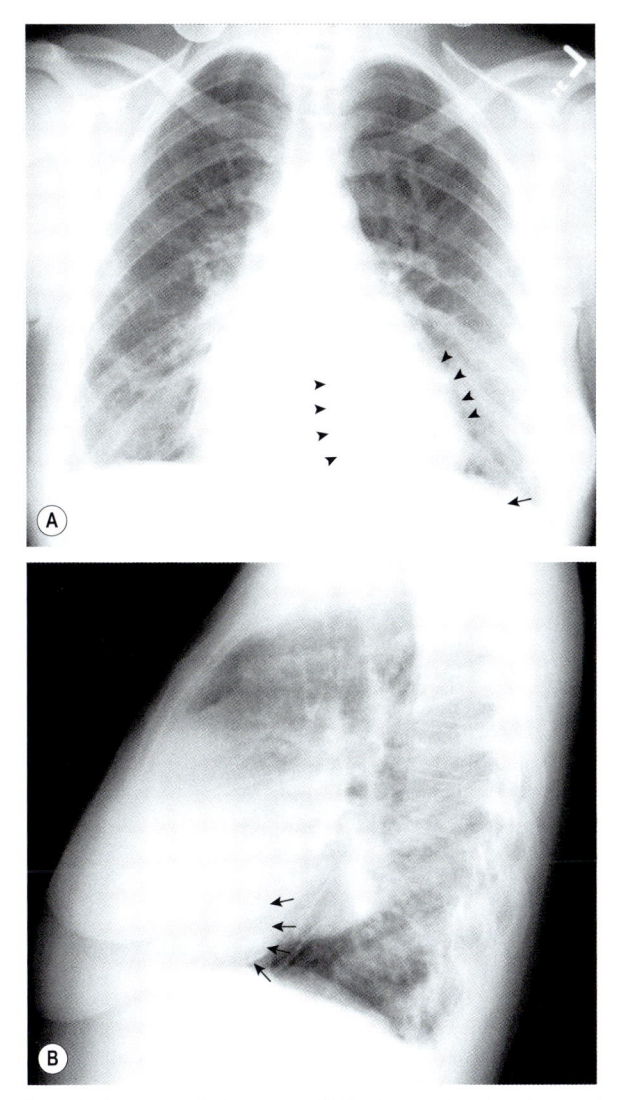

Fig. 19.2 Chest radiographs in severe mitral stenosis. **(A)** Posteroanterior view shows enlargement of the left atrium *(arrowheads)*, prominence of the hilar vessels, and pulmonary venous redistribution. Transverse angle of the apex suggests right ventricular enlargement *(arrow)*. **(B)** Lateral view confirms this, with filling in of the retrosternal airspace. Note also severe left atrial enlargement *(arrows)*. (With permission from Zipes, D.P., Libby, P., Bonow, R.O., Braunwald, E., 2007. Braunwald's Heart Disease. Saunders, Philadelphia, PA.)

- Kerley B lines (horizontal lines in the regions of the costophrenic angles)
- uncommonly the left bronchus may be horizontal as a result of an enlarged left atrium
- mottling caused by secondary pulmonary haemosiderosis.
- *Echocardiography*: two-dimensional and Doppler echocardiography is the diagnostic tool of choice for assessing the severity of mitral stenosis (2014 AHA/ACC Guideline for the Management of Patients with Valvular Heart Disease: A Report of the American College of Cardiology/American Heart Association Task Force on Practice Guideline)

for deciding routine management of the lesion and judging the applicability of percutaneous mitral balloon valvotomy. Advantages include:
- identifying restricted diastolic opening of the mitral valve leaflets caused by 'doming' of the anterior leaflet and immobility of the posterior leaflet
- assessment of the mitral valve apparatus and left atrial enlargement
- an accurate planimetric calculation of the valve area
- measurement of the mean transmitral gradient, using continuous wave Doppler signal across the mitral valve with the modified Bernoulli equation
- determining mitral valve area noninvasively from Doppler echocardiography
- estimation of the pulmonary artery systolic pressure from the tricuspid regurgitation velocity signal with Doppler and assess severity of concomitant mitral or aortic regurgitation.

- *Transoesophageal echocardiography* is not required routinely. It is used to exclude thrombus in the left atrial appendage before balloon valvotomy or cardioversion or after an embolic episode.
- *Cardiac catheterization* is indicated if echocardiography is not conclusive of the diagnosis or when there is a discrepancy between Doppler-derived haemodynamics and the clinical status of a symptomatic patient. It allows accurate measurement of chamber pressures:
  - shows raised right heart pressures and an end-diastolic gradient from pulmonary artery wedge pressure (or left atrium if transseptal puncture done to the LV)
  - left and right heart catheterization is indicated when percutaneous mitral balloon valvotomy is being considered.
- *Coronary angiography* may be required in selected patients who need intervention.
  - *Exercise haemodynamics* should be performed when the symptoms are out of proportion to the calculated mitral valve gradient area.

What is the normal cross-sectional area of the mitral valve?
It ranges from 4 to 6 cm^2, and turbulence of the flow occurs when this area is <2 cm^2.

How would you manage the patient?
All patients with mitral stenosis require regular follow-up with clinical assessment and echocardiography.

Follow-up: asymptomatic patients in sinus rhythm who do not develop symptoms even at stress testing will only require regular follow-up with history, clinical assessment, and echocardiography without any other medical or surgical intervention.

Anticoagulation: formal anticoagulation is recommended in all patients with atrial fibrillation, atrial thrombus, or previous thromboembolic event.

Note: Direct oral anticoagulants (DOACs) can now be used in atrial fibrillation with left heart valve diseases, with the exception of mitral stenosis.

Medical management: diuretics can be helpful to reduce left atrial pressure and, therefore, symptoms; beta-blockers can reduce the symptoms.

Atrial fibrillation: rate control is preferred to rhythm control strategies (digitalis, beta-blocker, or calcium channel blocker).

Intervention options: symptomatic patients will require some form of intervention. The timing of the intervention is crucial; too early can pose the patient unnecessary risks, but if

19—MITRAL STENOSIS

left too late, the development of complications may be irreversible. There are two kinds of intervention:
- Percutaneous mitral balloon valvotomy: patients with symptomatic stenosis, patients who would benefit from surgery but are too high risk to undergo surgery, and in asymptomatic patients with clinically significant stenosis that despite the lack of symptoms have high thromboembolic risk, or high risk of haemodynamic decompensation. For intervention to take place, a series of unfavourable patient characteristics have to be absent: unsuitable valve morphology or echocardiographic characteristics, patient's complication, and comorbid state.
- In severe stenosis that is symptomatic, patients who are assessed to be low risk for surgery where valvulotomy is contraindicated or has failed can undergo mitral valve surgery (repair or replacement).

What are the indications for surgery?
- Patients with severe symptoms of pulmonary congestion and significant mitral stenosis (mitral valve area ≤40.5 cm^2)
- Patients with pulmonary hypertension (pulmonary artery systolic pressure >50 mm Hg at rest or 60 mm Hg with exercise) or haemoptysis even if minimally symptomatic
- Patients with severe symptomatic stenosis who are undergoing cardiac surgery for another indication
- Patients with severe stenosis who are suffering from recurrent thromboembolic events despite therapeutic anticoagulation can undergo valve surgery combined with left atrial appendage excision.

What are the indications for mitral valve replacement?
Patients who are not good candidates for percutaneous balloon valvotomy or mitral valve repair who have:
- moderate to severe mitral stenosis and New York Heart Association class III–IV
- severe mitral stenosis (mitral valve area <1 cm^2) and severe pulmonary hypertension (pulmonary artery systolic pressure >60 mm Hg)
- severe mitral stenosis in patients who are undergoing cardiac surgery for another reason
- severe stenosis who would have been candidates for valvotomy, but have contraindications to the procedure
- recurrent thromboembolic episodes despite anticoagulation in conjunction with mitral stenosis.

Name some contraindications to percutaneous intervention.
- Left atrial thrombus
- Severe calcification
- Existence of other valve disease that requires surgery.

Mention some rarer causes of mitral stenosis.
- Calcification of mitral annulus and leaflets
- Rheumatoid arthritis
- Systemic lupus erythematosus
- Malignant carcinoid
- Congenital stenosis.

Which conditions simulate mitral stenosis?
- Left atrial myxoma

- Ball valve thrombus in the left atrium
- Cor triatriatum (a rare congenital heart condition where a thin membrane across the left atrium obstructs pulmonary venous flow).

Have you heard of Ortner syndrome?
It refers to the hoarseness of voice caused by left vocal cord paralysis associated with enlarged left atrium in mitral stenosis.

What are the haemodynamic changes in mitral stenosis?
It depends on the severity of mitral stenosis and includes an increase in left atrial pressure, an increase in pulmonary arterial pressure, and in severe cases, decreased cardiac output.

Further Information

N. Ortner (1865–1935), Professor of Medicine, Vienna, described the syndrome in 1897. He believed in laboratory research and its application to bedside clinical work and he said that the clinician's motto ought to be 'übers laboratorium dauernd zur Klinik' (translated: 'always via the laboratory to the clinic').

P.J. Kerley (1900–1978), British radiologist.

Elliott Cutler, in 1923 in Boston, USA, was the first to attempt surgical treatment of mitral stenosis by inserting a knife through the apex of the LV and blindly cutting the valve at right angles to its natural orifice.

Henry Souttar, in 1925, relieved mitral stenosis with a finger inserted through the atrial appendage.

In 1948, four surgeons working independently performed successful valvotomies: Horace Smithy, Charles Bailey, Dwight Harken, and Russell Brock.

In 1984, Kanji Inoue from Japan and, in 1985, James E. Lock and colleagues introduced balloon valvuloplasty for mitral stenosis.

R. Lutembacher, a French physician, described the Lutembacher syndrome in 1916.

CHAPTER 20

Mitral Valve Prolapse

Instruction
Examine this patient's heart.

Salient Features

HISTORY
- Palpitations associated with mild tachyarrhythmias
- Increased adrenergic symptoms
- Chest pain
- Anxiety or fatigue.

EXAMINATION
- Midsystolic click followed by late or midsystolic murmur
- Look for features of Marfan syndrome (high arched palate, arm span greater than height).
- Squatting will bring the midsystolic click closer to the second heart sound and decrease the duration of the murmur.
- A Valsalva manoeuvre and standing have the opposite effect.
- The midsystolic murmur begins after the first heart sound; the late systolic murmurs begin after the first heart sound but continue to or through the second heart sound (S_2). Both types of murmur may have a crescendo–decrescendo configuration.

Diagnosis
This patient has mitral valve prolapse (lesion) and a long pansystolic murmur, indicating significant mitral regurgitation.

Questions

What are eponyms for mitral valve prolapse?
Barlow syndrome, click–murmur syndrome, floppy mitral valve.

What is the prevalence in the normal population?
The new awareness that the mitral valve is saddle shaped rather than a planar valve has resulted in new echocardiographic definition for mitral valve prolapse as one or both mitral leaflets exhibit at least 2 mm displacement superior to the long-axis annular plane (a line connecting the annular hinge points), with or without leaflet thickening. With this new description, the prevalence of prolapse is estimated at 2% to 3% and is equally distributed between men and women.

What are the complications of mitral valve prolapse?
- Severe mitral regurgitation
- Arrhythmias: ventricular premature contractions, ventricular tachycardia, paroxysmal supraventricular tachycardia
- Atypical chest pain
- Transient ischaemic attacks, embolism
- Infective endocarditis in those with mitral regurgitation
- Sudden death.

Mention a few associated conditions.
- Marfan syndrome
- Chronic rheumatic heart disease
- Ischaemic heart disease
- Infective endocarditis
- Cardiomyopathies
- Atrial septal defects—secundum type
- Ehlers–Danlos syndrome
- Pseudoxanthoma elasticum
- Psoriatic arthritis
- Ebstein's anomaly
- Systemic lupus erythematosus.

How would you manage such patients?
- Reassure the asymptomatic patient.
- Relief of atypical chest pain with analgesics or beta-blockers (empiric treatment)
- Aspirin or anticoagulants in those with transient ischaemic attacks
- Antiarrhythmics in those with frequent tachyarrhythmias or ventricular premature contractions
- Consider surgery in those with severe mitral regurgitation.

What is the mechanism of click in the mitral valve prolapse?
Clicks result from sudden tensing of the mitral valve apparatus as the leaflets prolapse into the left atrium during systole.

What do you know about Carpentier's nomenclature of the mitral valve?
Anatomically, the posterior and anterior leaflets of the mitral valve each may be divided into three sections:
- Three posterior leaflet scallops: the lateral (P1), middle (P2), and medial (P3)
- Three anterior segments: lateral (A1), middle (A2), and medial (A3).

Which segments of the mitral valve commonly prolapse?
- Most cases of prolapse involve the posterior middle scallop (easily identified on long-axis echocardiographic images).
- Lateral scallop prolapse (not clearly seen on long-axis images; this aspect is best seen in the apical four-chamber view)
- Superior leaflet displacement in a four-chamber view should not be judged as diagnostic of prolapse. Therefore, transthoracic echocardiography can confirm the diagnosis of prolapse but may not be able to exclude lateral scallop prolapsed without taking into account several planes of imaging. Transoesophageal echocardiography is consequently very effective in identifying prolapsing segments.

Further Information

John Barlow, South African Professor of Cardiology.

The term mitral valve prolapse was introduced by Criley et al. (1966) and has been frequently used as a synonym for 'billowing mitral leaflet', which was used by Barlow et al. (1968) to describe the same condition.

The French surgeon Carpentier suggested that the term prolapse should be reserved to indicate that the free edge of the leaflet protrudes beyond the mitral annulus level during systole (Carpentier, 1983), whereas the term billowing should be used when the leaflet body bulges into the left atrium, overriding the mitral annulus plane and usually maintaining the free edge of the leaflets on the ventricular side (Barlow and Pocock, 1985), although the two conditions may coexist.

CHAPTER 21

Mixed Mitral Valve Disease

Instruction

Listen to this patient's heart.

Salient Features

- The patient will have signs of both mitral stenosis and regurgitation.
- The candidate will be expected to indicate the dominant lesion (see later).

Proceed as follows:
- Look carefully for surgical scars of mitral valvotomy in all patients (scars under the left breast in female patients are often missed). Patients with previous valvotomy may have regurgitation and restenosis.

	Dominant Mitral Stenosis	*Dominant Mitral Regurgitation*
Apex beat	Tapping, not displaced	Heaving and displaced
First heart sound	Loud	Soft
Third heart sound	Absent	Present

A third heart sound in mitral regurgitation indicates that any associated mitral stenosis is insignificant.

Diagnosis

This patient has mitral stenosis with mitral regurgitation (lesion), with the dominant lesion being stenosis caused by rheumatic heart disease (aetiology), and is in cardiac failure (functional status).

Questions

What is the cause of mitral stenosis with regurgitation?
Mixed mitral valve disease is usually caused by chronic rheumatic heart disease.

Which valves are most often affected by rheumatic heart disease?
The approximate frequencies are:
- Mitral valve disease: 80%
- Aortic valve: 50%
- Combined mitral and aortic valve lesion: 20%
- Tricuspid valve: 10%
- Pulmonary valve: <1%.

What is the significance of a diastolic rumble in mitral regurgitation?
It signifies the presence of coexistent mitral stenosis. In the absence of mitral stenosis, it suggests that there is high diastolic transmitral flow and severe mitral regurgitation. The presence of an opening snap suggests mitral stenosis as the cause of the diastolic rumble.

In patients with mitral regurgitation and a diastolic rumble, what does the presence of a giant left atrium indicate?
It indicates that there is no significant mitral stenosis.

CHAPTER 22

Mixed Mitral and Aortic Valve Disease

Instruction

This patient presents with shortness of breath on exertion. Please examine this patient's cardiovascular system.

Salient Features

- Pulse may be small volume (from either dominant aortic stenosis or mitral stenosis), regular, or irregularly irregular.
- Apex beat may be displaced.
- Left parasternal heave
- Middiastolic murmur of mitral stenosis
- Pansystolic murmur of mitral regurgitation
- Ejection systolic murmur of aortic stenosis at the base of the heart
- Early diastolic murmur of aortic regurgitation heard with the patient sitting forward on end expiration
- If the apex beat is not displaced in such mixed lesions, then mitral stenosis is the dominant lesion.
- In aortic stenosis, the murmur of mitral stenosis may be diminished or absent. The presence of the following features should alert the clinician to a coexisting mitral stenosis because they are not commonly associated with isolated aortic stenosis:
  - Atrial fibrillation
  - Absence of left ventricular (LV) hypertrophy in patients with left heart failure
  - Female sex
  - Giant-sized left atrium
  - Calcification of the mitral valve
  - Absence of aortic valve calcification in the symptomatic patient.

COMBINED MITRAL STENOSIS AND AORTIC STENOSIS

- Severe mitral stenosis and low cardiac output may mask moderate to severe aortic stenosis. A history of angina, syncope, or electrocardiographic evidence of LV hypertrophy or calcification of the aortic valve on the chest radiograph suggests the presence of aortic stenosis.
- The murmur of aortic stenosis is occasionally better heard at the apex than at the base, particularly in the elderly (Gallavardin phenomenon). When this occurs in younger individuals with a coexisting mitral stenosis, the murmur of aortic stenosis may be mistaken for mitral regurgitation.
- In patients with significant aortic stenosis and mitral stenosis, the physical findings of aortic stenosis generally dominate and those of mitral stenosis may be missed, whereas the symptoms are usually those of mitral stenosis. 'Combination stenosis' is almost always caused by rheumatic heart disease.

COMBINED MITRAL STENOSIS AND AORTIC REGURGITATION

The combination of severe mitral stenosis and severe aortic regurgitation may present with confusing pathophysiology and often leads to misdiagnosis. Mitral stenosis restricts LV filling and thus diminishes the impact of the aortic regurgitation on LV volume. Consequently, even severe aortic regurgitation may fail to cause a hyperdynamic circulation and the typical signs of aortic regurgitation will be absent during physical examination.

COMBINED MITRAL AND AORTIC REGURGITATION

Both lesions cause LV dilatation, but aortic regurgitation causes systolic hypertension and mild LV thickness. Treatment depends on the dominant lesion and to treat primarily that lesion.

COMBINED AORTIC STENOSIS AND MITRAL REGURGITATION

Aetiology includes rheumatic heart disease, congenital aortic stenosis with mitral valve prolapse in young patients, and degenerative aortic stenosis and mitral regurgitation in the elderly. When severe, aortic stenosis will worsen the degree of mitral regurgitation. Also, mitral regurgitation may cause difficulty in assessing the severity of aortic stenosis because of reduced forward flow. Mitral regurgitation will also enhance LV ejection performance, thereby masking the early development of LV systolic dysfunction caused by aortic stenosis.

Diagnosis

This patient has mixed mitral valve and aortic valve disease (lesion) of rheumatic aetiology with a dominant mitral regurgitation, as evidenced by the hyperdynamic circulation. The patient is in cardiac failure (functional status).

Questions

Mention a few causes of combined aortic and mitral valve disease.
- Rheumatic valvular disease
- Infective endocarditis
- Collagen degenerative disorder, e.g. Marfan syndrome
- Calcific changes in the aortic and mitral valve apparatus.

What are the indications for surgery?
- New York Heart Association (NYHA) class III status
- NYHA class II status where there is volume overload of the LV, e.g. in severe aortic regurgitation with moderate mitral valve disease or severe mitral regurgitation with moderate aortic stenosis and regurgitation.

What are some general rules when deciding on treatment of multiple valve disease?
- In terms of management decisions, the pathology should be considered severe, even if the two coexisting valve lesions are moderate clinically or echocardiographically.
- Management is generally decided upon the predominant valve lesion.
- The decision to surgically intervene on multiple valves should take into account the increased surgical risk of a double replacement, and the option of repair should be considered.
- The haemodynamic significance of the combination of the valve lesions should be taken into account when deciding on treatment options.

CHAPTER 23

Prosthetic Heart Valves

Instruction
Please examine this patient's heart and cardiovascular system.

Salient Features
- *Mitral* valve prostheses can be recognized by their site, metallic first heart sound, normal second heart sound, and metallic opening snap. Systolic murmurs are often also present and it is important to note that this does *not* indicate valve malfunction. Diastolic flow murmurs may be heard normally over the disc valves.
- *Aortic* valve prostheses may be recognized by their site, normal first heart sound, and metallic second heart sound.
- Both *mitral and aortic* valves may be replaced, and both the first and second heart sounds will be metallic. The presence of a systolic murmur does not indicate valve dysfunction. However, the presence of an early diastolic murmur indicates a malfunctioning aortic valve.
- Midsternal vertical thoracotomy scar and possible evidence of graft harvesting (arm or leg scar), as patients may have had coronary artery bypass grafting at the same time as the valve replacement.
- Often the metallic valve sounds are audible to the unaided ear.
- Lateral chest wall scars (in mitral valve replacement, a lateral scar may indicate a prior repair).

Diagnosis
This patient has both first and second heart sounds with a metallic quality (lesion), indicating that both mitral and aortic valves are artificial (aetiology) and the patient is not in heart failure (functional status).

Questions

What are the two different types of valves and when is each type preferred against the other?
Prosthetic heart valves can be either mechanical or bioprosthetic valves. The risk of long-term antithrombotic therapy is the main factor that is taken into consideration when deciding which type of valve prosthesis is most suitable for each patient. The major advantage of the mechanical valves is that their life expectancy is longer, but their major disadvantage is that they require long-term oral anticoagulation. The biological valves, on the other hand, do not require long-term anticoagulation, but their life expectancy is shorter when compared with mechanical valves.
   As such, *mechanical valves* are considered for patients who:
- are at risk of accelerated structural valve deterioration
- are already on lifelong anticoagulation for another reason
- have reasonable life expectancy and who would be high-risk surgical patients if future revision valve surgery is required.

Although age is not a strict cut-off anymore for valve-type choice, a general recommendation is that mechanical prosthesis is preferred in patients requiring aortic valve replacement and are younger than 60 years of age and patients requiring mitral valve replacement and are younger than 65 years of age.

Biological valves are considered for patients in cases when:
- bleeding risk from anticoagulation is high
- reoperation on a mechanical valve prosthesis is needed because of thrombosis
- there is either low likelihood of reoperation or low operating risk if a reoperation is required in the future.

Also, biological valves should be considered in young women who may wish to get pregnant because of the high risk of thromboembolism during pregnancy.

What are the complications of prosthetic valves?
- Thromboembolism
- Valve dysfunction, including valve leakage, valve dehiscence, and valve obstruction caused by thrombosis and clogging. Perivalvular leak is always abnormal. 'Built-in' transvalvular leakage should be <10 mL per beat. The loss of expected valve sounds is an important sign of mechanical valve thrombosis.
- Bleeding (such as upper gastrointestinal haemorrhage) caused by anticoagulants
- Haemolysis at valve causing anaemia
- Endocarditis, which carries a mortality rate of up to 60%; patients should be urgently referred to a tertiary cardiothoracic centre.
- Structural dysfunction: fracture, poppet escape, cuspal tear, calcification
- Nonstructural dysfunction: paravalvular leak, suture/tissue entrapment, noise.

What is the recommended follow-up after heart valve prosthesis?
- All patients with prosthetic valves should have an echocardiogram performed 1 month after surgery to establish baseline values, and annually after that.
- When prosthetic valve dysfunction is suspected, transoesophageal echocardiogram is the procedure of choice, but findings may be somewhat limited by acoustic shadowing and reverberations from prosthetic material.

What are the causes of anaemia in a patient with a prosthetic valve?
- Bleeding caused by anticoagulants
- Haemolytic anaemia
- Secondary to bacterial endocarditis.

What are the indications for valve replacement?
- Mitral stenosis
- Mitral regurgitation
- Aortic regurgitation
- Aortic stenosis.

If a patient with atrial fibrillation requires a prosthetic mitral valve, which kind of valve would you prefer?
A mechanical valve, as these patients need oral anticoagulation for atrial fibrillation.

If a patient with a mechanical aortic valve, on lifelong warfarin, undergoes coronary angiography with insertion of a bare metal stent, what should happen to his anticoagulation?
Prior to the procedure, if warfarin is stopped, bridging with heparin is required to protect against valve thrombosis. After the stent implantation, and irrespective of the type of stent used, triple

therapy with aspirin, clopidogrel, and warfarin is recommended for a month. Exceptions to this recommendation are:
- If the ischaemic risk is deemed high, then triple therapy may continue for more than a month and up to 6 months.
- If the bleeding risk is deemed high, then dual therapy with clopidogrel and warfarin should be the alternative to triple therapy for a month.

Further Information

The first aortic valve replacement (caged ball device) was performed by Dr Dwight Harken in March 1960 at Peter Bent Brigham Hospital in Boston. Shortly thereafter, Dr Nina Braunwald, at the National Institutes of Health, USA, performed a total mitral valve replacement with an artificial flexible leaflet valve.

CHAPTER 24

Tricuspid Regurgitation

Instruction

Examine this patient's heart.
Examine this patient's cardiovascular system.

Salient Features
HISTORY

- Intravenous drug abuse
- Trauma to the chest
- Rheumatic fever
- Chronic obstructive pulmonary disease.

EXAMINATION

- Peripheral cyanosis
- Large 'v' waves in the jugular venous pulse (Fig. 24.1)
- Left parasternal heave
- Palpable or loud P_2
- Pansystolic murmur at the left lower sternal border, which increases in inspiration (Carvallo's sign)
- Right ventricular third heart sound may be present.
- Atrial fibrillation may be present.
- Possible accompanying signs:
  - middiastolic murmur of mitral stenosis
  - systolic pulsations of an enlarged liver
  - ascites and ankle oedema.

Diagnosis

This patient has tricuspid regurgitation (lesion) secondary to chronic lung disease and cor pulmonale (aetiology) and is in cardiac failure (functional status).

Questions

What are the causes of tricuspid regurgitation?
- Most lesions (90%) are functional, due to dilation of right atrium, ventricle, and tricuspid annulus:
  - Primary pulmonary disease and pulmonary hypertension
  - Stenosis of pulmonary valve or pulmonary artery

93

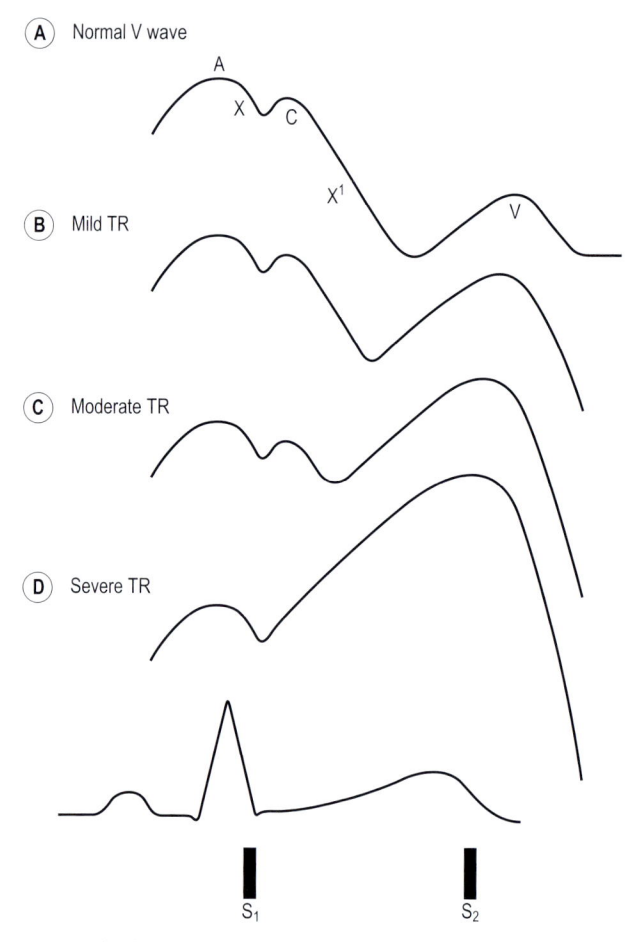

Fig. 24.1 Jugular venous pulse in tricuspid regurgitation (TR). The jugular venous pulse wave normally drops during ventricular systole. As TR becomes more severe, the CV wave becomes more obvious.

- Left-sided failure
- Increased right-sided pressures from left heart valve lesions (mitral stenosis).
- Rheumatic (associated with mitral and/or aortic valve disease)
- Right heart endocarditis
- Uncommon: carcinoid syndrome, Ebstein's anomaly, endomyocardial fibrosis, infarction of right ventricular papillary muscles, tricuspid valve prolapse, blunt trauma to the heart.

What are the indications for intervention in primary tricuspid regurgitation?
- Severe disease in patients undergoing left-sided valve surgery
- Severe and symptomatic disease
- Progressive right ventricular dilation or dysfunction.

How would you investigate this patient?
- *Electrocardiogram*: although there is no distinct electrocardiographic finding signifying tricuspid regurgitation, there may be findings of right ventricular hypertrophy in cases of pulmonary hypertension (right axis deviation, right bundle branch block, P pulmonale).

- *Chest X-ray*: enlarged heart silhouette with right ventricle dilation and right atrium enlargement.
- *Echocardiography* is used to establish and quantify the lesion (valve motion, right chamber dilation, Doppler colour flow for severity assessment, right ventricle function).
- *Cardiac magnetic resonance imaging* is rarely needed if the echocardiography is inconclusive.

CHAPTER 25

Pulmonary Stenosis

Instruction
Please examine this patient's cardiovascular system.

Salient Features
HISTORY
- Patients may be asymptomatic.
- Possible history of maternal rubella
- Dyspnoea on exertion or fatigability may occur (when the stenosis is severe); less often, patients may have retrosternal chest pain or syncope with exertion. Eventually, right ventricular failure may develop, with resultant peripheral oedema and abdominal swelling.
- Cyanosis and clubbing (If the foramen ovale is patent, shunting of blood from the right to the left atrium may occur.)

The presence or absence of symptoms, their severity, and the prognosis are influenced by the severity of stenosis, the right ventricular systolic function, and the competence of the tricuspid valve.

EXAMINATION
- Round plump facies
- Normal pulse
- Prominent 'a' wave in the jugular venous pressure
- Left parasternal heave
- Ejection click, which *decreases* on inspiration (This is the only right-sided sound that decreases with inspiration.)
- Soft P_2, with a wide split second sound
- Ejection systolic murmur in the left upper sternal border, best heard on inspiration. The murmur radiates to the left shoulder and left lung posteriorly. The more severe the stenosis, the longer the murmur, obscuring the second aortic sound A_2.
- If pulmonary stenosis is identified clinically, the clinician should look for central cyanosis and clubbing (Fallot's tetralogy).

Diagnosis
This patient has pulmonary stenosis (lesion), which is a congenital anomaly (aetiology), and the patient is severely limited by her symptoms (functional status).

Questions
What is the underlying cause of pulmonary stenosis?
- Congenital (commonest cause)
- Carcinoid tumour of the small bowel.

25 — PULMONARY STENOSIS

What is the normal valve area of the pulmonary valve?
The area of the pulmonary valve orifice in a normal adult is about 2.0 cm^2/m^2 body surface area, and there is no systolic pressure gradient across the valve.

How is the severity of pulmonary valve stenosis determined?
Pulmonary stenosis is classified into mild, moderate, and severe, and the quantification of the severity of the disease is made by echocardiography and Doppler flow studies, taking into account the length of the jet and the pressure gradient across the valve, as measured by Doppler studies.

How would you investigate this patient?
- *Electrocardiogram* may show right-axis deviation and right ventricular hypertrophy (Fig. 25.1).

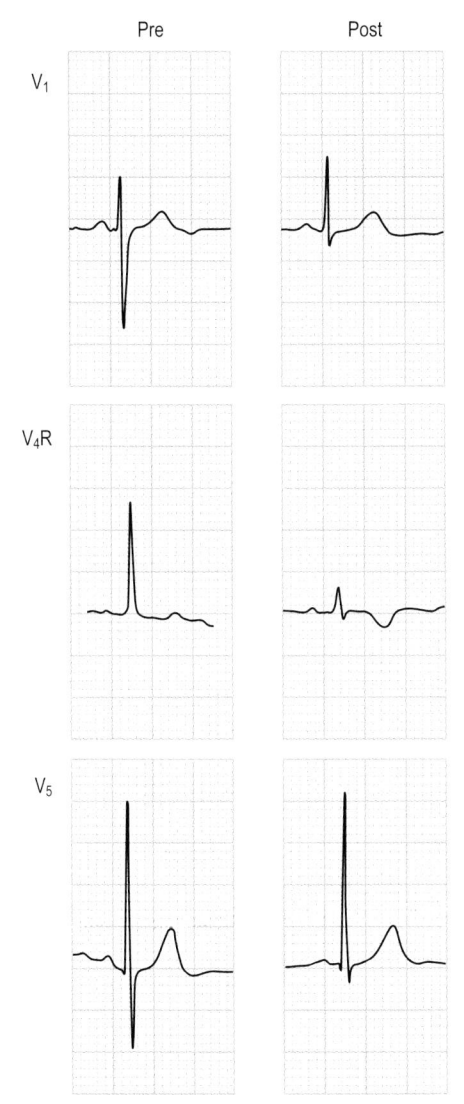

Fig. 25.1 Electrocardiogram in severe valvar pulmonary stenosis showing prehypertrophy before dilation and after QRS axis shift, and regression of hypertrophy after gradient reduction.

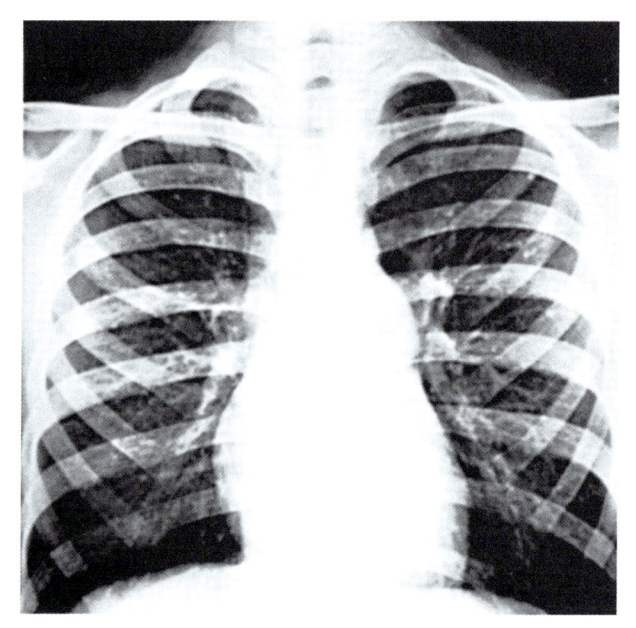

Fig. 25.2 Roentgenogram in valvular pulmonary stenosis with a normal aortic root. The heart size is within normal limits, but there is poststenotic dilatation of the pulmonary artery (usually the left branch). (With permission from Kliegman, R.M., Behrman, R.E., Jenson, H.B., Stanton, B.F., 2007. Nelson Textbook of Pediatrics, eighteenth edn. Saunders, Philadelphia, PA.)

- *Chest radiograph* shows a normal aortic knuckle, whereas the pulmonary conus is either normal or enlarged (caused by poststenotic dilatation of the main pulmonary artery) and the pulmonary vascular markings are diminished. The cardiac silhouette is usually normal in size or may be enlarged (when the patient has right ventricular failure or tricuspid regurgitation) (Fig. 25.2).
- *Echocardiography* can visualize the site of obstruction in most patients, but right ventricular hypertrophy and paradoxical septal motion during systole are evident. The leaflets of the valve will appear thickened and restricted in movement, creating a domed appearance in the images. Doppler flow studies accurately assess the severity of stenosis so that cardiac catheterization and angiography are usually unnecessary.
- *Cardiac catheterization* is reserved for patients in whom echocardiography is inconclusive or for candidates for intervention before the procedure takes place.

What are the complications of this condition?
- Cardiac failure
- Infective endocarditis: blood cultures are rarely positive; the emboli are entirely in the pulmonary circulation and not systemic.

What are the types of pulmonary stenosis?
- Valvular
- Subvalvular: infundibular and subinfundibular
- Supravalvular.

Do you know of any eponymous syndromes linked to pulmonary stenosis?
- *Noonan syndrome*: short stature, ptosis, downward slanting eyes, wide-spaced eyes (hypertelorism), low-set ears, webbed neck, developmental delay, and low posterior hairline.

About two-thirds of patients with Noonan syndrome have pulmonary stenosis caused by valve dysplasia.
- *Watson syndrome*: café-au-lait spots, developmental delay, and pulmonary stenosis
- *Williams syndrome*: infantile hypocalcaemia, elfin facies, and developmental delay, in addition to supravalvular pulmonary stenosis. Subvalvular pulmonary stenosis, which is caused by the narrowing of the right ventricular infundibulum or subinfundibulum, usually occurs in association with a ventricular septal defect.

How would you manage a patient with pulmonary stenosis?
Asymptomatic patients with pulmonary stenosis are closely monitored with clinical assessment and frequent echocardiography. When the peak gradient across the valve, as measured by Doppler studies, exceeds a specific limit (64 mm Hg according to the European Society of Cardiology), then intervention is indicated and the intervention of choice is balloon valvotomy, leaving valve replacement as a last resort in patients for whom balloon valvotomy is not effective. Otherwise, if the pressure gradient has not reached this limit in Doppler studies, the other indication to proceed to balloon valvotomy is the development of symptoms (symptoms of pulmonary stenosis, right ventricular dysfunction, arrhythmias, right-to-left shunt via a septal defect).

What is Erb's point?
The third left intercostal space adjacent to the sternum is Erb's point, and the murmur of infundibular pulmonary stenosis is best heard in this space and in the left fourth intercostal space.

CHAPTER 26

Atrial Septal Defect

Instruction
Examine this patient's heart.

Salient Features

HISTORY

Ostium Secundum Defect (Anatomically in the Region of the Fossa Ovalis)
- Asymptomatic particularly small defects with minimal left-to-right shunting; moderate or large defects often have no symptoms until the third or fourth decades despite substantial left-to-right shunting (characterized by a ratio of pulmonary to systemic flow of 1.5 or more)
- Fatigue
- Dyspnoea
- Palpitations indicating atrial arrhythmias
- Productive cough indicating recurrent pulmonary infections
- Symptoms of paradoxical emboli
- Right heart failure.

Ostium Primum Defect (Anatomically in the Lower Part of the Atrial Septum)
- Patients may develop symptoms and heart failure in childhood.
- Failure to thrive
- Chest infections
- Poor development
- In adults, in addition to the same symptoms as for secundum defect, the following occur:
  - Syncope: indicating heart block
  - Symptoms suggesting endocarditis.

EXAMINATION
- Diffuse or normal apical impulse
- Left parasternal heave
- Ejection systolic flow murmur in the left second and third intercostal space
- Wide, fixed, split second heart sound (occasionally a slight movement of P occurs) that does not vary with respiration (Fig. 26.1)
- Infrequently, a middiastolic murmur may be heard in the tricuspid area (indicating a large left-to-right shunt).

26—ATRIAL SEPTAL DEFECT

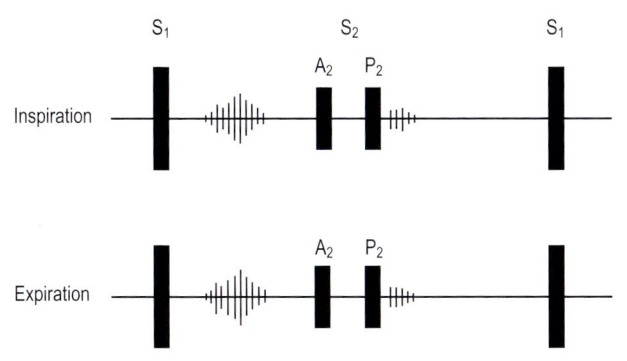

Fig. 26.1 Auscultatory findings resulting from an atrial septal defect. S_1, first heart sound; A_2, aortic valve closure; P_2, pulmonic valve closure.

- Proceed by looking for signs of:
    - pulmonary hypertension (Eisenmenger syndrome)
    - congenital defects of the thumb (Holt–Oram syndrome).

Note: Atrial secundum defect is often confused with pulmonary stenosis (P is soft and delayed and moves with respiration).

Diagnosis

This patient has an atrial septal defect (ASD) (lesion) that is congenital in origin (aetiology); she is not in cardiac failure and there is no reversal of shunt (functional status).

Questions

What are the types of atrial septal defect?
- *Ostium secundum defect* accounts for 70% of the cases. The defect is in the middle portion of the atrial septum and is usually 2 to 4 cm in diameter (incomplete right bundle branch block pattern, QRS axis rightward) (Fig. 26.2A,B).
- *Sinus venosus type* is a defect in the septum just below the entrance of the superior vena cava into the right atrium (leftward P wave axis so that P waves are inverted in at least one inferior lead).
- *Ostium primum type* is a defect in the lower part of the septum and clefts may occur in the mitral and tricuspid valves (QRS axis leftward) (Fig. 26.2C). A junctional or low atrial rhythm (inverted P waves in the inferior leads) occurs with sinus venosus defects.

Note: Although patent foramen ovale (PFO) is a communication between right and left atrium, it is not part of the ASD classification as there is no missing septal tissue.

What do you understand by the term patent foramen ovale?
In the fetus, the right and left atria communicate with each other through an oblique valvular opening, which is called the foramen ovale. The foramen ovale persists throughout fetal life. After birth, the left atrium receives blood from the lungs and the pressure in this chamber becomes greater than that in the right atrium; this causes the closure of the foramen ovale.

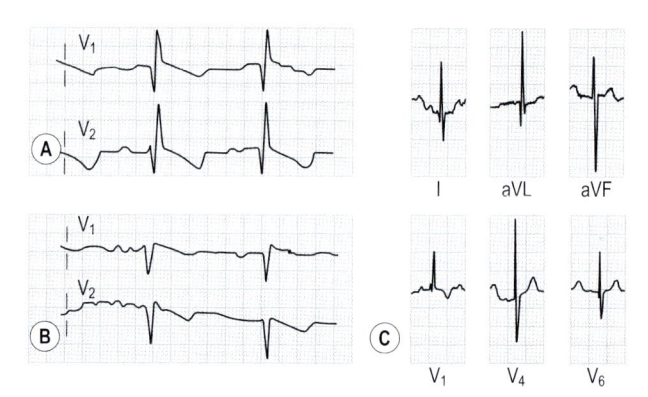

Fig. 26.2 Electrocardiography in atrial septal defect. (A, B) Ostium secundum defect right precordial leads V_1 and V_2 illustrate two variants of an incomplete right bundle branch block pattern, the rSrT pattern (A) and the rsR' pattern (B). (C) Ostium primum type: endocardial cushion defect—the QRS axis is leftward counterclockwise and superior.

What is the importance of patent foramen ovale?
PFO has been connected to cryptogenic stroke. Although data from studies are controversial, evidence has proven that treatment combination with both antiplatelets and closure of the PFO for cryptogenic stroke is more effective than antiplatelets alone in the prevention of recurrent strokes.

What is Holt–Oram syndrome?
This is an ostium secundum ASD with a hypoplastic thumb and an accessory phalanx. In addition, the thumb lies in the same plane as the other digits (ASD; Fig. 26.3). Cardiac conduction disturbances can also be part of this syndrome. The inheritance is autosomal dominant and it has been associated with mutations in chromosome 12q2.

At what age does the reversal of shunt occur?
Usually after the end of the second decade.

What is the mechanism of fixed split second sound?
In normal individuals on inspiration, there is a widening of the split between the two components of the second sound caused by a delay in closure of the pulmonary valve. In ASD, the effect of respiration is eliminated because of communication between the left and right sides of the heart.

In which conditions is an abnormally widely split second sound present?
- ASD, ventricular septal defect (VSD), pulmonary regurgitation (caused by increased right ventricular volume)
- Pulmonary stenosis (caused by increased right ventricular pressure)
- Right bundle branch block (caused by right ventricular conduction delay)
- Mitral regurgitation, VSD (caused by premature left ventricular emptying).

How would you investigate a patient with atrial septal defect?
- *Electrocardiogram (ECG):*
  - Often, there is right axis deviation and incomplete right bundle branch block (Fig. 26.2A,B).

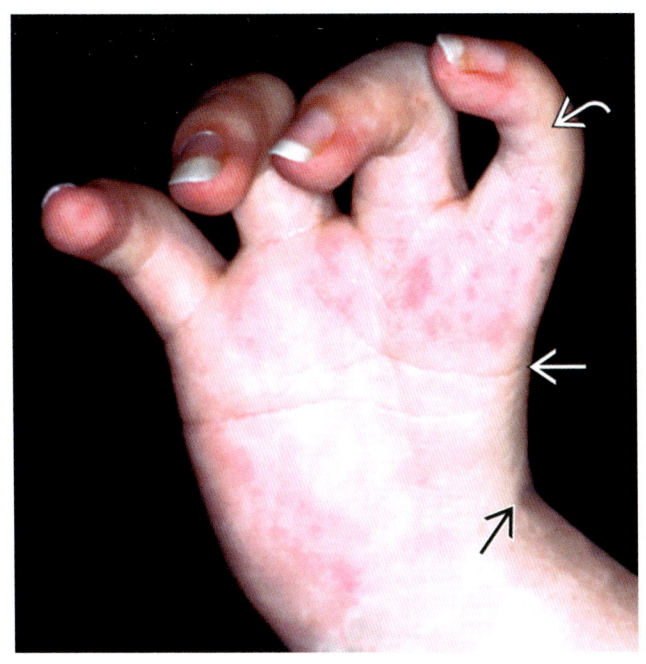

Fig. 26.3 Clinical photograph of the hand of a woman with Holt–Oram syndrome illustrates characteristic findings of radial deviation of the wrist due to a severely hypoplastic radius. The thumb is absent and only four digits are seen. Clinodactyly of the radial digit allows the finger some limited function as a thumb-like appendage. (With permission from Kennedy, A., Woodward, P.J., Sohaey, R., 2021. Diagnostic Imaging: Obstetrics, fourth edn. Elsevier.)

- In ostium primum defects, left axis deviation also occurs (Fig. 26.2C).
- In sinus venosus defects, a junctional or low atrial rhythm (inverted P waves in inferior leads) occurs.
- *Chest radiography:*
  - Prominent pulmonary arteries (large pulmonary conus)
  - A peripheral pulmonary vascular pattern of 'shunt vascularity' (in which the small pulmonary arteries are especially well visualized in the periphery of both lungs)
  - Small aortic knob
  - Enlarged right ventricle (RV) and right atrium.
- *Echocardiography:*
  - Transthoracic echocardiography visualizes ostium secundum and primum defects but usually does not identify sinus venosus defects.
  - Sensitivity can be enhanced by injecting microbubbles in the peripheral vein, after which the movement across the defect can be seen.
  - Transoesophageal and Doppler colour-flow echocardiography are useful in detecting and determining the location of ASDs and also in identifying anomalous venous drainage and sinus venosus defects.
- *Cardiac magnetic resonance imaging* is a reliable and accurate method to assess an ASD.
- *Cardiac catheterization* is often unnecessary in diagnosis but is useful in determining the magnitude and direction of shunting and to determine the severity and reversibility of pulmonary hypertension.

What are the complications of atrial septal defect?
- Atrial arrhythmias: atrial fibrillation is most common. Atrial fibrillation is often accompanied by the appearance of tricuspid regurgitation. Patients are usually in normal sinus rhythm in the first three decades of life, after which atrial arrhythmias including atrial fibrillation and supraventricular tachycardia may appear.
- Pulmonary hypertension with the development of right ventricular disease
- Eisenmenger syndrome with reversal of shunt
- Paradoxical embolus
- Infective endocarditis in patients with ostium primum defects only
- Recurrent pulmonary infections.

How is pregnancy tolerated in a woman with an atrial septal defect?
Pregnancy is usually well tolerated in women with uncomplicated ASDs. However, when complicated by significant pulmonary hypertension, there is increased maternal and fetal morbidity and mortality, and hence pregnancy should be avoided in Eisenmenger syndrome. Care should be given to prevent thromboembolic events during pregnancy and haemorrhage during delivery.

How would you manage an uncomplicated atrial septal defect in adulthood?
- In adults, small ASDs can be left alone, although many believe all ASDs must be closed. Those operated on before the age of 25 years have an excellent prognosis and one may anticipate normal long-term survival, but older patients require regular supervision. In a recent study, surgical repair of ASDs in middle-aged and elderly patients was found to improve longevity and reduce functional limitation caused by heart failure and was therefore superior to medical treatment. However, the risk of atrial arrhythmias, especially fibrillation and flutter, and the attendant risk of thromboembolic events were not reduced by closure of the defect.
- ASDs causing significant shunt require surgical closure to prevent right ventricular dysfunction.
- Other indications for surgery include evidence of pulmonary vascular reactivity when challenged with pulmonary vasodilators or a lung biopsy with pulmonary arterial changes being potentially reversible.
- A history of a cryptogenic cerebrovascular event in the presence of a small ASD with right-to-left shunting is also recommended for closure.
- Closure in adults results in a reduction in right ventricular size and improves symptoms.
- ASD closure should be avoided in Eisenmenger syndrome.

Is prophylaxis against infective endocarditis recommended in atrial septal defect?
Prophylaxis against infective endocarditis is not recommended for patients with ASDs (repaired or unrepaired).

What do you know about ostium primum defects?
They are associated with endocardial cushion defects often resulting in cleft mitral valve (usually anterior leaflet), causing mitral regurgitation. The ECG shows right bundle branch block and left axis deviation (Fig. 26.2C). Treatment is surgical closure with repair of cleft mitral valve, which generally involves simple interrupted suture repair of the cleft or the addition of a mitral annuloplasty for annular reduction and stabilization.

Further Information

Leonardo da Vinci's description in 1513 of a 'perforating channel' in the atrial septum is believed to be the first recorded account of a congenital malformation of the human heart.

Mary Holt, cardiologist, King's College Hospital, London.

Samuel Oram, cardiologist, King's College Hospital, London.

CHAPTER 27

Ventricular Septal Defect

Instruction
Listen to this patient's heart.

Salient Features

HISTORY
- Small defects are usually asymptomatic.
- Large defects with shunts: repeated respiratory tract infections, debilitating dyspnoea, and exercise intolerance
- Symptoms of infective endocarditis or past history of endocarditis
- Symptoms of Eisenmenger syndrome.

EXAMINATION
- There is a normal pulse.
- There are normal findings on palpation (there may be either left or right ventricular (RV) enlargement).
- With substantial left-to-right shunting and little or no pulmonary hypertension, the left ventricular impulse is dynamic and laterally displaced, and the RV impulse may not be felt. The murmur of a moderate or large defect is pansystolic, loudest at the lower left sternal border, and usually accompanied by a palpable thrill.
- A short middiastolic apical rumble (caused by increased flow through the mitral valve) may be heard.
- A decrescendo diastolic murmur of aortic regurgitation may be present if the ventricular septal defect (VSD) undermines the aortic valve annulus.
- Small, muscular VSDs may produce high-frequency systolic ejection murmurs that terminate before the end of systole (when the defect is occluded by contracting heart muscle) (Fig. 27.1).
- If pulmonary hypertension develops, an RV heave and a pulsation over the pulmonary trunk may be palpated. The pansystolic murmur and thrill diminish and eventually disappear as flow through the defect decreases, and a murmur of pulmonary regurgitation (Graham Steell murmur) may appear. Finally, cyanosis and clubbing are present.
- The second sound may be normal when the defect is small; A_2 is obscured by the pansystolic murmur of large defects. A single second sound indicates that the ventricular pressures are equal and a loud P indicates pulmonary hypertension.

Diagnosis

This patient has a VSD (lesion) of congenital origin (aetiology) and has pulmonary hypertension (functional status).

27 – VENTRICULAR SEPTAL DEFECT

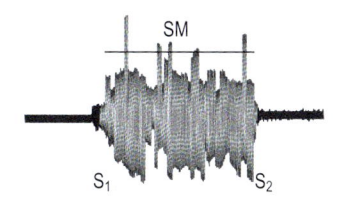

Fig. 27.1 Phonocardiogram showing the holosystolic murmur of isolated ventricular septal defect.

Questions

Is the loudness of the murmur related to the size of the defect?
No; in fact, very small defects (usually called 'maladie de Roger') cause loud murmurs.

What are the causes of a ventricular septal defect?
- Congenital
- Rupture of the interventricular septum as a complication of myocardial infarction.

Where is the defect usually situated?
In the membranous portion of the interventricular septum.

Can such defects close spontaneously?
Spontaneous closure usually occurs in a small defect, during early childhood in about 50% of patients.

What are the complications of a ventricular septal defect?
- Congestive cardiac failure
- RV outflow tract obstruction (muscular infundibular obstruction develops in about of 5% of VSDs)
- Aortic regurgitation
- Infective endocarditis
- Pulmonary hypertension and reversal of shunt (Eisenmenger complex)
- VSDs are associated with atrial and ventricular tachycardias.

How would you investigate this patient?
Electrocardiogram (ECG) and chest radiography provide insight into the magnitude of the haemodynamic impairment: with a small VSD, both ECG and chest radiograph are normal:
  - With a large defect, there is ECG evidence of left atrial and ventricular enlargement, and left ventricular enlargement and 'shunt vascularity' are evident on the chest radiograph (Fig. 27.2).
  - If pulmonary hypertension occurs, the QRS axis shifts to the right, and right atrial and ventricular enlargement are noted on the ECG; the chest radiograph shows marked enlargement of the proximal pulmonary arteries, rapid tapering of the peripheral pulmonary arteries, and oligaemic lung fields.

Doppler echocardiography can identify the presence and location of the VSD, and Doppler colour-flow mapping can identify the magnitude and direction of shunting.

Magnetic resonance imaging can provide an accurate assessment of the structure and the anatomy of the lesion.

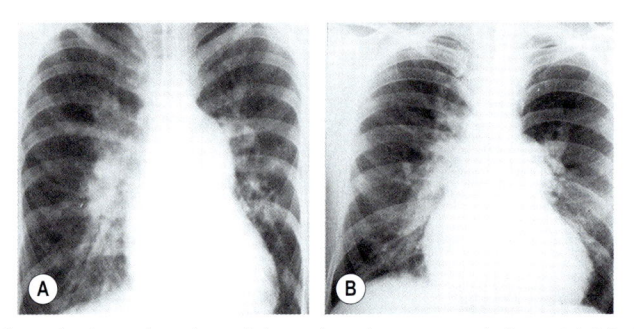

Fig. 27.2 (A) Radiograph of a moderately restrictive perimembranous ventricular septal defect (VSD) with left-to-right shunt. Pulmonary arterial vascularity is increased, the pulmonary trunk and its proximal branches are markedly dilated, and a moderately enlarged convex left ventricle (LV) occupies the apex. (B) Radiograph of a nonrestrictive perimembranous VSD and a bidirectional shunt. Pulmonary arterial vascularity is increased, the pulmonary trunk and its proximal branches are markedly dilated, an enlarged convex LV occupies the apex, and a prominent right atrium forms the right lower cardiac border. (With permission from Perloff, J.K., 2003. Clinical Recognition of Congenital Heart Disease, fifth edn. Saunders, Philadelphia, PA.)

Cardiac catheterization and angiography can be used in certain clinical situations, particularly when the haemodynamics of the shunt cannot be accurately assessed noninvasively and in the preoperative work-up.

What types of ventricular septal defect do you know?
- Type 1: The supracristal type (above the crista supraventricularis, a muscular ridge that separates the main portion of the RV cavity from the infundibular or outflow portion) is a high defect just below the pulmonary valve and the right coronary cusp of the aortic valve. The latter may not be adequately supported, resulting in aortic regurgitation and, occasionally, sinus dilation.
- Type 2: The membranous type is the commonest type of VSD and results from the membranous portion of the interventricular septum. If the defect extends to the muscular portion, then it is called a paramembranous defect.
- Type 3: The atrioventricular canal type results from the inlet septum below mitral and tricuspid valves.
- Type 4: Muscular defects are away from the cardiac valves, and can be small (maladie de Roger), large, or multiple small (Swiss cheese appearance). Gerbode defect (defect opening into the right atrium) is a rare type of VSD.

Mention other cardiac lesions that may be associated with a ventricular septal defect.
- Conditions in which VSD is an essential part of the syndrome:
  - Fallot's tetralogy
  - Truncus arteriosus
  - Double-outlet RV
  - Atrioventricular canal defects
- Conditions frequently associated with a VSD but not an essential part of the syndrome:
  - Patent ductus arteriosus
  - Pulmonary stenosis
  - Secundum atrial septal defects
  - Coarctation of aorta

- Tricuspid atresia
- Transposition of the great arteries
- Pulmonary atresia.

What is the effect of pregnancy in women with a ventricular septal defect?
- Small defects should present no problems.
- Repaired defects should present no problems either.
- Patients with moderate-sized defects and moderate pulmonary hypertension are at the risk of developing acute RV failure and rapidly worsening pulmonary hypertension in pregnancy.
- Pregnancy should be avoided in developed Eisenmenger syndrome.

What is the management of patients with a ventricular septal defect?
- The natural history of VSD depends on:
  - the size of the defect
  - pulmonary vascular resistance.
- Adults with small defects and normal pulmonary arterial pressure are usually asymptomatic, and pulmonary vascular disease is unlikely to develop. Such patients do not require surgical closure of their defect, but they are at risk for infective endocarditis and should receive antibiotic prophylaxis.
- Patients with large VSDs who survive to adulthood usually have left ventricular failure or pulmonary hypertension with associated RV failure. Surgical closure of such defects is recommended, if the magnitude of pulmonary vascular obstructive disease is not prohibitive. Once the ratio of pulmonary to systemic vascular resistance exceeds 0.7, the risk associated with surgery is excessive.

Which patients merit surgical attention?
Indications for a VSD closure are history of infective endocarditis and a pulmonary to systemic flow more than 2:1 and clinical evidence of left ventricular volume overload.

Closure can also be considered when there is a left-to-right shunt complicated with left ventricular dysfunction, without the development of severe irreversible pulmonary hypertension.

If the VSD is large enough to cause heart failure or pulmonary hypertension, it usually manifests in the first few years of life.

Further Information

Henri Roger (1809–1891), a French paediatrician, described maladie de Roger in 1879 in a paper entitled 'Clinical researches on the congenital communication of the two sides of the hearts, but failure of occlusion of the interventricular septum': 'A developmental defect of the heart occurs from which cyanosis does not ensue in spite of the fact that a communication exists between the cavities of the two ventricles and in spite of the fact that admixture of venous blood and arterial blood occurs. This congenital defect, which is even compatible with a long life, is a simple one. It comprises a defect in the interventricular septum'.

CHAPTER 28

Patent Ductus Arteriosus

Instruction

This patient was found to have a murmur on routine examination by his general practitioner. Please examine his cardiovascular system.

Salient Features

HISTORY

- Asymptomatic
- Exercise tolerance
- Symptoms of heart failure
- Take a maternal history of rubella, particularly in the first trimester.
- Determine whether the patient was a premature baby or had a low birth weight.
- Determine whether the patient was born in a place located at a high altitude.

EXAMINATION

- Collapsing pulse (caused by an aortic diastolic run-off)
- Wide pulse pressure
- Heaving and displaced apex beat
- Systolic and/or diastolic thrill in the left second interspace
- Loud, continuous 'machinery' murmur, i.e. pansystolic and extending into early diastole—known as Gibson murmur—is heard along the left upper sternal border and outer border of the clavicle. The murmur begins after the first heart sound, peaks with the second sound, and trails off in diastole (Fig. 28.1).
- If Eisenmenger syndrome has developed, then the murmur will diminish, and peripheral cyanosis will be evident.
- The second sound is not heard.

Diagnosis

This patient has a patent ductus arteriosus (PDA) (lesion), which is probably congenital in origin (aetiology); the patient is not in heart failure (functional status).

Questions

Mention a few causes of a collapsing pulse.
- Hyperdynamic circulation caused by:
  - aortic regurgitation
  - thyrotoxicosis

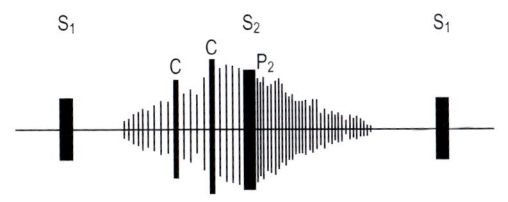

Fig. 28.1 The machinery murmur of patent ductus arteriosus is typically maximally loud at the time of the second heart sound (S_2); clicking noises (C) in systole contribute to the machinery sound.

- severe anaemia
- Paget disease
- complete heart block.

Mention a few causes of continuous murmurs.
- Venous hum
- Mitral regurgitation murmur with aortic regurgitant murmur
- Ventricular septal defect with aortic regurgitation
- Pulmonary arteriovenous fistula
- Rupture of the sinus of Valsalva
- Coronary arteriovenous fistula
- Arteriovenous anastomosis of intercostal vessels following a fractured rib.

What happens to the continuous murmur of patent ductus arteriosus in pulmonary hypertension?
It becomes softer and shorter, and P increases in intensity.

How would you investigate this patient?
- *Electrocardiogram (ECG)* may be normal or shows left ventricular hypertrophy. In pulmonary hypertension, ECG will show signs of right ventricular hypertrophy.
- *Chest radiograph* may be normal, or there may be left ventricular and left atrial enlargement. The chest film shows pulmonary plethora, proximal pulmonary arterial dilatation, and a prominent ascending aorta. The ductus arteriosus may be visualized as an opacity at the confluence of the descending aorta and the aortic knob. If pulmonary hypertension develops, right ventricular hypertrophy is noted.
- *Echocardiography* can usually visualize the ductus arteriosus. Doppler studies demonstrate continuous flow in the pulmonary trunk.
- *Cardiac magnetic resonance imaging*.

Mention a few associated lesions.
- Ventricular septal defect
- Pulmonary stenosis
- Coarctation of aorta.

What is differential cyanosis?
When Eisenmenger syndrome develops in PDA, cyanosis and clubbing develop on the toes of the feet rather than the fingers of the hand. This is called differential cyanosis and occurs because the ductus in the right-to-left shunt delivers unoxygenated blood distal to the left subclavian artery.

What are the complications of a patent ductus arteriosus?
- Congestive cardiac failure is the commonest complication.
- Infective endocarditis or endarteritis (involves the pulmonary side of the ductus arteriosus or the pulmonary artery opposite the duct orifice, from which septic pulmonary emboli may arise)
- Pulmonary hypertension and reversal of shunt
- Substantial left-to-right shunting through the ductus in infants may increase the risk of intraventricular haemorrhage, necrotizing enterocolitis, bronchopulmonary dysplasia, and death.
- The ductus may become aneurysmal and calcified, which may lead to its rupture.

What are the indications for closure of the patent ductus arteriosus?
- Patients with more than moderate defects who have developed symptoms of left-to-right shunt, clinical evidence of left overload, or reversible pulmonary hypertension
- Patients with history of infective endocarditis
- Small PDAs can be treated surgically or medically with regular follow-up.
- Once severe pulmonary vascular obstructive disease develops, surgical ligation or percutaneous closure is contraindicated.

Which congenital cardiac lesions are dependent on a patent ductus arteriosus?
- Hypoplastic left heart syndrome
- Complex coarctations of aorta
- Critical congenital aortic stenosis.

Further Information

Collapsing pulse is also called Corrigan's pulse, after Sir Dominic J. Corrigan (1802–1880), a Dublin-born physician who graduated from Edinburgh.

R.E. Gross was the first to report surgical closure of the PDA in 1939.

CHAPTER 29

Ebstein's Anomaly

Instruction
This patient has presented with palpitations. Please examine his cardiovascular system.

Salient Features
HISTORY
- An incidental cardiac murmur
- Ask the patient about palpitations (paroxysmal supraventricular tachycardia).
- Symptoms of right-sided heart failure
- History of maternal lithium ingestion.

EXAMINATION
- Raised jugular venous pulse; the large 'v' of tricuspid regurgitation is absent because the giant right atrium absorbs most of the regurgitant volume.
- Left parasternal heave
- Loud first heart sound produced by the sail-like anterior tricuspid leaflet
- Pansystolic murmur which increases on inspiration
- Hepatomegaly.

Proceed as follows:
- Ascertain whether the patient has exertional cyanosis or dyspnoea.
- Exclude an atrial septal defect.

Diagnosis
This patient has isolated tricuspid regurgitation (lesion) that is probably of congenital aetiology as there is no pulmonary hypertension. He has Ebstein's anomaly without cardiac failure (functional status).

Questions

What is the pathology in Ebstein's anomaly?
The tricuspid leaflets are abnormal and are displaced into the body of the right ventricle (RV). The septal leaflet is variably deficient or even absent. The posterior leaflet is also variably deficient and there is large 'sail-like' anterior leaflet, which is the hallmark of this condition. The anterior leaflet is rarely affected. The abnormally located tricuspid orifice produces a part of the RV lying between the atrioventricular ring and the origin of the valve, which is continuous with the right atrial chamber. This proximal segment is known as the 'atrialized' portion of the RV. Approximately 50% of the patients have either a patent foramen ovale or a secundum atrial septal defect, and 25% have one or more accessory atrioventricular conduction pathways. The anomaly is said to be associated with maternal lithium ingestion.

What are the mechanisms of cyanosis in these patients?
Right-to-left shunting at the atrial level, i.e. through a patent foramen ovale or atrial septal defect.

What are the poor predictors of outcome?
- The earlier the presentation, the higher the risk of mortality.
- A large right atrium or cardiothoracic ratio >60%
- Severe right outflow tract abnormalities.

How would you investigate such a patient?
- *Chest radiography* (Fig. 29.1) shows the large right atrium with oligaemic lung fields.
- *Electrocardiogram* shows right bundle branch block, prolonged PR interval, P pulmonale (indicating right atrial enlargement), large P waves (Himalayan P waves), and type B Wolff–Parkinson–White syndrome (where the QRS complex is downward in lead V_1) (Fig. 29.2). (Note: Wolff–Parkinson–White syndrome comprises a trial of short PR interval, delta wave, and wide QRS complex.) Approximately 10% of patients with Ebstein's anomaly have the Wolff–Parkinson–White syndrome.
- *Echocardiography* characteristic findings include the abnormal positional relation between the tricuspid valve and mitral valve with septal displacement of the septal tricuspid leaflet.
- *Cardiac catheterization* has no place in classic cases as in the past it has been associated with serious morbidity and mortality.

What are the indications for surgery?
- Reduced exercise tolerance
- Cyanosis
- Paradoxical embolism
- Severe tricuspid regurgitation.

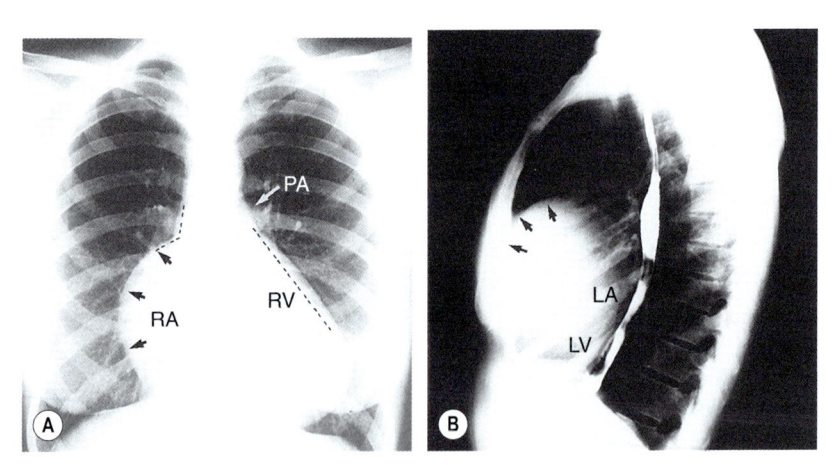

Fig. 29.1 Ebstein's anomaly. (A) A giant right atrium *(RA)* causes a shoulder along the right cardiac silhouette *(arrows)*. A giant RV outflow tract causes the left cardiac border to be straight; the pulmonary artery *(PA)* is very small. (B) The left atrium *(LA)* and left ventricle *(LV)* are essentially normal, but the RA and RV are filling in the retrosternal space *(arrows)*. (With permission from Mettler, F.A., 2004. Essentials of Radiology, second edn. Saunders, Philadelphia, PA.)

29 — EBSTEIN'S ANOMALY

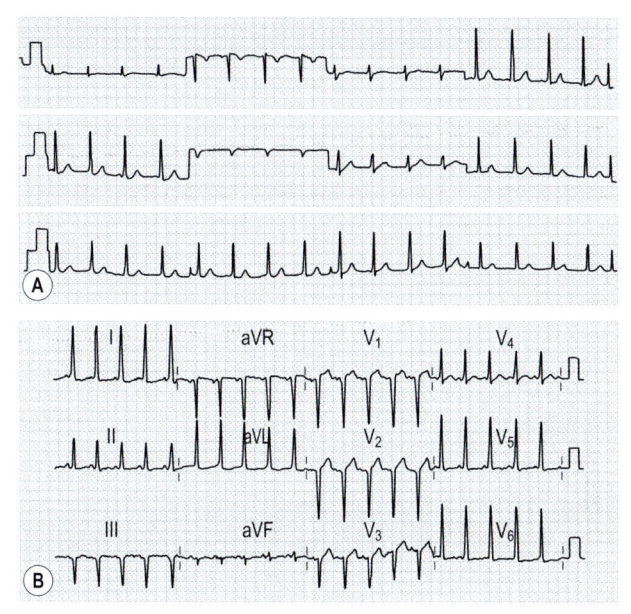

Fig. 29.2 Wolff–Parkinson–White syndrome. **(A)** Type A. The delta wave is recognized clearly in leads II, III, aVF, and V$_1$ through V$_4$. **(B)** Type B. The tracing also shows left ventricular hypertrophy. Tachycardia can be seen, which may be caused by a reentry phenomenon.

How are such patients treated?
- Management of heart failure
- Formal anticoagulation in atrial fibrillation or paradoxical embolus
- Endocarditis prophylaxis in cyanotic patients
- Appropriate treatment of arrhythmias
- Tricuspid valve replacement plus closure of atrial septal defect
- Tricuspid annuloplasty with plication of the atrialized portion of the RV.

Further Information

Wilhelm Ebstein (1836–1912), a German physician who also described the Armanni–Ebstein nephropathy (where there is glycogen vacuolation in the proximal convoluted tubules).
L. Armanni (1839–1903) was an Italian pathologist.

CHAPTER 30

Fallot's Tetralogy

Instruction

This patient with previous corrective heart surgery presents to the general medical clinic with shortness of breath on exertion. Please examine this patient's cardiovascular system.

Salient Features

HISTORY

Fallot's tetralogy has almost always been corrected by adulthood (as diagnosis takes place at birth and the first corrective surgery occurs before the first year of age), but if untreated (extremely rare), the symptoms of Fallot's tetralogy can be the following:
- Syncope (in 20% of cases)
- Tet spells and squatting to help with cyanosis
- Shortness of breath
- Decrease in exercise tolerance
- Growth restriction.

EXAMINATION

- Clubbing
- Central cyanosis
- Left parasternal heave with normal left ventricular (LV) impulse
- Second sound is single (absent second pulmonic sound)
- Ejection systolic murmur heard in the pulmonary area
- Signs indicating Blalock–Taussig shunt:
  - The left radial pulse is not as prominent as the right.
  - The arm on the side of the anastomosis (usually the left) may be smaller than the other arm.
  - Blood pressure is difficult to obtain because of the narrow pulse pressure in the arm supplied by the collateral vessels.
- Thoracotomy scar.

Diagnosis

- This patient has Fallot's tetralogy with a Blalock–Taussig shunt and is mildly cyanosed, indicating a right-to-left shunt (functional status).

Questions

What are the constituents of Fallot's tetralogy?
- Ventricular septal defect with a right-to-left shunt
- Pulmonary stenosis (infundibular or valvular)

- Right ventricular (RV) hypertrophy
- Dextroposition of the aorta with it overriding the ventricular septal defect.

What are the complications of Fallot's tetralogy?
- Cyanotic and syncopal spells
- Cerebral abscess (in 10% of cases)
- Endocarditis (in 10% of cases)
- Strokes: thrombotic secondary to erythrocytosis and hyperviscosity
- Paradoxical emboli.

What anomalies may occur in association with tetralogy of Fallot?
- Right aortic arch in 25% of patients
- Atrial septal defect in 10% (so-called pentalogy of Fallot)
- Coronary arterial anomalies in 10%.

What do you understand by a Blalock–Taussig shunt?
- It is the anastomosis of the left subclavian artery to the left pulmonary artery with the intention to increase pulmonary blood flow.

Why is a Blalock–Taussig shunt seen less frequently in adults in the recent past?
- With ready availability of cardiopulmonary bypass, such patients have total correction of their anomalies at an early age.

What is the survival rate of Fallot's tetralogy if left uncorrected?
- The rate of survival in uncorrected patients is as follows:
    - 66% at 1 year of age
    - 40% at 3 years of age
    - 11% at 20 years of age
    - 6% at 30 years of age
    - 3% at 40 years of age.
- The rate of survival 32 years after surgery in one series was 86% among patients with repaired tetralogy and 96% in an age-matched control population; the difference reflected the increased risk of sudden death.

What do you know about the embryological development of Fallot's tetralogy?
It arises from the anterior displacement of the conal septum, which leads to unequal partitioning of the conus at the expense of the RV infundibulum and results in the obstruction of the RV outflow tract and failure to close the intraventricular foramen.

What do you know regarding the relation between congenital heart disease and embryology of heart development?
In order of embryologic development, the steps in embryogenesis include the following:
1. Looping, laterality, and single-ventricle defects (e.g. double-inlet LV, situs inversus totalis)
2. Conotruncal defects (e.g. tetralogy of Fallot, double-outlet RV)
3. Atrioventricular canal defects (e.g. endocardial cushion defect, common atrioventricular canal defect)
4. RV outflow tract obstruction (e.g. pulmonary valve atresia or stenosis, Ebstein's anomaly)
5. LV outflow tract obstruction (e.g. aortic valve atresia or stenosis, hypoplastic left heart)
6. Septal defects (e.g. ventricular septal defect, atrial septal defect)
7. Total or partial anomalous pulmonary venous return.

What is the treatment for Fallot's tetralogy?
- Total correction under the age of 1 year when there is no need for an outflow transannular patch. A second-stage total correction can be performed when the child is over the age of 2 years. The mortality associated with surgery is <3% in children and 2.5% to 8.5% in adults.
- Blalock–Taussig shunting is performed nowadays only if the anatomy is unfavourable for a total correction.
- Modified Blalock–Taussig shunting is the interposition of a tubular graft between the subclavian and pulmonary arteries.
- The Waterston shunt involves anastomosis of the back of the ascending aorta to the pulmonary artery. It is used when surgery is required in a child younger than 3 months because the subclavian artery is too small for a good Blalock–Taussig shunt.
- The Potts shunt involves anastomosis of the descending aorta to the back of the pulmonary artery.
- The Glenn operation involves anastomosis of the superior vena cava to the right pulmonary artery. The bidirectional Glenn procedure involves anastomosis of the superior vena cava to both pulmonary arteries.
- Pulmonary balloon valvuloplasty is sometimes used as an alternative for surgery.

What cardiac lesions favour an initial shunt?
- Anomalous coronary artery
- Single pulmonary artery
- Hypoplastic pulmonary arteries
- Single pulmonary artery.

What is Fallot's triology?
- Atrial septal defect, pulmonary stenosis, and RV hypertrophy.

What is Fallot's pentalogy?
- Fallot's tetralogy with associated atrial septal defect.

What conditions are associated with Fallot's tetralogy?
- Right-sided aortic arch (in 30% of cases)
- Double aortic arch
- Left-sided superior vena cava (in 10% of cases)
- Hypoplasia of the pulmonary arteries
- Atrial septal defect.

Mention the common congenital heart diseases.
Ventricular septal defect, atrial septal defect of the secundum type, patent ductus arteriosus, and Fallot's tetralogy are the common congenital heart diseases, in order of frequency.

What are the findings from investigations?
Chest radiography:
- Boot-shaped heart (Fig. 30.1)
- Enlarged RV
- Decreased pulmonary vasculature
- Right-sided aortic arch (in 30% of cases).

Electrocardiogram:
- Right axis deviation RV hypertrophy (Fig. 30.2).

30—FALLOT'S TETRALOGY

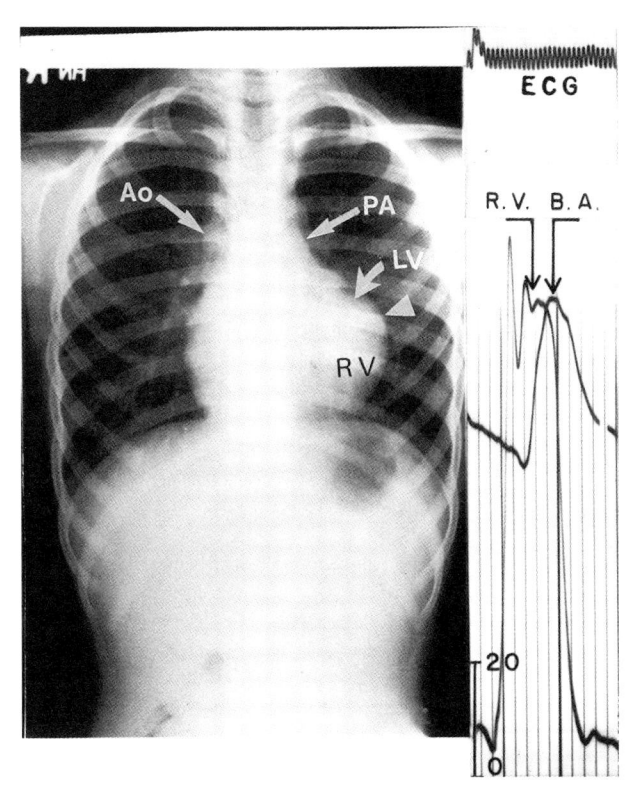

Fig. 30.1 Radiograph in classic cyanotic Fallot's tetralogy. The left ventricle *(LV)* is small and underfilled and lies superior to a relatively horizontal ventricular septum and an elevated interventricular sulcus *(arrowhead)* inferior to which lies the concentrically hypertrophied apex forming right ventricle *(RV)*. The ascending aorta *(Ao)* is prominent, the main pulmonary artery segment *(PA)* is concave, and the lungs are oligaemic. (With permission from Perloff, J.K., 2003. Clinical Recognition of Congenital Heart Disease, fifth edn. Saunders, Philadelphia, PA.)

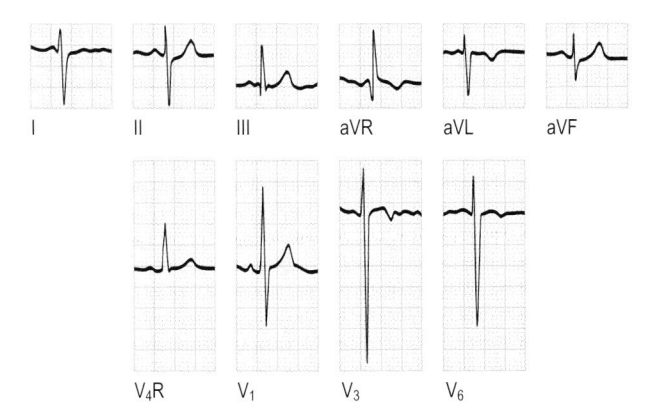

Fig. 30.2 Electrocardiogram in tetralogy of Fallot, with tall R waves in the right precordium, deep S waves in V_6, and positive T waves in V_4R and V_1 characteristic of right ventricular hypertrophy.

What are the arrhythmias detected with Holter monitoring with repaired tetralogy of Fallot?
- Ventricular arrhythmias can be detected in 40% to 50% of such patients and are most likely to occur in those who:
  - are older at the time of surgical repair
  - have moderate or severe pulmonary regurgitation
  - have systolic and diastolic LV dysfunction
  - have prolonged cardiopulmonary bypass
  - have prolongation of the QRS interval (to >180 ms).
- Atrial fibrillation or flutter, which may cause considerable morbidity.

What do you know about the Taussig–Bing syndrome?
In this condition, the aorta arises from the RV; the pulmonary trunk overrides both ventricles at the site of an interventricular septal defect.

What are long-term complications in patients with repaired tetralogy of Fallot?
- Pulmonary regurgitation may develop as a result of surgical repair of the RV outflow tract.
- Enlargement of the RV occurs, resulting in RV dysfunction, and repair or replacement of the pulmonary valve may be required.
- An aneurysm may form at the site where the RV outflow tract was repaired.
- Residual or recurrent obstruction of the RV outflow tract, requiring repeated surgery.
- Residual ventricular septal defects in approximately 10% to 20% of patients with repaired tetralogy of Fallot; such patients may require repeated surgery if the defects are of sufficient size.
- Right bundle branch block is common after repair of tetralogy of Fallot, but complete heart block is rare.
- Aortic root dilatation resulting in aortic regurgitation, usually mild.

Further Information

Etienne-Louis Arthur Fallot (1850–1911), Professor of Hygiene and Legal Medicine in Marseilles, published his 'Contribution to the pathologic anatomy of morbus coeruleus cardiac cyanosis' in 1888.

Helen Brook Taussig (1898–1986) is the founder of American paediatric cardiology. She collaborated with Alfred Blalock (1899–1964), a vascular surgeon, in the development of palliative surgery for Fallot's tetralogy (Taussig and Blalock, 1945).

The tetralogy was first described by Niels Stensen, Professor of Anatomy in Copenhagen, in 1672, but the term tetralogy of Fallot is attributed to Canadian Maude Abbott in 1924 (Fallot, 1888).

CHAPTER 31

Dextrocardia

Instruction
This patient presents to the general medical clinic for a routine check-up. Please examine his cardiovascular system.

Salient Features
HISTORY
- Asymptomatic
- Obtain history of cough with purulent expectoration (bronchiectasis) and sinusitis.

EXAMINATION
- Apex beat is absent on the left side and present on the right.
- Heart sounds are better heard on the right side of the chest.
- Ascertain whether the liver dullness is present on the right or left side.
- Examine the chest for signs of bronchiectasis.
- Proceed by telling the examiner that you would like to perform the following checks:
    - Chest radiograph (looking for right-sided gastric bubble; Fig. 31.1)
    - Electrocardiogram (inversion of all complexes in lead I; Fig. 31.2).

Notes:
- Dextrocardia without evidence of situs inversus is usually associated with cardiac malformation. It may occur with cardiac malformation in Turner syndrome.
- Situs solitus means normal position.

Diagnosis
This patient has dextrocardia (lesion) which is congenital (aetiology).

Questions

What is Kartagener syndrome?
It is a type of immotile cilia syndrome in which there is dextrocardia or situs inversus, bronchiectasis and dysplasia of the frontal sinuses.

Which other abnormality has been associated with dextrocardia?
Asplenia (blood smear may show Heinz bodies, Howell–Jolly bodies).

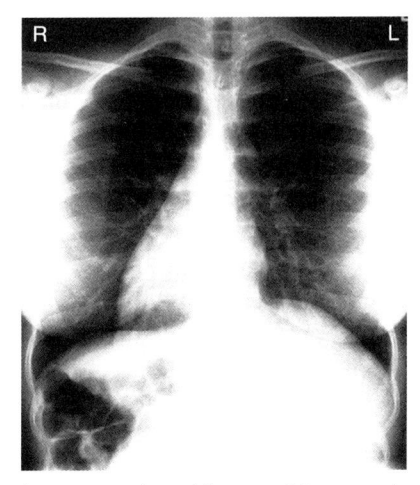

Fig. 31.1 Situs inversus. The heart, stomach, and liver are all in reversed positions (check that the right and left markers are placed correctly). (With permission from Mettler, F.A., 2004. Essentials of Radiology, second edn. Saunders-Elsevier, Philadelphia, PA.)

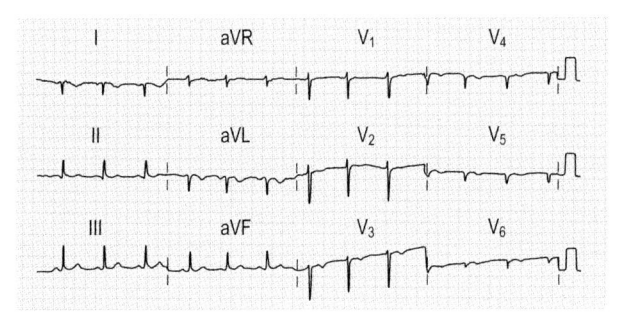

Fig. 31.2 Dextrocardia. Negative QRS wave on lead I and negative P, QRS, and T waves on leads I and aVL. Isoelectric aVR. Negative QRS and T waves in all the precordial leads.

What do you understand by the term situs inversus?
Right-sided cardiac apex, right stomach, right-sided descending aorta. The right atrium is on the left. The left lung has three lobes and the right lung has two.

What do you understand by the term dextroversion?
Right-sided cardiac apex, left-sided stomach, and left-sided descending aorta.

What do you understand by the term levoversion?
Left-sided apex, right-sided stomach, and right descending aorta.

Further Information
M. Kartagener (1897–1975), a Swiss physician, described this condition in 1933.

CHAPTER 32

Eisenmenger Syndrome

Instruction
Please examine this patient's cardiovascular system.

Salient Features
HISTORY
- Symptoms may not appear until late childhood or early adulthood.
- Cyanosis (appears as right-to-left shunting develops)
- Dyspnoea on exercise and impaired exercise tolerance
- Palpitations (common and usually caused by atrial fibrillation or flutter)
- Angina on exertion
- Haemoptysis (may occur as a result of pulmonary infarction or rupture of dilated pulmonary arteries or aorticopulmonary vessels)
- Syncope (owing to inadequate cardiac output or, less commonly, an arrhythmia)
- Symptoms of hyperviscosity including visual disturbances, fatigue, headache, dizziness, and paraesthesia
- Symptoms of heart failure are uncommon until the disease is in advanced stages.

EXAMINATION
- Clubbing of fingers and central cyanosis
- An 'a' wave in the jugular venous pressure (JVP); 'v' wave if tricuspid regurgitation also present
- Left parasternal heave and palpable P_2
- Loud P_2, pulmonary ejection click, early diastolic murmur of pulmonary regurgitation (Graham Steell murmur)
- Loud pansystolic murmur of tricuspid regurgitation
- Listen carefully to the second sound. The clinical findings from the underlying defect are as follows:
    - Ventricular septal defect (VSD): single second sound
    - Atrial septal defect (ASD): fixed, wide split second sound
    - Patent ductus arteriosus (PDA): reverse split of second sound and differential cyanosis where lower-limb cyanosis is marked.

Diagnosis
This patient has Eisenmenger syndrome with a shunt at the ventricular level (lesion) that is congenital in origin (aetiology). He has signs of severe pulmonary hypertension (functional status).

Questions

What do you understand by the term Eisenmenger syndrome?
Pulmonary hypertension with a reversed or bidirectional shunt due to congenital heart disease. It matters very little where the shunt happens to be (e.g. VSD, ASD, PDA, persistent truncus arteriosus, single ventricle, or common atrioventricular canal).

What do you understand by the term Eisenmenger complex?
Eisenmenger complex is a specific subtype of Eisenmenger syndrome caused by a VSD with a right-to-left shunt in the absence of pulmonary stenosis. The onset of Eisenmenger syndrome is often heralded by a softening of the murmur, a decrease in the left heart size, and an increase in P_2.

Mention some cyanotic heart diseases of infancy.
- Tetralogy of Fallot
- Transposition of the great vessels
- Tricuspid regurgitation
- Total anomalous pulmonary venous connection.

What is the age of onset of Eisenmenger syndrome?
In the case of PDA and VSD, about 80% occur in infancy, whereas in the case of ASD, over 90% occur in adult life.

What factors worsen pulmonary hypertension in these patients?
- Pregnancy
- Dehydration or acute vasodilation (e.g. sauna, hot tub)
- Increased fluid volume
- Worsened renal or hepatic function
- Chronic environmental hypoxia
- Increased left-sided filling pressure:
  - Left ventricular diastolic dysfunction
  - Obstructive congenital lesion
  - Myocardial restriction
  - Systemic hypertension with increased left ventricular afterload
- Erythrocytosis and increased blood viscosity; anaemia
- Hypercoagulability: thrombosis
- Acute infection
- Arrhythmias.

What are the complications of Eisenmenger syndrome?
- Haemoptysis
- Erythrocytosis
- Right ventricular (RV) failure
- Cerebrovascular accidents (as a result of paradoxical embolization, venous thrombosis of cerebral vessels, or intracranial haemorrhage)
- Sudden death
- Brain abscess
- Bleeding and thrombosis (patients at increased risks for both as a consequence of an abnormal haemostasis secondary to chronic arterial desaturation)
- Paradoxical embolization

- Infective endocarditis
- Hyperuricaemia
- Recurrent haemoptysis.

How would you investigate this patient?
- *Electrocardiogram* shows RV hypertrophy; atrial arrhythmias particularly in those with underlying ASD.
- *Chest radiograph* shows conspicuous dilatation of the pulmonary artery (Fig. 32.1) with narrowed 'pruned' peripheral vessels (caused by pulmonary hypertension); slight to moderate enlargement of the heart (predominantly RV) may be seen in ASD, whereas the size of the heart is normal in VSD or PDA.
- *Echocardiography* provides evidence of RV overload and pulmonary hypertension; the underlying cardiac defect can be visualized, although shunting may be difficult to demonstrate by colour Doppler imaging because of low-velocity jet; contrast echocardiography permits localization of shunt.
- *Cardiac catheterization* determines the extent and severity of pulmonary vascular disease and accurately quantifies the magnitude of the intracardiac shunting; assessment of reversibility of shunting is done using pulmonary vasodilators (e.g. oxygen, inhaled nitrous oxide, intravenous adenosine or epoprostenol).

What is the prognosis in these patients?
- Survival is 80% 10 years after diagnosis, 77% at 15 years, and 42% at 25 years.
- Death is usually sudden; other causes include heart failure, haemoptysis, brain abscess, or stroke.
- Poor prognostic factors include syncope, clinically evident RV systolic dysfunction, low cardiac output, and severe hypoxaemia.

Is pregnancy safe in this patient?
Pregnancy is associated with a high incidence of early spontaneous abortion and rarely results in the birth of a healthy child. Mortality of the mother is high (30%–60%) in those with

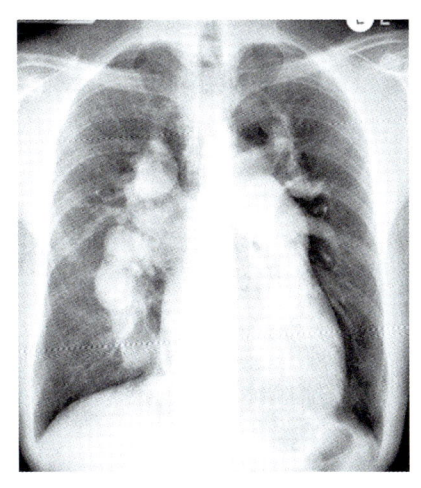

Fig. 32.1 Chest radiograph demonstrating gross dilatation of the main, left, and right pulmonary arteries in a patient with Eisenmenger atrial septal defect. (With permission from Adam, A., Dixon, A.K., Grainger, R.G., Allison, D.J., 2008. Grainger and Allison's Diagnostic Radiology, fifth edn. Churchill Livingstone, Edinburgh.)

underlying VSD, particularly in late pregnancy and the postpartum period. Pregnancy is therefore contraindicated and if occurs is best terminated at an early stage. If pregnancy proceeds to term, a vaginal delivery is the preferred route, with careful management of hydration, arrhythmias, and hypoxaemia. Epidural anaesthesia is preferred to general anaesthesia in complicated cases.

What treatment is available for Eisenmenger syndrome?
- Main treatment is towards pulmonary hypertension:
  - Long-term intravenous epoprostenol
  - Phosphodiesterase 5 inhibitors (e.g. sildenafil) have shown benefit in advanced pulmonary vascular disease.
  - Bosentan has shown a significant improvement in exercise capacity based on 6-min walk distance and reduction in pulmonary resistance, without serious safety concerns.
- Combined heart–lung transplantation or lung transplantation with intracardiac repair of the lesions.

Further Information

Victor Eisenmenger was a German physician who described this condition in an infant in 1897. His patient had cyanosis since infancy and a fairly good quality of life until he succumbed at the age of 32 years. The patient was active until the age of 29 years, when he developed right heart failure and died 3 years later following a massive haemoptysis. Postmortem revealed a large VSD (2.5 cm) with both the left ventricle and RV with equally thick walls. The pulmonary arteries revealed atheroma with multiple thrombi leading to pulmonary infarctions.

Paul Wood at the Brompton Hospital in 1958 published a study of 127 patients and was the first to suggest that Eisenmenger reaction occurred with defects other than the ventricular level (Wood, 1958).

CHAPTER 33

Hypertrophic Cardiomyopathy

Instruction
Examine this patient's cardiovascular system.

Salient Features
HISTORY
- Patients may be asymptomatic:
  - Generalized fatigue
  - Dyspnoea on exertion: in ~50% of patients
  - Chest pain: in ~50%; may be exertional or occur at rest
  - Syncope (in 15%–25%)
  - Dizziness and palpitations.
- Obtain a family history of the following:
  - Cardiomyopathy
  - Sudden cardiac death.

EXAMINATION
- Carotid pulse is bifid (Fig. 33.1):
  - 'a' wave in the jugular venous pulse
  - *Double apical impulse* (left ventricular (LV) heave with a prominent presystolic pulse caused by atrial contraction)
  - Pansystolic murmur at the apex caused by mitral regurgitation
  - Ejection systolic murmur along the left sternal border (across the outflow tract obstruction); accentuated by standing and Valsalva manoeuvre and softer on squatting (squatting increases LV cavity size and reduces outflow tract obstruction). Remember the Valsalva manoeuvre decreases the duration of murmur of aortic stenosis and increases the murmur of hypertrophic cardiomyopathy.
- Fourth heart sound.

Diagnosis
This patient has hypertrophic obstructive cardiomyopathy (HOCM) (aetiology) as evidenced by a double apical impulse and ejection systolic murmur along the left sternal border, which is heard better on standing (lesion); the patient is in cardiac failure (functional status).

Questions
How would you investigate this patient?
- *Echocardiogram* is useful for assessing LV structure and function, gradients (Fig. 33.2), valvular regurgitation, and atrial dimensions. Doppler echocardiography shows characteristic

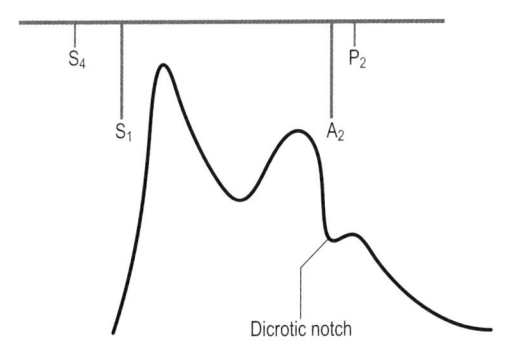

Fig. 33.1 Carotid pulse is bifid with two systolic peaks. The second peak (tidal or reflected wave) is of lower amplitude than the initial percussion wave.

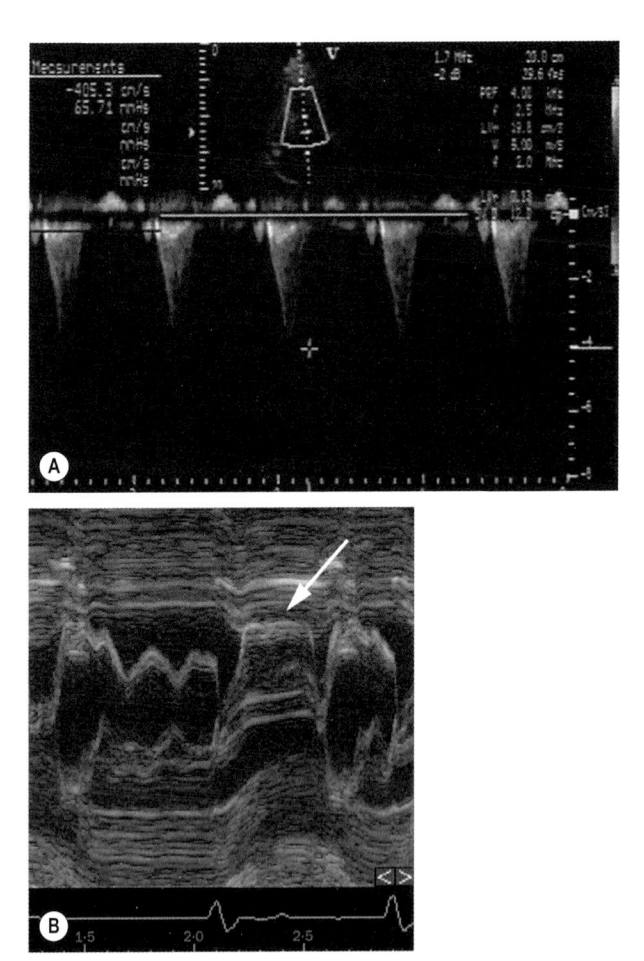

Fig. 33.2 Echocardiography. **(A)** Continuous wave Doppler in dynamic left ventricular outflow tract obstruction. Note the characteristic dagger-shaped velocity envelope. **(B)** M-mode shows the protracted contact between the anterior mitral valve leaflet and the interventricular septum in systole *(arrow)*. (With permission from Elliott, P., McKenna, W.J. 2007. Hypertrophic cardiomyopathy. *Lancet* 363, 1881–1891.)

high-velocity late-peaking or dagger-shaped spectral waveform (Fig. 33.2A). Characteristic findings include systolic anterior motion of mitral valve, asymmetric hypertrophy (ASH), and mitral regurgitation.
- *Electrocardiogram (ECG)* may be normal in about 5% of patients. Most patients, however, will have an abnormal ECG: abnormalities include LV hypertrophy, atrial fibrillation, left axis deviation, right bundle branch block, and myocardial disarray (e.g. ST-T wave changes, intraventricular conduction defects, abnormal Q waves); bizarre or abnormal findings in young patients should raise suspicion of hypertrophic cardiomyopathy (especially if family members also affected) (Fig. 33.3).
- *Chest radiograph* may be normal or show evidence of left or right atrial or LV enlargement.
- *Treadmill exercise test* is performed to risk-stratify patients diagnosed with HOCM and help with further management options.
- *Cardiac magnetic resonance imaging* is used to confirm diagnosis when echocardiography is not adequate, to assess the exact anatomy in order to risk-stratify patients, and before any planned procedure for HOCM. It shows patchy areas of hyperenhancement, the extent of which is greatest in patients with risk markers for sudden cardiac death and in those in whom progressive remodelling of the LV can be seen. The predominant site of hypertrophy is usually the 1-o'clock position in the short-axis view at the confluence of anterior septum and anterior wall.
- *48-hour Holter monitoring* should be performed in all patients diagnosed with HOCM. It identifies established atrial fibrillation (in about 10% of patients), paroxysmal supraventricular arrhythmias (in 30%), nonsustained ventricular tachycardia (in 25%), and ventricular tachycardia (in 25%); ventricular tachycardia is invariably asymptomatic during Holter monitoring but is a most useful risk marker of sudden death in adults; sustained supraventricular arrhythmias are often symptomatic and predispose to thromboembolic complications. More prolonged studies can be obtained for the detection of nonsustained ventricular arrhythmias.
- *Endomyocardial biopsy* is possibly necessary to exclude specific heart muscle disorder (amyloid, sarcoid) but has no role in diagnosis because of patchy nature of myofibrillar disarray.
- *Left heart catheterization* is rarely needed to make the diagnosis. In the presence of LV outflow obstruction, the LV-to-aortic late-peaking gradient is seen with characteristic aortic pressure tracing showing a rapid rise and fall followed by a plateau—the 'spike and dome' pattern.
- *Genetic testing* is not recommended for the diagnosis or risk stratification of HOCM and is not routinely performed.

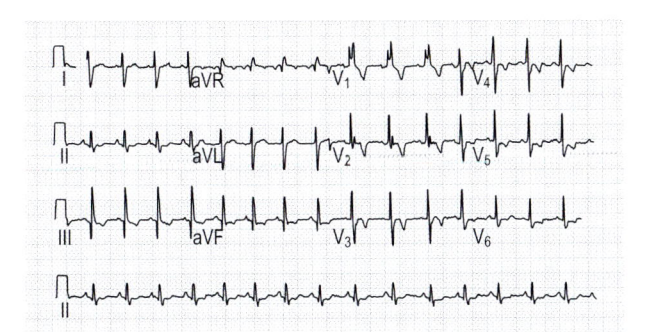

Fig. 33.3 Electrocardiographic patterns in hypertrophic cardiomyopathy. A 12-lead tracing, in concentric left ventricular hypertrophy, with T-wave inversion extending from V_1 to V_5, and deep Q waves in leads III and aVF.

What are the complications of hypertrophic cardiomyopathy?
- Sudden cardiac death
- Atrial and ventricular arrhythmias
- Heart failure
- Coronary artery disease
- Infective endocarditis
- Systemic embolization.

How would you manage such a patient?
- Relief of symptoms once they appear, prior to that, regular follow-up with yearly clinical assessment and echocardiography is adequate.
- Beta-blockers are used in symptomatic outflow obstruction, as they can reduce the obstruction because of their negative inotropic effect (propranolol up to 640 mg/day).
- Verapamil can be used as an alternative to propranolol if beta-blockers are contraindicated (up to 480 mg/day).
- Disopyramide can be added to beta-blockers if needed (up to 400–600 mg/day).
- Diuretics at small doses may be helpful with symptomatic relief of dyspnoea.
- In patients with outflow obstruction of more than 50 mm Hg, moderate to severe heart failure symptomatology, or recurrent syncopal episodes, invasive treatment should be considered.
- Cardiac pacing may be considered in patients with refractory symptoms who cannot undergo interventions.
- Implantable cardiac defibrillators to prevent sudden death
- Lifestyle modifications and treatment of coexisting disease and cardiovascular risk factors
- Cardioversion in patients with atrial fibrillation
- Digoxin and vasodilators should be avoided as they worsen outflow obstruction.

What is the most characteristic pathophysiological abnormality in hypertrophic cardiomyopathy?
Diastolic dysfunction.

What do you know about the genetics of hypertrophic cardiomyopathy?
Hypertrophic cardiomyopathy is an autosomal dominant heart muscle disorder. Mutations in the gene encoding contractile proteins cause disease in 50% to 60% of patients. At least 15 individual genes have been identified to date, with more than 1500 mutations in cardiac contractile proteins, including troponin T, troponin I, myosin, actin, tropomyosin, and titin. No matter the protein involved, the end result is dysfunction of the sarcomere.

What do you know about the Brockenbrough–Braunwald–Morrow sign?
Diminished pulse pressure in postextrasystolic beat occurs in hypertrophic cardiomyopathy/aortic stenosis.

What do you know about the epidemiology of this condition?
- The male-to-female ratio is equal, although the disease tends to affect younger men and older women.
- In children and adolescents, myocardial hypertrophy often occurs during growth spurts (a negative diagnosis made before adolescent growth does not exclude the condition and reassessment at a later age is important).
- Myocardial hypertrophy does not ordinarily progress after adolescent growth is completed.

- Sudden death can occur at any age (from childhood to over 90 years) and in subjects who have been asymptomatic all their life. The annual mortality from sudden death is 3% to 5% in adults and at least 6% in children and young adults.
- First-degree relatives of affected patients have a 50% chance of carrying the disease gene; they should be investigated by ECG and two-dimensional echocardiogram. Genetic counselling is therefore important.

What are the risk predictors of sudden death?

	Criteria	*Comment*
History	Exertional or recurrent syncope and presyncope	Risk greatest in children
	Family history of sudden death, known malignant genotype	Risk related to family size and number of members with sudden cardiac death
Diagnostic evaluation	Severe LV hypertrophy	Risk increases with an increase in wall thickness
	Nonsustained ventricular tachycardia	Higher predictive value in children and those with syncope
	Abnormal haemodynamic response to exercise (failure to augment systolic blood pressure by at least 20 mm Hg)	Less applicable to those >40 years

LV, Left ventricular.

Further Information

The pathology of hypertrophic cardiomyopathy was first described by two French pathologists in the mid-19th century and by a German pathologist in the early 20th century. The simultaneous reports of Sir Russel Brock, thoracic surgeon at Guy's and Brompton Hospitals (Brock, 1957), and of Teare (Teare, 1958) brought this to modern medical attention.

CHAPTER 34

Congestive Cardiac Failure

Instruction

This patient presented with bilateral ankle swelling and dyspnoea. Please examine this patient's cardiovascular system.

Salient Features

HISTORY

- Dyspnoea on exertion
- Orthopnoea, paroxysmal nocturnal dyspnoea
- Ankle oedema, abdominal distension
- Tiredness, fatigue, dizziness
- History of hypertension, ischaemic heart disease, or cardiomyopathy.

EXAMINATION

- Signs of fluid retention: raised jugular venous pressure, lung crepitations, pitting leg oedema, tender hepatomegaly
- Signs of impaired perfusion: cold clammy skin, low blood pressure
- Signs of ventricular dysfunction: displaced left ventricular (LV) apex, right ventricular heave, third or fourth heart sound, functional mitral or tricuspid regurgitation, tachycardia
- Look for the aetiology:
  - Valvular disease
  - Atherosclerotic vascular disease
  - Severe hypertension
  - Severe anaemia or volume overload, e.g. arteriovenous shunt
  - Pathological arrhythmia
  - Evidence of generalized myopathy or poisoning.

Diagnosis

This patient has congestive cardiac failure (lesion) probably caused by coronary artery disease (aetiology) and is severely limited with New York Heart Association (NYHA) class 4 dyspnoea (functional status).

Questions

How would you investigate this patient?
- *Serum B-type natriuretic peptide* should be sent as an initial screening test. It is particularly useful in the outpatient setting, where the diagnosis of heart failure is suspected but not established as it has a high negative predictive value.

- *Electrocardiogram* to look for underlying cause, e.g. ischaemia or infarction, LV hypertrophy, arrhythmia, other causes of pathological Q waves. Monitoring with 24-hour Holter can identify ventricular arrhythmias.
- *Transthoracic echocardiogram* is the investigation of choice to diagnose heart failure and decide on further treatment. It can also help with the aetiology of heart failure, as it detects valvular disease and determines whether LV function is globally impaired (e.g. idiopathic dilated cardiomyopathy) or whether there is segmental wall motion abnormalities (e.g. in ischaemic heart disease). It can assess the systolic and diastolic function of the LV, estimate the ejection fraction (EF) of the LV, and also assess the structure and function of the right ventricle.
- *Chest radiography* is more helpful in the acute setting and in patients presenting with acutely symptomatic decompensated heart failure. Findings on a chest X-ray (CXR) consistent with heart failure can be pulmonary oedema, bilateral pleural effusions, pulmonary vascular congestion with upper lobe diversion, and Kerley B lines. The presence of pulmonary oedema on chest radiograph suggests that LV end-diastolic pressure is 25 mm Hg (normal ~7 mm Hg). CXR in the outpatient setting is primarily useful to detect or exclude other pulmonary conditions that may contribute to the symptoms of dyspnoea, especially combined with other pulmonary investigations, such as computed tomography (CT) of the chest and lung function tests.
- *Cardiac magnetic resonance imaging* is useful when echocardiography cannot supply the answers about aetiology and myocardial structure and also in patients with complex congenital heart disease.
- *Cardiopulmonary exercise testing* is useful to determine functional capacity before cardiac rehabilitation and to determine eligibility for cardiac transplantation.
- *Blood tests* can identify associated disease: renal, liver, and electrolyte disturbances (common); metabolic causes (e.g. haemochromatosis, hypocalcaemic cardiomyopathy, thyroid heart disease, anaemia, heavy metal poisoning); amyloid (serum electrophoresis, rectal biopsy); sarcoid (serum angiotensin-converting enzyme (ACE)); and anaemia (full blood count, iron studies).
- *Noninvasive stress tests, cardiac CT, and invasive coronary angiography* are all used to identify or exclude ischaemic heart disease, each one with different indications, depending on the possibility or prior existence of existing coronary artery disease.
- *Ventricular biopsy* for specific myocarditis, especially viral, and to exclude infiltrative diseases such as cardiac sarcoidosis and amyloidosis.
- Right heart catheterization is considered for specific cases, such as patients with heart failure with preserved EF (HFpEF) to confirm diagnosis, or when the cause is thought to be constrictive pericarditis, restrictive cardiomyopathy or congenital heart disease.

What types of heart failure have you heard of?

Heart failure is divided according to the EF estimate on the echocardiography into HFpEF when the EF is less than 40% or heart failure with reduced EF (HFrEF) if the EF is normal (>50%). Patients with an EF between the earlier estimates have heart failure with mildly reduced EF, or HRmrEF. Both diagnosis and treatment of HFpEF are more difficult than diagnosis and treatment of HFrEF.

What is the pharmacologic treatment of symptomatic heart failure with reduced ejection fraction?

- ACE inhibitors (ACE-Is): have been shown to reduce mortality and hospitalization
- Angiotensin receptor blockers in patients who cannot tolerate ACE-I
- Beta-blockers: have been shown to reduce mortality and hospitalization

- Aldosterone receptor antagonists (MRA): when the patient remains symptomatic despite a combination of ACE-I and beta-blocker (has shown to reduce mortality and hospitalization)
- Angiotensin receptor-neprilysin inhibitor (ARNI): a replacement for ACE-I in patients who remain symptomatic despite the combination of the earlier-discussed medications
- Ivabradine: for patients in sinus rhythm with a resting heart rate more than 70 beats/min
- Diuretics for symptomatic control of fluid retention and oedema (loop diuretics, thiazide diuretics)
- ARNIs block the angiotensin–renin cycle and the cardiac remodelling.
- Verisiguat: a guanyl cyclase stimulator is used for prognostic benefit in patients who have needed hospitalization and intravenous diuretic therapy and has shown to reduce hospitalizations in patients with HFrEF.
- Others: digoxin, combination of hydralazine and nitrates.

What drugs should be avoided in heart failure?
- Antiarrhythmic drugs
- Nondihydropyridine calcium antagonists, e.g. verapamil, diltiazem in patients with systolic chronic heart failure
- Tricyclic antidepressants
- Nonsteroidal antiinflammatory drugs
- Cyclo-oxygenase 2 inhibitors
- Corticosteroids
- Doxorubicin and trastuzumab
- Thiazolidinediones.

Name an antidiabetic medication that has been proven to have a positive impact on heart failure prognosis.
The updated European guidelines for the treatment of heart failure recommend the use of sodium-glucose cotransporter 2 (SGLT2) inhibitors dapagliflozin or empagliflozin in patients with HFrEF due to their proven prognostic benefit.

What is heart failure with preserved ejection fraction?
It is the traditionally called diastolic heart failure, which is characterized by excessive stiffness of the heart muscle resulting in an inability of the LV to fill properly during diastole. This is in contrast to systolic dysfunction (HFrEF), where contractility is impaired. Patients have clinical features of left heart failure but normal systolic function by echocardiography or radionuclide ventriculography. It is a feature of hypertrophic cardiomyopathy, severe LV hypertrophy (e.g. aortic stenosis or hypertension), and restrictive cardiomyopathy (e.g. amyloidosis). Unlike HFrEF, trials of pharmacological treatments have failed to show positive impact on prognosis of HFpEF, hence the treatment is targeted towards reducing the cardiovascular risk factors and treating reversible underlying causes that have contributed to heart failure.

What is the role of devices in heart failure?
Three types of device have been found to be effective in treatment of systolic heart failure:
- Cardiac resynchronization therapy: patients who remain symptomatic despite optimal medical therapy for heart failure and have documented ventricular dyssynchrony electrocardiographically
- Implantable cardioverter defibrillators: for primary and secondary prevention of ventricular arrhythmias in patients with heart failure, as long as patients receive optimal medical therapy and do not have very poor prognosis with symptoms of stage NYHA IV
- LV assist devices may be considered in three situations:

- For individuals listed for transplantation but who need support before a suitable donor heart becomes available
- As a bridge to recovery in people with potentially reversible forms of heart failure, such as myocarditis or postpartum cardiomyopathy
- As 'destination therapy' for patients not judged candidates for transplantation.

What are the indications for heart transplantation?

When patients are refractory to treatment, both medical and surgical (such as valve replacement), and are in NYHA class IV, then they are unlikely to survive for 1 year and should be considered for heart transplantation. The candidates should be emotionally stable and capable of complying with the treatment needed after the operation.

Further Information

In 1967, Christiaan Barnard, a South African surgeon, was the first to perform cardiac transplantation in humans.

Sir Magdi Yacoub, professor of cardiology at University of London and Royal Brompton Hospital and Harefield Hospital, is an Egyptian-born surgeon who performed several pioneering cardiac surgeries.

Professor Shoumo Bhattacharya is Professor of Cardiovascular Medicine at Oxford. He is Fellow of Green Templeton College and his research interest includes cardiac development, congenital heart disease and myocardial homeostasis. His clinical interest is chemotherapy-induced cardiomyopathy.

CHAPTER 35

Constrictive Pericarditis

Instruction

Examine this patient's cardiovascular system.

Salient Features

HISTORY

- Dyspnoea
- Fatigue
- Ankle or abdominal swelling
- Nausea, vomiting, dizziness, and cough.

EXAMINATION

- The patient may appear cachectic.
- The pulse may be regular or irregularly irregular (one-third have atrial fibrillation).
- Prominent 'x' and 'y' descents in the jugular venous pulse (JVP) and the level of the JVP may rise with inspiration (Kussmaul's sign; Fig. 35.1)
- The apex beat is not palpable and there may be apical systolic retraction (Broadbent sign).
- Early diastolic pericardial knock along the left sternal border, which may be accentuated by inspiration
- Lungs are clear, but there may be pleural effusion:
  - Hepatomegaly and ascites, pitting leg oedema, oedema anasarca.

Diagnosis

This patient has constrictive pericarditis (lesion) caused by radiation therapy for previous Hodgkin disease (aetiology) and is now limited by dyspnoea and marked ascites (functional status).

Questions

Mention some causes of constrictive pericarditis.
- Idiopathic
- Viral
- Tuberculosis (TB)
- Connective tissue disorder
- Neoplastic infiltration
- Radiation therapy (often years earlier)
- Postpurulent pericarditis
- Haemopericardium after surgery (rare)
- Chronic renal failure.

35—CONSTRICTIVE PERICARDITIS

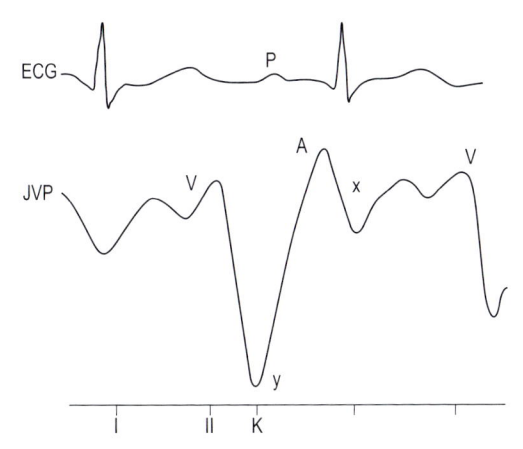

Fig. 35.1 Abnormal jugular venous waveform in constrictive pericarditis with a prominent 'y' descent. Note the timing of the pericardial knock (K) relative to S_2. The abrupt rise in pressure after the nadir of the 'y' descent is caused by the rapid rise in venous pressure with ventricular filling.

How does pericardial disease present and what is constrictive pericarditis?

Depending on the underlying aetiology, the duration of the pathology, and the haemodynamic consequences, pericardial disease can present as acute recurrent pericarditis, pericardial effusion, cardiac tamponade, constrictive pericarditis, and effusive-constrictive pericarditis. The normal pericardial sac contains about 20 to 50 mL of ultrafiltrated fluid, contributes to the haemodynamic interdependence of the ventricles, and can accommodate physiological differences in blood volume in the heart. In constrictive pericarditis the pericardium is fibrosed and calcified, and consequently the muscle of the heart is enclosed in a nonelastic shell. As a result, there is restriction in the blood volume the cardiac chambers can accommodate with increasing filling pressures and low cardiac output.

Constrictive pericarditis presents with symptoms of overload and low cardiac output, fatigue, dyspnoea, and oedema anasarca.

What is the mechanism for pericardial knock?

It is caused by the abrupt halting of rapid ventricular filling.

Mention the differential diagnosis of the early diastolic sound.

- Loud P_2
- S_4 gallop
- Opening snap (mitral stenosis)
- Pericardial sound
- Tumour plop (atrial myxoma).

What is Beck's triad?

The presence of low arterial blood pressure and high venous pressure and absent apex in cardiac tamponade is known as Beck's triad.

How would you clinically differentiate between constrictive pericarditis and restrictive cardiomyopathy?

Restrictive cardiomyopathy will present with the same symptoms as constrictive pericarditis, but they may have a few subtle changes in the history and clinical examination. For instance, the development of dyspnoea and fatigue on a background of amyloidosis would point towards restrictive cardiomyopathy, whereas oedema anasarca post cardiac surgery would suggest pericardial disease. On auscultation of the heart, patients with constrictive pericarditis may have a pericardial knock which is not a feature of restrictive cardiomyopathy. Patients with restrictive cardiomyopathy may have a third heart sound which is not expected to be found in constrictive pericarditis.

How would you investigate a patient with constrictive pericarditis?
- *Chest radiograph* typically shows normal heart size and pericardial calcification (note that the combination of pulsus paradoxus, pericardial knock, and pericardial calcification favours the diagnosis of constrictive pericarditis).
- *Electrocardiogram* shows low-voltage complexes, nonspecific T-wave flattening, or atrial fibrillation.
- *Echocardiogram* may reveal thickened pericardium, normal ventricular dimensions with enlarged atria, and good systolic and poor diastolic dysfunction. Doppler shows increased right ventricular systolic and decreased left ventricular systolic velocity with inspiration, expiratory augmentation of hepatic-vein diastolic flow reversal.
- *Computed tomography or magnetic resonance imaging* usually shows normal myocardial thickness and pericardial thickening and calcification.
- *Cardiac catheterization* typically shows identical left and right ventricular filling pressures and pulmonary artery systolic pressure usually <45 mm Hg, with normal myocardial biopsy: haemodynamic tracings show a rapid 'y' descent in atrial pressure and an early dip in diastolic pressure, with pressure rise to plateau in the mid or late diastole. Cardiac tamponade and constrictive pericarditis are basically similar in restricting the filling of the heart and raising the systemic and pulmonary venous pressures. The venous pressure waveforms differ, however, reflecting a single wave of forward flow (during systole) in tamponade, compared with a biphasic pattern (a lesser wave in systole and a greater wave in early diastole) in constrictive conditions.

How would you treat a patient with constrictive pericarditis?
- Surgery is the only satisfactory treatment: complete surgical resection of the pericardium (myocardial inflammation or fibrosis may delay symptomatic response).
- Patients with tuberculous pericarditis should be pretreated for TB; if the diagnosis is confirmed after pericardial resection, full antituberculous therapy should be continued for 6 to 12 months after resection.

What do you understand by the term effusive–constrictive pericarditis?
This is a clinical haemodynamic syndrome in which constriction of the heart by the visceral pericardium occurs in the presence of tense effusion in a free pericardial space. The hallmark is the persistence of elevated right atrial pressure after intrapericardial pressure has been reduced to normal levels by removal of pericardial fluid. Removing the pericardial fluid from a patient with effusive–constrictive pericarditis tends to change the venous waveform pattern from one more like that found in tamponade to one more like that associated with constriction.

Further Information

C.S. Beck (1894–1971), surgeon, Peter Bent Brigham Hospital in Boston.

W. Broadbent (1868–1951), English physician who qualified from St Mary's Hospital Medical School, London. He described the Broadbent sign in constrictive pericarditis, which is an indrawing of the 11th and 12th left ribs with a narrowing and retraction of the intercostal space posteriorly; this occurs as a result of pericardial adhesions to the diaphragm.

CHAPTER 36

Weight Loss

Instruction

This patient presented with fatigue, weight loss, and fever to his general practitioner. Initial tests including routine bloods, myeloma screen, and imaging have been negative for identifying malignancy or infection; autoimmune screen is negative; and the patient has been referred to the medical clinic for further assessment. Please assess.

Salient Features

HISTORY

- Onset and progression of the patient's symptoms
- Fever, malaise, anorexia, weight loss, and rigors may be nonspecific symptoms of inflammation.
- Pattern of weight loss; patients whose weight has always been stable and who present with progressive and unintentional weight loss of recent onset are more likely to have a sinister cause.
- Quantify the weight loss.
- Loss of appetite or other symptoms that hinder eating (dysphagia, odynophagia, postprandial pain)
- Systemic enquiry for symptoms that may point towards a specific system/organ pathology:
    - Altered bowel habit or bleeding per rectum (bowel malignancy)
    - Recent-onset dyspnoea with cough and haemoptysis in a chronic smoker (lung malignancy)
    - Joint pain, rash, eye symptoms (rheumatological and autoimmune conditions)
    - Constipation, dry skin, and cold intolerance (hypothyroidism)
- Social history including travel history, occupation (certain infections will be associated with specific risk factors and contacts), and alcohol consumption
- Medication and psychiatric history (Diuretic or laxative abuse can lead to weight loss.)
- Symptoms of heart failure, embolic events (stroke, pulseless limb, renal infarct, pulmonary infarct)
- Symptoms caused by immune-complex deposition (haematuria, arthralgia, loin pain)
- Risk factors for infective endocarditis (valvular heart disease, previous episodes of infective endocarditis, intravenous drug use).

EXAMINATION

- Look at the general appearance.
- Examine the abdomen for organomegaly and masses.
- Check for lymphadenopathy.
- Conduct respiratory and cardiovascular examination.

- Conduct neurological and musculoskeletal examination, including spine palpation for tenderness (discitis).
- Look particularly for peripheral stigmata of infective endocarditis:
  - Anaemia
  - Clubbing (seen in 20% of the cases)
  - Splinter haemorrhages in the nails (vasculitic phenomenon; probably caused by embolic phenomena in the nail bed) (Fig. 36.1)
  - Osler's nodes (vasculitic phenomenon): tender, erythematous, pea-sized nodules seen in the pulp of the fingers caused by inflammation around the site of the infected emboli lodged in distal arterioles (Fig. 36.2)
  - Janeway lesions (vasculitic phenomenon): flat, nontender red spots found on the palms and soles; they blanch on pressure
  - Petechiae: conjunctiva, palate, and skin
  - Digital infarcts
  - Maculopapular rash.
- Record the temperature.
- Listen to the heart for murmurs and look for signs of cardiac failure.
- Examine the fundus for Roth spots.
- Examine the abdomen for splenomegaly.
- Look for embolic phenomena: stroke, viscera, or occlusion of peripheral arteries.
- Test the urine for microscopic haematuria.

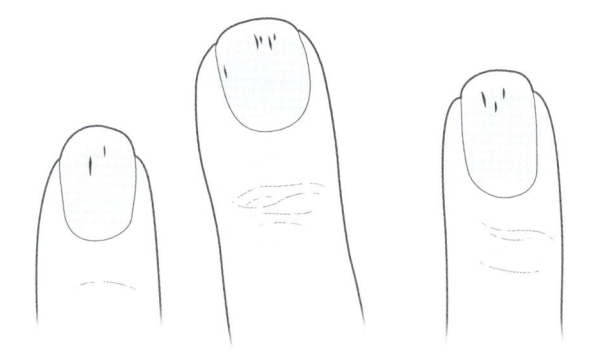

Fig. 36.1 Splinter haemorrhages: parallel streaks in the distal third of the finger.

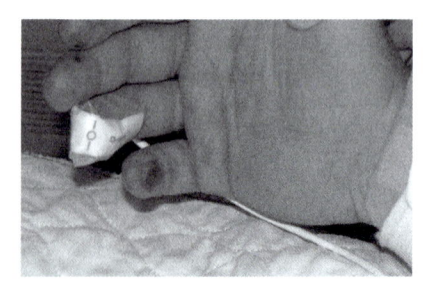

Fig. 36.2 Osler's nodes. (With permission from Goldman, L., Ausiello, D.A. 2007. Cecil Textbook of Medicine, twenty-third edn. Saunders, Philadelphia, PA.)

Diagnosis

This patient has a new murmur, Janeway lesions, and Roth spots (lesions), signifying a possible underlying diagnosis of infective endocarditis (aetiology) as a cause for his recent deterioration and weight loss (functional status).

Questions

How would you investigate such a patient?
- Blood tests: full blood count, biochemical profile including liver function tests, bone profile, and renal function. Inflammatory markers including C-reactive protein
- Autoimmune screen, myeloma screen, thyroid function, electrolytes including phosphate and magnesium
- Baseline viral screen including hepatitis virus screen and human immunodeficiency virus
- Other virology depending on the clinical suspicion
- Imaging to rule out occult malignancy or spinal abscess
- Urine dipstick and microscopy
- Blood culture: take three samples from different sites in 24 hours. It is the most important test for diagnosing endocarditis and cultures are negative in >50% of cases of fungal aetiology.
- Transthoracic echocardiography may show vegetations. A negative study does not rule out endocarditis as vegetations <3 to 4 mm in size cannot be detected. Furthermore, all the leaflets of the aortic, tricuspid, and pulmonary valves may not be visualized in every patient. Transoesophageal echocardiography is usually indicated in infective endocarditis.

What are some risk factors for infective endocarditis?
- Intravenous drug use
- Immunosuppression
- Preexisting heart disease (including valvular heart disease, congenital heart disease, and prosthetic valves)
- Previous episode of infective endocarditis
- Dental infection.

What do you know about the pathogenesis of infective endocarditis?
- The primary event is bacterial adherence to damaged valves. This occurs within minutes during transient bacteraemia and involves valve tissue and bacterial factors.
- The second step involves persistence and growth of bacteria within the cardiac lesions, usually associated with local extension and tissue damage.
- The third step is the dissemination of septic emboli to kidney, spleen, and brain.

What are the major manifestations of bacterial endocarditis?
- Manifestations of a systemic infection: fever, weight loss, pallor, splenomegaly
- Manifestations of vasculitic phenomena: cardiac failure, changing murmurs, petechiae, Roth spots, Osler's nodes, Janeway lesions, splinter haemorrhages, stroke, infarction of viscera, mycotic aneurysm
- Manifestations of immunological reactions: arthralgia, finger clubbing, uraemia.

A mnemonic to remember Duke's criteria for bacterial endocarditis is BE FEVER:

Major:
    B: blood culture positive at least twice, 12 hours apart (presence of typical microorganism)
    E: endocardial involvement from echocardiogram (vegetations)

Minor:
- **F**: fever
- **E**: evidence from microbiology (other than major)
- **V**: vascular findings
- **E**: evidence from immunology
- **R**: risk factors/predisposing factors, e.g. drug abuse, valvular diseases.

Name some common bacteria found in infective endocarditis.
- *Streptococcus viridans*
- *Staphylococcus aureus*
- Coagulase-negative staphylococcus
- Enterococcus (*Streptococcus faecalis*)
- *Streptococcus bovis*
- HACEK Gram-negative and non-HACEK Gram-negative bacteria (HACEK: *Haemophilus, Aggregatibacter, Cardiobacterium, Eikenella, Kingella*).

Mention a few poor prognostic factors for infective endocarditis.
- Heart failure, renal failure, septic shock, stroke
- Nonstreptococcal endocarditis (*S. aureus*, fungal endocarditis)
- Infection of prosthetic valve
- Elderly patients
- Existence of other medical comorbidities, diabetes
- Echocardiographic findings: severe left-sided valve regurgitation, low ejection fraction, large vegetations, prosthetic valve dysfunction, elevated diastolic pressures.

How would you manage this patient?
This patient needs to be admitted to hospital and will require a long course of intravenous antibiotics, preferably under joint care of infectious disease and cardiology teams.

The European Society of Cardiology has produced some guidance for antibiotic choice in treating bacterial endocarditis.
- Aminoglycosides are no longer recommended in the treatment of native valve endocarditis (NVE) caused by staphylococci.
- Rifampicin should be added only in foreign body infections after initial antimicrobial therapy of 3 to 5 days.
- Treatment of choice for oral streptococci and *S. bovis* is intravenous penicillin at a dose depending on the strain. Vancomycin is an alternative antibiotic in penicillin-allergic patients.
- Treatment of choice for staphylococcal NVE is intravenous flucloxacillin or vancomycin or daptomycin for resistant species or penicillin-allergic patients. In staphylococcal prosthetic valve endocarditis (PVE), rifampicin and gentamicin are added to the regimen.
- Treatment of enterococcal endocarditis is amoxicillin with gentamicin intravenously. Vancomycin is the recommended alternative to penicillin in case of allergy.

What do you know of prosthetic valve endocarditis?
It is a complication of prosthetic heart valves. Between 1% and 6% of patients with a prosthetic valve will develop PVE, with an incidence of 0.3% to 1.2% per patient per year.

Early PVE occurs within 1 year of surgery, with late PVE developing later than a year after valve surgery. Although this classification is convenient, the high prevalence of *Staphylococcus epidermidis* and diphtheroids among patients suggests that this division is not absolute. PVE accounts for a total of 20% of cases of infective endocarditis.

Duke's criteria are less sensitive for diagnosing this type of endocarditis, and the diagnosis in general is more challenging than the NVE with additional investigations needed to diagnose PVE. Staphylococcal and complicated PVE have a bad prognosis unless treated aggressively with surgery.

Antibiotic duration and choice may be different and more aggressive in PVE.

What are the complications of infective endocarditis?
- Congestive heart failure: may develop acutely or insidiously; it portends a grave prognosis
- Conduction disturbances caused by abscesses in the interventricular septum
- Valve destruction: acute regurgitation, pulmonary oedema, heart failure
- Embolism: occurs in 22% to 50% of cases, leading to infarction in any vascular bed including lungs, coronary arteries, spleen, bowel, renal (flank pain and haematuria), and extremities
- Local extension of infection: purulent pericarditis, aortic root abscess (may cause sinus Valsalva fistula), and myocardial abscess (conduction disturbance)
- Septic emboli to vasa vasorum: may lead to mycotic aneurysms anywhere in the vascular tree; most worrying in cerebral vessels, resulting in cerebral haemorrhage
- Distal infection (metastatic): caused by septic emboli, e.g. brain abscess, cerebritis
- Candidal endocarditis: may manifest as fungal endophthalmitis
- Glomerulonephritis: there are two types of renal lesion in subacute bacterial endocarditis: a diffuse proliferative glomerulonephritis and a focal embolic glomerulonephritis. This is associated with low complement levels and immune complexes.

What are the indications for surgery?
- Left heart valve endocarditis with severe regurgitation or obstruction causing heart failure or cardiogenic shock
- Uncontrolled infection (abscess formation, aneurysm formation, resistance to treatment, persistently positive blood cultures or relapse despite best available antibiotic treatment, PVE caused by staphylococci or non-HACEK Gram-negative bacteria)
- Left heart endocarditis with persistent large vegetations.

What do you understand by the term marantic endocarditis?
Marantic or Libman–Sacks endocarditis is seen in systemic lupus erythematosus and is a post-mortem diagnosis. It is rarely clinically significant.

What are MSCRAMMs?
MSCRAMMs (microbial surface component reacting with adhesive matrix molecules) are surface adhesives on microbial pathogens that promote attachment to damaged valves and vegetations. These include fibrinogen-binding protein (also called clumping factor) and fibronectin-binding proteins in *S. aureus*, protein M in streptococci; these proteins act as surface adhesions, platelet-activating factors, and exopolysaccharides.

What are the recommendations for prophylaxis?
The indications for infective endocarditis prophylaxis have narrowed in the recent years into a very-high-risk group of patients (patients with prosthetic valves, patients with previous episode of endocarditis, and patients with congenital cyanotic heart disease) and high-risk procedures that may cause bacteraemia (dental procedures that involve manipulation of gingiva, periapical region of the teeth, or perforation of the oral mucosa).

Further Information

Sir William Osler (1849–1919) was successively a Professor of Medicine in Montreal, Pennsylvania, Baltimore, and Oxford. He was reputed to be a brilliant clinician and educationalist.

M. Roth (1839–1914), Professor of Pathology in Basel, Switzerland.

E.G. Janeway (1841–1911) followed Austin Flint as Professor of Medicine at Bellevue Hospital, New York.

E. Libman (1872–1946), US physician.

B. Sacks (1873–1939), US physician who wrote on Hindu medicine.

SECTION III

Abdominal Cases

SECTION OUTLINE

37 Abdominal Case
38 Swallowing Difficulties
39 Diarrhoea
40 Crohn's Disease
41 Abdominal Mass
42 Ascites
43 Cirrhosis of the Liver
44 Jaundice
45 Hepatomegaly
46 Splenomegaly
47 Haemochromatosis
48 Wilson Disease
49 Felty Syndrome

CHAPTER 37

Abdominal Case

Instruction

Examine this patient's abdomen.

Salient Features

HISTORY

- Fever, loss of weight, fatigue, lassitude
- Gastrointestinal symptoms: dysphagia, nausea, vomiting, altered bowel movement, jaundice
- Renal symptoms: oliguria, history of renal failure
- History of diabetes, hypertension
- History of ascites, swelling of feet, abdominal mass.

EXAMINATION

- Ensure that the patient is lying flat (remove any extra pillows, if present, with the permission of the patient); the hands should by the patient's side with the abdomen exposed from the inframammary region to just above the genitalia. Do not expose the genitalia.
- Begin with the hands, looking for the following signs:
  - Clubbing, leukonychia (white chalky nails)
  - Palmar erythema
  - Dupuytren's contracture (feel for thickening of the fascia)
  - Hepatic flap.
- Examine the arms:
  - Look for arteriovenous fistula, haemodialysis catheters, spider naevi.
- Comment on the skin:
  - Pigmentation
  - Scratch marks.
- Examine the following:
  - Supraclavicular and cervical lymph nodes
  - Tongue for pallor
  - Eyes for anaemia, jaundice, xanthelasma
  - Upper chest and face for spider naevi
  - Axilla for hair loss, acanthosis nigricans
  - Breast for gynaecomastia.
- Inspect the abdomen, looking for the following signs:
  - Skin, e.g. ecchymosis (Fig. 37.1)
  - Movements
  - Any obvious mass
  - Visible veins (check direction of flow, which is usually away from the umbilicus)

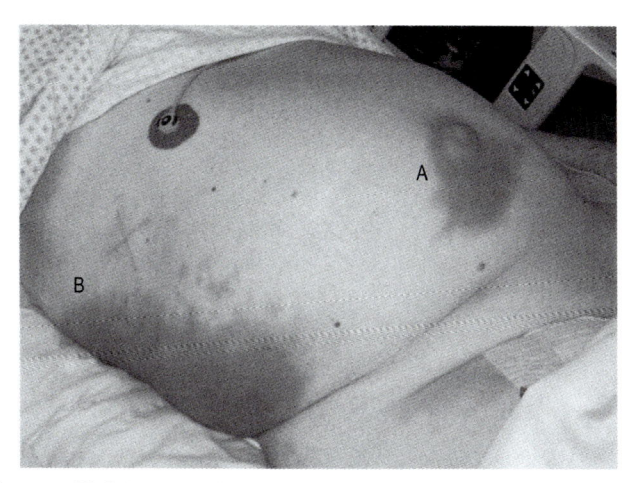

Fig. 37.1 Skin features. **(A)** Cullen's sign (periumbilical ecchymosis). **(B)** Grey–Turner's sign (ecchymosis on the abdominal flank). (With permission from Bosmann, M., Schreiner, O., Galle, P.R. 2009. Coexistence of Cullen's and Grey Turner's signs in acute pancreatitis. Am. J. Med. 122, 333–334.)

- Visible peristalsis
- Hernial orifices (ask the patient to cough at this stage)
- Expansile pulsations of aortic aneurysm.
- Ask the patient whether the abdomen is sore.
- Palpation: kneel on the floor or sit on a chair before you begin palpation. At all times, look at the patient's eyes to check whether he or she winces in pain. Begin with superficial pain and begin in the least tender area. Palpate in all the quadrants (remember that there are four quadrants). Palpate:
  - for mass, determine its characteristics
  - the liver (percuss for upper border using heavy percussion, for lower border using light percussion)
  - the kidneys (bimanual palpation, demonstrate ballottement) (Fig. 37.2)
  - the groin for lymph nodes
  - check hernial orifices
  - test for expansile pulsation of an aortic aneurysm.
- Percuss, looking for shifting dullness (at this stage, when the patient is lying on his or her right side, seize the opportunity to examine for a small spleen and for pitting oedema over the sacral region). Remember that abdominal percussion should follow adequate inspection and percussion.
- Auscultate:
  - over an enlarged liver for bruit
  - over a suspected aortic aneurysm
  - for bowel sounds.
- Tell the examiner that you would like to perform a rectal examination and examine the external genitalia.
- Examine the legs for oedema.
- Obtain a urine for dipstick examination.

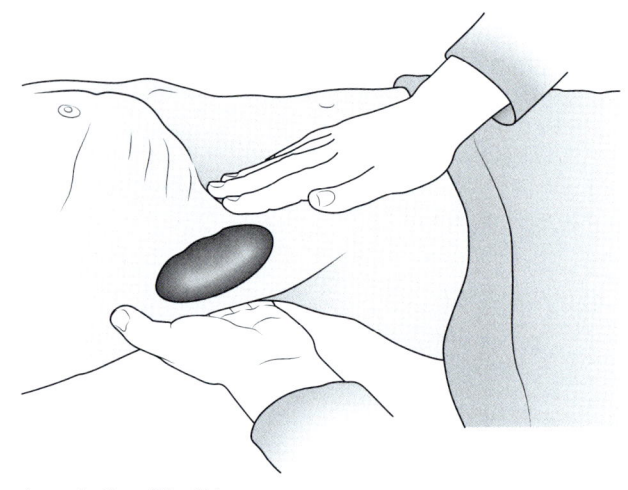

Fig. 37.2 Bimanual examination of the kidney.

Questions

Name some eponymous signs on abdominal examination.
- Cullen—ecchymosis of the subcutaneous fat of the periumbilical area, signifying major intraabdominal pathology
- Grey–Turner—ecchymoses in the flank, signifying retroperitoneal haemorrhage
- Giordano—tenderness over the costovertebral angle signifying pyelonephritis or other kidney pathology
- Murphy—tenderness on the right upper quadrant on inspiration while palpating the upper quadrant signifies acute cholecystitis
- Rovsing—tenderness on the right iliac fossa when palpating the left iliac fossa in appendicitis
- Blumberg—tenderness that is more marked on releasing the pressure after palpation compared to deep palpation is a sign of peritonitis
- Fox—internal thigh ecchymoses in intraabdominal haemorrhage
- Courvoisier—the combination of a palpable gallbladder and painless jaundice signify the possibility of biliary or pancreatic malignancy.

What are the main elements examined in a urine dipstick?
- Urinary pH—normal urinary pH is between 4.5 and 7.5; this is impaired in renal tubular acidosis.
- Glucose—glucosuria detected is an abnormal finding.
- Ketones—ketones are detected in diabetic ketoacidosis and also in severe starvation.
- Specific gravity—low specific gravity reflects inability to concentrate urine and indicates renal damage, whereas high specific gravity is seen in dehydration or reduced renal perfusion.
- Blood—haemoglobin and myoglobin are detected here.
- Protein—anything more than 'trace' indicates proteinuria and further investigations are warranted. Aside from renal disease, proteinuria can also occur in strenuous exercise, abdominal surgery, fever, orthostatic proteinuria, cold exposure, and congestive heart failure.
- Bilirubin—only detected in haemolysis or hepatobiliary disease.
- Nitrites—existence of nitrites signifies existence of gram negative bacteria.
- Leucocytes—seen in sterile pyuria, urinary tract infection, and inflammatory conditions.

CHAPTER 38

Swallowing Difficulties

Instruction

This elderly woman is coughing when drinking. Please take a history and examine any relevant systems.

Salient Features

HISTORY

- Is the problem with liquids, solids, or both? Oesophageal stricture (benign or malignant) often starts with solids and progresses to liquids.
- Location of food sticking (mouth/throat/midoesophagus/stomach)
- History of regurgitation. Is it immediate (stricture) or after minutes (gastric outlet obstruction)?
- Have there been any episodes of aspiration pneumonia? Is there cough or wheeze after eating or drinking?
- History of neurodegenerative disorder, stroke, previous stricture, Barrett's oesophagus
- Medication history: immunosuppressants (increased risk of oesophageal candidiasis)
- History of smoking or alcohol excess.

EXAMINATION

- Signs of stroke, cranial nerve lesions
- Evidence of weight loss
- Check for an epigastric mass and lymphadenopathy.
- Offer to watch the patient swallow a teaspoon of water.

Diagnosis

This woman has progressive oesophageal dysphagia (lesion) due to a probable oesophageal stricture (aetiology) causing weight loss and malnutrition (functional status).

Questions

Mention some causes for swallowing problems worse with solids.
- Oesophageal or gastric cancer
- Oesophageal stricture: causes include chronic reflux and oesophagitis, scleroderma, post radiotherapy.
- Oesophageal candidiasis
- Pharyngeal pouch
- Foreign bodies
- Hiatus hernia

- Gastroparesis: symptoms include early satiety and vomiting undigested food.
- External compression: cervical osteophyte, retrosternal goitre, lung tumour, aortic aneurysm.

How would you investigate this patient?
- Upper gastrointestinal endoscopy: diagnostic and therapeutic benefits
- Chest X-ray: looking for external compression and evidence of aspiration
- Barium swallow: to aid diagnosis if high risk of perforation with endoscopy but no therapeutic benefit.

Give a differential diagnosis for swallowing problems worse with liquids. And how would you investigate?
- Neurological disorders, including stroke (commonest), dementia, motor neurone disease, myasthenia gravis (look for fatiguability of swallow), multiple sclerosis, Parkinson disease, and Parkinson plus syndromes
- Oesphageal dysmotility including achalasia and oesophageal spasm

Initial investigations may include:
- videofluoroscopy
- oesophageal manometry
- computed tomography or magnetic resonance imaging of the brain, which may be required to investigate neurological causes.

How would you manage these conditions?
- Oesophageal stricture or cancer: dilatation or stenting. If benign stricture, start proton pump inhibitor
- Oesophageal candidiasis: oral fluconazole
- External compression: treatment of the underlying cause
- Gastroparesis: trial metoclopramide or erythromycin to stimulate gastric emptying
- Speech and language therapy: can advise on correct positioning, consistencies of food, and if thickened fluids are advisable
- Dietician for nutritional support
- For those with problems swallowing and malnutrition due to neurodegenerative problems such as advancing dementia, a palliative approach may be more appropriate following multidisciplinary discussions involving the patient, family, and carers.

What are the four stages of swallowing?
- Oral preparation: Food bolus is chewed and mixed with saliva.
- Oral phase: The tongue moves the food bolus backwards in the mouth.
- Pharyngeal phase: The pharynx and larynx are closed off, and peristalsis of the pharynx moves the bolus past the cricopharyngeal muscle in to the oesophagus.
- Oesophageal phase: Oesophageal peristalsis moves the food bolus down the oesophagus into the stomach.

What are the risk factors for oesophageal cancer?
- Smoking
- Dietary: red meat consumption, low intake of fresh fruit and vegetables, drinking hot tea, obesity
- Low socioeconomic status
- Barrett's oesophagus: this is an oesophagus in which any portion of the normal distal squamous epithelial lining has been replaced by metaplastic columnar epithelium, visible more than 1 cm above the gastro-oesophageal junction.

What is the role of screening in those with Barrett's oesophagus?
Due to the poor survival rates of invasive oesophageal cancer, endoscopic surveillance aims to detect cancer and the precancerous Barrett's oesophagus at a stage when curative options are available.
- For those without dysplasia, the annual risk of progression to oesophageal cancer is 0.25% per year and should be treated with acid suppression and endoscopic screening should be every 3 to 5 years.
- Those with high-grade dysplasia have a 6% risk of annual progression to oesophageal cancer and should be treated with endoscopic ablation therapy and screened endoscopically every 2 years.
- Those with low-grade dysplasia should have repeat endoscopy in 6 months. If low-grade dysplasia is found again, endoscopic ablation therapy should be offered. If declined, 6 monthly surveillance should continue.

What lifestyle advice should be given to people with chronic reflux?
- Lose weight.
- Stop smoking.
- Reduce alcohol and caffeine intake as these relax the lower oesophageal sphincter.
- Eat small but more frequent meals.
- Sleep propped up in bed at night.

What is achalasia and how is it managed?
- It is a rare, usually idiopathic, cause of oesophageal dysmotility.
- Symptoms include dysphagia, regurgitation, chest pain, and weight loss.
- Oesophageal manometry demonstrates abnormal or absent oesophageal peristalsis and impaired relaxation of the lower oesophageal sphincter. These changes can also be seen on barium swallow.
- Treatment:
    - Proton pump inhibitors
    - Endoscopic treatments, including injection of botulinum toxin to relax lower oesophageal sphincter, balloon dilatation of lower oesophageal sphincter, and peroral endoscopic myotomy (POEM)
    - Surgery: Heller myotomy: being increasingly replaced by POEM.

CHAPTER 39

Diarrhoea

PATIENT 1
Instruction

This patient has been complaining of diarrhoea for the last 2 weeks after returning from a work trip to Vietnam. Please take a history from the patient.

Salient Features
HISTORY

- Ask about the following:
  - Onset
  - Duration of diarrhoea
  - Frequency
  - Nocturnal symptoms
  - Blood (seen in ulcerative colitis, shigellosis, diverticulitis, carcinoma of the colon) and mucus in the stools; blood on the toilet paper
  - Nature of the stools (pale and bulky and difficult to flush away in steatorrhoea)
  - Associated pain in the abdomen
  - Appetite (increased in thyrotoxicosis)
  - Weight loss (marked in chronic diarrhoea)
  - Associated nausea and vomiting
  - Drug ingestion (including antibiotics and laxatives)
  - Foreign travel.

Diagnosis

- This patient presents with abdominal pain and loose nonbloody stool (lesion) following travel to South-East Asia. This is caused by infection with *Giardia lamblia* (diagnosis). His symptoms are slowly improving after starting a course of metronidazole (functional status).

PATIENT 2
Instruction

This patient presents with intermittent abdominal pains, general fatigue, and fever. The symptoms have persisted for a few months. The patient had noticed similar symptoms in the past but did not seek medical attention as they resolved spontaneously. She denies other systemic symptoms and has not been abroad recently. Please examine the patient.

Salient Features

EXAMINATION

- Look for the following signs:
  - Anaemia
  - Clubbing
  - Aphthous ulcers
  - Abdominal tenderness, abdominal masses
  - Fistulae.
- Tell the examiner that you would like to do a rectal examination and check for faecal occult blood and faecal calprotectin.

Diagnosis

- This patient has chronic diarrhoea with aphthous ulcers and abdominal tenderness (lesion) caused by inflammatory bowel disease (aetiology).

Questions

What do you understand by the term diarrhoea?
It implies passing of increased amounts of loose stool (stool weights >250 g/day).

How would you investigate a patient with diarrhoea?
- Full blood count, erythrocyte sedimentation rate (ESR)
- Coeliac screen
- Serum albumin
- Lower gastrointestinal endoscopy if symptoms persist
- Stool chart, stool cultures
- Faecal calprotectin
- Barium enema, small bowel barium studies.

What are the mechanisms of diarrhoea?
- Osmotic diarrhoea: the mucosa of the gut acts as a semipermeable membrane; the diarrhoea stops when the patient fasts (e.g. diarrhoea from magnesium sulfate, lactulose, malabsorptive states).
- Secretory diarrhoea: there is active secretion of intestinal fluid (e.g. *Escherichia coli* diarrhoea).
- Inflammatory diarrhoea: there is mucosal damage (e.g. shigellosis, ulcerative colitis).
- Increased gut motility (e.g. irritable bowel syndrome (IBS)).

What are the poor prognostic factors in ulcerative colitis?
Anaemia (haemoglobin <100 g/L), raised ESR (30 mm/hour), fever (37.5°C), increased frequency of stools (>6/day), tachycardia (>90 beats/min), and hypoalbuminaemia (<30 g/L).

What is irritable bowel syndrome?
- This is a diagnosis of exclusion and is a symptom cluster due to a variety of conditions, including alterations in the gut microbiome, intestinal permeability, gut immune function, motility, visceral sensation, brain–gut interactions, and psychosocial status.
- It can be predominantly diarrhoea, constipation, or mixed and may be associated with abdominal cramps and bloating.

- Treatment is through dietary and behavioural interventions. If predominantly IBS–diarrhoea, loperamide or codeine may be helpful. If predominantly constipation symptoms, laxatives can be used. Increasing interest in the importance of gut microbiome health and the interaction between the gut wall and this microbe population may pave the way to personalized treatment for IBS symptoms.

CHAPTER 40

Crohn's Disease

Instruction

This young male patient presents with chronic diarrhoea. He has lost some weight over the last 6 months and complains of general malaise and arthralgia. Examine this patient's abdomen.

Salient Features

HISTORY

- Loose stools or diarrhoea that is not usually bloody (unlike ulcerative colitis), but may contain copious mucus
- Abdominal discomfort or pain
- Anorexia, malaise, and weight loss
- Perianal inflammation and pain
- Joint pains, eye complaints, skin changes.

EXAMINATION

- Abdominal tenderness on palpation
- Mass in the right iliac fossa.

Proceed by examining:
- The mouth for aphthous ulcers
- Uveitis
- Anaemia
- Arthropathy
- Skin lesions (erythema nodosum, pyoderma gangrenosum)
- Liver disease.

Note: Crohn's disease may affect any part of the gastrointestinal tract from the mouth to the anus but has a tendency to involve the terminal ileum. The inflammation is transmural (extending through all layers of bowel) with relatively normal bowel in between (skip lesions).

Diagnosis

This patient has some mild tenderness in his right iliac fossa with no signs of peritonism (lesion). There is no guarding and in the absence of acute abdomen symptoms may be caused by inflammatory bowel disease, such as Crohn's disease (aetiology). He is currently unable to work due to his chronic diarrhoea (functional status).

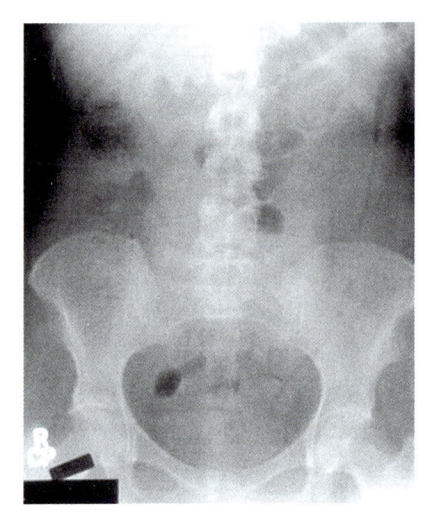

Fig. 40.1 Abdominal radiograph in toxic megacolon, showing oedematous haustral folds (thumbprinting) and a dilated transverse colon. (With permission from Marrero, F., Qadeer, M.A., Lashner, B.A., 2008. Severe complications of inflammatory bowel disease. Med. Clin. North Am. 92, 671–686.)

Questions

What are some potential complications of Crohn's disease?
- Toxic megacolon (Fig. 40.1)
- Iritis
- Arthritis
- Erythema nodosum
- Pyoderma gangrenosum.

Mention some associated diseases.
- Ankylosing spondylitis (HLA-B27 positive)
- Sacroiliitis
- Cholangitis, hepatitis, cirrhosis.

What are some ocular features of Crohn's disease?
Eye lesions are seen in about 5% of cases:
- Common: conjunctivitis, anterior uveitis
- Rare: scleritis, keratitis, keratoconjunctivitis sicca, choroiditis, retinal vasculitis, optic neuritis and orbital pseudotumour.

How would you investigate a patient with Crohn's disease?
- Full blood count, erythrocyte sedimentation rate, C-reactive protein, liver function tests, serum iron, vitamin B_{12}, red cell folate
- Autoantibody screen: antineutrophil cytoplasmic antibodies and anti-*Saccharomyces cerevisiae* antibodies, although there is no single autoantibody which is diagnostic of Crohn's disease. Increasing uses of antibody arrays may help in the diagnosis but histological examination of affected bowel is still the most accurate diagnostic tool available.

40 — CROHN'S DISEASE

- Stool sample for ova, cysts and parasites, as well as *Clostridium difficile* toxin
- Faecal calprotectin: can be useful as a screening test when trying to differentiate between inflammatory bowel disease and noninflammatory bowel pathology such as irritable bowel syndrome
- Colonoscopy with intubation of the terminal ileum
- Sigmoidoscopy and rectal biopsy as an initial test in a patient presenting with chronic diarrhoea
- Capsule endoscopy to determine extent of small bowel involvement
- Magnetic resonance imaging (MRI) of the pelvis to determine pelvic involvement and fistulae
- MRI of small bowel to determine disease activity and strictures.

Name two severity assessment systems used in Crohn's disease.
- Crohn's disease activity index
- Harvey–Bradshaw Index.

How would you treat Crohn's disease?
- Corticosteroids: monotherapy with oral steroids is the first-line treatment for inducing remission in patients with a first presentation and mild disease. Steroids should not be used for maintenance of remission.
- 5-Aminosalicylate (5-ASA): if steroid is not tolerated, then alternatives with fewer side effects but less efficacious are budesonide or 5-ASA. Many clinicians would prefer initiation of treatment with 5-ASA in mild disease to avoid steroid side effects.
- Immunotherapy: if weaning steroids is accompanied with recurrence of symptoms or if the patient has more than two exacerbations in a year, then consider adding azathioprine or mercaptopurine to the treatment. Thiopurine methyltransferase activity should be assessed in every patient before starting treatment with either of these agents, and if deficiency is found, methotrexate is an alternative.
- Biologics: biological treatment is reserved for patients with severe active disease or are intolerant to the initial treatment. If biologics are initiated, disease activity should be reassessed at the end of 12 months' treatment, and a trial of withdrawal should be considered in patients who are in clinical remission.
- Surgery: surgery is reserved for intestinal fistulae and intestinal obstruction that does not respond to medical management. Proctocolectomy and ileostomy are the standard operations.
- Colorectal cancer surveillance: colonoscopic surveillance should be offered to every patient who has had the disease for a duration of more than 10 years and the disease is not limited to one part of the colon.
- Antibiotics and probiotics: empirical clinical experience suggests that antibiotics are useful in the treatment of subgroups of patients. Metronidazole can be effective in those who have perianal fistulae. Ciprofloxacin and clarithromycin have been advocated as alternatives to metronidazole. The effectiveness of nonspecific antibiotics and experimental evidence of the central role of the luminal flora for the development of disease have led to the use of probiotic bacteria (the administration of 'healthy' bacteria). Patients with pouchitis or active Crohn's disease who were treated with a mixture of commensal bacteria had a positive therapeutic response. Local treatment with interleukin-10-secreting *Lactococcus lactis* is undergoing clinical evaluation.
- Lactose-free diet: lactose intolerance can coexist with Crohn's disease, and in patients with symptomatology suggesting lactose intolerance, dairy products should be avoided as a diagnostic trial.

What is the role of macroautophagy in this disease?

In Crohn's disease, there is an inability to eliminate intestinal bacteria by macroautophagy. The defect may be the primary cause of *ATG16L1*-associated Crohn's disease. Defective autophagy-related protein 16-1 in Paneth cells and reduced lysozyme in the intestinal lumen result in an increase in intestinal inflammation.

Macroautophagy is accompanied by the formation of double-membrane cytosolic vesicles (autophagosomes) that sequester cytoplasmic contents and deliver them to the lysosome for subsequent degradation. The process involves membrane expansion, which allows sequestration of particles of almost any size. The ability to remove invasive bacteria is probably an important role for these epithelial and immune cells that encounter a heavy microbial load.

Further Information

Burrill Bernard Crohn (1884–1983) was a physician in Mount Sinai Hospital, New York; he described the condition in 1932 and pointed out the nontuberculous aetiology (Crohn, Ginzburg and Gordon, 1932).

Anne Ferguson, formerly Professor of Gastroenterology at the Western General Hospital in Edinburgh, whose chief interest was inflammatory bowel disease. Sir Richard Thompson, President of Royal College of Physicians of London, trained in natural sciences and medicine at Oxford and St Thomas' Hospital Medical School. His chief interest was nutritional gastroenterology.

CHAPTER 41

Abdominal Mass

PATIENT 1
Instruction

This patient feels full after eating small amounts. Please examine their abdomen.

Salient Features
EXAMINATION

There is an epigastric mass.

Diagnosis

Differential diagnosis:
- Carcinoma of the stomach: look for supraclavicular lymph nodes, hepatomegaly; comment on pallor and asthenia.
- Carcinoma of the pancreas: look for jaundice.
- Aneurysm of the abdominal aorta: look for expansile pulsatile mass, check femoral and foot pulses, auscultate over the mass and the femoral pulses.
- Retroperitoneal lymphadenopathy (lymphoma).

PATIENT 2
Instruction

Examine this patient's abdomen.

Salient Features
EXAMINATION

There is a mass in the right iliac fossa.

Diagnosis

Differential diagnosis:
- Crohn's disease: look for mouth ulcers; tell the examiner that you would like to look for fistulae and take a history for chronic diarrhoea.
- Carcinoma of the caecum: look for hard mass, lymph nodes.
- Enlarged lymph node: look for enlarged nodes elsewhere, feel for liver and spleen, examine the drainage area of iliac lymph nodes (such as the leg, perianal area, external genitalia), and carry out a rectal examination.

- Transplanted kidney: comment on the laparotomy scars, stigmata of renal failure, and artificial arteriovenous fistulae.
- Appendicular abscess
- Ileocaecal abscess
- Ovarian tumours (must be mentioned as a differential diagnosis in female patients).

The less common causes of masses in the right iliac fossa are as follows:
- Amoebiasis
- Carcinoid (ileal)
- Actinomycosis
- Ectopic kidney.

PATIENT 3

Instruction

Examine this patient's abdomen.

Salient Features

EXAMINATION

There is a mass in the left iliac fossa.

Diagnosis

Differential diagnosis:
- Diverticular abscess: look for tender, mobile mass.
- Carcinoma of the colon: look for hepatomegaly; tell the examiner that you would like to do a per rectal examination.
- Faecal mass (The mass may be moulded by pressure.)
- Ovarian tumour (in females)
- Enlarged iliac lymph nodes: look for enlarged nodes elsewhere, feel for liver and spleen, examine the drainage areas.
- Transplanted kidney: comment on the laparotomy scar, look for signs of renal failure, arteriovenous fistulae.

Note: The investigation of first choice in such patients is abdominal ultrasonography. Computed tomography may be required. If a tumour is found, referral to the appropriate multidisciplinary team should follow.

Questions

Which diseases are most commonly associated with massive splenomegaly?
In the developed world, the most common causes are haematological tumour such as chronic myeloid leukaemia (CML), myelofibrosis, and lymphoma. Other causes include sarcoidosis and Gaucher disease. In the developing world, infectious causes are more common, such as visceral leishmaniasis (kala-azar) and malaria.

CHAPTER 42

Ascites

Instruction
This patient has noticed their abdomen is swollen. Please examine and present your findings.

Salient Features
HISTORY
- Abdominal distension, dyspnoea
- Abdominal pain: spontaneous bacterial peritonitis, malignancy
- Past history of heart failure, renal failure or liver disease
- Past history of tuberculosis (TB) (peritoneal TB), pancreatitis
- Past history of malignancy: mesothelioma, metastatic spread from primary tumours
- Alcohol or drug abuse.

EXAMINATION
- Full flanks and umbilicus (Fig. 42.1)
- Presence of shifting dullness (Always percuss with your finger parallel to the level of fluid.)
- If the ascites is gross, use the 'dipping' method of palpation to feel the liver and spleen.
- Look for stigmata of underlying disease (e.g. signs of cirrhosis, cardiac failure, renal failure or malignancy).

Proceed as follows:
- Check for sacral and peripheral oedema.

Diagnosis
- This patient has marked ascites and leg oedema with splenomegaly (lesions) caused by portal hypertension; the underlying cause needs to be investigated (aetiology).

Questions
What are the causes of a distended abdomen?
- Fat, fluid, faeces, flatus, and fetus.

What do you understand by the term ascites?
- It is the pathological accumulation of fluid in the peritoneal cavity.

What are the common causes of ascites?
- Portal hypertension with cirrhosis
- Abdominal malignancy
- Congestive cardiac failure.

161

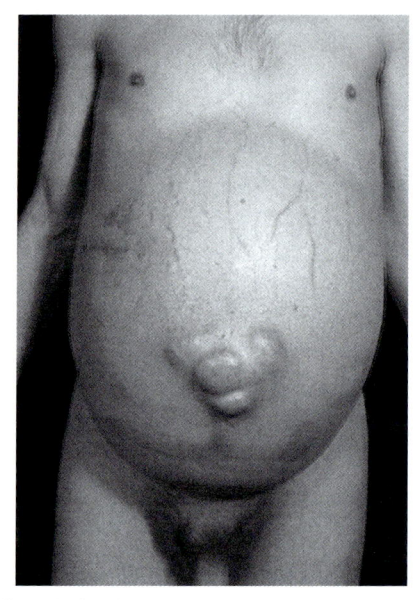

Fig. 42.1 Ascites, showing distended abdomen, dilated superficial collateral veins, haemorrhagic scratch marks, and umbilical varices. (With permission from Forbes, A., Misiewicz, J.J., Compton, C.C. (eds.), 2005. Atlas of Clinical Gastroenterology, third edn. Mosby, Oxford.)

What investigations would you do to determine the underlying cause?
- Diagnostic paracentesis for proteins, neutrophils, and malignant cells
- Ultrasonography of the abdomen
- Peritoneal biopsy or laparoscopy if the cause remains unclear.

What is the difference between an exudate and a transudate?
- An exudate has a protein content of >30 g/L.

What are the mechanisms of ascites formation in cirrhosis?
- It is caused by a combination of liver failure and portal hypertension. Altered hepatic architecture and reduced nitric oxide (NO) levels within the liver lead to an increase in intrahepatic resistance with resulting portal hypertension and increased portal flow.
- Bacterial translocation through the altered gut wall and reduced splanchnic and systemic vascular resistance due to increased levels of NO in the vasculature lead to activation of neurohumoral vasoconstrictor mechanisms.
- Secondary hyperaldosteronism caused by increased renin release and decreased metabolism of aldosterone by the liver
- Decreased metabolism of aldosterone and antidiuretic hormone
- Hypoalbuminaemia, which decreases colloid oncotic pressure
- Salt and water retention
- Lymphatic obstruction, resulting in a 'weeping' liver.

What is the relationship between ascites and chronic liver disease?
- Ascites indicates decompensation of previously asymptomatic chronic liver disease.
- Ascites occurs in about half of the patients within 10 years of a diagnosis of compensated cirrhosis.

42—ASCITES

- The development of fluid retention in patients with chronic liver disease is a poor prognostic sign: only half of these patients survive beyond 2 years.

What do you know about the serum:ascites albumin gradient?
- It is calculated by subtracting the ascitic fluid albumin concentration from the serum albumin concentration in samples obtained at the same time.
- This gradient correlates directly with portal pressure; those whose gradient is ≥11 g/L have portal hypertension (causes include cirrhosis, cardiac failure, Budd–Chiari syndrome) and those with gradients of <11 g/L do not (causes include peritoneal malignancy, pancreatitis, nephrotic syndrome).
- The accuracy of such determinations is 97%.

How would you manage a patient with cirrhosis and ascites?
- The most important treatments remain sodium restriction and diuretics.
- Sodium restriction to 87 to 113 mmol/day (5–6.5 g/day) through a no-added-salt diet and avoiding prepared food. Only 15% of these patients lose weight or have a reduction in ascitic fluid with this therapy alone. Effervescent drugs often have a high sodium content and should also be avoided where possible. Dietician advice should be sought.
- Fluid restriction is usually not necessary unless the person is euvolaemic with severe hyponatraemia and not on diuretic therapy.
- Diuretic therapy should be initiated immediately. The most effective diuretic regimen is a combination of spironolactone (up to 400 mg/day) and furosemide (up to 40 mg/day). More than 90% of patients respond to this therapy. 0.5 to 1 kg should be the maximum weight loss per day.
- Diuretic-resistant or tense ascites:
    - 5 L or more of ascitic fluid should be removed to relieve shortness of breath, to diminish early satiety, and to prevent pressure-related leakage of fluid from the site of a previous paracentesis. Human albumin solution should be used as a plasma expander during paracentesis. Diuretics should be restarted 1 to 2 days post paracentesis.
    - Transjugular intrahepatic portosystemic stent shunt (TIPSS) is a nonsurgical side-to-side shunt consisting of a stented channel between a main branch of the portal vein and the hepatic vein. The stent shunt is associated with an operative mortality rate of 1%.
    - Peritoneovenous shunting (e.g. Le Veen shunt); limited by the high rate of infection and disseminated intravascular coagulation.
    - Liver transplantation: in the UK and USA the Model for End-Stage Liver Disease is used to prioritize candidates for transplantation.

In patients with cirrhosis and refractory or recurrent ascites would you prefer paracentesis or transjugular intrahepatic portosystemic stent shunt?
- Once ascites is refractory to medical treatment, there is a 50% 6-month mortality rate. Meta-analyses comparing TIPSS versus regular paracentesis suggest that TIPSS results in improved ascites control, renal function, and nutritional status with a trend towards increased survival without liver transplant.
- Encephalopathy occurs in up to a third of patients post TIPSS and so should be avoided in those with recurrent hepatic encephalopathy.
- TIPSS was ineffective in patients with associated intrinsic renal disease and in those with advanced liver cirrhosis.
- Contraindications for TIPSS include heart failure, intrahepatic malignancy, and active infection.

What are the complications of ascites?
- Respiratory embarrassment may complicate large amounts of ascites.
- Spontaneous bacterial peritonitis is seen in cirrhotics: suspect when there is an ascitic neutrophil count of >250 × 10^6 cells/L. 70% of cases are due to *Escherichia coli, Streptococcus*, and *Enterococcus* species. Empirical therapy with a nonnephrotoxic broad-spectrum antibiotic should be initiated immediately. Improved diagnosis and management have reduced mortality from 90% to 20%.

Mention some uncommon causes for ascites.
- Nephrotic syndrome
- Constrictive pericarditis
- Tuberculous peritonitis
- Chylous ascites
- Budd–Chiari syndrome
- Meigs syndrome.

Further Information

G. Budd (1808–1882), Professor of Medicine at King's College, London.
H. Chiari (1851–1916), Professor of Pathology at the German University in Prague.
J.V. Meigs (1892–1963), Professor of Gynaecology at Harvard, Massachusetts General Hospital.
Le Veen, gastroenterologist at the Veterans Administration Hospital in New York.
Sometime during the rule of Tiberius (CE 25–50), the physician Celsus wrote about oedema, describing it as a chronic malady that may develop in patients who collect water under their skin. The Greeks called this hydrops. They described three types: water is all drawn within, ascites; body is rendered uneven by swellings arising here and there, hyposarka; and a tense belly filled with air or gas, tympanites (Diskin, 1999).

CHAPTER 43

Cirrhosis of the Liver

Instruction
This patient presents with abdominal distension. Please examine this patient's abdomen.

Salient Features
HISTORY
- Jaundice
- Abdominal distension and/or peripheral oedema
- Weight loss, fatigue
- Haematemesis or melaena
- Pruritus (often an early symptom of primary biliary cirrhosis)
- History of alcohol abuse
- History of chronic viral hepatitis (B or C)
- History of intravenous drug abuse
- Mental status changes such as confusion or drowsiness (hepatic encephalopathy)
- History of hepatotoxic prescribed medication
- History of Wilson disease, α_1-antitrypsin deficiency, type 2 diabetes.

EXAMINATION
- Hands:
    - Clubbing, leukonychia
    - Dupuytren's contracture (see Fig. 228.1), palmar erythema
    - Spider naevi (in distribution of superior vena cava), tattoos, hepatic flap, pallor
    - Scratch marks, generalized pigmentation
- Eyes and face:
    - Icterus, cyanosis, parotid enlargement, xanthomas (in primary biliary cirrhosis, fatty liver)
- Chest:
    - Spider naevi, loss of axillary hair, gynaecomastia (can be unilateral)
- Abdomen:
    - Splenomegaly (seldom >5 cm below the costal margin) a sign of portal hypertension
    - Ascites
    - Hepatomegaly (particularly in alcoholic liver disease)
    - Evidence of insulin injections
    - Obesity
- Legs:
    - Loss of hair on the shins
    - Oedema.

Tell the examiner that you would like to look for testicular atrophy.

Diagnosis

This patient has spider naevi, gynaecomastia, and hepatosplenomegaly (lesions) from cirrhosis caused by alcohol abuse (aetiology). The patient has hepatic flap, indicating liver cell failure (functional status).

Questions

What is cirrhosis?
Cirrhosis is defined pathologically as a diffuse liver abnormality characterized by necrosis of hepatocytes, fibrosis, and abnormal regenerating nodules.

Mention a few causes of cirrhosis.
- Alcohol excess
- Non-alcoholic fatty liver disease
- Hepatitis B infection (look for tattoos), hepatitis C
- Primary biliary cirrhosis
- Haemochromatosis
- Drugs: methotrexate, statins, antifungals
- Metabolic: Wilson disease, α_1-antitrypsin deficiency
- Budd–Chiari syndrome
- Idiopathic.

How would you investigate this patient?
- Full blood count
- Liver function tests including γ-glutamyltransferase (GGT) and albumin
- Prothrombin time
- Hepatitis B and C markers
- Liver-associated autoantibodies
- Serum iron and ferritin
- Serum α-fetoprotein
- Serum copper (if young)
- Ascitic fluid analysis
- Ultrasonography and elastography of the liver including portal and hepatic vein patency.

Why does this patient have a low serum albumin concentration?
Albumin is synthesized in the liver, and in cirrhosis, there is liver cell failure, causing impaired synthesis.

What are the major sequelae of cirrhosis?
- Portal hypertension (development of portosystemic collaterals)
- Variceal haemorrhage
- Hepatic encephalopathy
- Ascites and spontaneous bacterial peritonitis
- Hepatorenal syndrome
- Coagulopathy
- Hepatocellular carcinoma.

What are the important locations of the portosystemic collaterals?
- Oesophageal submucosal veins: supplied by the left gastric vein and drain into the superior vena cava via the azygous vein

- Paraumbilical veins: supplied by umbilical portion of the left portal vein and drain into abdominal wall veins near the umbilicus. These veins may form a caput medusae at the umbilicus.
- Rectal submucosal veins: supplied by the inferior mesenteric vein through the superior rectal vein and drain into the internal iliac veins through the middle and inferior rectal veins
- Short gastric veins: supplied by the oesophageal submucosal veins and drain into the splenic vein
- Splenorenal shunts: spontaneous or surgically created.

What are some poor prognostic factors in liver cirrhosis?
- Encephalopathy
- Low serum sodium concentration, <120 mmol/L (not caused by diuretic therapy)
- Low serum albumin level, <25 g/L
- Prolonged prothrombin time.

What is the utility of measuring serum ammonia level in patients with altered mental status?
- In patients with established hepatic encephalopathy, monitoring ammonia level during therapy is of limited value.
- In patients with acute liver failure, an elevated serum ammonia is a poor prognostic sign: an arterial ammonia level >2.0 mg/L is associated with cerebral herniation in acute liver failure.
- When there is no liver disease, search for an underlying cause such as total parenteral nutrition, gastrointestinal (GI) bleed, steroid use, portosystemic shunts, inborn errors of metabolism such as urea cycle disorders, drugs such as glycine, salicylates, and sodium valproate.

Remember: Altered mental status in a cirrhotic patient does not equal hepatic encephalopathy; for example, in patients with altered mental status due to alcohol dependence, consider Wernicke's encephalopathy.

What factors can precipitate hepatic encephalopathy in a patient with previously well-compensated cirrhosis?
- Infection
- Diuretics, electrolyte imbalance
- Diarrhoea and vomiting
- Sedatives
- Upper GI haemorrhage
- Abdominal paracentesis
- Surgery.

What are the laboratory changes seen in cirrhosis?
- Aminotransferases: alanine and aspartate aminotransferases normal or moderately elevated
- Alkaline phosphatase: usually slightly elevated
- GGT: usually slightly elevated, high in active alcoholics
- Bilirubin: elevates later in cirrhosis; predictor of death
- Albumin: decrease in advanced cirrhosis
- Prothrombin time: increases in advanced cirrhosis since the liver synthesizes clotting factors
- Immunoglobulins: increased, mainly immunoglobulin G (IgG)
- Serum sodium: hypernatraemia

- Thrombocytopenia: from both congestive splenomegaly and cirrhosis
- Leukopenia and neutropenia: from splenomegaly with splenic margination
- Coagulation defects: worsen in advanced cirrhosis.

What is the Cruveilhier–Baumgarten murmur?
This is a venous hum that can be auscultated in the abdomen in patients with portal hypertension. It is augmented by manoeuvres that increase intraabdominal pressure such as the Valsalva.

What do you know about the Model for End-Stage Liver Disease?
The Model for End-Stage Liver Disease is used to assess the prognosis of liver failure. This is used to prioritize candidates waiting for liver transplantation. The score assesses creatinine, bilirubin, international normalized ratio, sodium, and whether the person has required dialysis in the past week. A score of 12 or higher indicates a high risk of developing complications. The National Institute for Health and Care Excellence recommends the score is calculated every 6 months for someone with compensated liver cirrhosis.

How do you manage a patient with cirrhosis?

Complication	*Prevention*	*Treatment*
Itching		Medication
Constipation	Diet	Laxatives (e.g. lactulose)
Variceal bleeding	Nonselective beta-blockers (e.g. propranolol), variceal band ligation	Endoscopic band ligation, sclerotherapy, transjugular intrahepatic portosystemic shunts
Ascites	Salt restriction	Diuretics, therapeutic drainage
Renal failure	Avoid hypovolaemia	Rehydration, stop diuretics, albumin infusion
Hepatic encephalopathy	Avoid precipitants	Treat precipitating factors, bleeding, electrolyte imbalance, sedatives
Spontaneous bacterial peritonitis	Treat ascites	Antibiotics

How would you manage variceal bleeding in cirrhosis?
- Blood transfusion to replace falling hematocrit
- Other blood products if needed
- Somatostatin analogues like terlipressin
- Broad-spectrum antibiotics
- Early endoscopy to confirm the bleeding site and allow treatment endoscopically
- The two endoscopic treatments used are endoscopic band ligation and endoscopic sclerotherapy. Band ligation has almost completely replaced sclerotherapy.
- Balloon tamponade is effective in temporarily stopping bleeding while awaiting more definitive therapy.
- Transjugular intrahepatic portosystemic stent shunt.

Further Information

Cirrhosis comes from the Greek word *kirrhos* denoting a yellow/tan colour—the colour of the diseased liver.

Jean Cruveilhier was a French anatomist who was tempted into training as a doctor by Dupuytren, who was a friend of his father. He is credited with the likely first description of multiple sclerosis in the 1830s, before it was formally described by Charcot 30 years later.

Paul Clemens von Baumgarten was a German pathologist whose professional career was mostly devoted to the study of mycological disease.

CHAPTER 44

Jaundice

Instruction

This 65-year-old lady has noticed that her eyes are a yellow colour. Please examine her abdomen and present your findings.

Salient Features

HISTORY

- Age: hepatitis more common in the young, carcinoma more common in the elderly
- Abdominal pain: cholecystitis, gallstones, cholangitis, carcinoma of the pancreas
- Fever, rigors, and abdominal pain: suggests cholangitis
- Pruritus: cholestasis caused by hepatitis A and B, primary biliary cirrhosis
- Urine discolouration: dark, cola-coloured urine caused by renal excretion of conjugated bilirubin
- Colour of the stool: pale stools in obstructive jaundice
- Sore throat and rash: infectious mononucleosis
- Weight loss: malignancy
- Contact with jaundice: hepatitis A
- History: recurrent jaundice, as in Dubin–Johnson syndrome; recent surgery or other ischaemic insult
- Blood transfusions, injections, arthritis, urticaria: hepatitis B
- Drug history: oral contraceptives, phenothiazines, recent antibiotics, paracetamol
- Occupation: Weil disease in sewerage and farm workers
- Alcohol consumption.

EXAMINATION

- Hands: clubbing, palmar erythema, Dupuytren's contracture
- Sclera (to confirm the icterus)
- Conjunctiva for pallor
- Cervical lymph nodes
- Upper chest: spider naevi, loss of axillary hair, and gynaecomastia
- Abdomen: hepatomegaly, splenomegaly, Murphy's sign, palpable gallbladder, ascites
- Legs for pitting oedema.

Additional bedside tests:
- dipstick urinalysis
- digital rectal examination.

Remember: The most important question to answer in the evaluation of any jaundiced patient is 'Will this patient require surgery to relieve biliary obstruction?'

Diagnosis

This patient is markedly icteric and has spider naevi and gynaecomastia (lesions) caused by chronic liver disease (aetiology).

Questions

What do you understand by the term jaundice?
It is the yellowish discolouration of skin, sclera, and mucous membranes caused by the accumulation of bile pigments. Scleral icterus suggests a serum bilirubin of at least 51 µmol/L (3 mg/dL).

How would you differentiate jaundice from carotenaemia?
The discolouration of carotenaemia is differentiated from jaundice by the absence of yellow colour in the sclera and mucous membranes, normal urine colour, and the presence of yellow-brown pigmentation of carotenoid pigment in the palms, soles, and nasolabial folds.

What is Murphy's sign and what does it indicate?
It is the tenderness elicited on palpation at the midpoint of the right subcostal margin on inspiration. It is a sign of cholecystitis.

Have you heard of Courvoisier's law?
It states that in a patient with obstructive jaundice, a palpable gallbladder is unlikely to be caused by chronic cholecystitis.

What is Charcot's fever?
It is intermittent fever associated with jaundice and abdominal discomfort in a patient with cholangitis and biliary obstruction.

How would you investigate this patient?
- Urine for bile pigments
- Full blood count
- Serum haptoglobin, reticulocyte count, and Coombs' test, if you suspect haemolysis
- Liver function tests: serum albumin, bilirubin, enzymes
- Prothrombin time
- Viral studies: hepatitis antigen and antibodies, Epstein–Barr virus antibodies
- Ultrasonography of the abdomen, if you suspect cholestatic jaundice
- Special investigations: mitochondrial antibodies, endoscopic retrograde cholangiopancreatography, computed tomography of the abdomen, liver biopsy.

When would you admit someone with jaundice acutely to secondary care?
- They are acutely unwell or have signs of sepsis.
- The following are present: fever, right upper quadrant pain, signs of encephalopathy.
- Paracetamol overdose is suspected.
- Bilirubin level is >100 mmol/L.
- There is associated renal function impairment or coagulopathy.
- They are frail or have significant comorbidities.

What do you know about Gilbert syndrome?
Gilbert syndrome is very common, with a reported incidence of 3% to 7% of the population and with males predominating females by a ratio of 2–7:1. It is characterized by the impaired

conjugation of bilirubin caused by reduced activity of uridine diphosphate glucuronyltransferase. The patients typically have mild unconjugated hyperbilirubinaemia (<103 μmol/L or <30 mg/L).

What do you know about Dubin–Johnson syndrome?
It is a rare benign condition characterized by jaundice and pigmentation secondary to a failure of excretion of conjugated bilirubin. The defect in this syndrome is mutation in the gene for multiple drug resistance protein 2. The liver is stained by melanin in the centrilobular zone. Raised ratio of coproporphyrin I to coproporphyrin III is pathognomic of this condition.

Mention a few causes of postoperative jaundice.
The causes of postoperative jaundice (usually occurring in the first 3 postoperative weeks) include:
- resorption of haematomas, haemoperitoneum, haemolysis of transfused erythrocytes (particularly when stored blood products are used), haemolysis in glucose-6-phosphate dehydrogenase deficiency
- impaired hepatocellular function caused by halogenated anaesthetics, sepsis, hepatic ischaemia secondary to perioperative hypotension
- extrahepatic biliary obstruction caused by biliary stones, unsuspected injury to biliary tree.

How does estimation of serum bilirubin concentration help in discerning the aetiology of jaundice?
Normal serum bilirubin concentration is usually no greater than 1.5 mg/dL and is mainly unconjugated. If jaundice is primarily caused by haemolysis or a disorder of bilirubin conjugation, at least 85% of the bilirubin will be unconjugated. With normal liver function, haemolysis alone does not produce a serum bilirubin level >4 mg/dL. A rise in serum bilirubin levels of up to 2 mg/dL is compatible with extrahepatic cholestasis, but a greater rate indicates haemolysis, hepatitis, or hepatic cell necrosis. The serum bilirubin in pure biliary obstruction seldom exceeds 30 mg/dL; a greater value indicates that there is associated hepatocellular jaundice as well.

Discuss the metabolism of bilirubin.
Catabolism of the haem group in the blood gives rise to unconjugated bilirubin. Unconjugated bilirubin is not water soluble and does not pass into the urine. In the blood it is bound to albumin. Unconjugated bilirubin enters the hepatocytes, where it gets conjugated into mono- and diglucuronide bilirubin. Conjugated bilirubin is water soluble and is exported into the bile and from there goes to the small and subsequently the large bowel. Conjugated bilirubin is metabolized by colonic bacteria into stercobilinogen, a form that is excreted in the stool. A small amount of stercobilinogen is absorbed by the bowel and is excreted as urobilinogen in the urine.

Further Information

A. Gilbert (1858–1927), Professor of Medicine at l'Hôtel Dieu in Paris.
P.S.A. Weil (1848–1916), Professor of Medicine in Tartu, Estonia, and Berlin.
J.B. Murphy (1857–1916), Professor of Surgery at Northwestern University in Chicago.
J. Courvoisier (1843–1918), Professor of Surgery, Basel, Switzerland.
I.N. Dubin, Professor of Pathology, Pennsylvania, and F.B. Johnson, pathologist, Veterans Administration Hospital, Washington.

CHAPTER 45

Hepatomegaly

Instruction

Examine this patient's abdomen.

Salient Features

HISTORY

- Shortness of breath, leg oedema (heart failure)
- History of alcohol ingestion, cirrhosis
- History of malignancy (secondary lesions in the liver)
- History of haematological disease or blood cancer
- Social history, including occupation and foreign travel.

EXAMINATION

- Enlarged liver: comment on size, tenderness, surface (smooth or irregular)
- Percussion of the upper border (normally in the fifth intercostal space in the right midclavicular line) and auscultate for bruit.

> **Remember:**
> - How far the liver extends below the costal margin is of less importance than 'liver span', particularly in patients with emphysema or flattened diaphragms.
> - By percussion, the mean liver size is 7 cm for women and 10.5 cm for men, allowing for differences between ethnicities. A liver span 2 to 3 cm larger or smaller than these values is considered abnormal. The liver size depends on several factors, including age, sex, body size, ethnicity, shape, and the examination technique utilized (e.g. palpation versus percussion versus ultrasound).
> - Associated signs:
>   - Splenomegaly
>   - Signs of liver cirrhosis, including signs of decompensation of chronic liver disease
>   - Palpable lymphadenopathy
>   - Raised jugular venous pressure.
> - Request ultrasound of the abdomen and liver Doppler and elastography.
> - At this stage, if the underlying diagnosis is chronic liver disease secondary to alcohol excess, it is prudent to look for neurological signs of alcoholism (peripheral neuropathy, proximal myopathy, cerebellar syndrome, bilateral sixth cranial nerve palsy as in Wernicke encephalopathy, recent memory loss, and confabulation in Korsakoff psychosis).

Diagnosis

This patient has nodular and hard hepatomegaly, which indicates possible multiple lesions in the liver. A possible cause for that would be metastatic lesions of a primary malignancy elsewhere.

I would like to confirm my working diagnosis with an ultrasound scan of the abdomen and look for a primary source with further imaging.

Questions

How would you investigate hepatomegaly?
Once physical examination or radiography has suggested this diagnosis, the next step is abdominal ultrasound; this should distinguish a dilated biliary system, nodular liver, heterogeneity, fatty liver, or space-occupying lesion. Elastography can help to quantify the degree of fibrosis if present. Doppler ultrasound quantifies blood flow in the liver and can assess intrahepatic vascular lesions. Conditions to be excluded include viral hepatitis, alcohol- and drug-induced liver disease, fatty liver, autoimmune liver disease, and metabolic disorders, including haemochromatosis, Wilson disease, and α_1-antitrypsin deficiency. Systemic and infiltrative diseases include amyloidosis, lymphoma, sarcoidosis, and infectious processes such as disseminated tuberculosis and fungaemia.

What does a tender liver indicate?
A stretch of its capsule caused by a *recent* enlargement, as in cardiac failure or acute hepatitis.

What are the common causes of a palpable liver in the United Kingdom?
- Cardiac failure (firm, smooth, tender, mild to massive enlargement)
- Cirrhosis (nontender, firm; in later stages the liver decreases in size)
- Secondary metastasis in the liver (enlarged with rock-hard or nodular consistency).

Mention some less common causes of hepatomegaly.
- Leukaemia and other reticuloendothelial disorders
- Infections: glandular fever, infectious hepatitis
- Primary biliary cirrhosis
- Haemochromatosis
- Sarcoid, amyloid
- Tumours: hepatoma, hydatid cysts.

> **Note:** The liver may be felt without being enlarged in the following circumstances: increased diaphragmatic descent, presence of emphysema with an associated depressed diaphragm, thin body habitus with a narrow thoracic cage, presence of a palpable Riedel's lobe, and right-sided pleural effusion.

In which condition does a pulsatile liver occur?
Tricuspid regurgitation.

What does a hepatic arterial bruit over the liver indicate?
The hepatic arterial bruit has been described in alcoholic hepatitis, primary or metastatic carcinoma. Although reported to occur in cirrhosis, it is rare without associated alcoholic hepatitis.

What does the presence of an abdominal venous hum indicate?
It is virtually diagnostic of portal venous hypertension (usually caused by cirrhosis). When present together with the hepatic arterial bruit in the same patient, it suggests cirrhosis with either alcoholic hepatitis or cancer.

What does a hepatic friction rub indicate?
In a young woman, it could be caused by gonococcal perihepatitis (Fitz–Hugh–Curtis syndrome); in other cases, it could indicate hepatic neoplasm with inflammatory changes or infection in or adjacent to the liver. The presence of a hepatic rub with a bruit usually indicates cancer of the liver, whereas the presence of the hepatic rub, bruit, and abdominal venous hum indicates that a patient with cirrhosis has developed a hepatoma.

Further Information

Dame Sheila Sherlock (1918–2001), Emeritus Professor of Medicine, Royal Free Hospital, London, was a doyen of liver diseases with the liver unit at the Royal Free named after her.

Hans Popper (1903–1988), Professor of Pathology at Chicago and the founding dean of Mount Sinai School of Medicine in New York is regarded as the founding father of hepatology.

CHAPTER 46

Splenomegaly

Instruction

This man complains of fatigue; please examine his abdomen.

Salient Features

HISTORY

- Fatigue (from anaemia)
- Night sweats, low-grade fever: from hypermetabolic state caused by overproduction of white blood cells in chronic myeloid leukaemia. Infectious mononucleosis and infective endocarditis can also cause fever and lead to splenomegaly.
- Abdominal fullness: from splenomegaly
- Bleeding, bone pain: bone marrow infiltration in myeloproliferative disorders
- History of leukaemia or myelofibrosis
- History of residence in endemic areas of malaria, kala-azar
- Family history of Gaucher disease
- Blurred vision, respiratory distress, priapism (from leukostasis in chronic myeloid leukaemia)
- Occasionally, transverse myelitis (from myelopoiesis in epidural space).

EXAMINATION

- Massive spleen. There may be associated anaemia.
- Start low while examining for the spleen and be gentle during palpation. Even if you are certain it is the spleen, you must go through the motions of ruling out a palpable kidney: do a bimanual palpation and check for ballottement; feel for the splenic notch; auscultate for splenic rub.

Proceed as follows:
- Look for enlarged lymph nodes and anaemia.
- Remember that the spleen must be at least two or three times its usual size before it can be felt.
- Remember that the spleen normally does not extend beyond the anterior axillary line and lies along the 9th, 10th, and 11th ribs. The spleen percussion sign is a useful diagnostic technique.
- Comment on anaemia or facial suffusion.

Diagnosis

This patient has massive splenomegaly (lesion), probably caused by a myeloproliferative disorder (aetiology), and is short of breath because of severe anaemia (functional status).

Questions

What is your differential diagnosis?
- Myeloproliferative disorder
- Myelofibrosis, particularly in males
- Chronic myeloid leukaemia, particularly in females.

How would you confirm your diagnosis?
Bone marrow examination.

In what other conditions is a massive spleen palpable?
- Malaria
- Kala-azar
- Gaucher disease.

In which conditions can a moderately enlarged spleen (two to four finger-breadths or 4–8 cm) be felt?
- Portal hypertension secondary to cirrhosis
- Lymphoproliferative disorders such as Hodgkin disease and chronic lymphatic leukaemia.

In which common conditions would the spleen be just palpable?
- Lymphoproliferative disorders
- Portal hypertension secondary to cirrhosis
- Infection: infectious hepatitis, infectious mononucleosis, infective endocarditis, tuberculosis, brucellosis, schistosomiasis
- Sarcoid, rheumatoid arthritis, collagen disease, idiopathic thrombocytopenia, congenital spherocytosis, and polycythaemia rubra vera (95% of those with polycythaemia vera have a mutation affecting the JAK2 signalling molecule)
- Slender young women.

What do you know about the genetics of chronic myelocytic leukaemia?
The fusion of c-*abl* (normally present on chromosome 9) with *bcr* sequences on chromosome 22 is pathognomonic of the chronic phase of chronic myelocytic leukaemia (the Philadelphia chromosome). The p53 gene appears to be the culprit in myeloid blast transformation and there are structural alterations of *RB1* or N-*ras* in <10% of those with myeloid blast crisis.

What do you understand about the terms myeloid metaplasia and extramedullary haematopoiesis?
Myeloid metaplasia and extramedullary haematopoiesis are used interchangeably. They describe the process of ectopic haematopoietic activity that may occur in any organ system but predominantly affects the liver and spleen. It may or may not be associated with bone marrow fibrosis (myelofibrosis). 'Myelofibrosis with myeloid metaplasia' is usually used to describe idiopathic myelofibrosis or agnogenic myeloid metaplasia. Myelofibrosis is characterized by splenomegaly, teardrop poikilocytosis in peripheral smear, leukoerythroblastic blood picture and giant abnormal platelets, hypercellular marrow with reticulin, or collagen fibrosis (Fig. 46.1).

What do you understand by the term chronic myeloid disorders?
Chronic myeloid disorders include:
- chronic myeloid leukaemia: characterized by elevated white blood cell count, marked left-shift to myeloid series, but a low percentage of promyelocytes and blasts, presence of Philadelphia chromosome or *bcr/abl*

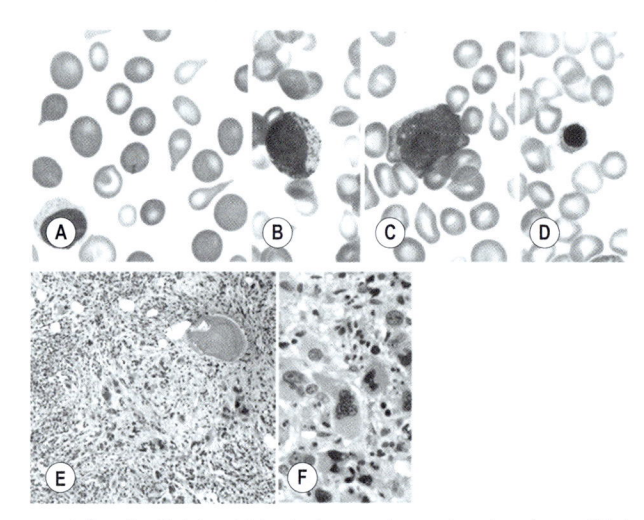

Fig. 46.1 Primary myelofibrosis. Peripheral blood: dacryocytes, or teardrop forms **(A)**, leukoerythroblastic profile with immature granulocytic precursors **(B)**, including blasts **(C)** and circulating nucleated red blood cells **(D)**. Bone marrow biopsy is frequently hypercellular **(E)** with atypical megakaryocytic and granulocytic proliferation **(F)**. (With permission from Hoffman, R., Benz, E., Shattil, S., Furie, B., Cohen, H., 2008. Hematology: Basic Principles and Practice, fifth edn. Churchill Livingstone, Philadelphia.)

- myelodysplastic syndromes: characterized by cytopenias with a hypercellular bone marrow, morphologic abnormalities in two or more haematopoietic cell lines
- atypical chronic myeloid disorder
- chronic myeloproliferative disease: polycythaemia vera, essential thrombocythaemia, myelofibrosis with myeloid metaplasia
- essential thrombocythaemia, in turn, includes agnogenic myeloid metaplasia, postpolycythaemic myeloid metaplasia and postthrombocythaemic myeloid metaplasia.

What is the treatment of Gaucher disease?
Enzyme replacement therapy with intravenous recombinant glucocerebroside. After 6 months of treatment, there may be a 25% reduction in spleen volume.

An alternative includes substrate reduction therapy with miglustat.

Further Information
P.C.E. Gaucher (1854–1918), Professor of Dermatology in France.

The 1902 Nobel Prize was awarded to Sir Donald Ross (1857–1932; born in Almora, India), University of Liverpool, for his work on malaria, in which he showed how the parasite enters the organism. This laid the foundation for successful research on this disease and methods of combating it.

CHAPTER 47

Haemochromatosis

Instruction

This patient has recently developed diabetes. Please examine their abdomen.

Salient Features

HISTORY

- Family history
- Early cases usually asymptomatic, symptoms rarely present before 40 years of age in men or before the menopause in women
- Initial symptoms vague: fatigue, weakness, weight loss, erectile dysfunction in men
- Joint pain (present in 50% of cases): pseudogout usually affects the second and third metacarpophalangeal joints. Any small joints may be involved (Fig. 47.1).
- Advanced disease presents with:
  - skin tan
  - shortness of breath (cardiac failure)
  - diabetes (pancreatic involvement).
- Melaena, haematemesis (secondary to variceal bleeding).

EXAMINATION

- Bronze skin pigmentation typically in a male over 30 years of age
- Palmar erythema, spider naevi
- Jaundice
- Ascites, hepatomegaly (firm, regular)
- Loss of secondary sexual hair.

Proceed as follows:

Tell the examiner that you would like to investigate as follows:
- Look for testicular atrophy (caused by iron deposition affecting hypothalamopituitary function).
- Examine the heart for dilated cardiomyopathy, cardiac failure.
- Check urine for sugar, looking for evidence of diabetes mellitus (present in 80% of cases).

Remember: Patients with haemochromatosis develop cirrhosis and hepatocellular carcinoma.

Diagnosis

This male patient has generalized hyperpigmentation, hepatomegaly, and signs of liver disease (lesions) caused by haemochromatosis, which may be hereditary (aetiology).

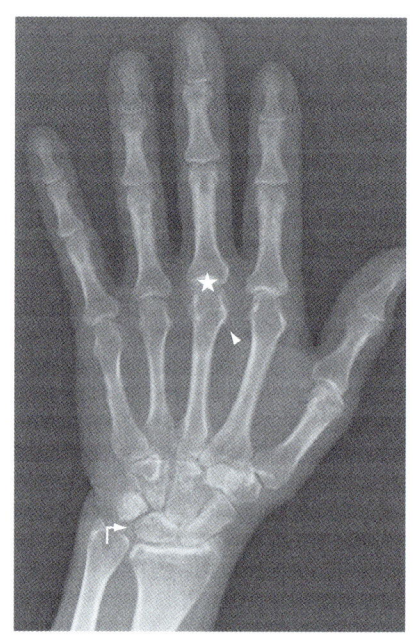

Fig. 47.1 Haemochromatosis. Hooklike osteophyte *(arrowhead)* at the third metacarpal head with cartilage loss at metacarpophalangeal joints *(star)* and chondrocalcinosis of triangular fibrocartilage *(bent arrow)*. (With permission from Firestein, G.S., Budd, R.C., Harris, E.D., Jr. et al., 2008. Kelley's Textbook of Rheumatology, eighth edn. Saunders, Philadelphia, PA.)

Questions

Does this disease run in families?
Yes, with autosomal recessive heritability. At least four different genes encoding proteins involved in iron metabolism have been described: *HJV*, *HAMP*, *TfR2*, and *HFE*. *HFE* is on chromosome 6. Two mutations (845A (C282Y) and 187C (H63D)) account for 90% of cases in those of European extraction. *HFE* is closely associated with *HLA-A3* and, to a lesser extent, with *HLA-B14*. The responsible alleles are on the short arm of chromosome 6. Asymptomatic close relatives of patients with hereditary haemochromatosis, in particular siblings, should be advised to undergo screening (measurements of serum ferritin and iron and saturation of iron-binding capacity. If raised should proceed to testing for C282Y and H63D polymorphisms). Hereditary haemochromatosis can occur in adults who do not have pathogenic mutations affecting chromosome 6. A substantial number of homozygous relatives of these patients (more commonly men) have disease-related conditions such as cirrhosis, hepatic fibrosis, elevated aminotransferase, and haemochromatotic arthropathy that may not have been detected clinically.

However, 10% or more of the patients with clinically severe hereditary haemochromatosis do not have these mutations, and this limits the value of diagnostic DNA testing. Ferroportin-associated iron overload, currently classified as hereditary haemochromatosis type 4, was clinically recognized in 1999 and was linked to *SLC40A1*, which encodes ferroportin, a protein involved in cellular iron export.

What is the mechanism of increased iron uptake?
Iron absorption is mediated by the duodenal metal transporter DMT-1 (also called NRAMP-2). It has been suggested that increased expression of mRNA for NRAMP-2 in the duodenal mucosa

of patients with hereditary haemochromatosis may promote duodenal uptake of iron and result in iron overload.

What is the benefit of early identification?
Early venesection has shown benefits, particularly in those who have not developed diabetes mellitus or cirrhosis. Early venesection prevents progression of hepatic disease and may consequently prevent the complication of hepatocellular carcinoma. Other complications that should be monitored for include arthropathy, hypogonadism, hypothyroidism, osteoporosis, cardiac disease, and porphyria cutanea tarda.

How would you confirm your diagnosis?
- Transferrin saturation is increased.
- Serum ferritin levels are raised.
- C282Y mutation of the HFE gene should be tested for if liver biopsy to measure iron stores is to be a definitive test.
- Magnetic resonance imaging (MRI) is now the modality of choice for noninvasive quantification of iron storage in the liver. It allows repeated measurements and reduces sampling (Fig. 47.2).

How would you manage such a patient?
- Avoid supplements containing iron, including cereals highly fortified in iron.
- Avoid alcohol and food prepared in cast iron cookware.
- Avoid large doses of vitamin C, which will increase the amount of iron absorbed.
- Encourage drinking tea with meals to reduce the absorption of iron.
- Avoid uncooked shellfish and marine fish, since these patients are susceptible to fatal septicaemia from the marine bacterium *Vibrio vulnificus*.
- Phlebotomy: venesection prolongs life and often reverses tissue damage. Initially, weekly venesection (400–500 mL blood per week or fortnight) for 2 years (as 50 g iron or more is removed) and then once every 3 months. Iron depletion is confirmed by serum ferritin <50 μg/L and transferrin saturation <40%. Many manifestations improve (insulin requirements often diminish), except for testicular atrophy and chrondrocalcinosis.

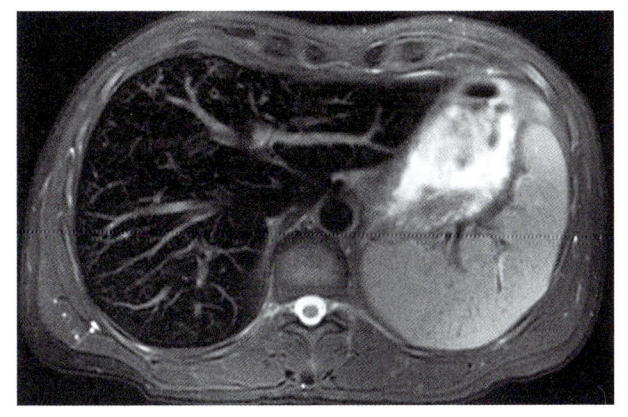

Fig. 47.2 T_2-weighted magnetic resonance image demonstrating abnormally low liver signal in haemochromatosis. (With permission from Adam, A., Dixon, A.K., Grainger, R.G., Allison, D.J., 2008. Grainger and Allison's Diagnostic Radiology, fifth edn. Churchill Livingstone, Edinburgh.)

- Desferrioxamine, an iron chelating agent, is used when haemodynamics do not permit venesection.
- Screening of family members by measuring fasting transferring saturation and ferritin levels. Counselling for HFE testing should occur with risks (insurance) and benefits discussed.

What is the commonest cause of death in patients with hereditary haemochromatosis?
The most common cause of death is hepatocellular carcinoma, for which the risk is 200-fold greater than that of the general population. Depletion of iron, and even reversal of cirrhosis, does not totally prevent the occurrence of this fatal neoplasm. Patients diagnosed in the subclinical, precirrhotic stage and treated by regular phlebotomy have a normal life expectancy.

Mention a few causes of generalized pigmentation.
Common causes are sun exposure and ethnic background.
  Uncommon causes are:
- liver disease: haemochromatosis in males; primary biliary cirrhosis in females
- Addison disease
- uraemia
- chronic debilitating conditions such as malignancy.

Further Information

The term haemochromatosis was first used by von Recklinghausen in 1889 to describe postmortem findings in men with cirrhosis associated with massive deposition of iron in the hepatocytes (von Recklinghausen, 1889).

The inherited nature of haemochromatosis was first recognized by Sheldon in 1935.

CHAPTER 48

Wilson Disease

Instruction

This patient has developed abdominal distension. Look at this patient's eyes.

Salient Features

HISTORY

- History of consanguinity
- In a young adult or child: hepatitis, haemolytic anaemia, portal hypertension, or neuropsychiatric abnormalities
- In adolescents: presents as liver disease
- In adults <40 years of age: consider chronic or fulminant hepatitis.

EXAMINATION

- Look for greenish-yellow to golden-brown pigmentation at the limbus of the cornea (Kayser–Fleischer ring).
- Look for:
    - jaundice (look at the sclera)
    - sunflower cataracts
    - hepatomegaly
    - signs of liver cell failure.
- Look for neurological manifestations: tremor, chorea, mask-like facies with a vacuous smile.

Diagnosis

This patient has a classic Kayser–Fleischer ring with jaundice and hepatomegaly (lesions) caused by Wilson disease (aetiology) and does not have a hepatic flap (functional status).

Questions

What is a Kayser–Fleischer ring?
Deposition of copper in Descemet's membrane. The ring is most marked at the superior and inferior poles of the cornea. It is often apparent only on slit-lamp examination. It may be absent in patients with only hepatic manifestations, but it is present in those with neuropsychiatric disease.

Is a Kayser–Fleischer ring pathognomonic of Wilson disease?
No, it is also seen in primary biliary cirrhosis, chronic active hepatitis with cirrhosis, cryptogenic cirrhosis, and long-standing intrahepatic cirrhosis of childhood.

At what age do neurological manifestations usually present?
They usually appear between 12 and 30 years of age. The most frequent first neurological symptom is difficulty in speaking or writing while in school. Asymmetric tremor is also common and can be resting, postural, or kinetic. Other signs include ataxia and personality changes.

Late neurological signs include dystonia, spasticity, seizures, progressive personality changes such as disinhibition and emotional lability. Fortunately, these late signs are rare now due to earlier diagnosis and effective treatment.

What do you know about the inheritance of the disease?
Autosomal recessive inheritance with the gene *ATP7B* located on chromosome 13, often associated with a family history of consanguinity. It is caused by mutations encoding a copper-transporting P-type ATPase (Wilson disease protein, WNDP). More than 400 mutations have been reported; the most common, leading to the substitution H1069Q, is present in about a third of patients of European extraction.

What do you know about the pathophysiology of this disease?
The precise defect is not known. The major aberration is excessive absorption of copper from the small intestine, with decreased excretion of copper by the liver, resulting in an increase in tissue deposition, particularly in the brain, cornea, liver, and kidney.

What are the biochemical changes in Wilson disease?
- Abnormal liver biochemistry
- Haemolytic anaemia, Coomb's negative
- Low serum caeruloplasmin level (caeruloplasmin is the copper-carrying protein)
- Serum copper concentration may be high, low, or normal.
- Orally administered radiolabelled copper is incorporated into caeruloplasmin.
- Increased urinary excretion of copper.

How is the diagnosis of Wilson disease made?
The diagnosis of Wilson takes into account clinical symptoms and signs characteristic of the disease, abnormal biochemistry, liver biopsy, and mutation analysis.

How would you treat such a patient?
- Copper-chelating agents:
  - Penicillamine, which removes and detoxifies deposits of copper; treatment is lifelong and continuous and is given with pyridoxine to minimize side effects.
  - Penicillamine should never be given as initial therapy in those with neurological manifestations.
  - In patients intolerant to penicillamine, trientine dihydrochloride is an acceptable alternative.
- Zinc salts
- Tetrathiomolybdate with zinc salts is the treatment of choice in those with neurological symptoms.
- Those who develop decompensated liver failure may require transjugular intrahepatic shunting or liver transplant.

Research is ongoing for cures, including gene and cell therapies, as well as liver X receptor agonists, which would not require copper chelation.

What are the clinical stages of Wilson disease?
Wilson disease progresses through four clinical stages.
1. There is asymptomatic accumulation of copper in the liver, which begins when the patient is born.
2. The patient is either asymptomatic or manifests with haemolytic anaemia or liver failure.
3. Copper accumulates in the brain.
4. There is progressive neurological disease.

What are the radiographic features of Wilson disease?
- Osteopenia: most apparent in the hands, feet, and spine
- Arthropathy
- Articular abnormalities: subchondral bone fragmentation, cyst formation and cortical irregularities, most commonly identified in the wrist, hand, foot, hip, shoulder, elbow, and knee. Irregularity and indistinctness of the subchondral bone may form a characteristic 'paintbrush' appearance.
- Osteomalacia and rickets have been reported. Radiologic signs of rickets, delay of skeletal maturation, and pseudofractures may be observed.
- Additional characteristic radiographic findings are small, distinctly corticated ossicles around the affected joint and periosteal bone formation at the attachment sites of tendons and ligaments.
- Chondrocalcinosis is rare, usually limited to the knees.

Further Information
Samuel Alexander Kinnier Wilson (1877–1937) qualified in Edinburgh and worked at the National Hospital, Queen Square, London, as a neurologist (Wilson, 1912).
Bernard Kayser (1869–1954) and Bruno Fleischer, both German ophthalmologists, described the same condition in 1902 and 1903, respectively.

CHAPTER 49

Felty Syndrome

Instruction
Examine this patient's abdomen.

Salient Features
HISTORY
- Fever, weight loss
- Recurrent infections
- Rheumatoid arthritis
- Leg ulcers, hyperpigmentation.

EXAMINATION
- Mild to moderate splenomegaly
- Rheumatoid arthritis.

Proceed as follows:
- Look for the following signs:
  - Anaemia
  - Vasculitis
  - Diffuse pigmentation
  - Leg ulcers.

Diagnosis
This patient has moderate splenomegaly with rheumatoid arthritis (lesions) caused by Felty syndrome (aetiology).

Questions
What is Felty syndrome?
It is a rare complication of rheumatoid arthritis in which there is leucopenia with selective neutropenia and splenomegaly. The bone marrow is typically hyperplastic. The disease typically manifests late in the course of 'burnt-out' joint disease. The prognosis is poor because of recurrent Gram positive infections. The 'large granular lymphocyte syndrome' (Fig. 49.1), a premalignant disorder of the T lymphocyte, occurs in one-third of patients with Felty syndrome in rheumatoid arthritis.

Note: Splenectomy does not prevent sepsis and may hasten the onset of malignancy.

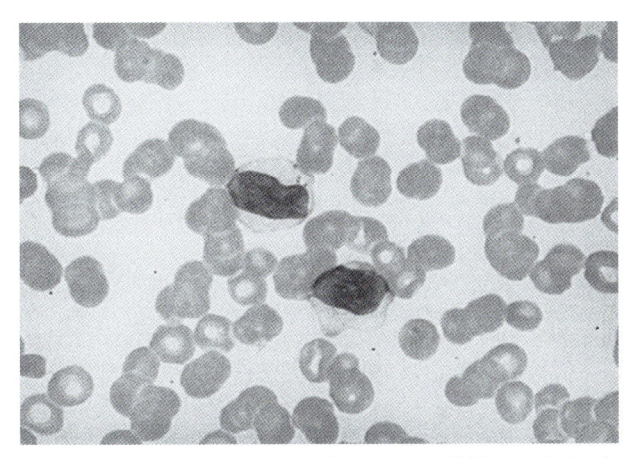

Fig. 49.1 Peripheral blood smear with large granular lymphocytes. (With permission from Firestein, G.S., Budd, R.C., Harris, E.D., Jr. et al., 2008. Kelley's Textbook of Rheumatology, eighth edn. Saunders, Philadelphia, PA.)

What do you understand by the term hypersplenism?
It implies removal of erythrocytes, granulocytes, or platelets from the circulation by the spleen. Removal of the spleen is indicated when the underlying disorder cannot be corrected.
  Criteria for hypersplenism include:
- enlarged spleen
- destruction of one or more cell lines in the spleen
- normal bone marrow.

What are the indications for splenectomy?
- Hereditary spherocytosis in children
- Autoimmune thrombocytopenia or haemolytic anaemia not controlled by steroids
- To ameliorate hypersplenism in Gaucher disease, thalassaemia, hairy cell leukaemia
- For symptom control in massive organomegaly
- Trauma.

What are the characteristic cells in a peripheral blood smear following splenectomy?
The presence of Howell–Jolly bodies (in all) (Fig. 49.2), siderocytes, and spur cells (in 25% of patients).

What are the causes of asplenia?
- *Diminished function:* sickle cell disease, thalassaemia, coeliac disease, systemic lupus erythematosus, lymphoma, leukaemia, amyloidosis
- *Surgical removal:* hereditary spherocytosis, thalassaemia, lymphoma, idiopathic thrombocytopenia, traumatic rupture.

To which infections is the asplenic patient susceptible?
- *Streptococcus pneumoniae*, *Haemophilus influenzae* B, *Neisseria meningitidis*, and malaria parasites cause significant risk.
- Less common infections are babesiosis, caused by tick-borne protozoa, and infection with *Capnocytophaga canimorsus* following a dog bite.

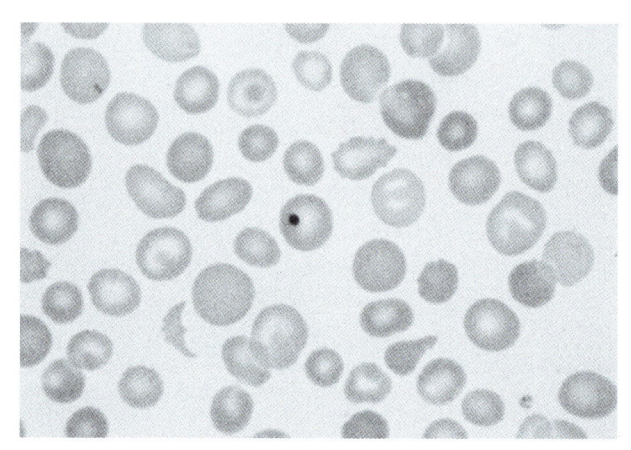

Fig. 49.2 Howell–Jolly body in an erythrocyte. (With permission from Goldman, L., Ausiello, D.A., 2007. Cecil Textbook of Medicine, twenty-third edn. Saunders, Philadelphia, PA.)

What precautions would you advise an asplenic patient to take in the outpatient clinic?
- Vaccination:
    - Pneumococcal vaccine: a single injection; booster doses at 5- to 10-year intervals
    - Hib vaccine: a single dose at the same time as pneumococcal immunization
    - Meningococcus groups A and C vaccine (although the majority of infections are caused by group B strains, for which there is no vaccine of proven efficacy).
- Antibiotic prophylaxis lifelong: phenoxymethylpenicillin or amoxicillin
- Foreign travel: antimalarial chemoprophylaxis, other precautions (insect repellants, screens at night).

Further Information
Augustus R. Felty (1895–1964) was a physician at Hartford Hospital, Hartford, Connecticut. He described this syndrome while he was working at the Johns Hopkins Hospital, Baltimore.

SECTION IV

Renal Cases

SECTION OUTLINE

50 Unilateral Palpable Kidney
51 Polycystic Kidney Disease
52 Nephrotic Syndrome
53 Transplanted Kidney
54 Hypertension

CHAPTER 50

Unilateral Palpable Kidney

Instruction

Examine this patient's abdomen.

Salient Features

HISTORY

- Nephrectomy
- Congenital absence of kidney
- History of azotaemia, dialysis.

EXAMINATION

- One kidney is palpable (bimanually ballotable; there is a transverse band of colonic resonance on percussion and you will be able to insinuate your fingers between the mass and costal margin).

Proceed as follows:
- Look carefully for arteriovenous fistulae in the arms, haemodialysis catheters in the subclavian region.

Diagnosis

This patient has a unilateral palpable kidney (lesion), which may be caused by either polycystic kidney disease or renal neoplasm (aetiology).

Questions

What are the common causes of a palpable kidney?
- Polycystic kidney disease
- Renal carcinoma
- Hydronephrosis
- Renal cyst
- Hypertrophy of the solitary functioning kidney.

What changes can occur in a kidney when the other is removed?
Long-term renal function remains stable in most patients with a reduction in renal mass of >50%. However, these patients are at increased risk for proteinuria, glomerulopathy, and progressive renal failure. Hence, it is important to monitor patients with remnant kidneys. Problems are most frequent in those in whom the amount of renal tissue removed is greatest and who have survived the longest. Survival and the risk of end-stage renal disease in carefully screened kidney donors appear to be similar to those in the general population. Most donors who were studied had a preserved

glomerular filtration rate, normal albumin excretion, and an excellent quality of life. Renal failure has gradually developed in a small proportion of donors, and according to the United Network for Organ Sharing, 56 of >50,000 previous kidney donors have ultimately been listed for transplants themselves. Although some donors develop hypertension over time, hypertension is common in the general population. Occasionally, microalbuminuria develops in donors who should be screened annually for this as well as with blood pressure and glomerular filtration rate.

What are the short-term risks of donation?
- The short-term physical risks are small: the death rate is 0.03%, which is similar to or lower than that for any operation involving the use of general anaesthesia.
- There is risk of bleeding during or after the procedure.
- There are risks of infection or other perioperative problems.
- Donors will lose time from work. Most return to work within 4 to 5 weeks.
- It can take a few weeks to recover fully from surgery, although the increasing use of laparoscopic donation means that a donor may now be released from the hospital in just a few days.

CHAPTER 51

Polycystic Kidney Disease

Instruction
This patient gives a history of intermittent haematuria. Obtain a brief history and examine this patient's abdomen.

Salient Features
HISTORY
- Acute loin pain and/or haematuria (from haemorrhage in a cyst, cyst infection, or urinary stone formation)
- Loin or abdominal discomfort, caused by increasing size of kidneys
- Family history of polycystic kidney disease (as the condition is autosomal dominant with nearly 100% penetrance)
- Complications of hypertension
  - Stroke (as a result of ruptured berry aneurysm)
  - Family history of brain aneurysm: the prevalence of intracranial aneurysms increases from 5% to 20% when there is a family history.

EXAMINATION
- Arteriovenous fistulae in the arms or subclavian dialysis catheter (polycystic kidneys constitute the third most common cause for chronic renal failure in the United Kingdom after glomerulonephritis and pyelonephritis)
- Palpable kidneys: confirm by bimanual palpation and ballottement; there is a resonant note on percussion from overlying colon; the hand can get between the swelling and the costal margin.

Proceed as follows:
- Look for the following signs:
  - Enlarged liver as a result of cystic disease
  - Transplanted kidney: may be palpable in either iliac fossa
  - Third nerve palsy (berry aneurysms are associated with polycystic kidneys)
- Signs of anaemia (chronic renal failure) or polycythaemia (increased erythropoiesis)
- Check the blood pressure (BP) (hypertension develops in 75%)

Tell the examiner you would like to investigate as follows:
- Electrocardiogram to look for left ventricular hypertrophy (this appears to occur to a greater degree for a given rise in BP in autosomal dominant polycystic kidney disease (ADPKD) than in other renal disorders, and with essential hypertension)
- Microscopic haematuria

Polycystic kidney disease is a misnomer as it is a systemic disorder affecting many organs, including the liver, pancreas, and, in some rare cases, the heart and brain. Polycystic kidney disease is the most common genetic life-threatening disease, affecting an estimated 12.5 million people worldwide.

Diagnosis

This patient has polycystic kidney disease (lesion and diagnosis) and is currently on dialysis as evidenced by the arteriovenous fistula in the arm (functional status).

Questions

How may polycystic disease present?
Haematuria, hypertension, urinary tract infection, pain in the lumbar region, uraemic symptoms, subarachnoid haemorrhage associated with berry aneurysm, and complications of associated liver cysts. Kidney stones (more likely to be uric acid rather than calcium oxalate stones) are twice as prevalent as in the general population.

Is the kidney involvement usually unilateral or bilateral?
The disease is universally bilateral; unilateral cases reported probably represent multicystic renal dysplasia.

What do you know about the prevalence of this disease?
ADPKD is one of the most common hereditary disorders, being 10 times more common than sickle cell disease, 15 times more common than cystic fibrosis, and 20 times more common than Huntington disease. It has a worldwide distribution. In the White population, the disease appears to occur in about 1 in 3000 people. Although the disease is rare in Africa and less common in Black Americans than White Americans, the incidence of end-stage renal disease caused by ADPKD is similar in Black and White people. ADPKD is an important cause of renal failure, with 50% needing renal replacement therapy.

In which other conditions may bilateral renal cysts be observed on ultrasound?
Multiple simple cysts, autosomal recessive polycystic kidney disease in children, tuberous sclerosis, and von Hippel–Lindau syndrome.

What are the criteria for diagnosis of polycystic kidney disease using ultrasonography?
- Individuals at risk and those <30 years of age: the presence of at least two renal cysts (unilateral or bilateral) is sufficient to establish a diagnosis in those with a positive family history; five cysts bilaterally in those with no such history
- 30 to 60 years of age: at least two cysts in each kidney in those with a positive family history; five cysts bilaterally in those with no such history
- ≥60 years of age: at least four cysts in each kidney regardless of family history.

How would you like to manage this patient?
- Full blood count, urea and electrolytes, serum creatinine, urine microscopy, urine culture.
- Ultrasonography of the kidneys to confirm the diagnosis. Ultrasound may be equivocal in subjects under the age of 20 years. Ultrasound or renal magnetic resonance imaging (MRI) can also be used to determine total kidney volume, a measure of disease progression.
- MRI should not be used routinely to screening for intracranial aneurysms but may be offered for those with a family history of intracranial aneurysms or subarachnoid haemorrhage due to increased incidence.

In which other organs are cysts seen in this condition?
Liver (in 30% of cases), spleen, pancreas, lungs, ovaries, testes, epididymis, thyroid, uterus, broad ligament, and bladder. Women with hepatic cysts. Women with ADPKD may have massive cystic

enlargement of the liver, a complication attributed to the role of oestrogens in promoting the growth of cysts. Exogenous oestrogens and repeated pregnancies are also risk factors for this complication; therefore oral contraceptives and hormone replacement therapy should be avoided.

What are the neurological manifestations of this condition?
Subarachnoid haemorrhage from an intracranial berry aneurysm, causing death or neurological lesions in about 9% of patients. About 8% of patients with ADPKD have an asymptomatic intracranial aneurysm, and the prevalence is twice as high with a family history of such aneurysms or of subarachnoid haemorrhage. Typically, intracranial aneurysms present as a 'sentinel' or 'thunderclap' headache.

What is the pathology?
Cysts develop in Bowman's capsule and at other levels in the nephron, displacing kidney tissue. In the normal kidney, polycystin 1 is an integral membrane glycoprotein involved in cell–cell and/or cell–matrix interaction; polycystin 2 is similar to a subunit of voltage-activated calcium and sodium channels, which suggests a role in regulating calcium entry. The polycystins interact through their C-terminal cytoplasmic tails, which suggests that they may function through a common signalling pathway. As activation of the intracellular calcium pathways inhibits cell proliferation, in ADPKD, with insufficient or abnormal polycystins and impaired calcium entry, the proliferative pathways dominate, resulting in cyst formation and, ultimately, renal failure. Renal function remains stable until kidney volumes reach a critical size.

What cardiovascular manifestations have been reported in these patients?
- Mitral valve prolapse in 26%
- Other lesions commonly seen are mitral, aortic, and tricuspid valve regurgitation: adult polycystic disease of kidney with involvement of liver.

What are the renal manifestations of this disease?
- The main structural change is the formation of cysts. Cysts enlarge, lose their tubular connection, and become isolated from the glomerulus, requiring transepithelial transport of solutes and fluids for further expansion. Cyst fluids have different sodium compositions, some high and others low.
- One of the earliest and most consistent functional abnormalities is a decrease in renal concentrating ability.
- There may be altered endocrine function, as reflected by increased secretion of both renin (causing increased predilection to hypertension) and erythropoietin (resulting in better maintained haematocrit in renal failure, unlike in renal failure from other causes; rarely can result in polycythaemia).

What are the causes of abdominal pain in this disease?
Infected cyst, haemorrhage into cyst, or diverticular perforation.

What are the complications of polycystic kidney disease?
Renal complications:
- Hypertension (Intrarenal activation of the renin–angiotensin system is said to be the main mechanism and, hence, angiotensin-converting enzyme (ACE) inhibitors are first-line agents to control BP; diuretics should be avoided because hypokalaemia promotes cyst formation.)
- Pain: back pain or abdominal pain (Cyst decompression may help to relieve pain but does not alter the rate of progression.)

- Gross or microscopic haematuria
- Cyst infection (Lipophilic antibiotics against Gram-negative bacteria such as co-trimoxazole; fluoroquinolones penetrate the cysts better and are preferred to standard antibacterial agents.)
- Renal calculi (seen in 10%–20% with ADPKD and are frequently radiolucent and composed of uric acid)
- Urinary tract infection including pyelonephritis
- Proteinuria
- Renal failure (once the glomerular filtration rate (GFR) is <50 mL/min, the rate of progression is more rapid than in other primary renal disorders and there is a reduction in GFR of about 5 mL/min every year). About one-half of the patients have adequate renal function the rest require renal replacement therapy by a median age of 55 years.

Extrarenal manifestations:
- Cystic: cysts in the liver, ovary, pancreas, spleen, and central nervous system. Unlike renal cyst formation, liver cysts seem to be influenced by female hormones. Whilst men and women have the same frequency of liver cysts, massive liver cysts are almost exclusively found in women.
- Noncystic:
    - Cardiac valvular abnormalities: mitral valve prolapse (seen in ~20% of ADPKD), aortic valve abnormalities
    - Intracranial saccular aneurysm or berry aneurysm: magnetic resonance (MR) angiography is the most reliable technique of noninvasive screening among such patients.
- Gastrointestinal: colonic diverticula, herniae of the anterior abdominal wall.

What do you know about the genetic transmission of this disease?
Polycystic kidney disease is an autosomal dominant disorder. Mutations in at least three different genes can lead to ADPKD. The *PKD1* gene (encoding polycystin-1) is located on chromosome 16. The *PKD2* gene (encoding polycystin-2) is situated on chromosome 4.

Among the European ADPKD population, *PKD1* is the cause in about 85% of families and *PKD2* is the cause in about 15%. Compared with individuals affected by *PKD2*, those with *PKD1* have more severe disease, with a higher prevalence of hypertension, an increased risk of progression into renal failure, and shorter life expectancy.

What do you know about screening in this condition?
- The children and siblings of patients with established ADPKD should be offered screening.
- Affected individuals should have their BP checked regularly and offered genetic counselling:
    - Genetic linkage analysis can be utilized in many families. Ultrasound is usually not useful before the age of 20 years.

What are some poor prognostic factors in autosomal dominant polycystic kidney disease?
Patients are liable to progress more rapidly if they are male or have *PKD1* mutations, early-onset hypertension, episodes of gross haematuria, or a family history of hypertension in an unaffected person; however, these only account for a fraction of the variability of disease progression.

What are the causes of death in these patients?
One-third of adult patients die of renal failure; another one-third die of the complications of hypertension (including heart disease, intracerebral haemorrhage, and rupture of berry aneurysm). The remaining third die from unrelated causes.

Are there any special treatments for this condition?
Patients should be advised to:
- increase their water intake to 3 L a day (to reduce antidiuretic hormone and cyclic adenosine monophosphate (AMP) stimulation)
- limit their sodium intake (to control hypertension or kidney cyst formation)
- avoid caffeine or methylxanthine derivatives (since they block phosphodiesterase, thereby resulting in more cyclic AMP to stimulate cyst formation)
- avoid situations that could carry a high risk of abdominal trauma, such as high-impact contact sports

Aggressive BP control as evidenced by the HALT PKD (Halt Progression of Polycystic Kidney Disease) study
- Tolvaptan is a selective vasopressin antagonist. It inhibits the binding of vasopressin to the V2 receptors, so reducing cell proliferation, cyst formation, and fluid excretion. It is recommended for those with chronic kidney disease stage 2 or 3 with rapidly progressing disease
- Studies of mammalian target of rapamycin inhibitors and somatostatin did not show reduction in progression of renal disease.

What do you know about hypertension in a pregnant woman with autosomal dominant polycystic kidney disease?
Although ACE inhibitors or an angiotensin receptor blocker are the best choice for hypertension in ADPKD, these drugs are contraindicated in pregnancy. Normotensive women with ADPKD and creatinine <12 mg/L typically have uncomplicated pregnancies, but 16% get new hypertension and are more likely to develop chronic hypertension. Pregnant patients with ADPKD have a higher frequency of maternal complications (particularly hypertension, oedema, and preeclampsia) than patients without ADPKD (35% vs. 19%, $P < 0.001$).

Further Information
Sir W. Bowman (1816–1892), Surgeon at the Royal London Ophthalmic Hospital.

E.L. Potter (1901–1993), US pathologist. She also described Potter syndrome, with renal agenesis and characteristic epicanthic folds, receding jaw and low set ears with less cartilage than usual.

O.Z. Dalgaard's study in 1957 clarified the autosomal dominant pattern of inheritance of the disease.

CHAPTER 52

Nephrotic Syndrome

Instruction
This patient presents to the medical clinic with recent onset of generalized and facial oedema. Please examine.

Salient Features
HISTORY
- Facial and bilateral periorbital oedema
- Generalized peripheral oedema
- Lethargy, fatigue, generalized weakness
- Muscle weakness and muscle loss
- Frothy urine
- Weight gain
- Venous thromboembolic disease
- Medical history—kidney disease, autoimmune conditions, thyroid disease, diabetes, malignancy, amyloidosis
- Drug history
- Recent or previous infections, hepatitis B, malaria, hepatitis C, HIV.

EXAMINATION
- Periorbital oedema
- Peripheral pitting oedema
- Muscle wasting
- Absence of signs of heart failure or cirrhosis.

Proceed as follows:
- Check the blood pressure for hypertension
- Test the urine for protein.

Diagnosis
This young man presents with generalized oedema and weakness (lesions) in keeping with the nephrotic syndrome, likely caused by membranous nephropathy (aetiology).

Questions
How is nephrotic syndrome defined?
Nephrotic syndrome is comprised by the triad of heavy proteinuria with more than 3.5 g of protein in a 24-hour urine collection, hypoalbuminaemia, and peripheral oedema.

197

Why do patients with nephrotic syndrome develop oedema?

Oedema in nephrotic pressure was traditionally attributed to the decreased oncotic pressure caused by the hypoalbuminaemia which is caused by urinary loss of albumin. However, this is not the main mechanism believed to account for the generalized oedema in such patients, as decrease in oncotic pressure in nephrotic syndrome is concurrent with a decrease in the interstitial protein concentration, and as such the oncotic pressure gradient remains unchanged. Alternative mechanisms are believed to give rise to severe oedema. Elevated tumour necrosis factor α (TNF-α) levels seen in nephrotic syndrome activate protein kinase C, which increases vessel permeability. In addition, in nephrotic syndrome there is renal sodium retention in the cortical collecting duct, where the Na-K-ATPase activity is doubled or tripled in nephrotic syndrome. This sodium retention would normally be counteracted by increased sodium secretion in the medullary collecting duct, but in nephrotic syndrome this is stopped by enhanced cyclic GMP activity. Aside from the primary sodium retention and inability of the kidney to compensate with increased secretion, there is also secondary sodium retention by activation of the renin–aldosterone system due to the reduced filling pressure intravascularly caused by hypoalbuminaemia.

What is the treatment of nephrotic syndrome?
- High-dose loop diuretics in combination with low sodium intake. If the oedema does not respond to loop diuretics then thiazide diuretics can be added in the regime.
- Angiotensin-converting enzyme inhibitors or angiotensin II receptor blockers to reduce the progression of kidney function loss
- Specified treatment towards the underlying cause (immunosuppressants, corticosteroids)
- Prophylactic low-molecular-weight heparin
- Statins for patients with hyperlipidaemia and high cardiovascular risk.

What is the treatment of nephrotic syndrome in pregnancy?
Treatment of nephrotic syndrome in pregnancy may differ from the nonpregnant population, as caution has to be taken using specific drugs:
- Diuretics may decrease placenta perfusion so if not avoided they should be used with caution in pregnancy.
- Once nephrotic syndrome is confirmed, low-dose aspirin has to be used prophylactically after the first trimester to prevent eclampsia.
- Specific immunosuppressive medications are safe to use in pregnancy; the initiation of immunosuppressants must be overseen by an expert.
- Prophylactic anticoagulation is encouraged depending on the individual patient, but statins are not used in pregnancy.

Name some complications of nephrotic syndrome.
- Thromboembolic disease
- Acute kidney injury
- Infections by encapsulated bacteria
- Vitamin D deficiency
- Anaemia
- Hyperlipidaemia.

What are the most common renal causes of primary nephrotic syndrome?
- Minimal change glomerulonephritis
- Focal segmental glomerulonephritis
- Membranous nephropathy
- Membranoproliferative glomerulonephritis.

Name some renal causes that can cause a mixed nephrotic and nephritic picture
- Mesangiocapillary glomerulonephritis
- Mesangial proliferative glomerulonephritis.

What is preeclampsia?
Preeclampsia is the new onset of hypertension and proteinuria after 20 weeks of gestation or postpartum in a previously normotensive woman.

Eclampsia is defined when a woman with preeclampsia develops seizures.

The combination of haemolysis, elevated liver enzymes, and low platelets (HELLP) is a severe form of pre-eclampsia.

Why is there hyperlipidaemia in nephrotic syndrome?
Albuminuria leads to low plasma albumin, which in turn causes increase of lipoprotein synthesis. As a result, there is an increase in low-density lipoprotein (LDL), very-low-density lipoprotein, and intermediate-density lipoprotein which results in increased LDL/high-density lipoprotein (HDL) ratio.

CHAPTER 53

Transplanted Kidney

Instruction

Examine this patient's abdomen.

Salient Features

HISTORY

- History of chronic renal failure: determine duration, aetiology (diabetes, hypertension, glomerulonephritis)
- History of haemodialysis
- History of arteriovenous fistula
- History of transplanted kidney.

EXAMINATION

- Laparotomy scar (comment on the scar)
- Arteriovenous fistulae in arms
- Transplanted kidney felt in either right or left iliac fossa.

Proceed as follows:
- Tell the examiner that you would like to look for other signs of uraemia.
- Know the differential diagnosis for masses in the right/left iliac fossa.

Diagnosis

This patient has a transplanted kidney (lesion), probably required because of diabetic nephropathy, as evidenced by the sugar-free drinks by the bedside (aetiology). He is euvolaemic and appears well (functional status).

Questions

Mention a few indications for renal transplantation.
End-stage renal disease: the most common diseases that result in referral of patients for transplantation include:
- Diabetes mellitus with renal failure
- Hypertensive renal disease
- Glomerulonephritis.

Would you refer a patient for renal transplantation before instituting haemodialysis?
Referral for renal transplantation need not be delayed until the patient has begun dialysis. It is acceptable and, in fact, usually preferable to refer the patient to a renal transplant unit before

dialysis is required. With judicious planning on the part of the general practitioner, renal physician, and transplant surgical team, transplantation can be performed even before dialysis is required.

Renal transplant should be considered for patients with chronic kidney disease stage 5 who are fit for major surgery and chronic immunosuppression.

In which age group is transplantation preferred to dialysis?
Infants and children have a high morbidity rate on long-term haemodialysis or peritoneal dialysis. Therefore, renal transplantation from parents or siblings improves growth and allows a more normal lifestyle.

Is there any advantage to human leukocyte antigen matching before transplantation?
Kidneys from living-related donors who are human leukocyte antigen (HLA) identical and also red blood cell ABO matched have a 90% survival rate at 1 year; less identical grafts tend to have a somewhat lower survival rate. Kidney transplants from matched cadaver donors survive nearly as long, especially if the recipient does not contain antibodies to donor antigens.

There is some evidence that HLA mismatching has a greater effect on living-related transplantation than it does on cadaveric donor kidney transplantation. Recent evidence has shown that HLA-matched kidneys, particularly for HLA-DR, HLA-B, and HLA-A antigens, are associated with long-term survival of the patient. Complete matching of HLA-DR, HLA-B, and HLA-A is associated with the best chance of success. HLA-DR matching appears to have the greatest impact on survival, followed by HLA-B and, lastly, HLA-A.

Should repeated blood transfusions be avoided in a patient waiting for a renal transplant?
If the anaemia is well tolerated and is caused by the renal failure per se, blood transfusion should be avoided as it carries a risk of HLA sensitization.

What other factors are known to cause sensitization to HLA antigens?
Pregnancy, previously failed transplant.

What drugs are used for posttransplant immunosuppression?
Steroids, azathioprine, ciclosporin, tacrolimus, rapamycin, sirolimus, mycophenolate mofetil, and basiliximab: used independently or in combination.

What are the contraindications for kidney transplantation?
- A positive cross-match by cytotoxicity testing between recipient serum and donor cells is considered to be a contraindication for transplantation.
- Presence of medical condition limiting life expectancy to less than 5 years.

What are the complications of renal transplantation?
- Opportunistic infection, e.g. cytomegalovirus, *Pneumocystis*
- Premature coronary artery disease
- Hypertension: primarily with ciclosporin therapy
- Lymphomas and skin cancers
- De novo glomerulonephritis in the transplanted kidney
- Complications of steroid therapy, e.g. aseptic necrosis of bone.

What do you know about warm ischaemic time?
Shorter warm ischaemic time of the transplanted kidney is associated with longer survival of the recipient. However, a slight increase in the duration of cold ischaemia justifies HLA matching before kidney transplantation because of higher rates of survival, a lower incidence of the episodes of rejection, and lower risk of loss as a result of rejection.

What is the survival rate following kidney transplant?
The 2-year kidney graft survival rate for living-related donor transplantation is 90%, whereas in cadaveric donor transplantation, it is about 85%.

What do you know about rejection of the transplanted kidney?
Rejection may be acute or chronic and must be suspected when the graft is tender, the urine output is falling, or the creatinine concentration is rising. It is a complex process in which both cell-mediated immunity and circulating antibodies play a role. Evaluation of a suspected rejection usually requires graft biopsy.
- Acute rejection is characterized by a lymphocytic interstitial infiltrate with destruction of epithelial cells. It usually responds to treatment, which includes high-dose methylprednisolone, antilymphocytic immunoglobulin, and anti-T-cell monoclonal antibody (OKT3)
- Chronic rejection shows histological features of interstitial fibrosis, atrophy of tubules, and proliferation of the arterial intima. There is no specific treatment, and general management of chronic renal failure should be reinstituted.

Is there any advantage of renal transplantation compared with long-term dialysis in end-stage renal disease?
The benefits of renal transplantation include better quality of life, reduced medical expenses, and about a 68% reduction in the long-term risk of death.

What is the role of pancreas–kidney transplantation in patients with diabetes mellitus and end-stage renal failure?
Pancreas transplantation in type 1 diabetes can reverse the lesions of diabetic nephropathy but reversal requires >5 years of normoglycaemia. Simultaneous pancreas–kidney transplantation prolongs survival in patients with diabetes and end-stage renal failure and should be the treatment of choice for these patients.

Does acute myocardial infarction influence long-term survival among patients on long-term dialysis?
Patients on dialysis who have an acute myocardial infarction have high mortality from cardiac causes and poor long-term survival.

Further Information

In the 1920s, Alexis Carrel developed the technique of vascular anastomoses, which made possible the human allograft attempts by David Hume and Joseph Murray in the early 1950s.

Joseph E. Murray (1919–2012), Professor of Surgery, Brigham and Women's Hospital and Harvard Medical School, was awarded the 1990 Nobel Prize for Medicine for his pioneering work on organ transplantation along with Thomas E. Donnall (1920–2012) of the Fred Hutchinson Cancer Research Center, Seattle, Washington, USA (Murray et al., 1963).

In 1966, Terasaki and coworkers reported the association between HLA matching and outcome in patients receiving cadaveric organs (Terasaki et al., 1966).

The observation by Schwartz and Damasheck that 6-mercaptopurine was effective in blocking primary but not secondary antibody response in rabbits paved the way for drug-induced immunosuppression in the late 1950s (Schwartz and Dameshek, 1959).

CHAPTER 54

Hypertension

Instruction

This 39-year-old patient, who was recently diagnosed with hypertension, has presented to the general medical clinic for a routine review. Please take a focused history, examine the patient, and advise on further management.

Salient Features

HISTORY

- Chest pain or shortness of breath
- Intermittent claudication
- Headaches or visual disturbances (in accelerated or severe hypertension)
- Family history of hypertension
- Ask about hypertension during pregnancy
- Medication history.

EXAMINATION

Look for aetiology:
- Comment on Cushingoid facies if present.
- Look for radio-femoral delay of coarctation of aorta.
- Examine blood pressure (BP) in both upper arms (the arm with the higher BP is used for serial follow-up of patients).
- Listen for renal artery bruit of renal artery stenosis and feel for polycystic kidneys.

Look for target organ damage (heart, kidney, nervous system, eyes):
- Palpate the apex for left ventricular hypertrophy.
- Look for signs of cardiac failure.
- Examine the fundus for changes of hypertensive retinopathy.
- Tell the examiner that you would like to check urine for protein (renal failure) and glucose (associated diabetes): increases risk of cardiovascular disease.

Explore cardiovascular risk factors for the patient:
- Use the Q-Risk2 risk assessment tool to calculate the patient's cardiovascular risk, in order to offer primary prevention appropriately.

Diagnosis

This patient has retinopathy (lesion) caused by hypertension, which is probably renovascular (aetiology) as evidenced by the renal artery bruit. She likely has damage to other target organs (functional status).

Questions

What are the causes of blood pressure discrepancy between the arms or between the arms and legs?
- Coarctation of aorta
- Patent ductus arteriosus
- Dissecting aortic aneurysm
- Arterial occlusion or stenosis of any cause
- Supravalvular aortic stenosis
- Thoracic outlet syndrome.

How would you investigate a patient with hypertension in outpatients?
All newly diagnosed patients with hypertension will need to have some baseline routine investigations:
- Full blood count
- Urine for a routine urine dipstick to test for presence of haematuria and proteinuria and estimation of the albumin:creatinine ratio
- Urea, electrolytes, and serum creatinine
- Fasting lipids, fasting blood sugar
- Fundoscopy for presence of hypertensive retinopathy
- 12-lead electrocardiogram.

How would you record the blood pressure?
- Use a device whose accuracy has been validated and also recently calibrated.
- The patient should be seated for 5 min before the BP measurement and during the measurement the arm and cuff should be at the level of the heart.
- The BP cuff should be appropriate for the size of the arm and the cuff should be deflated at 2 mm/s and the diastolic BP is measured to the nearest 2 mm Hg. Systolic BP is recorded at phase I and diastolic BP is recorded as disappearance of the sounds (phase V).
- If there is a discrepancy of BP measurement between the two arms, use the arm with the highest recording.
- At least two recordings of BP should be made during the same consultation, 1 to 2 min apart.

What are the stages of hypertension?
The National Institute for Health and Care Excellence (NICE) UK has provided three stages for hypertension:
- Stage 1 hypertension: clinic BP more than 140/90 mm Hg, and subsequent ambulatory monitoring average of more than 135/85 mm Hg
- Stage 2: clinic BP more than 160/100 mm Hg, and subsequent ambulatory monitoring average more than 150/95 mm Hg
- Stage 3 or severe hypertension: clinic BP of systolic more than 180 mm Hg or diastolic more than 110 mm Hg

The European Society of Cardiology guidelines are in accordance with the aforementioned staging.

The American College of Cardiology and American Heart Association have defined the stages slightly differently with lower measurement cut-offs for diagnosing hypertension.

Who would you screen for hypertension?
All adults 18 years old and above should be screened for hypertension. This recommendation follows the United States Preventive Services Task Force 2021 and is in agreement with the UK national recommendations.

What are the indications for ambulatory blood pressure recording?

Any suspicion of high BP measured in a single clinic appointment that is above 140 mm Hg systolic and 90 mm Hg diastolic needs further investigation in order to establish a diagnosis of hypertension and decide on the most appropriate treatment. In other words, all patients with a clinic BP of more than 140/90 mm Hg and not severe hypertension will need ambulatory BP monitoring (ABPM). If the patient cannot tolerate the 24-hour monitor, then home BP monitoring is an alternative. In this case the patient has to be instructed how to appropriately monitor their BP: an oscillometer that measures BP in the branchial artery has to be used, the patient has to be relaxed and seated in a calm environment before and during the BP measurement, for each BP recording two measurements have to take place, one after the other at least 1 min apart. For each day the patient needs to perform two recordings, in the morning and in the evening. The monitor and recording of the BP has to continue for a week.

> **Note:** If a person has severe hypertension in the clinic appointment, then ABPM is not needed and antihypertensive therapy should be initiated without a need for further confirmation.

Name some causes of hypertension.
- Primary or idiopathic (in 90% of cases)
- Renovascular: glomerulonephritis, diabetic nephropathy, renal artery stenosis, pyelonephritis, fibromuscular dysplasia
- Endocrine: Cushing syndrome, steroid therapy, phaeochromocytoma, primary aldosteronism
- Others: coarctation of aorta, contraceptives, pregnancy related.

What special investigations would you do to screen for an underlying cause?
- If renovascular disease is suspected: magnetic resonance angiography
- If phaeochromocytoma is suspected: urinary catecholamines: 24-hour collection of at least three samples
- If Cushing syndrome is suspected: cortisol levels and dexamethasone suppression test.

What are the treatment targets for blood pressure according to the National Institute for Health and Care Excellence?
- BP below 135/85 mm Hg for patients younger than 80 years old
- BP below 145/95 mm Hg for patients older than 80 years old.

What are the National Institute for Health and Care Excellence guidelines for initiating hypertensive agents?

The treatment of hypertension should be as follows:
- Lifestyle measures should be offered initially and continually apply to all stages of hypertension.
- Antihypertensive medications should be offered to patients with stage 1 hypertension and end-organ damage, cardiovascular or renal disease, diabetes, or estimated 10-year cardiovascular risk more than 10% and all patients with hypertension of stage 2 and above.
- If a drug needs to be added to the above therapy, then the choice is between an angiotensin converting enzyme inhibitor (ACE-i)/angiotensin II receptor blocker (ARB), a thiazide diuretic, and a calcium channel blocker (CCB). There is a stepwise approach on treatment, so if a single agent has failed to provide adequate control further medication can be added on to the treatment regime.
- In resistant hypertension that three agents have failed to control, then a higher diuretic dose or the addition of aldosterone antagonist should be the next step, but specialist advice should be sought for further investigations.

What are the National Institute for Health and Care Excellence recommendations for follow-up of a patient with well-controlled blood pressure?

Conduct annual review of care to monitor BP, provide patients with support, and discuss their lifestyle, symptoms, and medication. Patients may become motivated to make lifestyle changes and want to stop using antihypertensive drugs. If at low cardiovascular risk and with well-controlled BP, patients should be offered a trial reduction or withdrawal of therapy with appropriate lifestyle guidance and ongoing review.

What are the lifestyle modifications that have an impact on reducing blood pressure?

- Diet: weight reduction in obese patients, low-cholesterol diets for associated hyperlipidaemia, salt restriction (2–3 g sodium/day), increased consumption of fruit and vegetables. Diets like the Mediterranean and the DASH (dietary approaches to stop hypertension) have a positive effect in treating hypertension.
- Regular physical exercise that should be predominantly dynamic (for example brisk walking) rather than isometric (weight lifting)
- Limit alcohol consumption (<14 units/week for women and <21 units/week for men)
- Stop smoking.

Why are beta-blockers no longer recommended as first-line agents in the management of hypertension?

- Beta-blockers are no longer routinely recommended as first-line agents in hypertension because of an increased long-term risk of diabetes, particularly when used with diuretics
- The Conduit Artery Function Evaluation study showed that beta-blocker-based treatment was significantly less effective than regimens based on CCBs at lowering aortic systolic BP and pulse pressure despite identical brachial BP in both treatment groups (pseudohypertensive effects).

In head-to-head clinical trials, beta-blockers were usually less effective than comparator antihypertensive medications at reducing major cardiovascular events, in particular stroke. Atenolol was the beta-blocker used in most of these studies, and, in the absence of substantial data on other agents, it is unclear whether this conclusion applies to all beta-blockers. It has been proposed that in the case of atenolol, insufficient duration of action leaves night-time BP untreated, which is one reason for its lack of efficacy. However, when hypertension is accompanied by coronary artery disease, congestive heart failure, increased sympathetic activity, and arrhythmia, beta-blocker therapy could be beneficial.

What is the role of alpha-blocker-based regimens in the control of blood pressure?

The Antihypertensive and Lipid Lowering Treatment to Prevent Heart Attack trial showed that an alpha-blocker-based regimen is less effective than a diuretic-based regimen in preventing heart failure. Additionally, there was a marginally significant excess of stroke and cardiovascular risk in the alpha-blocker group. Although poorer BP control might account for the higher risk of stroke, it does not entirely explain the two-fold greater risk of heart failure. However, an alpha-blocker may be appropriate treatment option for subgroup of patients (e.g. with coexistent benign prostate hyperplasia).

Why are thiazide-like diuretics preferred to traditional thiazide diuretics in the treatment of hypertension?

They are more potent and longer acting, and as a result, lower doses are needed to produce desirable antihypertensive effects with a better side effect profile.

They have shown to have an effect in reducing cardiovascular risk when compared to thiazide diuretics.

What are the indications for specialist referral?
- Hypertensive emergency: malignant hypertension, impending complications
- To evaluate therapeutic problems or failures
- Special circumstances: unusually variable BP, possible white-coat hypertension, pregnancy.

What do you understand by resistant hypertension?
Resistant or refractory hypertension is defined as BP persistently greater than target (i.e. >140/90 mm Hg for most patients and >130/80 mm Hg in those with diabetes or renal disease) despite therapy with three different antihypertensive medication classes, including a diuretic. True resistant hypertension can occur in volume overload, use of contraindicated drugs, or exogenous substances and with some associated conditions (e.g. smoking, obesity, pain, excessive alcohol intake). Resistant hypertension can occur secondary to Conn's adenoma, sleep apnoea, and chronic kidney disease.

What do you understand by the term 'malignant hypertension' and how do you treat it?
Malignant or accelerated hypertension is a BP of more than 180 mm Hg systolic and more than 120 mm Hg diastolic with papilloedema or retinal haemorrhage and often associated with other organ damage. When the BP increases, arteries and arterioles vasoconstrict in order to protect the smaller vessels, but as the BP increases even further vasoconstriction fails to provide enough protection. As such, the increased pressure is transferred to the capillaries with an immediate consequence damage to their wall. This leads to retinal haemorrhages and papilloedema. The aim of treatment is to reduce the BP by 10% within the first hour of treatment, but by no more than 25% within the first 24 hours of treatment. For that reason, an intravenous infusion is preferred as the initial treatment, so that the rate of infusion can be set according to the variations of the BP. After BP has fallen slowly into a safe range, oral medications can be started, following appropriate guidelines. The agents preferred for the treatment of accelerated hypertension are different in each setting. Sodium nitroprusside, nitroglycerin, and labetalol are amongst the most commonly used ones.

SECTION V

Haematology Cases

SECTION OUTLINE

55 Anaemia
56 Bruising
57 Multiple Myeloma
58 Myelodysplastic Syndrome
59 Chronic Lymphocytic Leukaemia
60 Chronic Myeloid Leukaemia
61 Acute Leukaemia
62 Lymphadenopathy

CHAPTER 55

Anaemia

Instruction
This patient presented to the ambulatory care unit with dyspnoea on exertion. Please examine.

Salient Features
HISTORY
- Fatigue and lethargy
- Generalized weakness—the patient finds it hard to perform activities that were easy tasks a few months prior to presentation.
- Exertional chest pain and dyspnoea
- Palpitations—anaemia can affect both the oxygen delivery to the tissues and cause arrhythmias.
- Dizziness, orthostatic hypotension
- Presyncope and collapse
- Headaches—it is not uncommon for patients to present with headaches of new onset, undergo a series of investigations, including brain imaging and lumbar puncture, being treated for presumed syndromes with no effect and the headaches to disappear once anaemia is diagnosed and treated.

Tell the examiner that you would like to enquire about specific symptoms or clues in the history which may lead to an underlying cause for the anaemia.
- Dietary history—a vegan diet can be a cause of dietary iron-deficiency anaemia or B_{12}-deficiency anaemia.
- Onset of symptoms (Abrupt onset may point towards acute bleeding or acute haemolysis.)
- Family history and ethnic background (A family history of haemoglobinopathies may point towards an inherited cause, Mediterranean descent can point towards thalassaemia, or African descent can point towards sickle cell disease.)
- Neurological problems may point towards B_{12} deficiency.
- Pica syndrome, beeturia, pagophagia, angular cheilitis, and metallic taste in mouth are associated with iron-deficiency anaemia.
- Dark urine and jaundice is associated with haemolytic anaemias.
- Travel history (parasitic infections)
- Medication history—specific medications are associated with different types and causes of anaemia—a detailed drug history should be obtained.
- Past medical history (for identifying conditions that may be causing anaemia of chronic disease, such as hypothyroidism, kidney disease, cardiac failure, malignancy, chronic infections, rheumatological conditions).

EXAMINATION
- Pallor—pallor is the most commonly reported sign in anaemia, but it should be looked for with caution, as the underlying skin colour and pigmentation of the patient may pose

- difficulties in detecting it or interpreting it. Deeply pigmented skin may hide pallor so careful inspection of areas such as the palms of the hands, soles of the feet, oral mucosa, and conjunctivae is needed. Equally, when detecting pallor in a fair-skinned individual, they should be asked to compare their skin colour with how it was previously.
- Cardiac signs—systolic flow murmur is associated with hyperdynamic circulation in anaemia. Other additional sounds can also be heard in severe anaemia, such as a venous hum in the neck and Cabot–Locke diastolic murmur. Detection of a new murmur in an anaemic patient should be interpreted carefully as anaemia can give rise to flow murmurs, but the opposite is also true; anaemia can be caused by valvular disease (e.g. Heyde syndrome in aortic stenosis).
- Tachycardia, arrhythmias, postural hypotension, signs of cardiac failure—anaemia can cause dilated cardiomyopathy and cause heart failure symptoms, but can also exacerbate cardiac failure in patients with established heart failure.
- Koilonychia—spoon-shaped soft nails associated with iron deficiency anaemia
- Facial and skull bone deformities in thalassaemia major
- Leg ulcers in sickle cell disease
- Plummer–Vinson (Patterson–Brown–Kelly) syndrome with dysphagia and glossitis in iron deficiency anaemia
- Peripheral neuropathy or subacute combined degeneration in B_{12} deficiency
- Bruising and ecchymoses, mouth blisters, bleeding gums and epistaxis, lymphadenopathy, and hepatosplenomegaly in aplastic anaemia
- Jaundice, organomegaly, and abdominal tenderness in haemolytic anaemias.

Diagnosis

This young Nigerian man presents with chest pain and shortness of breath (lesion). This is caused by anaemia secondary to sickle cell disease (aetiology). Prompt administration of oxygen has alleviated his symptoms (functional status).

Questions

Name some causes of haemolytic anaemia.
- Inherited red cell membrane defects—hereditary spherocytosis and hereditary elliptocytosis
- Haemoglobinopathies—thalassaemia, sickle cell disease
- Inherited metabolic defects—G6PD deficiency, pyruvate kinase deficiency, pyrimidine kinase deficiency
- Infections—mycoplasma, Epstein–Barr virus (EBV), parvovirus, SARS-CoV-2, hepatitis C
- Drug induced—methyldopa, dapsone, penicillins, nonsteroidal antiinflammatory drugs
- Disseminated intravascular coagulation (DIC)—burns, sepsis, trauma
- Autoimmune haemolysis—warm, cold, transfusion related, post-allogenic bone marrow or organ transplantation
- Acquired nonimmune—microangiopathic haemolytic anaemia, prosthetic valve related, haemolytic–uraemic syndrome, systemic disease.

What do you know of G6PD deficiency?
Glucose-6-phosphate dehydrogenase (G6PD) deficiency is the most common enzyme disease of red blood cells. The enzyme G6PD is responsible for oxidizing glucose-6-phosphate to 6-phosphoglycerate, a reaction that happens within the red blood cells protecting them from oxidative stress. Deficiency of the enzyme is usually an X-linked inherited disorder that results in haemolytic anaemia in male patients. The severity of the haemolysis and the phenotypic

disease depends on the degree of the deficiency. The major symptoms include drug-induced haemolysis, favism, acute haemolysis in the context of acute illness or acute infections and chronic haemolytic anaemia in severe cases. In some countries screening for enzyme deficiency is part of their newborn screening test programmes. In countries where enzyme deficiency screening is not part of their routine newborn screening, screening of at-risk individuals prior to administering specific drugs that may cause severe haemolysis in the context of enzyme deficiency should be sought.

What are the main types of autoimmune haemolytic anaemias?
Haemolytic anaemias can be categorized into different groups dependent on:
- Where the red cell destruction takes place—intravascular or extravascular
- How long does the haemolytic episode last for—acute or chronic
- Whether they are linked to a genetic cause—inherited or acquired
- Whether they are immune related—autoimmune or nonimmune.

Autoimmune haemolytic anaemias (AIHA) are caused by antibodies that react with red blood cells causing cellular disruption in blood vessels or in the reticuloendothelial system, predominantly the spleen. There are two main types of autoimmune haemolytic anaemias: warm and cold such as chronic cold haemagglutinin disease and paroxysmal cold haemoglobinuria. Direct Coomb's test (DAT) is positive. Warm autoimmune haemolytic anaemia is due to antibodies—usually IgG—that are active at body temperature. Cold autoimmune haemolytic anaemia is due to antibodies—usually IgM—which do not attach to red blood cells in normal body temperature but do so at lower temperatures causing haemolysis. Conditions associated with warm AIHA are rheumatological disorders and SLE, lymphomas and CLL, certain drugs (methyldopa, quinine, interferon), and infections (COVID-19). Conditions associated with cold AIHA are infections (mycoplasma, EBV) and lymphomas.

What is Evan syndrome?
Evan syndrome is the concurrence of an autoimmune haemolytic anaemia with immune thrombocytopenia. Some patients may also have immune neutropenia or lymphopenia. It can be primary or secondary due to underlying malignancy or an autoimmune condition.

How do you confirm haemolysis?
Haemolysis as the underlying process of an identified anaemia is confirmed with blood tests. If a patient is found to be anaemic, primary investigations are a biochemical profile, a coagulation screen, iron and haematinic studies, and a blood film. These investigations will initially point towards the underlying pathophysiological process that has led to anaemia. Once metabolic causes have been excluded (iron, B_{12}, folate deficiency) and the initial screening suggests haemolysis (increased bilirubin, normal or low MCV, increased reticulocytes), then further tests can provide further light into the diagnosis of a haemolytic anaemia and the underlying cause for it. Haptoglobins are expected to be low in haemolysis, LDH should be raised, and DAT will be positive in AIHA. Blood film will confirm destruction of the red cells with specific forms seen in different kinds of anaemias (schistocytes, tear drop cells, intracellular organisms, etc.) (Fig. 55.1).

How is iron deficiency treated?
Iron deficiency is treated with iron replacement and tackling the underlying cause for the iron deficiency. Iron replacement can be given orally or parenterally with the route of replacement individualized to the patient. Oral iron replacement is not associated with any major risk or adverse reaction but it takes months, can lead to gastrointestinal side effects that can in turn affect compliance, and it cannot be absorbed well enough by patients suffering from bowel inflammation. Iron infusion replenishes the iron in the blood and iron stores quickly; it is effective in almost all patients receiving it but can lead to infusion-related and anaphylactic reactions and can only be

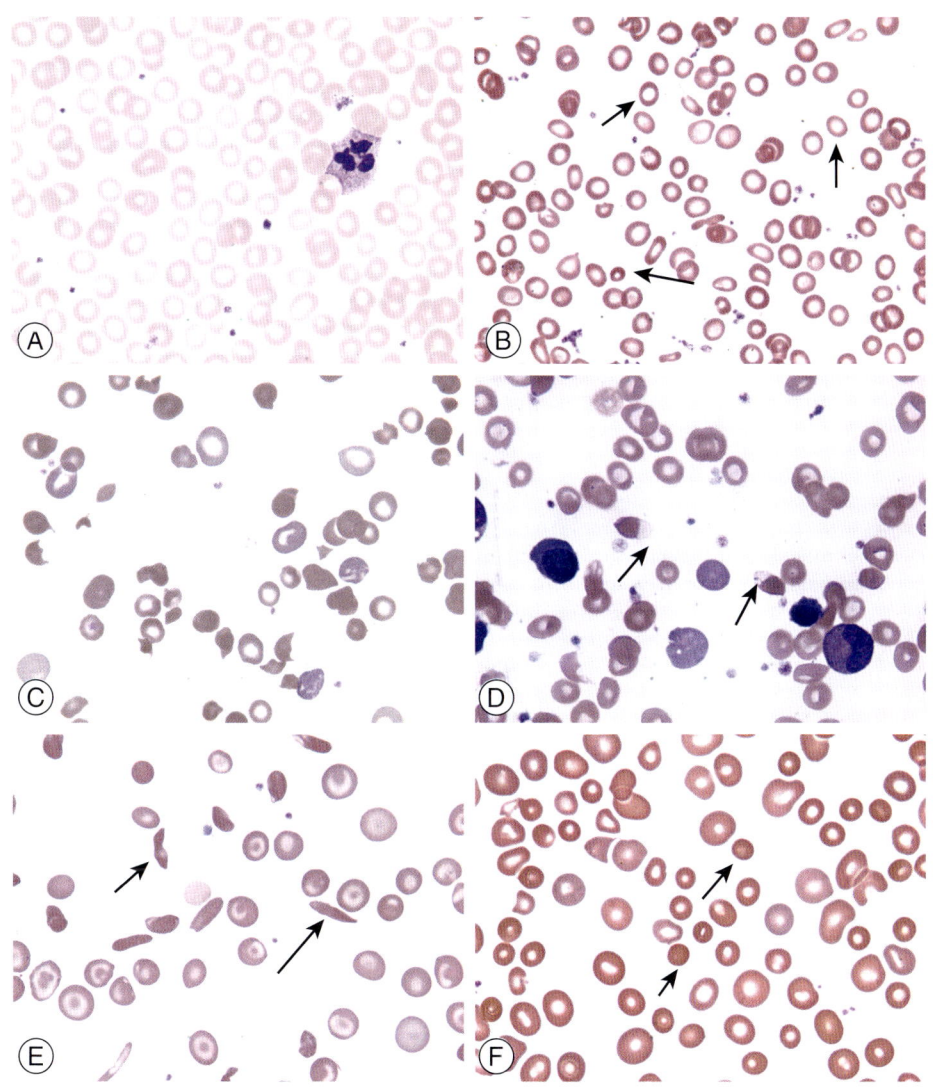

Fig. 55.1 Morphologic abnormalities of the red blood cell. **(A)** Normal, **(B)** hypochromic microcytes (iron deficiency), **(C)** schistocytes (haemolytic uremic syndrome), **(D)** blister cells (G6PD deficiency), **(E)** sickle cells (haemoglobin SS disease) and **(F)** spherocytes (autoimmune haemolytic anaemia). (*Courtesy* Trost B., Scott, J.P., 2016. In: Marcdante, K.J., Kilegman, R.M. (eds.), Mishra, O.P., Prabhu, S., Singh, S. (adaptation eds.), Nelson Essentials of Pediatrics, South Asia Edition. Elsevier, Gurgaon.)

done in a hospital environment. As well as replacing iron with oral or intravenous iron, patients have to be advised and investigated for the underlying cause of iron deficiency. Dietary advice regarding iron-rich foods should be given. Specific groups such as pregnant women will have physiologically increased iron requirements and these should be discussed with the patient. Adults with a normal diet who present with new iron-deficiency anaemia with no history of evident bleeding should undergo coeliac disease and thyroid function screening, and upper and lower endoscopy to identify or exclude gastrointestinal causes of blood loss.

Why may patients on vegan diet be depleted of vitamin B_{12} and how can the deficiency be prevented?

Cobalamin (vitamin B_{12}) is found in foods of animal origin—poultry, fish, meat, eggs, dairy products, clams. It is not found in plant-based foods. People who are vegan can have B_{12} intake from fortified foods like cereal or yeasts or by supplements. B_{12} supplements are oral tablets, lozenges, or sublingual sprays; all three similar in efficacy and absorption.

Name some complications of sickle cell disease.

- Sickle cell crises—occlusion of the small vessels caused by cell sickling resulting in bone pain accompanied by fever, splenic or hepatic sequestration crises with acute painful organ enlargement and acute chest syndrome with acute respiratory distress, pain, fever, and pulmonary infiltrates
- Anaemia—chronic haemolytic anaemia with a low but steady baseline haemoglobin around 8 g/dL, with episodes of acute drop in haemoglobin due to acute haemolytic crisis, splenic sequestration crisis, and aplastic crisis
- Infections—patients with sickle cell anaemia develop functional hyposplenism so they are at risk of infections with encapsulated bacteria. Patients with sickle cell disease are also at high risk for developing severe symptoms from SARS-CoV-2 viral infection.
- Thrombosis—patients with sickle cell disease are at increased risk of stroke and pulmonary thrombotic episodes. Patients with sickle cell disease are at risk of developing other intracranial complications apart from stroke, such as haemorrhage and seizures.
- Chronic complications—leg ulcers, cholelithiasis, tubulointerstitial nephritis, priapism, retinopathy, avascular necrosis of the hips, osteoporosis, diastolic dysfunction of the left ventricle, and pulmonary hypertension.

Further Information

Linus Pauling (1901–1994) is truly one of the greatest scientists of the 20th century and is the only person to receive two unshared Nobel prizes in different disciplines. Although he is perhaps most famous for his work in determining the properties of chemical bonds, he published the molecular genetic basis for sickle cell disease in 1949, the first description of a human disease caused by an abnormal protein.

CHAPTER 56

Bruising

Instruction
This 22-year-old man presented to his general practitioner with easy bruising. Please assess the patient and discuss further management.

Salient Features

HISTORY
- Associated trauma
- Systemic or other associated symptoms (detailed systemic enquiry of cardiovascular, neurological, and gastrointestinal symptomatology)
- Social history and sensitive enquiry of nonaccidental injury
- Location of bruising (significant if more than five lesions of more than 1 cm each)
- Recent operations or procedures
- Onset of symptoms/pattern of symptoms
- Other bleeding sites (haematemesis, haemarthrosis, haemoptysis, melaena, haematuria, epistaxis)
- Detailed drug history, including alcohol intake
- Medical history, including autoimmune conditions
- Family history of bleeding diathesis.

EXAMINATION
- Inspect the bruises and record:
  - Location (location of bruising is really important, as it helps to rule out nonaccidental trauma, as well as nontraumatic bruising)
  - Number and size (e.g. less than five lesions on one occasion with a small diameter less than 1 cm is not significant bruising, and possibly signifies minor trauma that the patient has no recollection of)
  - Age of bruises (the colour of the bruise can reveal the age)
- Differentiate from other forms of skin rashes that patients may refer to as bruises (telangiectasias, purpura, petechiae, pigmentation)

After inspection of the bruising, a general examination has to be performed, especially looking to elicit or exclude specific signs:
- Lymphadenopathy
- Organomegaly
- Stigmata of steroid use or Cushingoid features
- Stigmata of chronic liver disease
- Phenotypic features of disorders associated with increased bruising (Marfan, osteogenesis imperfecta)
- Systemic features of connective tissue disorders

- Signs of joint effusion or arthritis especially in large joints such as the knee
- Thyroid goitre
- Signs of cytopenias; pale sclera, recurrent infections.

Diagnosis

This patient has multiple bruises over his trunk and upper limbs with a history of spontaneous haemarthrosis (lesion), which makes a clotting disorder the most possible underlying cause (aetiology). He needs additional investigations to establish a diagnosis.

Questions

How would you investigate the patient?
The causes of bruising can be broadly classified into three main categories:
- Mechanical causes including blood vessel trauma
- Platelet dysfunction and cytopenias
- Coagulation problems.

To determine the cause, after careful history and examination, initial blood tests include full blood count with blood film, biochemical profile, and coagulation screen. Depending on the suspected cause or the abnormality revealed from the initial screening, further tests may need to follow.

Name some possible causes of thrombocytopenia associated with microangiopathic haemolytic anaemia.
- Thrombotic thrombocytopenic purpura (TTP)
- Haemolytic–uraemic syndrome
- Drug-induced thrombotic microangiopathy
- Disseminated intravascular coagulation
- Systemic illness (infection, autoimmune condition, malignancy).

What are the causes of prolonged prothrombin time with a normal activated partial thromboplastin time (APTT)?
As prothrombin time (PT) is used to evaluate the extrinsic and common pathway of clotting, it is raised in isolation in situations that affect the factors involved in the extrinsic pathway such as warfarin use, vitamin K deficiency, factor VII deficiency, and liver disease.

What do you know about von Willebrand disease?
This is the most common inherited bleeding disorder, affecting 1% of the population and is due to dysfunction of von Willebrand factor causing disturbed platelet adhesion. This leads to bleeding in the form of easy bruising, skin bleeding, and excessive mucosal bleeding. Von Willebrand factor consists of multimers and plays a major role in bridging between platelets and subendothelial tissue after an injury. Most affected patients will never express symptoms, but if the disease is symptomatic the treatment is with desmopressin, topical antifibrinolytic therapy, or von Willebrand replacement therapy.

What is haemophilia and what can you tell me about the genetics of this condition?
Haemophilia A is deficiency of factor VIII and haemophilia B is deficiency of factor IX (also known as Christmas disease), Both of these diseases are inherited in an X-linked recessive pattern and therefore present almost exclusively in males. Haemophilia C is a rare condition caused by deficiency of Factor XI inherited in an autosomal dominant pattern. Haemophilia A is the most

common type amongst all inherited haemophilias with approximately four times the incidence of Haemophilia B. Haemarthrosis is the most common site of bleeding and accounts for about 80% of all bleeding presentations. Currently, factor replacement therapy is the mainstay of treatment but recent developments mean that gene therapy delivered by viral vector is close to being a reality.

What are inhibitors in the context of bleeding disorders?
Inhibitors are neutralizing antibodies that often develop after repeated exposure to factor infusion, reducing the effectiveness of treatment. Treatment of inhibitor development is directed at reducing the production of inhibitors by immune tolerance induction with or without immunosuppression or, in Haemophlia A, the use of emicizumab, a biological monoclonal antibody.

Further Information

Queen Victoria (1819–1901) was a carrier of the haemophilia gene and passed it on to many of the Royal families of Europe via her daughters. Her son, Prince Leopold, had haemophilia and died following a fall.

John Otto, a physician from Philadelphia, first formally described a bleeding disorder which affected males, though clearly haemophilia was known for years before. The Talmud, a Jewish text, suggests not circumcising boys if two of his brothers had already died from the procedure, presumably due to the likelihood of the third son also having haemophilia and coming to harm at the end of a surgeon's knife.

CHAPTER 57

Multiple Myeloma

Instruction
This elderly patient presented with back pain and confusion. Please examine.

Salient Features

HISTORY
- Confusion, altered mental status, memory problems, bone pains, kidney stones, abdominal pains (symptoms suggesting hypercalcaemia)
- Dizziness, tiredness, fatigue, chest pains, palpitations (symptoms suggesting anaemia)
- Loss of height, bone pain, back pain, shoulder pain, sternal pain (symptoms from osteolytic lesions)
- Frequent infections (dysfunctional lymphocytes).

EXAMINATION
- Pallor
- Postural hypotension
- Peripheral neuropathy
- Confusion
- Abdominal and bony tenderness
- Splenomegaly, hepatomegaly
- Cachexia.

Questions

What is Castleman disease?
Castleman disease, also known as giant cell lymph node hyperplasia, is a group of lymphoproliferative disorders associated with infection with human herpesvirus 8 (HHV-8). Clinical features of the disease are fevers, weight loss, fatigue, night sweats, lymphadenopathy, organomegaly, oedema, skin changes, pulmonary disease. Patients have pancytopenia with polyclonal hypergammaglobulinaemia.

What is POEMS?
POEMS syndrome is a rare monoclonal gammopathy with a series of symptoms and signs that give rise to its name: **P**olyneuropathy, **O**rganomegaly, **E**ndocrinopathy, **M**onoclonal protein, and **S**kin changes. It is a monoclonal plasma disorder with overproduction of cytokines that lead to microangiopathy, neovascularization, and increased vascular permeability. All cases are associated with neuropathy, which is usually a peripheral symmetrical sensorimotor demyelinating neuropathy, increased protein in the CSF, and osteosclerotic bone lesions. The other features of the acronym are present in about 60% of the patients. Other clinical features of the

57 — MULTIPLE MYELOMA

syndrome can be weight loss, oedema, papilloedema, and Castleman disease. Immunofixation shows increased M protein with lambda light chain.

How is kidney disease caused in multiple myeloma?
Light chains form casts resulting in light-chain cast nephropathy. Light chains are excreted in the glomerulus and reabsorbed in the proximal tubule. When the rate of production and subsequent excretion of light chain is increased and resorptive capacity is exceeded, light chains remain in the tubules and form dense casts that obstruct the tubules. This in turn leads to inflammation and fibrosis. Resorbing large amounts of toxic light chains can directly harm the tubules and cause tubular dysfunction and interstitial nephritis. Deposition of light chains within the kidney can lead to amyloidosis and proteinuria or nephrotic syndrome. Medications used in multiple myeloma can be nephrotoxic causing a range of kidney pathology. All the aforementioned pathophysiologies can lead to kidney failure.

Name some complications of multiple myeloma that present as medical emergencies.
- Spinal cord compression and cauda equina syndrome
- Severe hypercalcaemia
- Symptomatic hyperviscosity
- Bacterial infection.

How can the anaemia of multiple myeloma be explained?
- Bone marrow is infiltrated with the clonal plasma cells.
- Kidney failure can cause reduction of erythropoietin.
- Some patients get a concurrent megaloblastic anaemia from B_{12} deficiency. It is not fully understood why this is the case, but it is probably multifactorial; clonal plasma cells with high turnover may be using a large proportion of the B_{12} needed for normal erythropoiesis, free light chains in the proximal tubule may interfere with B_{12} reabsorption, or free light chains may play an anti-intrinsic factor role, hence reducing the body's absorption of B_{12}.

A patient diagnosed with multiple myeloma reports that they are shorter than the information mentioned in their ID card. How would you explain that?
Osteolytic lesions in the vertebras can cause vertebral collapse and loss of height. One-fifth of patients with multiple myeloma will suffer from osteoporosis.

What do you know of IgM multiple myeloma?
Multiple myeloma is usually an IgG gammopathy (50%). Less frequently multiple myeloma is associated with non-IgG heavy chain paraprotein (IgA 20%) or light chain kappa or lambda detected as free light chains in urine electrophoresis (Bence Jones). Multiple myeloma with IgM paraprotein is very rare (<1%). IgM paraproteinaemia is caused by Waldenstrom's macroglobulinaemia (WM), unless it is associated with osteolytic lesions or translocation t(11;14) where a diagnosis of IgM multiple myeloma is given. The differentiation of the two conditions can be done by cytogenetic analysis.

WM is an IgM monoclonal gammopathy. Clinical features are due to bone marrow infiltration, hyperviscosity syndrome due to IgM paraprotein, constitutional symptoms, and infections. Patients with WM usually have pancytopenia with elevated LDH, β-2 microglobulin, and IgM paraprotein in the serum electrophoresis and immunofixation and bone marrow aspirate shows infiltration by small lymphocytes with plasma cell differentiation.

The diagnosis of WM is established with the combination of an IgM paraprotein in the blood with lymphoplasmacytic lymphoma in the bone marrow. Treatment of WM is indicated in symptomatic disease in order to control symptoms. Hyperviscosity requires plasmapheresis.

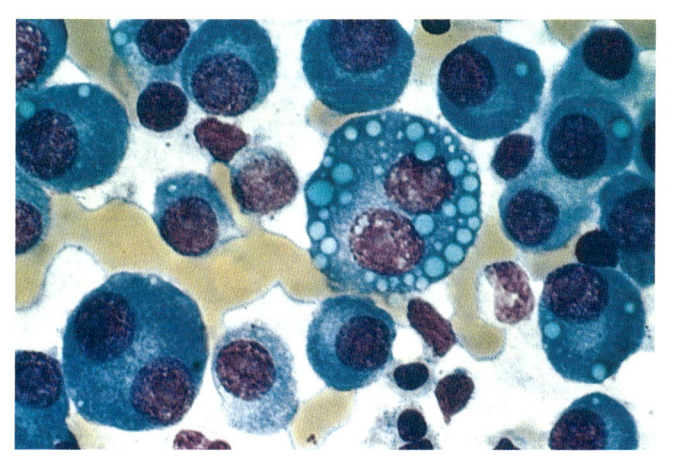

Fig. 57.1 Multiple myeloma. (With permission from Abbas, A.K., Aster, J.C., Kumar, V., 2021. Robbins & Cotran Pathologic Basis of Disease, tenth edn. Elsevier.)

What does the bone marrow of patients with multiple myeloma look like?
Bone marrow aspirate demonstrates clonal plasma cells in a concentration of >10% (multiple myeloma Fig. 57.1).

What are the diagnostic criteria for multiple myeloma?
According to the Revised International Myeloma Working Group diagnostic criteria are:
Clonal bone marrow plasma cells >10% or biopsy proven plasmacytoma (bony or extramedullary) and any of the:
- End-organ damage that can be attributed to multiple myeloma (CRAB—raised **c**alcium, **r**enal failure, **a**naemia, **b**one osteolytic lesions) *or*
- Any of these criteria; plasma cell percentage in the bone marrow >60%, involved:uninvolved serum-free light-chain ratio >100, more than one focal lesion on MRI of 5 mm or more.

What is MGUS?
When a paraprotein is detected but in quantities <30 g/L, the bone marrow infiltration is less than 10% and there is no evidence of end-organ damage, then the gammopathy is not called multiple myeloma but monoclonal gammopathy of undetermined significance (MGUS).

How does hyperviscosity syndrome present?
Blurring of vision, deafness, tinnitus, gingival bleeding, vertigo, ataxia, diplopia, confusion, stroke, coma, papilloedema, bleeding.

What is the treatment for multiple myeloma?
Autologous haematopoietic cell transplantation or chemotherapy (bortezomib, lenalidomide, daratumumab) or a combination is given to patients with multiple myeloma and the choice of treatment will depend on the patient's comorbid state, frailty, and functional status, as well as patient choices.

What depositions can occur in multiple myeloma?
- Light chain deposition disease (fragments of light chains)

- Heavy chain deposition disease (abnormal heavy chains without the light component of the immunoglobulin)
- Amyloid light chain (AL) amyloidosis (primary amyloidosis, monoclonal light chains form fibrils).

How are the different organs affected in AL amyloidosis?
In primary amyloidosis small fragments of monoclonal light chains form fibrils which in turn deposit in different tissues causing multiorgan damage. Depending on the site of deposition, AL amyloidosis can affect a number of organs creating a series of clinical pictures. Some examples are:
- Kidneys—proteinuria or nephrotic syndrome
- Heart—restrictive cardiomyopathy
- Peripheral nerves—peripheral neuropathy
- Liver—coagulopathy and liver failure
- Muscles and joints—hypertrophy and arthropathy
- Skin—subcutaneous nodules.

Further Information

POEMS syndrome was given this name by Bardwick in 1980 after a report of two monoclonal gammopathy cases with the same characteristics.

CHAPTER 58

Myelodysplastic Syndrome

Instruction

This patient presents with recurrent infections and easy bruising. Please examine.

Salient Features

HISTORY

- Recurrent infections—most commonly bacterial infections, skin infections, and throat infections
- Symptoms of anaemia—fatigue, tiredness, reduced exercise tolerance, orthostatic hypotension, palpitations, angina, exertional chest pain, exertional dyspnoea, syncopal episodes, dizziness, memory problems, cognitive impairment, lethargy, exhaustion
- Constitutional symptoms—fatigue, night sweats, fevers, unintentional weight loss.

EXAMINATION

- Cachexia, pallor, tachycardia
- Signs of anaemia, thrombocytopenia, and neutropenia
- Skin involvement with ulcerations, bruising, petechiae, cutaneous rashes, mucosal ulceration, Sweet syndrome
- Organomegaly
- Autoimmune phenomena with pericardial effusion, pleural effusions, rheumatoid arthritis.

Diagnosis

This elderly gentleman presents with pallor, large ecchymoses, and splenomegaly (lesions) which may be caused by myelodysplasia (aetiology). He is short of breath, likely due to anaemia (functional status).

Questions

What does the blood film show in myelodysplastic syndrome (MDS)?

The peripheral blood shows anaemia, leucopenia, and thrombocytopenia. Almost all patients have anaemia which may be normocytic or macrocytic with low reticulocyte count. If reticulocyte count is elevated, that may represent an accompanying autoimmune haemolytic anaemia or pseudoreticulocytosis. Half of patients have leucopenia and neutropenia with immature neutrophils in the peripheral blood. One-quarter of patients have thrombocytopenia with morphologically normal or small platelets, while specific mutations (JAK2 and SF3B1) are associated with thrombocytosis.

58—MYELODYSPLASTIC SYNDROME

What does the bone marrow look like?
Bone marrow aspirate shows hypercellular dysplasia with increased myeloblasts and myeloid cells at different stages of maturation with abnormal localization of immature precursors, different stages of erythroid cells in increased numbers, abnormally big or abnormally small megakaryocytes, and bone marrow fibrosis.

How is MDS classified according the WHO?
MDS in the adult population is classified against specific criteria:
- number of dysplastic lineages
- percentage of blasts in bone marrow and the number of blasts in peripheral blood
- specific cytogenetic findings
- percentage of ring sideroblasts
- cell type affected causing cytopenia (neutrophils, platelets, and red blood cells).

How do you establish the diagnosis of MDS?
The diagnosis is established by the clinical picture, the laboratory findings in the peripheral blood showing cytopenia and the bone marrow aspirate demonstrating dysplasia. Cytochemistry can help with classifying the specific MDS abnormality.

Which other conditions can cause myelodysplasia?
Other conditions that can cause myelodysplasia are different haematological malignancies (AML), B_{12} and folate deficiency, HIV infection, lead poisoning, alcohol abuse, drug toxicity (antibiotics, immunosuppressants, antivirals), sideroblastic anaemias.

What is Sweet syndrome?
Sweet syndrome is characterized by abrupt onset of painful erythematous skin plaques or nodules with accompanying pyrexia in the background of an underlying haematological malignancy (MDS Fig. 58.1).

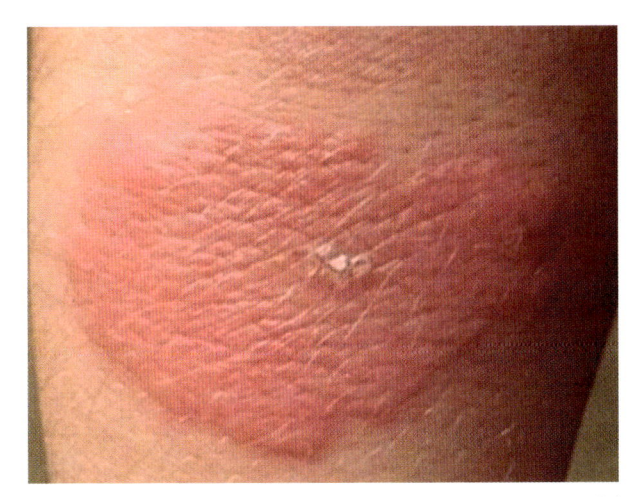

Fig. 58.1 Sweet syndrome, also known as acute febrile neutrophilic dermatosis, is an inflammatory disease that clinically presents with fever and an abrupt onset of neutrophil-rich skin lesions. (With permission from Lebwohl, M.G., Coulson, I.H., James, W.D., Gowda, A., Wanat, K.A., Murrell, D.F., Heymann, W.R., 2022. Treatment of Skin Disease: Comprehensive Therapeutic Strategies, sixth edn. Elsevier.)

What is the prognosis in MDS?

Prognosis of MDS varies amongst patients and depends on clinical and molecular factors. Increased age with poor performance status on diagnosis is a bad prognostic factor. A worse outcome is expected when more blood cell lines are affected and the more severe the cytopenia the worse the prognosis. Aside from clinical and laboratory factors, specific cytogenetic and molecular characteristics are paired with bad or good outcomes in MDS. There are several prognostication models used to predict outcomes in MDS. One of the most widely used is the IPSS-R model (international prognostic scoring system—revised), taking into account the factors described earlier. Each factor adds 0–2 points on a scale and then prognostication is based on median survival from diagnosis.

Further Information

R.D. Sweet (1917–2001), a British dermatologist who described what came to be known as Sweet syndrome in 1964.

CHAPTER 59

Chronic Lymphocytic Leukaemia

Instruction
Perform a general examination of this patient.

Salient Features
HISTORY
- Asymptomatic in 50% of patients, onset is insidious
- Palpable lymph nodes
- Left upper quadrant abdominal discomfort or early satiety secondary to splenomegaly
- Predisposition to infections
- Bleeding or bruising is rare
- Symptoms of anaemia are uncommon
- Weight loss, fever, and night sweats are unusual.

EXAMINATION
- Usually men over the age of 40 years (male:female ratio is 2:1)
- Symmetrical, painless, rubbery lymph nodes
- Liver or spleen may be palpable
- Leukaemia cutis can present as painless papules or different form of skin lesions.

Proceed as follows:
- Tell the examiner that you would like to do a full blood count and examine the peripheral smear (lymphocytosis >15 × 10^9 cells/L, with mature appearance of small lymphocytes) (CLL Fig. 59.1).

Remember that chronic lymphocytic leukaemia manifests clinically with organ infiltration with lymphocytes, immunosuppression (hypogammaglobulinaemia), and bone marrow failure.

Diagnosis
This elderly male patient with painless enlargement of lymph nodes probably has chronic lymphocytic leukaemia (lesion). He has severe pallor indicating Binet stage C (functional status).

Questions
What are the causes of anaemia in chronic lymphocytic leukaemia?
- Bone marrow infiltration
- Autoimmune (Coombs' positive) haemolysis
- Increased tumour necrosis factor leading to suppressed red cell production.

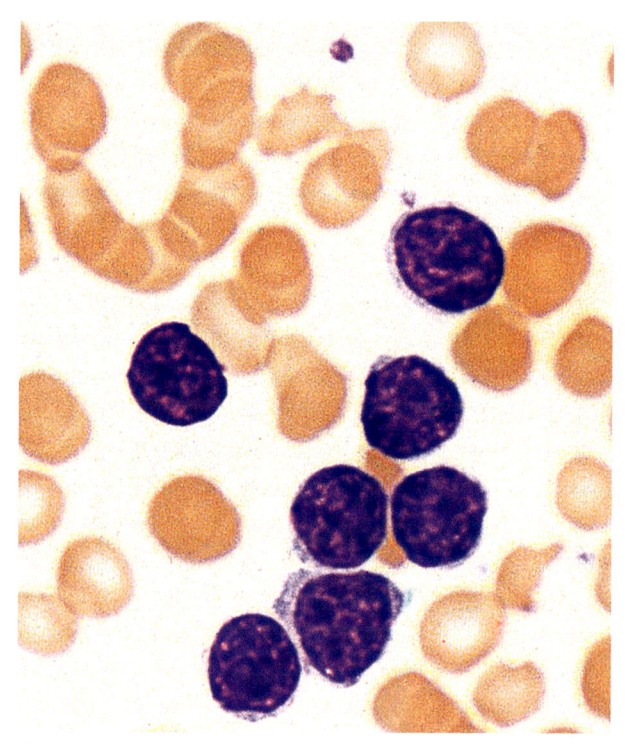

Fig. 59.1 Peripheral blood smear demonstrating lymphocytosis: small lymphocytes with condensed chromatin, imparting a 'soccer ball' pattern, and scant cytoplasm (Wright stain). (With permission from Hsi, E.D., 2009. The leukemias of mature lymphocytes. Hematol./Oncol. Clin. North Am. 23, 843–871.)

How may a patient with chronic lymphocytic leukaemia present?
- About 50% of cases are asymptomatic; some complain of generalized malaise, weight loss, night sweats, and loss of appetite; others complain of bleeding.

What is the prognosis in chronic lymphocytic leukaemia?
About one-third of the patients will not require treatment and die from unrelated causes; in another third, the disease is initially indolent followed by rapid progression. In the remaining third the disease is very aggressive from the outset and needs immediate treatment.

How is chronic lymphocytic leukaemia staged?
- Binet staging (evaluates the enlargement of spleen, liver, and lymph nodes in the head and neck, axillae, and groin) has three stages, A–C:
  A: no anaemia or thrombocytopenia and less than three areas of lymphoid enlargement
  B: no anaemia or thrombocytopenia, with three or more involved areas
  C: anaemia and/or thrombocytopenia, regardless of the number of areas of lymphoid enlargement.
- Rai staging has five stages, 0–IV:
  0: lymphocytosis only (in blood and bone marrow)
  I: lymphocytosis plus lymphadenopathy
  II: lymphocytosis with hepatic and/or splenic enlargement
  III: lymphocytosis with anaemia
  IV: lymphocytosis with thrombocytopenia.

The primary role of the Rai and Binet staging systems is to help clinicians to decide when to initiate treatment.

How is staging and overall prognosis related?
The Binet and Rai staging systems are very helpful tools based on clinical examination and help clinicians to decide when it is appropriate to initiate treatment. When used in isolation they cannot predict the clinical course with precision and therefore are less helpful in predicting long-term prognosis. There are multiple factors associated with aggressive disease, such as determination of immunoglobulin variable gene (*V*-gene) mutation status, lymphocyte doubling duration, raised β-2 microglobulin, expression of CD38, and zeta-chain-associated protein 70 (ZAP-70) levels.

As the prognosis of the disease and the treatment combination available vary, clinicians need to be able to predict prognosis with specific treatment given. Efforts have been made in this direction and the "four-factor" prognostic model is an example. The model is used to predict outcome in patients starting treatment with ibrutinib. This model takes into consideration Del(17p), TP53 mutation, raised β2 microglobulin, raised lactate dehydrogenase (LDH), and relapse or refractory disease and puts patients into three risk groups (low, intermediate, and high) with different rates of progression free survival and overall survival.

What do you know about the pathogenesis of chronic lymphocytic leukaemia?
Chronic lymphocytic leukaemia is a heterogeneous disease that originates from B-lymphocytes, which may differ in activation, maturation state, or cellular subgroup. The B-lymphocytes are antigen experienced (differ in the level of immunoglobulin *V*-gene mutations). The accumulation of leukaemic cells occurs because of survival signals delivered to a subgroup of leukaemic cells from the external environment through a variety of receptors (e.g. B-cell receptors and chemokine and cytokine receptors) and their cell-bound and soluble ligands.

How are patients with chronic lymphocytic leukaemia treated?
- Stage A. Specific treatment may not be indicated until stage B or C. Patients with stage A disease should be reassured that, despite the frightening diagnosis of leukaemia, they will be able to live a normal life for many years, with a median survival of 10 years.
- Stage B and C. Patients will require specific and supportive therapy: correction of anaemia and folic acid deficiency, and correction of bone marrow infiltration initially with prednisolone and oxymetholone and subsequently with chemotherapeutic agents.

Standard treatment currently is with fludarabine, cyclophosphamide, and rituximab. For elderly or frail patients, a combination or chlorambucil with an antiCD20 antibody (obinutuzumab, rituximab, or ofatumumab) or ibrutinib is used. Refractory disease may be treated with bendamustine (plus rituximab), alemtuzumab, lenalidomide, ofatumumab, ibrutinib, idelalisib, or venetoclax. Those relapsing with TP53 mutations or deletions of 17p may be considered for allogeneic stem cell transplant.

What is Richter syndrome?
This is when chronic lymphocytic leukaemia is transformed into an aggressive large cell lymphoma. There is a median survival of <1 year after its appearance.

Which lymphomas can convert to leukaemias?
- Small cell lymphoma (chronic lymphocytic leukaemia)
- Burkitt lymphoma (B cell acute lymphoblastic leukaemia)
- Lymphoblastic lymphoma (T cell acute lymphoblastic leukaemia).

CHAPTER 60

Chronic Myeloid Leukaemia

Instruction

This patient was found to have an abnormal full blood count with basophilia and neutrophilia. Please examine.

Salient Features

HISTORY

- Unintentional weight loss
- Fevers and night sweats
- Abdominal fullness
- Abdominal pain
- Fatigue
- Bleeding.

EXAMINATION

- Pallor (anaemia)
- Splenomegaly
- Abdominal tenderness (splenomegaly)
- Gout tophi (overproduction of uric acid)
- Sternum tenderness on palpation (bone marrow expansion).

Questions

What is the underlying genetic involved in the pathophysiology of chronic myeloid leukaemia (CML)?
The Philadelphia chromosome. In CML a translocation between two genes—BCR on chromosome 22 and ABL on chromosome 9—results in the creation of the fusion gene BCR:ABL and the new chromosome 22 with the fusion gene is called Philadelphia chromosome (Ph).

The end result of the fusion gene is the creation of a tyrosine kinase that is not regulated and leads to uncontrolled production of myeloid cells.

What is the prognosis in chronic myeloid leukaemia?
The mean life expectancy of patients with the disease is almost normal compared to the general population. However, there are good and bad prognostic factors that are taken into account at diagnosis and affect the general prognosis and life expectancy.

Do you know of any prognostic models for survival in CML?
There are several risk stratification scores used in clinical practice to guide treatment. Most of them take into account the age of diagnosis, the immature myeloblasts seen in the peripheral blood smear, the size of the spleen, and the number of platelets in the peripheral blood count.

60 – CHRONIC MYELOID LEUKAEMIA

What are some poor prognostic factors for CML?
- Increasing white cell count in blood
  - >10% blast cells in the peripheral blood film
  - >20% basophils in the peripheral blood firm
- Thrombocytopenia in the peripheral blood film
- Progressing splenomegaly
- Development of chromosomal abnormalities additional to the Philadelphia chromosome (e.g. trisomy 19, trisomy 8, second Philadelphia).

All aforementioned are features of the accelerated phase of CML and response to treatment is poor.

What are the phases of CML?
- Chronic phase
- Accelerated phase
- Blast crisis.

Which haematological malignancies come under the umbrella of myeloproliferative disorders?
- Chronic myeloid leukaemia
- Polycythaemia rubra vera
- Essential thrombocythaemia
- Myelofibrosis.

They are all clonal disorders of the stem cells with tendency to progress to acute leukaemia.

How do the peripheral blood film and the bone marrow aspirate look under direct microscopy?
The blood film shows leucocytosis with all series of neutrophils present, from blasts to mature myelocytes and basophilia (CML Fig. 60.1). The bone marrow aspirate shows granulocytic hyperplasia also with all series present (CML Fig. 60.2).

What do you know of the Pelger–Huet neutrophils?
Pelger–Huet anomaly is an inherited nonsignificant blood dyscrasia where neutrophilic nuclei are unusually shaped (peanut or dumbbell shaped). In the accelerated phase of CML Pelger–Huet-like neutrophils can be seen in the peripheral blood film.

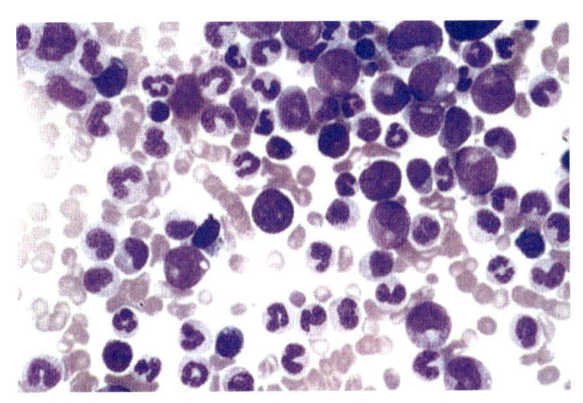

Fig. 60.1 Blood film in chronic myeloid leukaemia. Note the large numbers of granulocytic cells, in particular neutrophils, at all stages of development. (Parveen, K., Michael, C., 2020. Kumar & Clark's Cases in Clinical Medicine, fourth edn. Elsevier.)

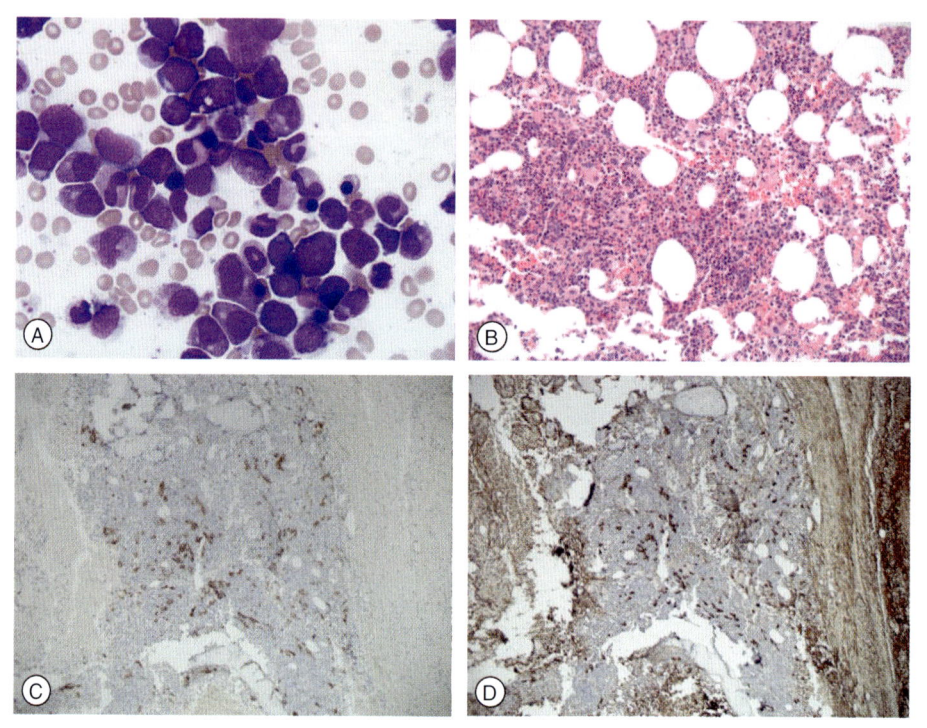

Fig. 60.2 Representative views of **(A)** bone marrow aspirate and **(B)** trephine demonstrating changes of chronic myeloid leukaemia in accelerated phase; **(C)** kappa staining and **(D)** CD138.

Can the Philadelphia chromosome be found in other types of leukaemia?
Rarely patients with other myeloproliferative disorders other than CML or lymphomas can have the Philadelphia chromosome. Patients with acute leukaemia may also have the chromosome, but that is probably because CML was undiagnosed and the patient was diagnosed during a blast crisis (acute leukaemia).

What are the treatment options for CML?
- Allogenic haematopoietic cell transplantation
- Tyrosine kinase inhibitors (imatinib).

Further Information
Philadelphia chromosome was discovered and linked with malignancy in 1960 by Peter Nowell (University of Pennsylvania School of Medicine) and David Hungerford (Fox Chase Cancer Centre) and it was named after the city of Philadelphia where it was discovered.

Huet—Dutch paediatrician who discovered the eponymous condition in 1931.

CHAPTER 61

Acute Leukaemia

Instruction

This 65-year-old man is referred to you with pancytopenia. Please examine him and advise on further management.

Salient Features

HISTORY

- Weakness, fatigue, malaise
- Dyspnoea, dizziness
- Headache
- Spontaneous bleeding
- Easy or spontaneous bruising
- Fever
- Weight loss
- Night sweats
- Rashes
- Recurrent infections
- Abdominal pain
- Gum hypertrophy.

EXAMINATION

- Pale sclera
- Pallor
- Gingival hyperplasia and haemorrhages
- Lymphadenopathy
- Organomegaly
- Leukaemia cutis or other skin manifestations
- Petechiae, ecchymoses
- Focal neurological findings.

Diagnosis

This usually fit and well man presents with widespread ecchymoses and spontaneous severe epistaxis (lesions). Blood examination shows pancytopenia caused by acute myeloid leukaemia (AML) (aetiology).

231

Questions

Which is the commonest acute leukaemia in adults?
AML—80% of acute leukaemias.

What is the pathognomonic cell found in peripheral blood film of patients with AML?
The peripheral blood film of a patient with AML shows myeloblasts with increased nucleus:cytoplasm ratio. Some of the myeloblasts have a red rod-like structure in the cytoplasm called an Auer rod (Fig. 61.1). The Auer rods are a pathognomonic finding of AML.

How is AML diagnosed?
The diagnosis of AML is established when bone marrow aspirate and peripheral blood film confirm presence of blasts of myeloid origin or a specific genetic abnormality has been confirmed by cytogenetic analysis.

What do you know about acute promyelocytic leukaemia (APML)?
APML is a distinct variant of AML. Some 92% of patients with APML have a characteristic cytogenetic abnormality; translocation t(15;17). This translocation is between the RAR (retinoic acid receptor) alpha gene and the promyelocytic leukaemia (PML) gene and results in the creation of two fusion genes. APML is a medical emergency, as patients present with severe coagulopathy, disseminated intravascular coagulation, and life-threatening bleeding. It is characterized by the presence of atypical promyelocytes in the blood film and bone marrow (Fig. 61.2). It is treated with all-trans retinoic acid (ATRA) with potential cure.

Name some causes of gingival hyperplasia.
- AML
- Poor dental hygiene
- Smoking
- Diabetes
- Scurvy
- Autoimmune conditions
- Ciclosporin, phenytoin, calcium channel blockers
- HIV, Kaposi sarcoma.

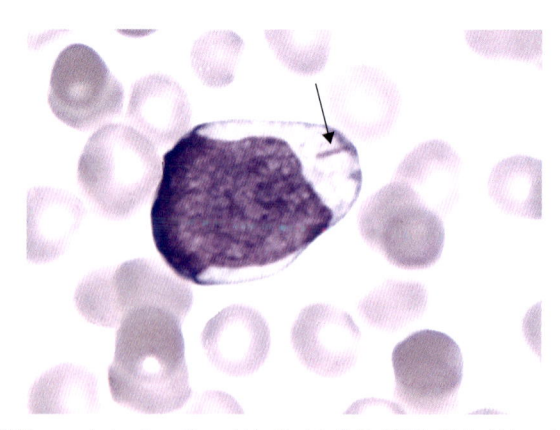

Fig. 61.1 Auer rod. (With permission from Carr, J.H., Rodak, B.F., 2009. Clinical Hematology Atlas, third edn. Saunders, St Louis, MO.)

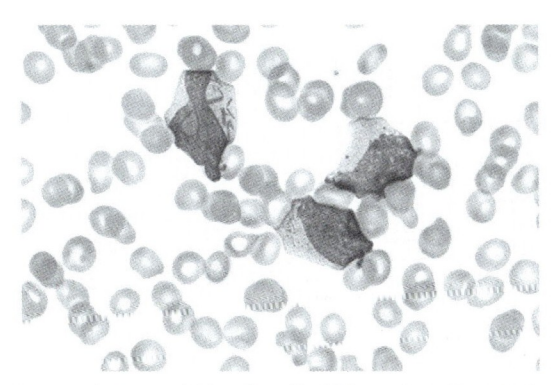

Fig. 61.2 Promyelocytes are large myeloid cells with high nucleus to cytoplasmic ratio, prominent nucleoli, and violet granules in the cytoplasm. The cells of acute promyelocytic leukemia (APL) are Pelger–Huet-like cells. (With permission from Isaacs, D., Anazodo, A., O'Brien, T., South, M., South, M., 2012. Practical Paediatrics, seventh edn. Elsevier.)

Name some life-threatening complications of AML.
- Tumour lysis syndrome—this is caused by rapid cell death following chemotherapy. The lymphocyte cell death is accompanied by phosphate and potassium release and purine nucleic acids in the blood causing hyperkalaemia, hyperphosphataemia, and hyperuricaemia.
- Bleeding—bleeding occurs in acute leukaemia because of thrombocytopenia, platelet dysfunction, and disseminated intravascular coagulopathy.
- Neutropenic sepsis—as with all malignancies treated with chemotherapy, neutropenic sepsis needs to be suspected even with mild symptoms, and appropriate treatment must be given while waiting for investigation and culture results. Neutropenic patients are at risk of bacterial, fungal, and viral infections that may not cause problems in the immunocompetent adult.
- Leukostasis with respiratory failure—this is one of the complications of an extremely elevated lymphocyte number in the bloodstream and can lead to death if left untreated.

How common is acute lymphoblastic leukaemia (ALL) in the adult population?
ALL is not common in adults. It represents less than 20% of the acute leukaemias overall.

What are the cytogenetics of ALL?
Myeloperoxidase (MPO) negative
Periodic acid-Schiff (PAS) positive.

Name some causes of lymphocytosis.
- Chronic lymphocytic leukaemia
- ALL
- Lymphoma
- Viral infection (EBV, CMV, HIV)
- Smoking
- Lead toxicity
- Autoimmune disorders
- Toxoplasmosis
- Pertussis.

How can leukostasis present?
Leukostasis is a complication of hyperleukocytosis in leukaemias, most commonly occurring in acute leukaemias. The combination of an increased number of lymphocytes with the existence of rigid blast cells in the blood can lead to hyperviscocity and cell plugging in the microcirculation of different organs, most commonly causing respiratory and neurological complications. Leukostasis can lead to death. The treatment consists of reduction of the lymphocytes with chemotherapy while supportive measures such as hydration and prevention of tumour lysis syndrome are essential.

Why are patients with acute leukaemia prone to bleeding and bruising?
Patients with acute leukaemia may have a low platelet count, and their platelets may be immature and not functioning correctly. The combination of a low platelet level with the remaining cells dysfunctional leads to bleeding diathesis. In addition, there are types of acute leukaemia, e.g. APML, that are complicated with DIC.

How does the differentiation syndrome present?
Differentiation syndrome usually occurs in the days or weeks after receiving chemotherapy with ATRA in APML. The symptoms are usually water retention with peripheral oedema and pleural effusions, accompanied with fever and circulatory collapse. It is complicated with acute respiratory and renal failure. Treatment is with supportive care and systemic steroids.

What are the types of AML according to the WHO 2016 classification?
- AML with recurrent genetic abnormalities
  - AML with t(8;21)(q22;q22.1);*RUNX1-RUNX1T1*
  - AML with inv(16)(p13.1q22) or t(16;16)(p13.1;q22);*CBFB-MYH11*
  - Acute promyelocytic leukemia (APL) with *PML-RARA*
  - AML with t(9;11)(p21.3;q23.3);*MLLT3-KMT2A*
  - AML with t(6;9)(p23;q34.1);*DEK-NUP214*
  - AML with inv(3)(q21.3q26.2) or t(3;3)(q21.3;q26.2);*GATA2, MECOM*
  - AML (megakaryoblastic) with t(1;22)(p13.3;q13.3);*RBM15-MKL1*
  - AML with mutated *NPM1*
  - AML with biallelic mutations of *CEBPA*.
- AML with myelodysplasia-related changes
- Therapy-related myeloid neoplasms
- AML, NOS (not otherwise specified)
  - AML with minimal differentiation
  - AML without maturation
  - AML with maturation
  - Acute myelomonocytic leukaemia
  - Acute monoblastic/monocytic leukaemia
  - Pure erythroid leukaemia
  - Acute megakaryoblastic leukaemia
  - Acute basophilic leukaemia
  - Acute panmyelosis with myelofibrosis.

CHAPTER 62

Lymphadenopathy

Instruction

This woman presents with fever. Perform a general examination.
Examine this patient's neck.

Salient Features

HISTORY AND EXAMINATION

Use the mnemonic ALL AGES to approach a patient with lymphadenopathy:
- ALL:
  - **A**ge at presentation (e.g. infectious mononucleosis is commoner in younger age groups, Hodgkin disease has a bimodal peak)
  - **L**ocation(s) of enlarged lymph nodes: those outside the inguinal regions (enlarged for >4 weeks and measuring 1 cm² or larger without an obvious diagnosis should be considered for biopsy)
  - **L**ength of time the lymph nodes are present.
- AGES:
  - **A**ssociated symptoms and signs including fever ('B' symptoms: temperature >38°C, drenching night sweats, unexplained weight loss >10% body weight)
  - **G**eneralized lymph node enlargement
  - **E**xtranodal organ involvement
  - **S**plenomegaly: consider infectious mononucleosis, lymphoma, chronic lymphocytic leukaemia, and acute leukaemia; rare in metastatic cancer.
- As soon as you feel a group of lymph nodes, examine drainage areas for obvious pathology. For example:
  - Inguinal lymph nodes: examine the lower limbs and external genitalia
  - Axillary lymph nodes: examine the chest, breasts, and upper limbs
  - Upper cervical lymph nodes: examine the chest, breast, and upper limbs; also, perform an ear, nose, and throat examination for nasopharyngeal carcinoma
  - Lower cervical and supraclavicular lymph nodes: examine the thyroid, chest, abdomen for gastric carcinoma (Virchow nodes), and testes.
- Examine other lymph node areas in a systematic manner: submental, submandibular, deep cervical (upper and lower), occipital, posterior triangle, supraclavicular, axillary, epitrochlear, and inguinal.
- Examine the mouth for the following signs:
  - Oral and oropharyngeal tumours
  - Palatal petechiae and pharyngitis (glandular fever).
- Examine the abdomen for liver and spleen
- Examine the chest and do chest radiography for lung cancer and tuberculosis (TB).

Diagnosis

This patient has generalized lymphadenopathy, probably a lymphoma—either Hodgkin or non-Hodgkin (aetiology)—and has severe disease, as evidenced by alopecia, presumably caused by chemotherapy (functional status). I would like to discuss other causes of generalized lymphadenopathy.

Questions

What are the causes of regional lymphadenopathy?
- Cervical lymphadenopathy—causes include infections and malignancies. Infectious causes include bacterial pharyngitis, dental abscess, otitis media, infectious mononucleosis, cytomegalovirus, gonococcal pharyngitis, toxoplasmosis, hepatitis, and adenovirus. Malignancies include non-Hodgkin disease, Hodgkin disease, and squamous cell carcinoma of head and neck.
- Virchow node (anterior left supraclavicular lymph node; also known as Troiser ganglion)—enlargement suggests the presence of a thoracic or abdominal neoplasm. Common causes include carcinoma of breast, bronchus, lymphomas, and gastrointestinal neoplasms.
- Delphian node (a midline prelaryngeal lymph node)—heralds thyroid disease, laryngeal malignancy, or lymphoma
- Axillary lymphadenopathy—causes include infections and malignancies. Infectious causes include staphylococcal, streptococcal infections of the arm, cat-scratch fever, tularaemia, and sporotrichosis. Malignant causes, including Hodgkin disease, non-Hodgkin lymphoma, carcinoma of breast, and melanoma, are common.
- Epitrochlear lymphadenopathy—the most common causes are lymphoma/chronic lymphatic leukaemia and infectious mononucleosis. Other diagnoses include HIV, sarcoidosis, and connective tissue disorders. In developing countries, secondary syphilis, lepromatous leprosy, leishmaniasis, and rubella are important causes.
- Inguinal lymphadenopathy—in adults, some degree of lymph node enlargement is not uncommon. In those who walk outdoors with footwear, benign reactive lymphadenopathy is common. Malignant causes include lymphoma, malignant melanoma, and carcinoma of external genitalia. Benign causes include cellulitis, syphilis, chancroid, genital herpes, and lymphogranuloma venereum.
- Node of Cloquet (also known as Rosenmüller node)—a deep inguinal lymph node located near the femoral canal. When palpable, it may be mistaken for an inguinal hernia.

What are the causes of generalized lymphadenopathy?
- Lymphomas, chronic lymphatic leukaemia, acute lymphoblastic leukaemia
- Glandular fever, cytomegalovirus
- HIV infection, toxoplasmosis
- Systemic lupus erythematosus, rheumatoid arthritis, sarcoid
- Chronic infections such as TB, secondary syphilis, brucellosis
- Drugs: phenytoin.

(Use the mnemonic CHICAGO: **c**ancers, **h**ypersensitivity, **i**nfections, **c**onnective tissue disorders, **a**typical lymphoproliferative disorders, **g**ranulomatous disorders, **o**ther unusual causes.)

What do you understand by the term Hodgkin disease?

Hodgkin disease is a group of neoplasms characterized by Reed–Sternberg cells in an appropriate reactive cellular background. It is divided into several subtypes histologically: lymphocyte predominance, nodular sclerosis, mixed cellularity, and lymphocyte depletion. The Reed–Sternberg cell is a giant cell with two or more nuclear lobes and huge eosinophilic inclusion-like nucleoli.

62 – LYMPHADENOPATHY

The classic Reed–Sternberg cell has a symmetrical, mirror image nucleus that creates an 'owl-eye' appearance.

What is the cause of egg-shaped calcification in hilar lymph nodes?
Silicosis.

What do you know of Sister Joseph nodule?
It is a classic sign of gastric adenocarcinoma in the umbilical area and may represent a metastatic deposit or an enlarged anterior abdominal wall lymph node (Fig. 62.1).

What is the mode of presentation of Hodgkin disease?
- Usually as a painless lymphadenopathy
- Other presenting symptoms: systemic symptoms such as fever, weight loss, drenching night sweats, generalized pruritus, or pain in the affected lymph node following the ingestion of alcohol.

How is Hodgkin disease staged?
The staging system has four stages (I–IV) plus a system of letters to indicate symptoms, bulk, lymph node involvement.
  Stage I: one lymph node region involved
  Stage II: more than two lymph node regions involved on one side of the diaphragm
  Stage III: lymph nodes involved on both sides of the diaphragm
    3.1: with splenic hilar, coeliac, or portal nodes
    3.2: with paraaortic, iliac, or mesenteric nodes
  Stage IV: involvement of extranodal sites(s) beyond that designated as 'E' later
  Systemic symptoms:
    A: absent
    B: significant weight loss >10% in 6 months, fever, or night sweats.
  Disease bulk and spread:
    X: bulky disease: greater than a third widening of mediastinum, >10 cm maximum diameter of nodal mass
    E: involvement of single, contiguous, or proximal extranodal site.
  Clinical stage (CS) is determined by history, physical examination, radiological studies, isotope scans, laboratory tests of urine and blood, and the initial biopsy results.
  Pathological stage relates to the tissue sampled and the results of histopathological examination.

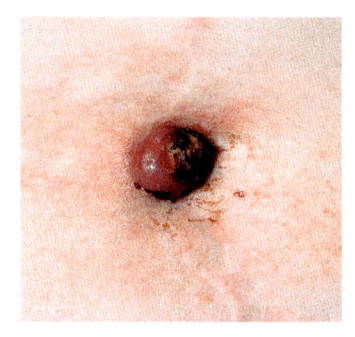

Fig. 62.1 Sister Mary Joseph nodule. (With permission from James, W.D., Elston, D.M., Treat, J.T., Rosenbach, M.A, Neuhaus, I.M. M.D., 2020. Andrews' Diseases of the Skin, thirteenth edn. Elsevier.)

How is a patient with Hodgkin disease treated?
- Localized disease (i.e. stages IA and IIA) is treated with radiotherapy or combination radiotherapy and chemotherapy consisting of doxorubicin, bleomycin, vinblastine, and dacarbazine (ABVD). Five-year cure rates are over 90%. Positron electron tomography (PET) scanning can help test tumour sensitivity to therapy, assisting in prognostication.
- Stages IIB, III, and IV are treated with combination chemotherapy. Five-year survival rates are 50% to 80%. Patients who relapse after initial chemotherapy may be cured with autologous bone marrow transplantation.

What do you understand by the term non-Hodgkin lymphomas?
These are a heterogeneous group of cancers of lymphocytes. They are variable in their presentation and natural history, varying from a slow indolent course to a rapidly progressive illness.

How are non-Hodgkin lymphomas classified?
A working classification is as follows:
- Low grade or favourable—there is a slow, indolent course with good response to minimal therapy and long survival. These include small lymphocytic, plasmacytoid, follicular small cleaved cell, and follicular mixed cell. Patients are usually treated with alkylating agents such as chlorambucil or a cyclophosphamide, vincristine, and prednisolone regimen.
- High grade or unfavourable—this includes immunoblastic, small noncleaved (Burkitt and non-Burkitt), lymphoblastic, and true histiocytic lymphoma. The mainstay of therapy is combination chemotherapy; traditionally, the cyclophosphamide, doxorubicin, vincristine, and prednisolone regimen is used. In highly aggressive lymphomas, autologous bone marrow transplantation may increase the chances of cure.
- Intermediate grade—this includes follicular large cell, diffuse small cleaved cell, diffuse mixed cell, and diffuse large cell.
- Others—this includes cutaneous T cell (mycosis fungoides, adult T-cell leukaemia/lymphoma).

What symptoms of non-Hodgkin lymphoma merit urgent referral to an oncologist?
Symptoms of non-Hodgkin lymphoma needing urgent referral include the following:
- Lymphadenopathy (>1 cm persisting for 6 weeks)
- Hepatosplenomegaly
- Three or more of the following symptoms:
  - Fatigue
  - Night sweats
  - Weight loss
  - Itching
  - Breathlessness
  - Bruising
  - Recurrent infection
  - Bone pain.

What are the risk factors in localized Hodgkin lymphoma?
European Organisation for the Research Treatment of Cancer risk factors in localized disease:
- Favourable: patients must have all features:
  - CS 1 and 2
  - Maximum of three nodal areas involved
  - Age younger than 50 years
  - Erythrocyte sedimentation rate (ESR) <50 mm/hour without B symptoms or ESR <30 mm/hour with B symptoms
  - Mediastinal/thoracic ratio <0.35.

- Unfavourable: patients have any features:
    - CS 2 with involvement of at least four nodal areas
    - Age >50 years
    - ESR >50 mm/hour if asymptomatic or ESR >30 mm/hour if B symptoms
    - Mediastinal/thoracic ratio >0.35.

What are the poor prognostic factors of advanced Hodgkin lymphoma?
The Hasenclever index is an international prognostic score including the following seven factors:
- Age >45 years
- Male sex
- Serum albumin <40 g/L
- Haemoglobin concentration <105 g/L
- Stage IV disease
- Leukocytosis (white-cell count ≥15 × 10^9/L)
- Lymphopenia (<0.6 × 10^9/L or <8% of the total white-cell count).

These factors individually reduced predicted 5-year freedom from progression rate by around 8%.

What are the late effects of Hodgkin lymphoma and its treatment?
- Second malignancies
- Cardiac disease
- Endocrine dysfunction
- Psychological trauma
- Lung damage (usually subclinical)
- Hyposplenism (after splenectomy or splenic irradiation)
- Dental caries.

What are the investigations done before initiation of treatment on non-Hodgkin lymphoma?
Essential procedures:
- A full history, recording growth rate, symptoms present, performance status
- A detailed physical examination, with special attention to all node-bearing areas
- Adequate surgical biopsy specimen, allowing immunophenotyping and examined by a skilled pathologist
- Laboratory procedures:
    - Full blood count, including ESR
    - Serum lactate dehydrogenase, calcium, uric acid, protein and electrophoresis, alkaline phosphatase
    - Assessment of renal and liver function.
- Radiological studies:
    - Chest radiograph
    - Thoracic and abdominal–pelvic computed tomography scan.
- Bone marrow aspirate and trephine, to include molecular genetic analysis if available

Optional procedures, depending on clinicasl picture:
- β_2-Microglobulin
- Endoscopy, e.g. for gastric mucosa-associated lymphoid tissue lymphoma
- Plain radiographs, bone scan, or magnetic resonance imaging (MRI)
- PET
- Head or spinal MRI for neurological symptoms
- Cerebrospinal fluid analysis in patients at risk.

Further Information

Thomas Hodgkin (1798–1866), an English physician at St. Thomas's Hospital, London. He was the curator of the Pathology Museum at Guy's Hospital before this.

R.L.K. Virchow (1821–1902), successively Professor of Pathology at Würzberg and Berlin. He also described Virchow cell (lepra cell), Virchow space (perivascular space of Virchow–Robin), and Virchow triad of the pathogenesis of thrombosis.

Dorothy Reed (1874–1964) graduated from Johns Hopkins Hospital, Baltimore, and worked successively in New York and Wisconsin.

K. Sternberg (1872–1935), an Austrian pathologist who described the cells in 1898. Burkitt lymphoma was described by Dennis Burkitt in children in West Africa who presented with a lesion in the jaw, extranodal abdominal involvement, and ovarian tumours. Most patients have Epstein–Barr antibodies in the serum.

The disease was first described in China in 1937 by Kim and Szeto but became more widely known as Kimura disease after a description in 1948 by Kimura and co-workers.

SECTION VI

Rheumatology Cases

SECTION OUTLINE

63 Rheumatology Case
64 Ankylosing Spondylitis
65 Charcot Arthropathy
66 Ehlers–Danlos Syndrome
67 Gout
68 Osteoarthritis
69 Psoriatic Arthritis
70 Rheumatoid Hands
71 Dermatomyositis—Proximal Muscle Weakness
72 Scleroderma
73 Systemic Lupus Erythematosus
74 Small-Vessel ANCA-Associated Vasculitis

CHAPTER 63

Rheumatology Case

Instruction

Examine this patient's joints.

HISTORY

Ask the patient whether he or she has any pain, stiffness, or difficulty in dressing or walking.

EXAMINATION

- *Look* at posture, gait, and joint deformity
- *Feel* for temperature, tenderness, joint fluid, and crepitus of movement of the joints
- *Move*: check passive and active movements of the joints; test stability of the joints
- *Measure* muscle wasting and shortening of the limb.

Examination of the Hands

Fig. 63.1 shows patterns of peripheral joint disease and Fig. 63.2 gives a useful template on which to mark joint disorders.
1. Ask the patient, 'Are your hands painful?'
2. Inspect for joint deformity:
    - Swan-neck deformity (flexion at the distal interphalangeal joints and hyperextension of the proximal interphalangeal joints)
    - Boutonnière deformity (flexion of the proximal interphalangeal joints and hyperextension of the distal interphalangeal joint)
    - Z deformity of the thumb
    - Ulnar deviation of the fingers.
3. Examine the nails:
    - Nailfold infarcts (rheumatoid arthritis)
    - Nail pitting, onycholysis, ridging, hyperkeratosis, discoloration (psoriasis).
4. Comment on the following:
    - Wasting of small muscles of the hand, in particular those on the dorsum of the hand
    - Heberden's nodes, i.e. bony nodules at the distal interphalangeal joints (osteoarthroses)
    - Bouchard's nodes, i.e. bony nodules at the proximal interphalangeal joints (osteoarthroses)
    - Spindle-shaped deformity of the fingers
    - Gouty tophi.
5. Examine the palms:
    - Wasting of the thenar or hypothenar eminence
    - Thickening of the palmar fascia: Dupuytren's contracture (rheumatoid arthritis)
    - Palmar erythema (rheumatoid arthritis)
    - Tap over the flexor retinaculum to detect median nerve entrapment (Tinel's sign).

63 — RHEUMATOLOGY CASE

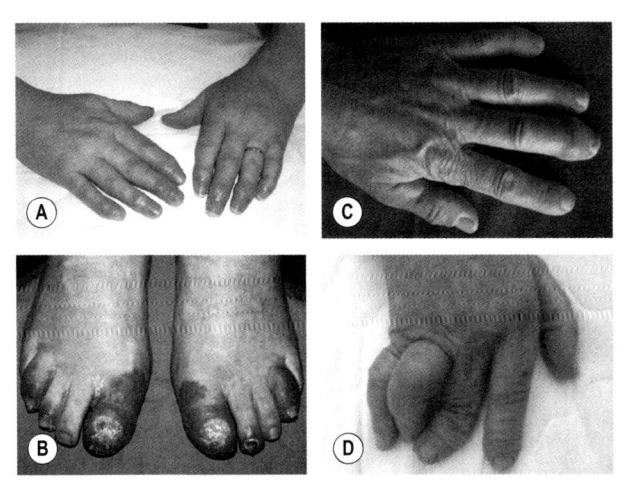

Fig. 63.1 Asymmetric polyarticular disease. **(A)** Distal interphalangeal joint involvement and forearm lymphoedema. **(B)** Toe dactylitis with skin and nail changes. **(C)** Predominant distal interphalangeal joint involvement. **(D)** Arthritis mutilans. (With permission from Firestein, G.S., Budd, R.C., Harris Jr, E.D., et al., 2008. *Kelley's Textbook of Rheumatology*, eighth edn. Saunders, Philadelphia, PA.)

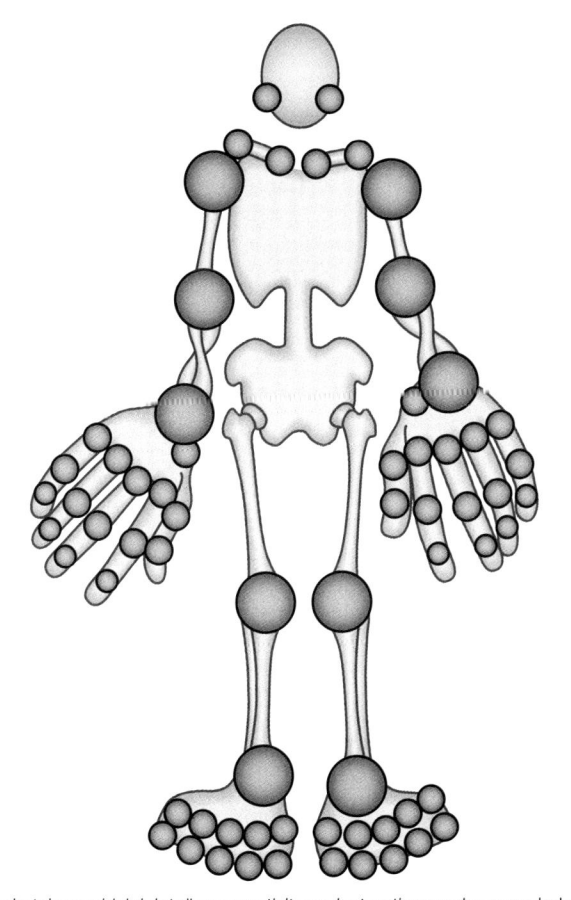

Fig. 63.2 An outline sketch on which joint disease activity or destruction can be recorded at each assessment.

6. Get the patient to perform the following movements:
   - Unbuttoning of clothes
   - Pincer movements
   - Hand grip
   - Abduction of the thumb
   - Writing.
7. Test sensation of the index and little fingers.
8. Examine the elbows for the following signs:
   - Rheumatoid arthritis
   - Gouty tophi
   - Psoriatic plaques.
9. Tell the examiner that you would like to examine the other joints.

Note: When asked to examine the hands, consider the possibility of arthropathy, myopathy, neuropathy, a peripheral nerve lesion, or acromegaly.

Examination of the Knees

- Ask the patient if the joints are sore.
- Expose both knees and lower thighs fully with the patient lying supine.
- Look for:
  - quadriceps wasting
  - swelling of the joint.
- Feel for:
  - temperature
  - synovial thickening.
- Do the patellar tap (ballottement): fluid from the suprapatellar bursa is forced into the joint space by squeezing the lower part of the quadriceps and then the patella is pushed posteriorly with the fingers; this test indicates fluid in the synovial cavity (Fig. 63.3).
- Assess movement:
  - Test passive flexion and extension: make a note of the range of movements and feel for crepitus
  - Gently extend the knee and examine for fixed flexion deformity
  - Test the medial and lateral ligaments by steadying the thigh with the left hand and moving the leg with the right laterally and medially when the knee joint is slightly flexed: movement of >10 degrees is abnormal
  - Test the cruciate ligaments by steadying the foot with your elbow and moving the leg anteriorly and posteriorly with the other hand: laxity of >10 degrees is abnormal.
- Ask the patient to lie on his or her stomach and feel the popliteal fossa when the knee is extended.

Examination of the Feet

- Look:
  - for skin rash, scars
  - at the nails for changes of psoriasis
  - at the forefoot for hallux valgus, clawing, and crowding of the toes (rheumatoid arthritis)
  - at the callus over the metatarsal heads, which may occur in subluxation
  - at both the arches of the foot, in particular medial and longitudinal (flat foot, pes cavus).

63 – RHEUMATOLOGY CASE

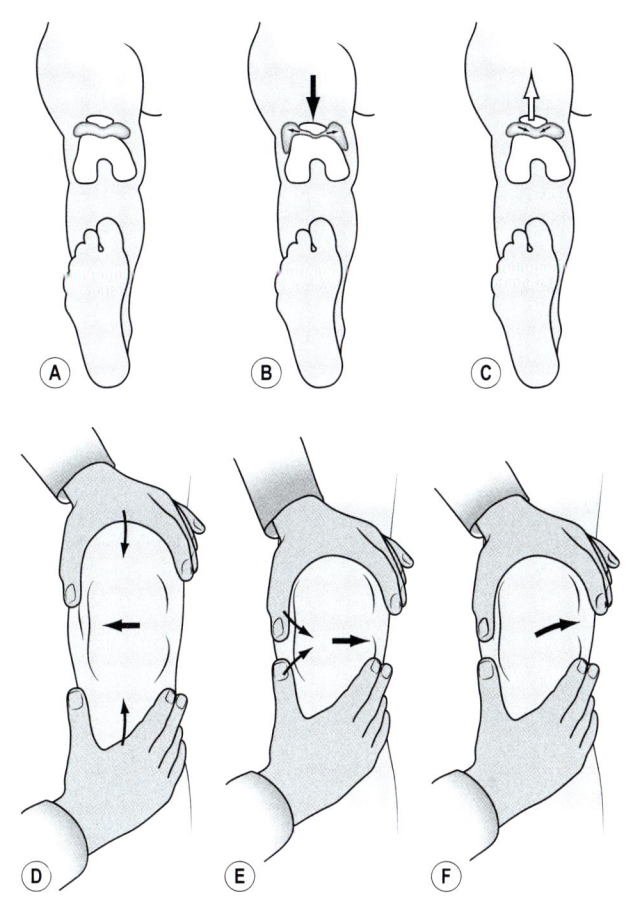

Fig. 63.3 Detection of effusions. **(A–C)** Large effusions can be detected by 'ballotting' the patella with the knee in extension. **(D–F)** Small effusions can be identified by the 'bulge' test, where fluid is 'milked' into the suprapatellar pouch and then pressed so that it can be seen bulging below the medial edge of the patella.

- Palpate:
    - ankles for synovitis, effusion, passive movements at the subtalar joints (inversion and eversion) and talar joint (dorsiflexion and plantar flexion); remember that tenderness on movement is more important than the range of movement
    - the metatarsophalangeal joints for tenderness
    - individual digits, for synovial thickening
    - bottom of heel, for tenderness (plantar fasciitis), and Achilles tendon for nodules.

Questions

Name some eponymous extraarticular diseases that are associated with arthritis or arthralgia.
- Felty syndrome—splenomegaly, neutropenia, lymphadenopathy, and rheumatoid arthritis
- Still disease—juvenile idiopathic arthritis with salmon pink skin rash

- Crohn's disease—inflammatory bowel disease can be associated with arthritis
- Christmas disease—haemarthrosis is a common complication of haemophilia
- Reiter syndrome—anterior uveitis, conjunctivitis, and arthritis.

Further Information

W. Heberden, Sr (1710–1801), an English physician.
C.J. Bouchard (1837–1915), a French physician.

CHAPTER 64

Ankylosing Spondylitis

Instruction
Examine this patient's back.

Salient Features
HISTORY
- Back stiffness and back pain: worse in the morning, improves on exercise, and worsens at rest
- Symptoms in the peripheral joints (in ~40%), particularly shoulders and knees
- Onset of symptoms is typically insidious and in the third to fourth decade
- Extraarticular manifestations: red eye (uveitis), diarrhoea (gastrointestinal involvement), history of aortic regurgitation, pulmonary apical fibrosis (worse in smokers).

EXAMINATION
- 'Question mark' posture (as a result of loss of lumbar lordosis, fixed kyphoscoliosis of the thoracic spine with compensatory extension of the cervical spine)
- Protuberant abdomen.

Proceed as follows:
- Ask the patient to look to either side: the whole body turns
- Examine the cervical, thoracic, and lumbar spines (remember that cervical spine involvement occurs later in the disease and results in pain and crepitus on neck movement).
- Measure the occiput-to-wall distance (inability to make contact when heel and back are against the wall indicates upper thoracic and cervical limitation).
- Perform Schober test. This involves marking points 10 cm above and 5 cm below a line joining the 'dimple of Venus' on the sacral promontory. An increase in the separation of <5 cm during full forward flexion indicates limited spinal mobility.

Finger–floor distance is a simple indicator but is less reliable because good hip movement may compensate for back limitation.
- Examine for distal arthritis (occurs in up to 30% of patients and may precede the onset of the back symptoms). Small joints of the hand and feet are rarely affected
- Measure chest expansion with a tape (<5 cm suggests costovertebral involvement)
- Tell the examiner that you would like to examine the following:
    - Eyes for iritis, anterior uveitis (seen in 20% of patients)
    - Heart for aortic regurgitation (seen in 4% of patients who have had the disease for over 15 years), cardiac conduction defects
    - Lungs for mild restrictive disease, apical fibrosis, apical cavities, and secondary fungal infection; look for cyanosis (patients with rigid spine syndrome often have underlying hypoventilation).

- Central nervous system, such as tetraplegia, etc.
- Foot for Achilles tendinitis and plantar fasciitis.
- The four A's of ankylosing spondylitis (AS): apical fibrosis, anterior uveitis, aortic regurgitation, and Achilles tendinitis
- Psoriasis and Reiter syndrome can also cause sacroiliitis.

Diagnosis

This patient has fixed kyphoscoliosis of the thoracic spine with loss of lumbar lordosis (lesion) caused by a spondyloarthropathy (SpA), possibly AS (aetiology). On examination, spinal movements are severely diminished (functional status).

Questions

What are the diagnostic criteria for AS?
Modified New York criteria 1984 for AS: definite AS is present if the radiological criterion is associated with at least one clinical criterion:
Clinical criteria:
- Low-back pain and stiffness for longer than 3 months, which improve with exercise but are not relieved by rest
- Restriction of motion of the lumbar spine in both the sagittal and frontal planes
- Restriction of chest expansion relative to normal values correlated for age and sex

Radiological criterion:
- Sacroiliitis grade ≥2 bilaterally, or grade 3 to 4 unilaterally.

What other classification models are you aware of for spondyloarthropathies?
Since the New York criteria were established, the classification of The European Spondyloarthropathy Study Group criteria and The Assessment of Spondyloarthritis International Society criteria for peripheral and axial spondyloarthropathy, many attempts for classification of SpAs have taken place and multiple models have been developed for diagnostic criteria for SpAs including AS. However, all models have limitations when used in clinical practice, and as such they are limited to use for research purposes. When it comes to diagnosis, this should be made on the basis of clinical, radiological, and biochemical findings for each individual patient without the restriction of strict diagnostic criteria.

What investigations would you like to do in this patient?
Anteroposterior view of sacroiliac joints and lateral radiographs of lumbar spine (Fig. 64.1A): the earliest changes are erosions and sclerosis of the sacroiliac joints. Later in the disease, syndesmophytes may be found in the lumbosacral spine. In severe disease, involvement progresses up the spine, leading to a 'bamboo spine' (Fig. 64.1B). Although the New York criteria require a combination of clinical and radiographic features, the diagnosis should be suspected on the basis of inactivity, spinal stiffness, and pain, with or without additional features.

In which other seronegative arthritic disorders is low-back pain a feature?
Sacroiliitis is often seen in Reiter syndrome, psoriatic arthritis, juvenile chronic arthritis, and intestinal arthropathy.

How would you manage a patient with AS?
- Encourage exercise, particularly physical therapy, to preserve back extension.

64 — ANKYLOSING SPONDYLITIS

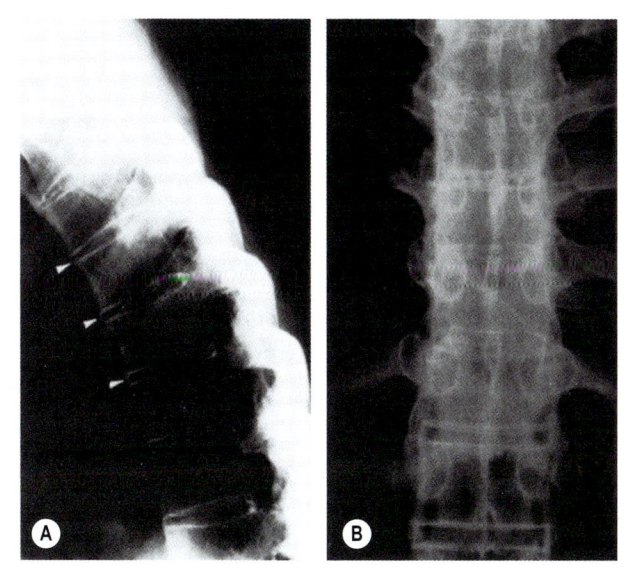

Fig. 64.1 Ankylosing spondylitis. **(A)** Bone erosion of dorsal aspect of thoracic spine. **(B)** Bamboo spine. (With permission from Kelley, W.N., Harris, E.D., Ruddy, S., et al. (eds.), 1997. Textbook of Rheumatology, fifth edn, vol. 1. Saunders, Philadelphia, PA.)

- Nonsteroidal antiinflammatory drugs (NSAIDs), either nonselective or COX2 inhibitors are used. This is usually the first-line treatment and for many patients the only treatment required. Other analgesics are not as effective as NSAIDs; however, they can be considered for residual pain, despite continuous maximum treatment with NSAIDs.
- Sulfasalazine has some evidence in peripheral arthritis associated with AS but there is no evidence for methotrexate in axial spine disease. Methotrexate use has shown no benefit in AS, either as monotherapy or in combination with other disease-modifying agents.
- Tumour necrosis factor (TNF) antagonists: etanercept, adalimumab, infliximab, and golimumab. Anti-TNF therapy has been proven to improve disease activity and patient symptoms as well as disease progression if treatment is started in very early disease.
- Surgical therapy, consisting of vertebral wedge osteotomy, is occasionally indicated.
- Refer to an ophthalmologist when anterior uveitis occurs.

What genetic counselling would you give this patient?
In HLA-B27-positive patients, the siblings have a 30% chance of developing this disease. Hence, children of such patients who develop symptoms such as joint pains or sore eyes should be referred to a rheumatologist.

What is the natural history of the disease?
About 40% go on to develop severe spinal restriction; about 20% have significant disability. Early peripheral joint disease, particularly of the hip, indicates a poor prognosis.

What is the risk in those with a 'bamboo' cervical spine when driving?
Increased susceptibility to whiplash injury and restricted lateral vision.

What therapy may the patient have received in the past if the blood film shows a leukaemic picture?
In the past, patients were treated with irradiation of the spine. However, those treated tend to develop leukaemia several years after therapy.

In anti-TNF treatment for AS, what are the predictors of response to treatment?
Anti-TNF treatment will result in improvement of greater than 50% in more than two-thirds of patients. Possible factors that have been identified as positive in predicting improvement are increased inflammatory markers at initiation of treatment, young patients, and short disease duration prior to treatment.

What criteria predict that lower-back pain is a precursor of AS?
New criteria for inflammatory back pain in young to middle-aged adults (<50 years) with chronic back pain are as follows:
- Morning stiffness >30 min
- Improvement in back pain with exercise but not with rest
- Awakening because of back pain during the second half of the night only
- Alternating buttock pain
- Diagnosis is confirmed if at least two of the four the parameters are present (sensitivity 70.3%, specificity 81.2%).

Further Information

Keat, A., 1995. Spondyloparthopathies. Brit. Med. J. 310, 1321–1324 (classic review).

The term ankylosing spondylitis derives from the Greek words *ankylos* (bent or crooked) and *spondylos* (vertebra). Past names have included Marie–Strümpell disease and von Bechterew disease.

The first clinical report of AS (1831) concerned a man from the Isle of Man. Vladimir von Bechterew of St. Petersburg, Russia, described a series of cases between 1857 and 1927. Adolf Strümpell (1853–1926) of Erlangen and Pierre Marie (1853–1940) of Paris independently described this condition in 1897 and 1898, respectively.

H.C. Reiter (1881–1969), a German physician.

Achilles is a figure from Greek mythology who was a hero of the Trojan war. His mother dipped him into the river Styx, holding him by his heel, to make him invulnerable to the attack. He slew Hector in this war but was himself slain, wounded in his vulnerable heel by Paris.

CHAPTER 65

Charcot Arthropathy

Instruction

This patient presented with a 2-day history of right foot swelling and redness. Examine the locomotor system in this patient.

Salient Features

HISTORY

- History of diabetes
- History of minor or no trauma preceding the presentation
- Recurrent, acute, or insidious onset of oedema, erythema, and warmth
- Gait deformity
- Loss of pain threshold (painless arthropathy)
- Atrophy of muscles of the joint.

EXAMINATION

- Enlargement of the affected joint (compare with the other side)
- Instability of the joint, in particular hypermobility of the joint
- May be warm, swollen, and tender in the early stages
- Enlargement and crepitus may be present in the later stages.
- Collapse of the longitudinal arch resulting in a 'rocker-bottom' deformity
- Atrophic ulcers may coexist.

Proceed as follows:
- Check sensation in the affected limb.
- Tell the examiner that you would like to investigate as follows:
  - Do a thorough neurological examination, looking for loss of proprioception and/or pain sensation and vibratory sensation with a 128-Hz tuning fork.
  - Examine the urine for sugar (looking for evidence of diabetes mellitus).
- Ask for lancinating pains, check posterior column signs, and look for Argyll Robertson pupil (tabes dorsalis).
- Check for dissociated sensory loss (syringomyelia).
- Test muscle strength.

Diagnosis

This patient has Charcot joint (lesion) caused by diabetes mellitus (aetiology) and has marked deformity of the joint with restricted movement, probably belonging to Rogers and Bevilacqua class 3C or 3D (functional status) (Fig. 65.1).

The six Ps of prevention of neuropathic foot are: podiatry, pulse examination, protective shoes, pressure reduction, prophylactic surgery, and preventive education.

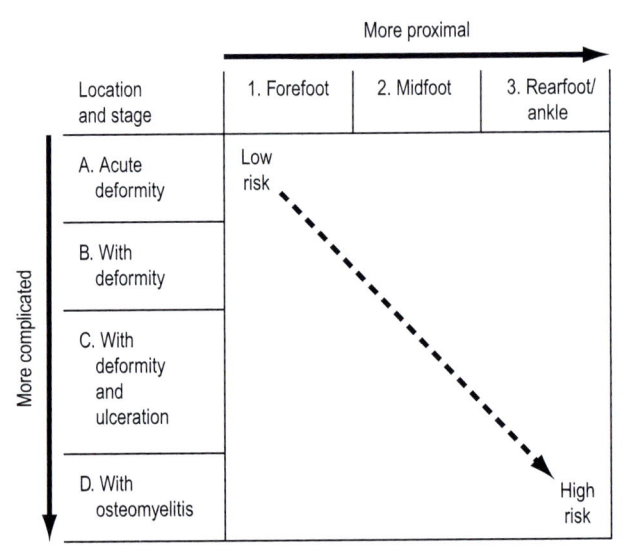

Fig. 65.1 Rogers and Bevilacqua classification. Moving towards a more complicated Charcot joint or proximally in the foot increases the risk of extremity amputation. (Adapted from Rogers, L.C., Bevilacqua, N.J., 2008. The diagnosis of Charcot foot. Clin. Podiatr. Med. Surg. 25, 43–51.)

Questions

What do you understand by the term Charcot joint?
It is a chronic progressive degenerative arthropathy resulting from a disturbance in the sensory innervation of the affected joint. It is a neuropathic arthropathy that is a complication of various disorders affecting the nervous system. It results in gross deformity, osteoarthrosis, and new bone formation from repeated trauma.

Mention a few conditions responsible for the development of Charcot joints.
- Diabetic neuropathy: affecting the tarsal joints, tarsometatarsal, metatarsophalangeal joints
- Tabes dorsalis: affecting the knee, hip, ankle, lumbar, and lower dorsal vertebrae
- Syringomyelia: affecting the shoulder, elbow, cervical vertebra
- Myelomeningocoele: affecting the ankle, tarsus
- Miscellaneous: hereditary sensory neuropathies, peripheral nerve injury, congenital insensitivity to pain, leprosy, paraplegia (hips).

What is the advantage of measuring skin temperature in Charcot foot?
Skin temperature difference between feet, measured with a contact or noncontact thermometer, may be significant. The average difference between the acute Charcot foot and the unaffected side is as much as 9°F (5°C). A difference of 4°F (2°C) is considered significant.

How is Charcot foot classified?
The Rogers and Bevilacqua classification (Fig. 65.1) combines the features of the clinical examination, radiography (Fig. 65.2), and anatomy. The graph indicates increasing risk for amputation as the Charcot foot becomes 'more complicated'.

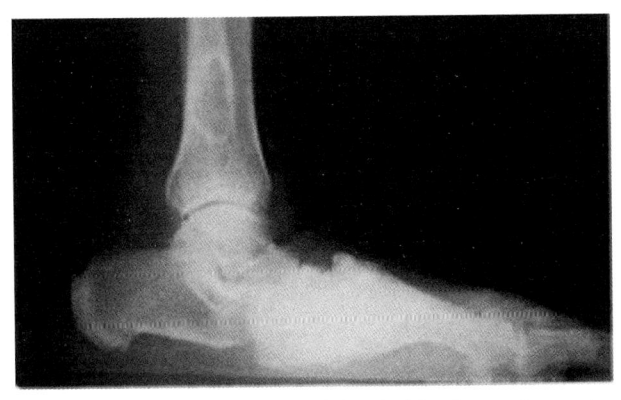

Fig. 65.2 Lateral radiograph showing equinus, tarsometatarsal subluxation, and a prominent cuboid plantarly in Charcot foot. (With permission from Rogers, L.C., Bevilacqua, N.J., 2008. The diagnosis of Charcot foot. Clin. Podiatr. Med. Surg. 25, 43–51.)

What is the pathogenesis of acute Charcot foot in diabetics?

It has been suggested that an initial insult triggers an inflammatory cascade through increased expression of proinflammatory cytokines (including tumour necrosis factor-α and interleukin-1β). This cascade results in increased expression of the nuclear transcription factor, NF-κB, which results in increased osteoclastogenesis. Osteoclasts cause progressive bone lysis, leading to further fracture; this, in turn, potentiates the inflammatory process.

Further Information

Jean Martin Charcot (1825–1893) was a French neurologist. He was a Professor of Pathology in 1872 and Professor of Nervous Diseases in 1882. Other conditions that bear his name include Charcot fever (intermittent fever from cholangitis), Charcot triad (intention tremor, nystagmus, and scanning speech in multiple sclerosis), Charcot–Leyden crystals (seen in the sputum of asthmatics), Charcot–Marie–Tooth disease (peroneal muscular atrophy), and Charcot–Wilbrand syndrome (visual agnosia). Charcot acknowledged that the neuropathic arthropathy had been first reported by the American physician John Kearsley Mitchell (1798–1858) in 1831. Mitchell's cases were secondary to spinal damage caused by tuberculosis, whereas Charcot's were the result of tertiary syphilis.

CHAPTER 66

Ehlers–Danlos Syndrome

Instruction

Examine this patient's joints.

Salient Features

HISTORY

- Family history
- Hypermobile joints (Fig. 66.1)
- Fragile skin with impaired wound healing
- Bleeding diathesis.

EXAMINATION

- The skin over the neck, axillae, and groin is smooth and elastic (Fig. 66.2). It can be stretched and, when released, it returns immediately to its normal position. Late in the disease, it becomes lax and wrinkled and hangs in folds.
- Look at bony prominences for bruising, haematomas, and gaping wounds. Wounds heal forming tissue-paper or papyraceous or 'cigarette-paper' scars. Haematomas heal, forming pseudotumours or nodules.
- Kyphoscoliosis
- Hypermobile joints (Fig. 66.3).

Proceed as follows:
Tell the examiner that you would like to examine the following:
- The hernial orifices
- The heart for mitral valve prolapse and aortic regurgitation
- The eyes for myopia, retinal detachment.

Note: The three basic clinical criteria are fragile skin, bleeding diathesis, and hypermobile joints.

Diagnosis

This patient has hypermobile joints (lesion) caused by Ehlers–Danlos syndrome (aetiology).

Questions

What are the gastrointestinal manifestations of this syndrome?
- Marked tendency to herniate
- Achalasia cardia

66 — EHLERS–DANLOS SYNDROME

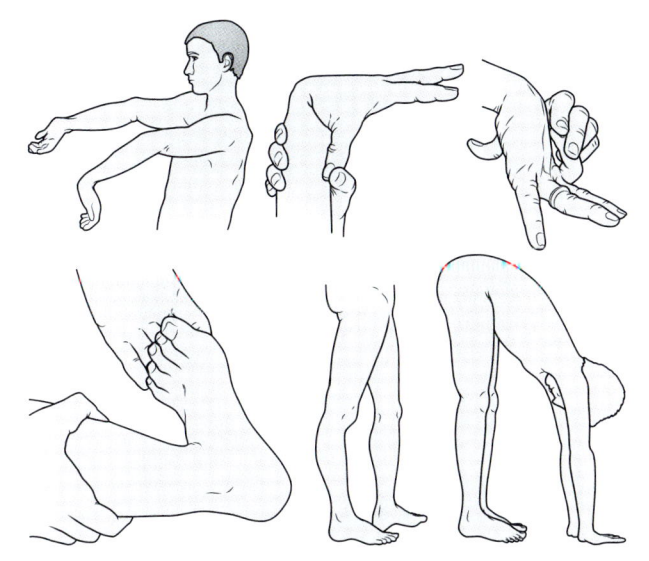

Fig. 66.1 Manoeuvres that may establish clinically significant joint laxity.

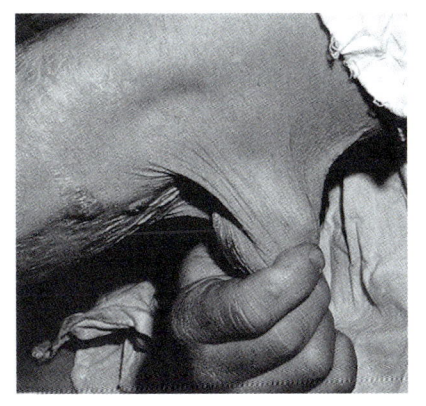

Fig. 66.2 The skin over the neck, axillae, and groin is smooth and elastic; it can be stretched and, when released, it returns immediately to its normal position. Late in the disease it becomes lax and wrinkled and hangs in folds.

- Eventration of the diaphragm
- Megacolon.

What are the cardiovascular manifestations?
- Mitral valve prolapse
- Aortic dissection.

What precautions would you take in managing skin wounds?
As the skin wounds tend to be gaping, they should be approximated with care; removable sutures are usually left in place for twice the usual time.

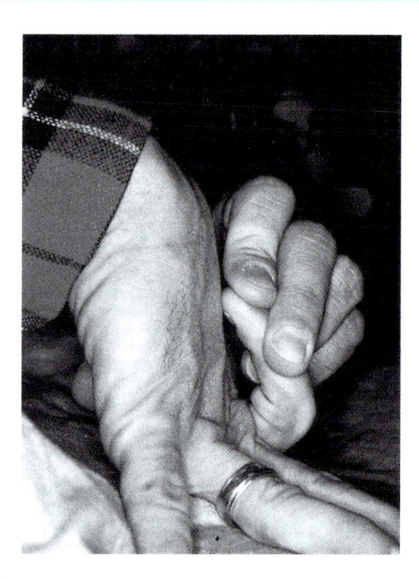

Fig. 66.3 Hypermobile joints.

What do you know about Ehlers–Danlos syndrome?
It comprises a group of heterogeneous disorders that result from defects in collagen synthesis and vary genetically and clinically from one another. Some molecular defects are known.
- Type VI (kyphoscoliotic type)—the most common and autosomal recessive form of inheritance. There is a defect in the enzyme lysyl hydroxylase, which is necessary for hydroxylation of lysyl residues during collagen synthesis. Only collagen types 1 and 3 are affected, and collagen types 2, 4, and 6 are normal. The predominant clinical features are ocular fragility with rupture of the cornea and retinal detachment. Some of these patients respond to ascorbic acid.
- Type IV ('vascular type')—this is caused by a defect in the structural gene for collagen type 3 (*COL3A1*) and is inherited as an autosomal dominant trait. As type 3 collagen is present largely in blood vessels and intestines, the typical features of this syndrome include easy bruising; thin skin with visible veins; characteristic facial features; rupture of the large arteries, uterus, or colon; and reduced life expectancy. This is the most severe form of Ehlers–Danlos syndrome. Loeys–Dietz syndrome overlaps with this type.
- Type VII—a defect in the conversion of procollagen to collagen, caused by the mutation that affects one of the two type 1 collagen genes (*COL1A1* and *COL1A2*). Although in the single mutant allele, only 50% of type 1 collagen chains are affected, heterozygotes manifest the syndrome because these abnormal chains interfere with the formation of normal collagen helices.
- Type IX—this is caused by a defect in copper metabolism, with high levels of copper in the cells but low levels of serum copper and caeruloplasmin. Because the gene influencing copper metabolism is on the X chromosome, it is inherited as an X-linked recessive trait. This disease illustrates how copper metabolism can affect connective tissue.
- Classic or types I and II—null alleles of the *COL5A1* gene encoding type V collagen are a cause of the classic form. A single base mutation in *COL5A2* causes type II. Mutations in a gene that encodes tenascin-X, which is neither a collagen nor a collagen-modifying protein, can result in a variation of the classic form of the Ehlers–Danlos syndrome.

Patients with type I, II, and IV disease are often investigated for bleeding diathesis before the correct diagnosis is made. Because of joint instability and laxity, many patients with types I, II, III, VI, and VII disease are investigated for developmental delay before it is recognized that they have this syndrome.

Over 35 collagen genes have now been identified and these encode the chains of >20 types of collagen: types 1, 2, and 3 are the interstitial or fibrillar collagen, whereas types 4, 5, and 6 are amorphous and are present in the interstitial tissue and basement membranes.

In which other condition is there a defect in collagen metabolism?
Osteogenesis imperfecta.

What are the criteria for diagnosis of joint hypermobility?
Beighton nine-point scoring for joint hypermobility assigns two points for each of the following four paired manoeuvres:
- Hyperextension of the fifth metacarpophalangeal joint to 90 degrees
- Apposition of the thumb to the volar aspect of the forearm
- Hyperextension of the elbow beyond 10 degrees
- Hyperextension of the knee to beyond 10 degrees.

One point is assigned for the ability to place the palms of the hands on the floor with the knees extended.

It is not unusual to find extreme laxity in small joints and less laxity in large joints. Laxity decreases with age, so the dominant nature of most of these syndromes may not be appreciated when examining older family members.

Is hypermobility advantageous to musicians?
Lax fingers and wrists are good for flautists and string players, but lax knees and spines are bad for tympanists and others who stand while they play. It can be advantageous to some types of swimmers, such as the fin swimmers.

Further Information

The Ehlers–Danlos Society (https://www.ehlers-danlos.com): a global community of patients, caregivers, healthcare professionals, and supporters, dedicated to saving and improving the lives of those affected by the Ehlers–Danlos syndromes, hypermobility spectrum disorders, and related conditions.

Ehlers–Danlos Support Group (www.ehlers-danlos.org): UK patient support group.

Edvard Ehlers (1863–1937), a Danish dermatologist, and H. A. Danlos, a French dermatologist, described this condition independently in 1901 and 1908, respectively. Tschernogobow in Moscow first described this syndrome in 1892 (Pyeritz, 2000).

It is widely believed that the outstanding virtuosity of the violinist Niccolò Paganini (1782–1840) was the result of remarkable flexibility of the joints of his left hand: he could span three octaves with little effort (Smith, 1982).

Robert James Gorlin (1923–2006) described Gorlin's sign, which is the ability to touch the tip of the nose with the tongue in Ehlers–Danlos syndrome.

CHAPTER 67

Gout

Instruction

Examine this patient's hands and feet.

Salient Features
HISTORY

- Acute pain at the base of great toe, worse at night and associated with redness
- Occasionally, multiple joints involved
- Systemic symptoms, e.g. low-grade fever.

EXAMINATION

- Chronic tophaceous deposit with asymmetrical joint involvement.

Proceed as follows:

Tell the examiner that you would like to examine the:
- helices of the ears
- elbow for olecranon bursae
- Achilles tendons for tophi
- feet and hands
    - Uric acid crystals are negatively birefringent and needle shaped and may be deposited in bursae and bone marrow. They are demonstrable in synovial fluid within leukocytes and free in the fluid during attacks of gouty arthritis. Identification of tissue or synovial fluid monosodium urate crystals is considered pathognomonic and the gold standard for diagnosis.
    - Be prepared to discuss the differences between the clinical features of typical gout and gout in the elderly. It has a more equal gender distribution, frequent polyarticular presentation with involvement of the joints of the upper extremities, fewer acute gouty episodes, a more indolent chronic clinical course, and an increased incidence of tophi.

Diagnosis

This patient has a painful great toe with swelling of the joint (lesion) caused by gout (aetiology) and is unable to walk because of the pain (functional status).

Questions

What is the basic pathophysiology of gout?
Gout is a metabolic disorder of purine metabolism. It is characterized by hyperuricaemia caused by either overproduction or underexcretion of uric acid.

67 — GOUT

What are the different clinical manifestations of gout?
- Asymptomatic hyperuricaemia
- Acute arthritis
- Chronic arthritis
- Chronic tophaceous gout (Figs. 67.1 and 67.2).

How would you treat an acute attack of gout?
Amongst the preferred treatment options are nonsteroidal antiinflammatory drugs (NSAIDs), selective cyclooxygenase-2 inhibitors like etoricoxib, colchicine, and steroids (intraarticular or systemic).

What factors may precipitate acute gouty arthritis?
Drugs (diuretics, aspirin), copious consumption of alcohol, dehydration, surgery, fasting, food high in purines (sweetbreads, liver, kidney, and sardines).

Under what circumstances would you treat hyperuricaemia?
Frequent attacks of acute arthritis, renal damage, and consistently raised serum uric acid levels. Before attempting to lower serum uric acid levels, it is prudent to use colchicine to treat acute attacks. Colchicine should be given within 24 hours of the onset of symptoms to abort a severe attack.

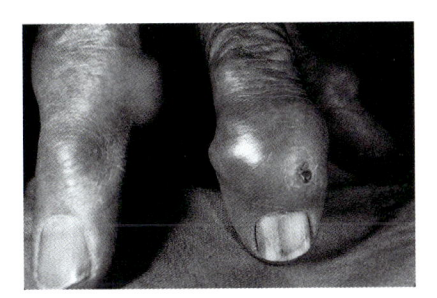

Fig. 67.1 Gouty tophi.

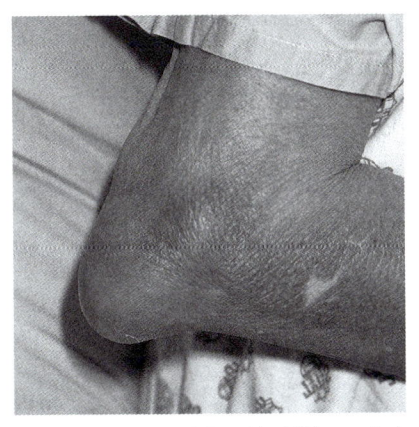

Fig. 67.2 Painful olecranon bursitis resembling septic bursitis. (With permission from Roberts, J.R., Hedges, J.R., 2009. Clinical Procedures in Emergency Medicine, fifth edn. Saunders, Philadelphia, PA.)

What is the drug of choice for controlling hyperuricaemia?
Allopurinol (a xanthine oxidase inhibitor). The goal of therapy is to reduce serum uric acid to <6 mg/dL (350 µmol/L). At this level, monosodium urate crystals within joints and in soft tissue tophi are reabsorbed. Febuxostat, a novel nonpurine xanthine oxidase inhibitor, may be a useful alternative medication in patients with renal insufficiency.

What are the diagnostic criteria for acute gout?
Multiple criteria are in existence and have been validated over the years, using mainly clinical features of gout including time of attack, onset of attack (within 24 hours), type of arthritis (monoarthritis), joint involvement (first metatarsophalangeal joint), associated symptoms (swelling and erythema), tophus, increased uric acid levels, crystals in the aspirate, and characteristic radiographic findings.
- These criteria have recently been reviewed by an expert panel and having been accepted by both the American College of Rheumatology and the European League Against Rheumatism, a universal scoring system has been introduced to reach a diagnosis of gout.
- Any patient who presents with an episode of swelling, pain, or tenderness over a peripheral joint or bursa satisfies the entry criterion, and further use of the criteria given later should be applied.
- Fluid aspirate of a symptomatic joint, bursa, or tophus-containing crystals at microscopy is sufficient to make a diagnosis of gout (sufficient criterion) with no need for further criteria application.
- If crystals are not seen, the scoring system has to be applied based on a list of clinical, biochemical, and radiographic criteria. The scoring system has both negative and positive scores; the total sum of the individual criteria scoring will determine a diagnosis of gout. Fluid negative for crystals carries a negative score of minus 2. The total calculated score of equal to or more than 8 makes a diagnosis of gout.
- Each set of criteria has an individual weighting into the total calculation and online calculators can aid with the diagnosis. Criteria include the following:
  - Pattern of joint/bursa involvement: ankle, midfoot, first metatarsophalangeal joint
  - Characteristics of symptomatic episodes: erythema, pain to touch, difficulty walking
  - Time course or episode: time to maximum pain less than a day, resolution of symptoms of an attack in less than 14 days, and symptom free in between attacks
  - Clinical evidence of tophus
  - Serum urate level: different scores achieved, even negative scoring, depending on the serum urate level
  - Imaging: urate deposits in symptomatic joint, gout-related joint damage (erosions in hand/feet).

What drugs would you use if the patient was allergic to allopurinol?
Uricosuric drugs such as probenecid and sulfinpyrazone.

How would you determine whether a patient with elevated uric acid is an overproducer or an underexcretor?
An overproducer is one whose 24-hour urinary uric acid level >750 mg.

What is pseudogout?
Pseudogout is an acute arthritis resulting from the release of calcium pyrophosphate dihydrate crystals (deposited in the bone and cartilage) into the synovial fluid.

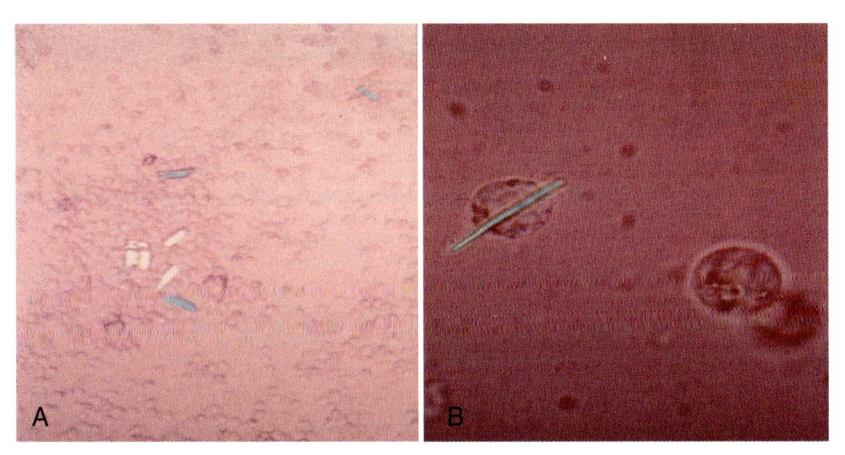

Fig. 67.3 Compensated polarized light microscopy of synovial fluid. **(A)** Positively birefringent crystals of calcium pyrophosphate dihydrate (CPPD) from patient with pseudogout. **(B)** Negatively birefringent crystal of monosodium urate monohydrate from a patient with gout. (With permission from Luqmani, R., Porter, D., Nuki, G., Robb, J., Keating, J.F., 2008. Textbook of Orthopaedics, Trauma and Rheumatology. Elsevier.)

Name some clinical differences between gout and pseudogout.

In monoarthritic cases, acute inflammation of the great toe of the foot is more commonly seen in gout, whereas inflammation of the knee is more commonly seen in pseudogout. Risk factors differ (trauma would usually precede an attack of pseudogout, hyperuricaemia is associated with gout). Different medication can precipitate the two conditions (bisphosphonate initiation can be complicated with pseudogout, lead toxicity is associated with gout).

How do you differentiate gout with pseudogout?

With synovial fluid analysis. Monosodium uric acid crystals are negatively birefringent and needle shaped, while calcium pyrophosphate crystals are positive birefringent or not birefringent, rhomboid- or cubic-shaped crystals (Fig. 67.3).

How is a pseudogout attack treated?

As most commonly it presents as acute monoarthritic inflammatory arthritis of a large joint like the knee, intraarticular steroid injection is the most appropriate treatment. In cases that this is not feasible, all antiinflammatory options given in gout, NSAIDs or colchicine, can be given.

Further Information

Gout was recognized as early as the 4th century BCE. Two concepts have prevailed: that it occurs mainly in sexually active mature men and that gastronomic and sexual excesses may precipitate acute attacks.

Antonie van Leeuwenhoek (1632–1723) described the microscopic appearance of urate crystals from gouty tophus.

In 1847, Alfred Garrod, in London, identified uric acid in the serum of a gouty man.

Michelangelo's gout has been depicted in a fresco by Raphael (Espinel, 1999).

CHAPTER 68

Osteoarthritis

Instruction

Look at this patient's hands.
Examine this patient's joints.

Salient Features

HISTORY

- Age
- Pain in the joints, which usually gets worse with activity and is relieved by rest
- Stiffness after a period of inactivity
- Impairment of gait as a result of joint pain
- Knees: pain on activities such as climbing stairs, getting out of a chair, and walking long distances (Morning stiffness usually lasts <30 min. Ask the patient whether their knees 'give way', a so-called instability symptom.)
- Hip: morning stiffness and pain (lasting <30 min) and pain at rest or at night are common. However, nocturnal hip pain may reflect inflammatory arthritis, infection, tumours, or crystal diseases.

EXAMINATION

- Heberden's nodes (bony swellings) at the terminal interphalangeal joints
- Squaring of the hands as a result of subluxation of the first metacarpophalangeal joint.

Proceed as follows:
- Tell the examiner that you would like to examine the hips and knees as these joints are usually involved. Clinical signs that can be elicited from joint examination are tenderness on palpation and motion, reduced range of movement of the joint, and joint deformity in advanced osteoarthritis.
- Knee: feel for crepitus: it may be red, warm, tender and have an effusion.
- Hip: the strongest clinical indicator of osteoarthritis of the hip is pain, exacerbated by internal or external rotation of the hip while the knee is in full extension. An assessment of the range of motion of the knee joint and lower lumbar spine may help to determine whether hip pain is referred from these other joints rather than the hip.

Diagnosis

This elderly patient has Heberden's nodes and squaring of the hands with involvement of the interphalangeal joints of the hands (lesions) caused by osteoarthritis (aetiology) and is unable to button his clothes (functional status).

68 — OSTEOARTHRITIS

Questions

Which joints are most frequently involved?
Spine, in particular cervical and lumbar spines, knees, hips, interphalangeal joints, carpometacarpal joints.

Mention the types and a few causes of osteoarthritis.
- Primary
- Secondary, caused by:
    - trauma: affects athletes, pneumatic drill workers, anyone doing work involving heavy lifting
    - inflammatory arthropathies: rheumatoid arthritis, septic arthritis, gout
    - neuropathic joints: diabetes mellitus, syringomyelia, tabes dorsalis
    - endocrine: acromegaly, hyperparathyroidism
    - metabolic: chondrocalcinosis, haemochromatosis.
- Osteoarthritis is classified into single-joint, multiple-joint, or generalized osteoarthritis, depending on the clinical picture and the distribution/number of joints involved in the disease process, as well as the presence of Heberden's nodes.

What are Heberden's nodes?
Bony swellings seen at the terminal interphalangeal joints in osteoarthrosis (Fig. 68.1).

What are Bouchard's nodes?
Bony swellings at the proximal interphalangeal joints in osteoarthrosis (Fig. 68.1).

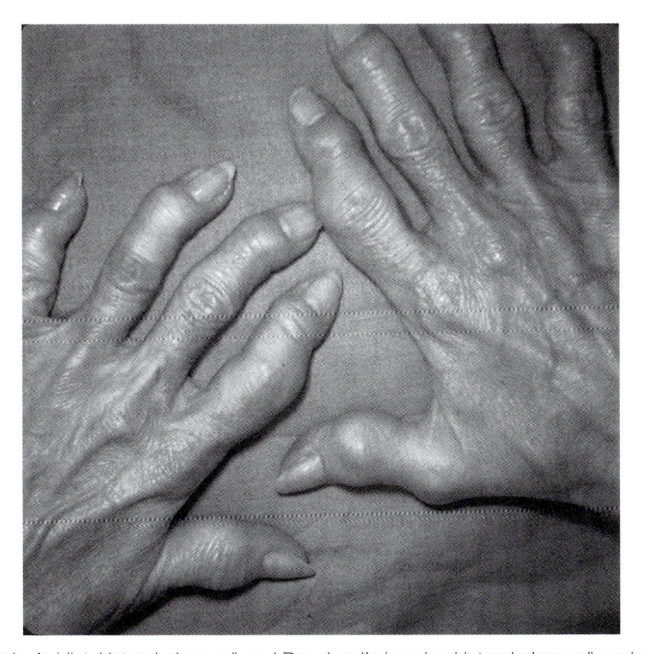

Fig. 68.1 Heberden's (distal interphalangeal) and Bouchard's (proximal interphalangeal) nodes on both index fingers and thumbs. Note angular changes at distal joints as result of loss of joint cartilage and instability. (With permission from Canale, S.T., Beaty, J.H. (eds.), 2007. Campbell's Operative Orthopaedics, eleventh edn. Mosby, Philadelphia, PA.)

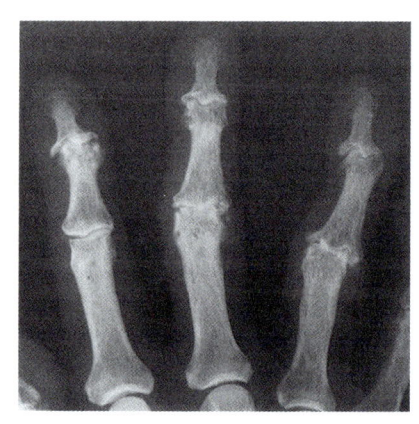

Fig. 68.2 Primary osteoarthritis of the fingers, with characteristic cartilage loss, deviations, and spurs of the proximal (Bouchard's nodes) and distal (Heberden's nodes) interphalangeal joints. (With permission from Grainger, R.G., Allison, D., 2001. Grainger & Allison's Diagnostic Radiology: A Textbook of Medical Imaging, fourth edn. Churchill Livingstone, Edinburgh.)

What are the typical radiological features?
- Subchondral bone sclerosis and cysts
- Narrowing of joint space
- Osteophytes (Fig. 68.2).

> **Note:** Radiological findings correlate poorly with the severity of pain. The European League Against Rheumatism have published guidelines on imaging recommending avoidance of radiological imaging if clinical features are consistent and adequate to reach a diagnosis, and if imaging is required, then simple films should be adequate.

What will the synovial aspirate show?
White blood cell count of $<100 \times 10^3$ cells/L.

What do you understand by the term nodal osteoarthrosis?
Nodal osteoarthrosis is a primary generalized osteoarthrosis with characteristic features. It occurs predominantly in middle-aged women with genetic predisposition. It characteristically affects the terminal interphalangeal joints, with the development of Heberden's nodes. The arthritis may be acute, and, although there may be marked deformity, there is little disability. It can also affect the carpometacarpal joints of the thumbs, spinal apophyseal joints, knees, and hips.

How would you manage a patient with osteoarthritis?
The approach in treatment, as with every chronic condition, should be within a multidisciplinary team and tailored to individual patients' needs:
- Patient education is paramount in optimizing treatment benefits.
- Change in lifestyle: maintain optimal weight, use appropriate footwear, encourage exercise to strengthen muscles (range-of-motion exercise that does not strengthen muscles is generally ineffective). An exercise programme of water aerobics, Pilates, or with a physical therapist at a frequency of twice a week for at least 2 months should improve muscle strength; nonpharmacologic therapy should not be ignored in the treatment of osteoarthritis, as

interventions such as exercise and weight loss have been proven to be as efficacious as pharmacologic options.
- Drugs: simple analgesics, rubefacients, nonsteroidal antiinflammatory drugs (NSAIDs), and cyclooxygenase-2 inhibitors for acute flare-ups; intraarticular corticosteroid injections for acute flare-ups or patients unfit for surgery. Topical NSAIDs are preferred as first line prior to oral treatments.
- Chondroitin, glucosamine, and their combination do not have a clinically relevant effect on perceived joint pain or on joint space narrowing, but they do not cause any significant side effects.
- Surgery: arthroscopic removal of loose body, arthroscopic washout, or radioisotope synovectomy for persistent synovitis; joint replacement for hip and knee. A recent study suggests that arthroscopic surgery for osteoarthritis of the knee provides no additional benefit to optimized physical and medical therapy.

What is the role of aggrecan in osteoarthritis?
In osteoarthritis, the degeneration of the cartilaginous extracellular matrix far exceeds its synthesis. The extracellular matrix of cartilage wears away, exposing articular cartilage, and eventually, bone. The two important components of this extracellular matrix are a type II collagen-rich collagenous network (which provides tensile strength) and a cartilage-specific proteoglycan called aggrecan (which is highly hydrated and thereby allows cartilage to resist a compressive load). Experimental studies suggest that the loss of aggrecan is the primary event leading to the destruction of cartilage. Three enzymes capable of degrading aggrecan have been identified: ADAMTS 1, ADAMTS 4, and ADAMTS 5. ADAMTS 5 is the main aggrecanase in mouse articular cartilage and is a possible pharmacologic target to prevent osteoarthritis.

Further Information

William Heberden (1710–1801) was a London physician who described the nodes as 'little hard knobs' and this was first published posthumously in 1802.

J.K. Spender (1886), of Bath, introduced the term osteoarthritis. Archibald E. Garrod, from London, established the modern usage and clinical differentiation from rheumatoid arthritis in 1907.

In 1884, C.J. Bouchard (1837–1915) described nodes adjacent to the proximal interphalangeal joints identical to those at the distal interphalangeal joints.

CHAPTER 69

Psoriatic Arthritis

Instruction

Examine this patient's hands.

Salient Features

HISTORY

- Cutaneous psoriasis with itching in a fifth of patients
- Joint pain, joint stiffness worse in the morning.

EXAMINATION

- Distal interphalangeal joint involvement.

Proceed as follows:
- Tell the examiner that you would like to:
  - examine the nails, looking for pitting, onycholysis, discoloration, thickening (nails are involved in 80% of patients with psoriatic arthritis)
  - look for psoriatic plaques in the extensor aspects of elbows, scalp, submammary region, umbilicus, and natal cleft; describe these as reddish plaques with well-defined edges and silvery white scales (Fig. 69.1)
- Comment on the fingers, which are sausage shaped because of tenosynovitis (called dactylitis) (Fig. 69.2).

Diagnosis

This patient has nail pitting, psoriatic plaques, and distal interphalangeal arthropathy (lesion) caused by psoriasis (aetiology) and has good hand function (functional status).

Questions

What are the patterns of joint involvement seen in psoriasis?
The patterns include:
- asymmetrical terminal joint involvement
- symmetrical joint involvement as seen in rheumatoid arthritis
- sacroiliitis: this differs from ankylosing spondylitis, most notably in that the syndesmophytes tend to arise from the lateral and anterior surfaces of the vertebral bodies and not at the margins of the bodies
- arthritis mutilans: complicated by the 'telescoping' of digits.

69 — PSORIATIC ARTHRITIS

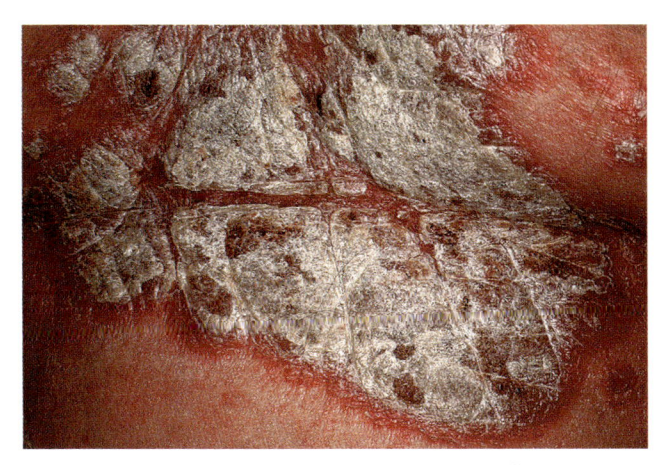

Fig. 69.1 Psoriatic plaque. Note the sharp demarcation and silvery scale. (Courtesy Bolognia, J.L., Schaffer, J.V., Duncan, K.O., 2022. Dermatology Essentials, second edn, Elsevier.)

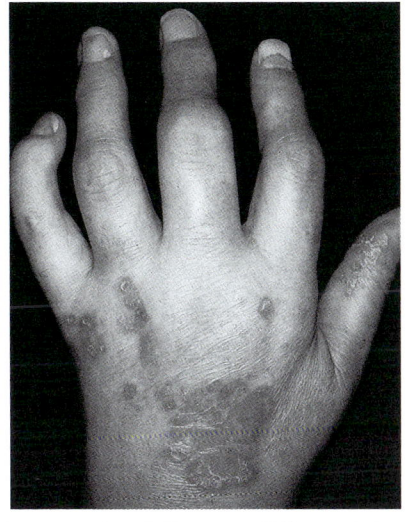

Fig. 69.2 Psoriatic arthritis with asymmetric arthritis pattern. (With permission from Habif, T.P., 2009. *Clinical Dermatology*, fifth edn. Mosby, Philadelphia, PA.)

What are the radiological features of psoriatic arthritis?
- 'Fluffy' periostitis
- Destruction of small joints
- 'Pencil and cup' appearance, osteolysis, and ankylosis in arthritis mutilans (Fig. 69.3)
- Nonmarginal syndesmophytes in spondylitis.

What is the prognosis?
Deforming and erosive arthritis is present in 40% of cases and 11% are disabled by their arthritis.

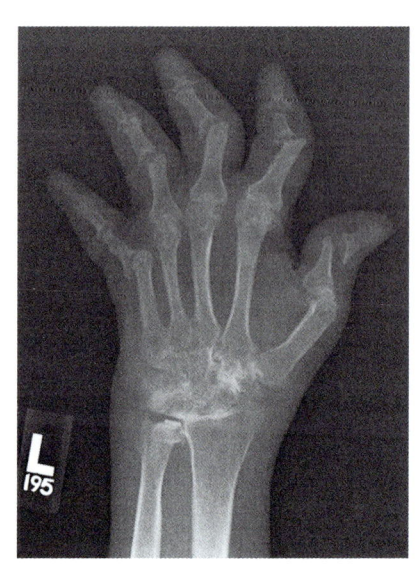

Fig. 69.3 Arthritis mutilans with destructive changes, joint deformity of the hand and pancompartmental ankylosis of the wrist. (With permission from Firestein, G.S., Budd, R.C., Harris Jr., E.D., et al., 2008. Kelley's Textbook of Rheumatology, eighth edn. Saunders, Philadelphia, PA.)

What are the management options?
- Nonsteroidal antiinflammatory drugs, e.g. indomethacin
- Selective cyclooxygenase-2 inhibitors
- Intraarticular corticosteroids
- Disease-modifying agents: sulfasalazine, hydroxychloroquine, leflunomide, tumour necrosis factor-α (TNF-α) blockers (adalimumab, etanercept, infliximab), newer agents including ustekinumab, certolizumab pegol, secukinumab, and PDE4 inhibitors—apremilast.

What do you know about the pathogenesis of psoriasis and therapy to mitigate it?
T-cell activation—inhibition by drugs of molecules involved in the formation of the immunologic synapse

Pathogenic T cells—depletion achieved by targeting molecules expressed specifically by activated T cells, such as the high-affinity interleukin-2 receptor or CD4

Release of inflammatory cytokines (e.g. TNF-α)—targeted by several biologic agents, the monoclonal antibodies infliximab and adalimumab, and the fusion proteins etanercept

Predominance of helper T cells (Th) type 1—induction of shift in immune balance to a milieu weighted with Th2 cells, thus alleviating psoriasis, e.g. using interleukin-10 and interleukin-4.

CHAPTER 70

Rheumatoid Hands

Instruction
This 67-year-old woman complains of painful hands. Please examine her.

Salient Features
HISTORY
- Painful swollen joints
- Morning stiffness.

EXAMINATION
- Ask the patient for permission to examine her hands and then ask whether the hands are sore.

Proceed as follows:
- Comment on deformities (Fig. 70.1), such as the following:
  - Subluxation at the metacarpophalangeal joint
  - Swan-neck deformity
  - Boutonnière deformity (hyperextension at the distal interphalangeal joint and flexion at the proximal interphalangeal joint)
  - Z deformity of the thumb
  - Dorsal subluxation of the ulna at the carpal joint.
- Comment on the following signs:
  - Nailfold infarcts and vasculitic skin lesions
  - Palmar erythema
  - Wasting of the first dorsal interosseous and other small muscles of the hand.
- Test grip and pincer movements. Quickly test for abductor pollicis brevis and interossei and pinprick sensation over index and little fingers. The median nerve may be involved if there is associated carpal tunnel syndrome.
- Examine the elbow for rheumatoid nodules.
- Ask the patient to perform simple tasks involving hand function, such as unbuttoning clothes or writing.
- Ask the patient their concerns about their symptoms and the impact of the disease on their activities of daily living.

Tell the examiner that you would like to examine other joints
- Highlight the following points:
  - Whether distal interphalangeal joints are spared or affected
  - Whether the arthritis is active (if the joints are inflamed) or inactive
  - Be prepared to discuss the radiological features.

269

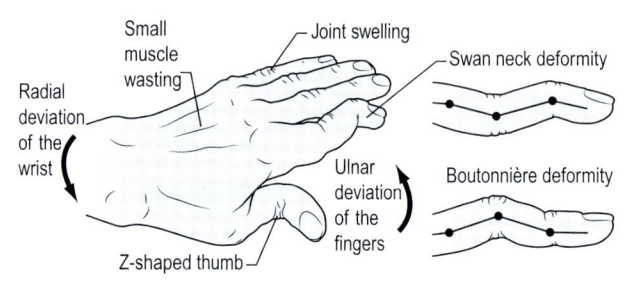

Fig. 70.1 Deformities of the hands in rheumatoid arthritis.

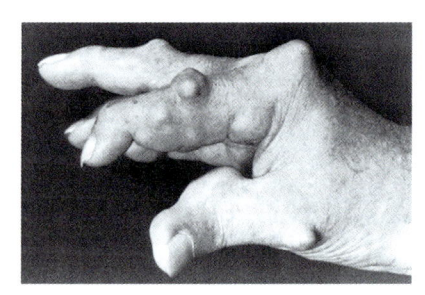

Fig. 70.2 Hand in seropositive rheumatoid arthritis, showing fixed deformities and gross rheumatoid nodules. (With permission from Canoso, J.J., 1997. Rheumatology in Primary Care. Saunders, Philadelphia, PA.)

Diagnosis

This patient has swan-neck deformity of the fingers (lesions) caused by rheumatoid arthritis (aetiology) with marked active arthritis of the interphalangeal joints and is unable to button her clothes (functional status).

Questions

What is the significance of nodules in rheumatoid arthritis?
The presence of nodules indicates seropositive and more aggressive arthritis (Fig. 70.2).

Where are nodules found?
Flexor and extensor tendons of the hand, sacrum, Achilles tendon, sclera, lungs, and myocardium.

Other than nodules, which other cutaneous manifestations are seen in rheumatoid arthritis?
Vasculitis, palmar erythema, nailfold infarcts, clubbing, venous and arterial ulcers, pyoderma gangrenosum, painful erythematous plaques (in Sweet syndrome—raised neutrophils, fever, and characteristic skin lesions), Cushingoid skin features (iatrogenic).

What are the causes of anaemia in rheumatoid arthritis?
- Anaemia of chronic disease
- Megaloblastic anaemia from folate deficiency or associated pernicious anaemia
- Felty syndrome
- Drugs.

70 — RHEUMATOID HANDS

What factors have been implicated in anaemia of chronic disease?
- Decreased production of red blood cells:
  - Inadequate iron: impaired absorption and transport, failure to release iron stores
  - Decreased concentration or marrow resistance to erythropoietin
- Ineffective erythropoiesis
- Abnormal development of erythroid progenitor cells
- Increased destruction of red cells.

What are the pulmonary manifestations of rheumatoid arthritis?
- Pleural effusion or pleurisy (seen in 25% of men with rheumatoid arthritis)
- Rheumatoid nodules
- Fibrosing alveolitis
- Caplan syndrome (rheumatoid arthritis coexisting with rounded fibrotic nodules 0.5 to 5.0 cm in diameter, mainly in the periphery of lung fields in coal-worker's pneumoconiosis).

What are the eye manifestations of rheumatoid arthritis?
- Episcleritis
- Scleritis
- Scleromalacia, scleromalacia perforans
- Keratoconjunctivitis sicca
- Sjögren syndrome.

What precautions are necessary before upper gastrointestinal endoscopy or general anaesthesia?
It is prudent to take a cervical spine radiograph to rule out atlantoaxial subluxation.

Which joints are commonly affected in rheumatoid arthritis?
Wrists, proximal interphalangeal joints and metacarpophalangeal joints of the hands, metatarsophalangeal joints, and knees.

What is palindromic rheumatoid arthritis?
Palindromic onset is seen in some patients with recurrent episodes of joint stiffness and pain in individual joints lasting only a few hours or days. Hydroxychloroquine may be of value in preventing recurrences.

How would you treat the arthritis?
One basic tenet of treating any arthritis is to control pain with analgesia. Nonsteroidal antiinflammatory drugs (NSAIDs) should be the first line of treatment and should be prescribed with gastroprotection, usually in the form of a proton pump inhibitor.

At the time of diagnosis, treatment of rheumatoid arthritis should be directed at inducing remission of the disease with initiation of disease-modifying antirheumatic drugs (DMARDs). There are a number of DMARDs: methotrexate, hydroxychloroquine, sulfasalazine, azathioprine, mycophenolate mofetil, and cyclosporine. Low-dose methotrexate together with another DMARD and a short course of corticosteroids is the initial treatment of choice. If the disease is severe, calculated by the disease severity score (DAS28), biological agents should be considered. Commonly used biological agents include anti-tumour necrosis factors (adalimumab, etanercept, infliximab) and rituximab (antibody to CD20). Common side effects of biological agents are local reactions at the injection site (particularly with etanercept), hypersensitivity reactions (particularly with infliximab), and immunosuppression with risk of infection (a shared common side effect of

DMARD use). All DMARDs used in the treatment of rheumatoid arthritis require appropriate monitoring, and various national and international best practice guidelines exist.

What do you know of thiopurine methyltransferase (TPMT) and azathioprine treatment?
Azathioprine is commonly used as a DMARD in the treatment of rheumatoid arthritis. One of its common side effects, in common with all thiopurine drugs, is myelosuppression. TPMT is involved in the metabolism of azathioprine. Patients with low levels of TPMT run a high risk of azathioprine myelotoxicity. Thioguanine nucleotide metabolites precipitated by low TPMT activity in azathioprine use can cause life-threatening bone marrow toxicity. Hence, TPMT levels should be assessed prior to initiating treatment with azathioprine.

What are the neurological manifestations of rheumatoid arthritis?
- Peripheral neuropathy: glove-and-stocking sensory loss
- Mononeuritis multiplex
- Entrapment neuropathy, e.g. carpal tunnel syndrome
- Cervical disease or atlantoaxial subluxation may cause cervical myelopathy.

What are the causes of proteinuria in patients with rheumatoid arthritis?
- Drug therapy
- Amyloidosis.

What is Sjögren syndrome?
- The association of keratoconjunctivitis sicca (lack of lacrimal secretion) and xerostomia (dry mouth as a result of lack of salivary gland secretion) in association with a connective tissue disorder, usually rheumatoid arthritis. This syndrome may be associated with autoimmune thyroid disease, myasthenia gravis, or autoimmune liver disease.
- Anti-Ro (SSA) and anti-SS-B antibodies may be seen in this syndrome.
- Treatment is symptomatic with artificial tears (hypromellose drops or 1% methylcellulose), artificial saliva, and NSAIDs for the arthritis.
- The Schirmer filter paper test provides a crude measure of tear production. Filter paper is hooked over the lower eyelid and in normal people at least 15 mm is wet after 5 min, whereas in patients with keratoconjunctivitis sicca, it is <5 mm.

What is the role of anti-cyclic citrullinated peptide (CCP) antibodies?
The presence of autoantibodies to CCP is specific to rheumatoid arthritis. Their detection contributes both to the differential diagnosis and to a prediction of the severity of joint destruction. It is the antibody of choice in diagnosing and monitoring disease progression, as it combines the high sensitivity of rheumatoid factor (RF) with a far better specificity for rheumatoid arthritis; they both have a sensitivity of around 88%. However, anti-CCP antibodies have a sensitivity of 95% compared to a sensitivity of 85% for RF.

What are the American College of Rheumatology/European League Against Rheumatism criteria for rheumatoid arthritis?
Patients are definitively diagnosed with rheumatoid arthritis if they score 6 or more points on the following series of assessments:

Joint involvement:
- 1 medium–large joint: 0 points
- 2 to 10 medium–large joints: 1 point
- 1 to 3 small joints: 2 points
- 4 to 10 small joints: 3 points
- >10 small joints: 5 points.

Serology:
- Not positive for either RF or anti-citrullinated protein antibody: 0 points
- At least one of these two tests is positive at low titre (more than the upper limit of normal but not higher than three times the upper limit of normal): 2 points
- At least one test is positive at high titre (more than three times the upper limit of normal): 3 points.

Duration of synovitis:
- Lasting fewer than 6 weeks: 0 points
- Lasting 6 weeks or longer: 1 point.

Acute phase reactants:
- Neither C-reactive protein nor erythrocyte sedimentation rate (ESR) abnormal: 0 points
- Abnormal C-reactive protein or abnormal ESR: 1 point.

Patients receive the highest point level they fulfil within each domain. For example, a patient with five small joints involved and four large joints involved scores 3 points.

What are the poor prognostic factors?
- Systemic features: weight loss, extraarticular manifestations
- Insidious onset
- Rheumatoid nodules
- Presence of RF >1:512
- Persistent activity of the disease for over 12 months
- Early bone erosions.

What are the factors leading to ulnar deviation of the hands?
In the normal grip, the fingers move to ulnar deviation; this is caused by:
- Weakening of radial side of the joint capsule and the radial insertion of the interossei ligaments
- The volar supports of the flexor tendon sheath are weakened by inflammation, allowing the tendon to bow in the direction of the ulna during gripping.
- Ulnar displacement of the extensor tendons in early deviation makes them slip if the dorsal metacarpophalangeal joint is taut, and this exacerbates the development of ulnar deviation by acting as a bowstring.
- Joint capsules of metacarpophalangeal joints are weaker on radial sides than on ulnar sides

What is the role of cadherins in the pathogenesis of rheumatoid arthritis?
Fibroblast-like synoviocytes mediate cartilage damage in rheumatoid arthritis (rheumatoid inflammation causes damage to both articular cartilage and periarticular bone). Cadherin-11 deficiency protects mice from cartilage damage but not from bone erosion, probably because cadherin-11 seems to mediate the migration of fibroblast-like synoviocytes over the articular cartilage and its subsequent damage.

What is the role of phosphatidylinositol 3′-kinase-γ in the pathogenesis of rheumatoid arthritis?
A novel inhibitor of phosphatidylinositol 3′-kinase has been shown to be effective in blocking inflammation and joint destruction in mouse models of rheumatoid arthritis.

Further Information
A.B. Garrod coined the term rheumatoid arthritis in 1858.
H.S.C. Sjögren, a Swedish ophthalmologist, described his eponymous condition in 1933.

- A. Caplan, a British physician, was an industrial medical officer in the Welsh coal mines when he identified the association between rheumatoid arthritis and pneumoconiosis and went on to describe Caplan syndrome in 1953.
- In 1931, Philip S. Hench (1896–1965) of the Mayo Clinic observed that arthritic pain temporarily decreased in pregnant women. He then studied the phenomena for the next 8 years, finding that allergic conditions such as asthma, hay fever, and food sensitivity were also lessened in the presence of jaundice or pregnancy. He reasoned that a steroid hormone may be responsible, since levels of steroid hormones are high in the blood during pregnancy (Hench, 1953).
- Edward Kendall (1886–1972), Chief of the Division of Biochemistry, suggested the name 'corsone' on a piece of paper but Hench amended this to 'cortisone', and thus, the steroid hormone was 'baptized'. The 1950 Nobel Prize for Medicine was jointly awarded to Kendall, Hench, and Tadeus Reichstein (1897–1996) of Basel University, Switzerland, for their discoveries relating to the hormones of the adrenal cortex, their structure and biological effects (Raju, 1990).
- Sir John Vane showed that inhibition of prostaglandin synthesis was central to both the actions and side effects of aspirin (Maiden and McLaren, 2000).

CHAPTER 71

Dermatomyositis — Proximal Muscle Weakness

Instruction

Examine this patient.

Salient Features

HISTORY

- Adult form usually occurs after the age of 40 years
- Weakness of proximal muscles evolving over weeks or months: difficulty in getting up from a low chair or squatting position, climbing stairs, lifting and running
- Inability to raise head
- Dysphagia (caused by weakness of the muscles of the pharynx)
- Dysphonia
- Muscle pain and tenderness
- Raynaud phenomenon
- Rash is made worse by exposure to sunlight (photosensitivity)

EXAMINATION

- Skin features (Fig. 71.1):
  - Heliotrope rash or purplish-blue rash around the eyes, back of the hands, dilated capillary loops at the base of fingernails, erythema of knuckles accompanied by a raised violaceous scaly eruption (Gottron's sign); the erythema spares the phalanges (unlike that of systemic lupus erythematosus in which the phalanges are involved and the knuckles are spared)
  - Erythematous rash may be present on the neck and upper chest (often in the shape of a V), shoulders (shawl sign), elbows, knees, and malleoli
  - Cuticles may be irregular, thickened, and distorted; the lateral and palmar areas of the fingers become rough and cracked with irregular 'dirty' horizontal lines, resembling those in a mechanic's hands
- Muscle features:
  - Proximal muscle weakness and tenderness of muscles (muscle wasting absent or minimal)
  - Weakness of neck flexors in two-thirds of cases
  - Intact or absent deep tendon reflexes
- If the patient is >40 years of age, an underlying neoplasm should be sought
- Signs of interstitial lung disease (occurs in 5%–10% of patients with polymyositis or dermatomyositis, especially in those with anti-Jo-1 antibody).

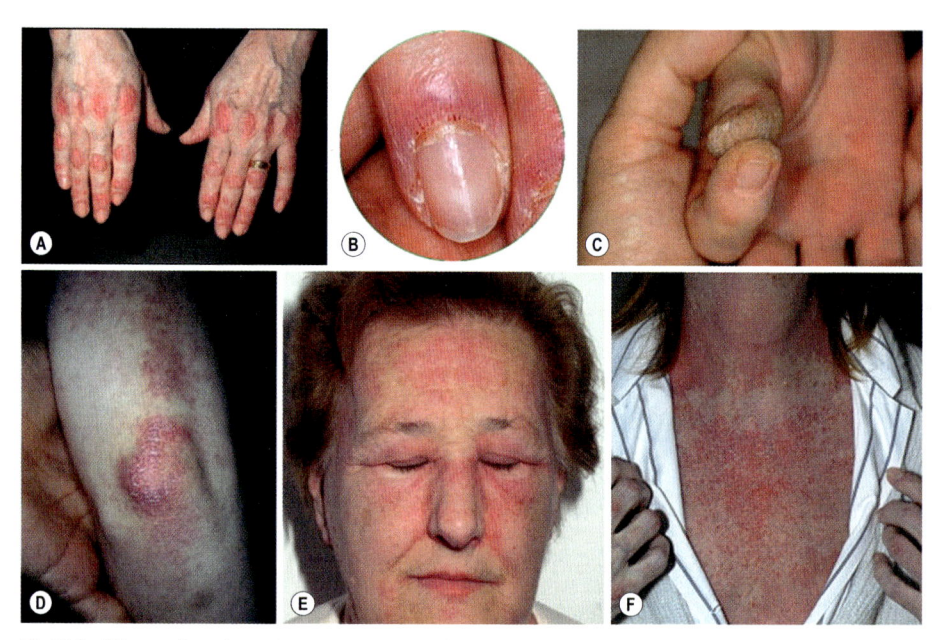

Fig. 71.1 Skin manifestations of dermatomyositis: **(A)** Gottron papules, **(B)** periungual telangiectasia with cuticular hemorrhage and dystrophy, **(C)** mechanic's hand, **(D)** Gottron sign, **(E)** heliotrope rash, **(F)** poikilodermatomyositis. (With permission from Laccarino, L., Ghirardello, A., Bettio, S., Zen, M., Gatto, M., Punzi, L., Doria, A., 2014. The clinical features, diagnosis and classification of dermatomyositis. J. Autoimmun. 48–49, 122–127.)

Diagnosis

This patient has Gottron's papules and proximal muscle weakness (lesion) caused by dermatomyositis (aetiology).

Questions

What investigations would you like to do?
- Estimate serum creatine kinase (also known as creatine phosphokinase) levels
- Electromyography shows myopathic changes (spontaneous fibrillation, salvos of repetitive potentials, and short duration of polyphasic potentials of low amplitude)
- Perform muscle biopsy (will show necrosis and phagocytosis of muscle fibres and interstitial and perivascular infiltration of inflammatory cells)
- Magnetic resonance imaging and magnetic resonance spectroscopy of affected tissue may show abnormal signals in striated muscle and abnormalities of muscle metabolism.

In which other conditions is there proximal muscle weakness with high serum creatine kinase levels?
Proximal muscle weakness can be a manifestation of a variety of myopathies, such as autoimmune conditions (dermatomyositis), endocrinopathies (Cushing disease), drug-induced myositides (statins), rheumatological diseases (polymyalgia rheumatica), inherited myopathies (muscular dystrophy), metabolic disorders and conditions that cause rhabdomyolysis. The main differential for a proximal weakness with high creatine kinase (CK) levels is drug-induced myopathy. Causative medications can be statins, chloroquine, and colchicine, especially in patients on chronic haemodialysis, and rhabdomyolysis.

How would you treat a patient with an inflammatory myopathy?
- Most patients respond to steroids; prednisolone is the first-line drug for the empiric treatment of polymyositis and dermatomyositis. It is started as soon as possible, with an average duration of a year, depending on the patient's response.
- Steroid-resistant dermatomyositis will benefit from a steroid-sparing agent such as methotrexate or azathioprine.
- Other agents may be used for resistant disease, like intravenous immunoglobulin or rituximab.
- Those with an underlying neoplasm may see the dermatomyositis remit after treatment of the tumour.

Mention some side effects of chronic systemic use of steroids.
- Skin changes
- Cushingoid features, adrenal insufficiency on stopping, diabetes mellitus
- Peptic ulcers, gastritis, ileus, or visceral perforation
- Weight gain, osteoporosis, myopathy
- Increased risk of infections
- Neuropsychiatric disorders.

What are the inflammatory myopathies?
Inflammatory myopathies are a group of myopathies that are classified into five categories, based on their features on histology:
- Dermatomyositis
- Polymyositis
- Necrotizing myositis
- Inclusion body myositis
- Overlap myositis.

Mention a few disorders associated with myositis.
Sarcoid myositis, focal nodular myositis, infectious polymyositis (Lyme disease, toxoplasma), inclusion body myositis, eosinophilic myositis.

What do you know about inclusion body polymyositis?
Inclusion body myositis usually occurs in men >50 years of age. It is characterized by indolent, progressive proximal muscle weakness, which may be asymmetric, that eventually also involves distal muscles. Both myopathic and neuropathic changes can be seen on electromyography studies. Muscle biopsy reveals mononuclear infiltrates and vacuoles in the muscle cells that contain inclusion bodies. Inclusion body myositis often responds poorly to conventional therapy with steroids.

What do you understand by the term overlap syndrome?
Overlap syndrome indicates that the characteristics of two different disorders are common to both. Dermatomyositis overlaps with systemic sclerosis and mixed connective tissue disease. Specific signs of systemic sclerosis and mixed connective tissue disease, such as sclerotic thickening of the dermis, contractures, oesophageal hypomotility, microangiopathy, and calcium deposits, are present in dermatomyositis. Patients with the overlap syndrome of dermatomyositis and systemic sclerosis may have a specific anti-nuclear autoantibody, anti-PM/Scl, directed against a nucleolar protein complex.

A patient presents to the acute medical take with acute onset dyspnoea. They were seen in the medical clinic a week prior to the presentation with symptoms consistent with dermatomyositis and a muscle biopsy result and autoimmune screen are pending. On examination you note fine bibasal inspiratory crackles, mechanic's hands bilaterally, and joint tenderness. Which antibodies would you suspect to come back positive?

The description of possible dermatomyositis, pulmonary fibrosis, mechanic's hands, and arthritis would suggest antisynthetase syndrome and you would expect the anti-Jo antibodies to be positive. Antisynthetase syndrome is a group of inflammatory myopathies with antibodies against RNA synthetases.

Further Information

Heinrich Adolf Gottron (1890–1974), a German dermatologist.

CHAPTER 72

Scleroderma

Instruction
Look at these hands, examine, and proceed.

Salient Features
HISTORY
- Tight skin over face and joints
- Raynaud's phenomenon
- Puffy hands and feet
- Fatigue
- Dry eyes
- Shortness of breath (lung involvement, cardiac fibrosis), dry cough
- Gastrointestinal (GI) symptoms: dysphagia, diarrhoea, bloating, and indigestion
- History of renal failure
- Personal or family history of autoimmune disorders.

EXAMINATION
- Thickening and tightening of the skin over fingers, sclerodactyly (finger pulp atrophy) (Fig. 72.1), beaking of nails (pseudoclubbing), atrophic nails, telangiectasia (nailfold capillaries) (Fig. 72.2)
- Raynaud's phenomenon
- Subcutaneous calcification (fingers, elbows, and extensor aspect of the forearms)
- Vitiligo or pigmentation.

Proceed as follows:
- Assess hand function: pincer movements, handgrip, unbuttoning of clothes, abduction of thumb, and writing
- Examine:
  - the joints for arthralgia or arthritis
  - the face for microstomia, difficulty in opening the mouth, beak-like or pinched appearance of the nose, blotchy telangiectasia
  - the abdomen for liver (primary biliary cirrhosis).

Diagnosis
This patient has sclerodactyly, tightening of the skin over hands and face (lesion) caused by scleroderma (aetiology). He has difficulty in buttoning his clothes and has marked dysphagia as a result of oesophageal involvement (functional status).

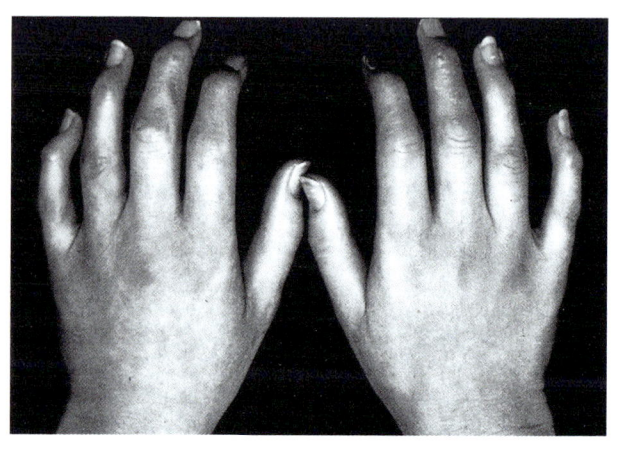

Fig. 72.1 Hands in scleroderma.

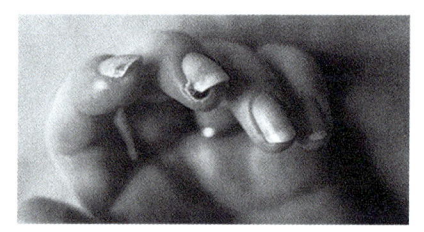

Fig. 72.2 Digital ulcers. (With permission from Charles, C., Clements, P., Furst, D.E., 2006. Systemic sclerosis: hypothesis-driven treatment strategies. Lancet 367, 1683–1691.)

Questions

What other organ systems are involved?
- Skin: Raynaud's phenomenon, localized morphoea, local or generalized oedema, hyperpigmentation, telangiectasia, subcutaneous calcification, ulceration, particularly at the fingertips. Ten-year survival rate is 71%, with skin tightness limited to fingers but 21% with diffuse truncal skin involvement. Iloprost, a prostacyclin analogue, helps to heal digital ulceration. Penicillamine improves the skin and prolongs survival in patients with early, rapidly progressive, systemic sclerosis.
- Musculoskeletal system: arthritis, myositis, myopathy, bone ischaemia with resorption of the phalanges
- GI tract: dysphagia, reflux oesophagitis, large or small bowel obstruction
- Lung: fibrosis, atelectasis, pulmonary hypertension, pneumonia
- Kidney: glomerulonephritis, malignant hypertension (poorest prognosis with renal involvement). Angiotensin-converting enzyme inhibitors dramatically improve renal crisis.
- Heart: myocardial fibrosis.

Remember: The prognosis is worse in those with renal disease and in males. Patients with skin and/or gut involvement without other organ disease have the best prognosis. Severely debilitating oesophageal dysfunction is the most common visceral complication, and lung involvement is the leading cause of death.

72 — SCLERODERMA

What are the variants of scleroderma?
CREST syndrome (see later), eosinophilic fasciitis, Thibierge–Weissenbach syndrome.

What is 'CREST' syndrome?
Calcinosis, Raynaud's phenomenon, oesophageal dysmotility, sclerodactyly, and telangiectasia. It has a more favourable prognosis than systemic sclerosis and is associated with the anticentromere antibody. CREST syndrome is also known as limited cutaneous systemic sclerosis.

What are the criteria for diagnosis of scleroderma?
The following criteria have been developed by the American College of Rheumatology and the European League Against Rheumatism

Item	Subitem	Points
Skin thickening of the fingers of both hands extending proximal to the metacarpophalangeal (MCP) joints		9 (this is sufficient criterion on its own; if not present, apply the following items)
Skin thickening of the fingers	Puffy fingers	2
	Sclerodactyly of the fingers (distal to MCP joints but proximal to the interphalangeal joints)	4 (only count the higher score)
Fingertip lesions	Digital tip ulcers	2
	Fingertip pitting scars	3 (only count the higher score)
Telangiectasia		2
Abnormal nailfold capillaries		2
Lung involvement	Pulmonary arterial hypertension	2
	Interstitial lung disease	2 (max score 2)
Raynaud phenomenon		3
Systemic sclerosis (SSc)-related autoantibodies	Anti-centromere	3
	Anti-topoisomerase I (anti-Scl-70)	
	Anti-RNA-polymerase III	

A total score of 9 or more has a 91% sensitivity and 92% specificity for a diagnosis of scleroderma.

What are the subsets of scleroderma?
- Limited cutaneous scleroderma: where the skin is affected only at the extremities
- Diffuse cutaneous scleroderma: skin of trunk and extremities affected
- Scleroderma sine scleroderma: skin not affected, patients present with pulmonary fibrosis, scleroderma renal crisis, cardiac failure or malabsorption, and pseudoobstruction. The presence of anticentromere, scleroderma-70, and antinuclear antibodies can be helpful.

What are the causes of anaemia in such a patient?
- Iron deficiency from chronic oesophagitis
- Folate and vitamin B deficiency from malabsorption
- Anaemia of chronic disease
- Microangiopathic haemolytic anaemia.

What are the phases of skin changes in scleroderma?
- An early oedematous phase (with pitting oedema of hands and possibly forearms, legs, and face)
- The dermal phase
- An atrophic phase, followed by contracture
- Other skin changes, e.g. depigmentation.

What do you know about the pathogenesis of these skin changes?
- Endothelial damage caused by a circulatory protein factor has been implicated as an early component of the 'inflammatory' phase; this endothelial damage may result in the capillary and arteriolar abnormalities seen as well as affecting local access of circulating proteins acting on fibroblast-enhancing collagen secretion.
- The profibrotic phenotype of fibroblasts in scleroderma is maintained by at least three factors:
  - Abnormal signalling by transforming growth factor-β (TGF-β) results in an increased level of platelet-derived growth factor receptor (PDGFR) (TGF-$β_1$ mediates fibrosis).
  - Amplification of the Ras–ERK1/2–ROS signalling loop, perhaps as a result of the upregulation of PDGFR
  - Stimulation of autoantibodies against PDGFR that initiate and maintain the Ras–ERK1/2–ROS cascade.

How would you manage a patient with scleroderma?
- Educational and psychological support
- Stop smoking.
- Treat vascular abnormalities such as Raynaud's phenomenon.
- Screening for pulmonary artery hypertension and interstitial lung disease and renal disease
- Early phase of diffuse form: immunosuppressive drugs (cyclophosphamide, methotrexate, mycophenolate mofetil, rituximab)
- Those at risk of severe organ involvement may be considered for autologous stem cell transplant.
- Later stages: antifibrotic drugs to reduce collagen production (penicillamine, interferon)
- Treat pulmonary hypertension with endothelin receptor antagonist, phosphodiesterase type 5 inhibitors, or riociguat. Consider intravenous epoprostenol for those with severe pulmonary artery hypertension.
- Treat renal disease with angiotensin-converting enzyme inhibitors.
- Symptomatic GI involvement: treat oesophagitis with proton pump inhibitors for oesophagitis; prokinetics for reflux and dysphagia; intermittent antibiotics for small bowel overgrowth.

What is the role of prednisone in the treatment of scleroderma?
Prednisone has little or no role in the treatment of scleroderma.

What are the common fatal events in this disease?
In most cases, death results from cardiac, renal, or respiratory failure.

Further Information
The first reports of scleroderma were by W. D. Chowne in 1842 and James Startin, both from London, in 1846. The term sclerodermie was suggested by E. Gintrac (1791–1877) of Bordeaux; Italian physician G. B. Fantonetti introduced the term sklerodarma in 1836.

Maurice Raynaud commented on the presence of Raynaud's phenomenon in scleroderma in 1863.

Heirich Auspitz (1835–1886) reported, in 1863, on death from renal failure in scleroderma; this was proved to be a more than chance association by H. Moore and H. Sheehan of Liverpool in 1952.

CHAPTER 73

Systemic Lupus Erythematosus

Instruction
This young patient presented with a facial rash of recent onset. Please examine her face.

Salient Features
HISTORY
- Fatiguability and tiredness: suggests anaemia
- Joint symptoms: particularly small joints (90% of patients)
- Gangrene of the digits: vasculitis
- Skin rash (butterfly rash on face; Fig. 73.1) in sun-exposed areas, livedo reticularis, alopecia, Raynaud's phenomenon
- Mouth ulcers
- Hypertension, oedema (suggesting renal involvement)
- Fever, enlargement of lymph nodes
- Bleeding from gums, excessive menstrual bleeding, purpura (caused by thrombocytopenia)
- Neuropsychiatric symptoms, seizures
- History of remissions and exacerbations
- Drug history (hydralazine, procainamide, minocycline).

EXAMINATION
- Butterfly rash: follicular plugging, scales, telangiectasia, and scarring affecting the bridge of the nose and cheeks (the patient may be cushingoid because of steroids)
- Examine the following:
  - Conjunctiva for anaemia (often Coombs' test positive)
  - Mouth ulcers (seen in one-third of cases; Fig. 73.2)
  - Scalp for alopecia
  - Sun-exposed areas and elbows for vasculitic rash, subcutaneous nodules
  - Nails for splinter haemorrhages, nailfold capillaries, and periungual infarcts
  - Hands for palmar erythema, Raynaud's phenomenon, arthritis
  - Knees for vasculitic rash
  - Feet for secondary oedema (secondary to nephrotic syndrome)
- Tell the examiner that you would like to examine the urine for proteinuria.

Note: Systemic lupus erythematosus (SLE) principally affects skin, joints, kidney, and serosal membranes.

73—SYSTEMIC LUPUS ERYTHEMATOSUS

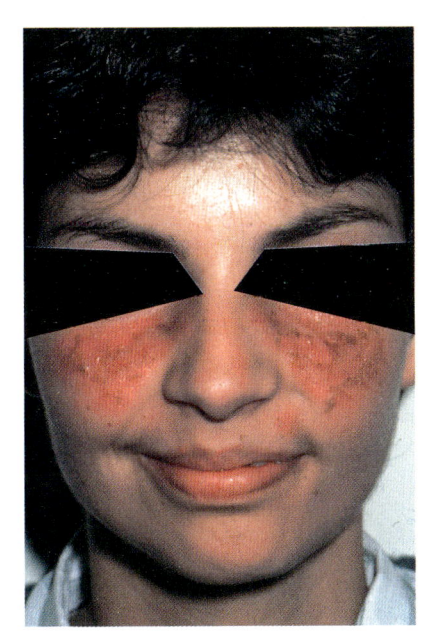

Fig. 73.1 Malar rash in a patient with systemic lupus erythematosus. Note that the rash does not cross the nasolabial fold. (With permission from Klippel, J.H., Dieppe, P.A. (Eds.), 1998. Rheumatology, second edn. Mosby, London.)

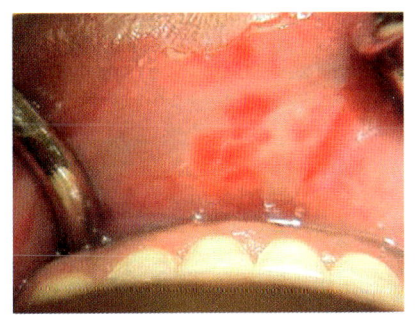

Fig. 73.2 Oral mucosal ulcerations: generally painless and can present on other cutaneous tissues. (With permission from Powers, D.B., 2008. Systemic lupus erythematosus and discoid lupus erythematosus. Oral Maxillofac. Surg. Clin. North. Am. 20, 661–662.)

Diagnosis

This patient has a butterfly rash on the face with telangiectasia (lesion) caused by SLE (aetiology) and has renal failure, probably caused by lupus nephritis as evidenced by the haemodialysis catheter (functional status).

Questions

What is the histology of the skin rash in SLE?
- Liquefactive degeneration of the basal layer of the epidermis together with oedema at the dermoepidermal junction. Immunofluorescence microscopy shows deposition of immunoglobulin and complement along the dermoepidermal junction.
- Oedema of the dermis accompanied by infiltrates of perivascular mononuclear cells
- Vasculitis with fibrinoid necrosis of the vessels.

What are the skin manifestations of SLE?
Butterfly rash, periungual erythema, nailfold telangiectasia, alopecia, livedo reticularis, hyperpigmentation, urticaria, purpura, scarring eruption of discoid lupus.

What are the criteria for diagnosis of SLE?
The entry criterion is a positive antinuclear antibody (ANA) at a titre of >1:80.

The European League Against Rheumatism (EULAR)/American College of Rheumatology (ACR) criteria, updated in 2019, are at least one clinical criterion and a total score of at least 10.

Clinical domains: fever, haematologic (leukopoenia, thrombocytopenia, autoimmune haemolysis), neuropsychiatric (delirium, psychosis, seizure), mucocutaneous (nonscarring alopecia, oral ulcers, cutaneous or discoid lupus), serosal (pleural/pericardial effusion, pericarditis), musculoskeletal (joint involvement), and renal (proteinuria, nephritis on renal biopsy).

Immunological domains: antiphospholipid antibodies, low complement, SLE-specific antibodies.

> **Note:** It is often possible to be reasonably confident about a diagnosis of SLE on clinical grounds. A diagnosis of SLE is usually made when patients have three or four typical manifestations, such as a characteristic skin rash, thrombocytopenia, serositis or nephritis, and ANA. Polyarthritis and dermatitis are the most common manifestations. It should be noted that antibodies to double-stranded DNA and the so-called Smith antigen (Sm) are virtually diagnostic of SLE.

The Systemic Lupus International Collaborating Clinics revised the aforementioned criteria and developed a more comprehensive list in order to increase sensitivity. The final diagnostic criteria are 17 in total, and for a diagnosis to be established, a patient has to have at least four of them, of which one has to be clinical and one has to be immunological, or the patient must have biopsy-proven lupus nephritis with ANAs or anti-double-stranded DNA antibodies.
- Acute cutaneous lupus
- Chronic cutaneous lupus
- Nonscarring alopecia
- Oral or nasal ulcers
- Joint disease
- Serositis
- Proteinuria
- Neurological symptoms
- Anaemia
- Thrombocytopenia
- Leucopenia
- Low complement levels
- Antiphospholipid antibodies
- Anti-smooth muscle antibodies

- Anti-double-stranded DNA antibodies
- ANAs
- Direct Coomb's test positive.

What do you know about SLE in older patients?

The initial presentation of idiopathic SLE usually occurs between the first and fourth decades of life. However, about 10% may first occur in patients >60 years of age. Patients with SLE after the age of 50 years less often present with malar rash, arthritis, and nephritis.

Diagnosis of SLE in older patients must be one of exclusion. The frequency of low titres on ANA tests increases with advancing age, and a positive test may be associated with malignant disease or chronic infection.

What do you know about drug-induced lupus erythematosus?

- Procainamide is responsible for the majority of the cases. Other causes include hydralazine, quinidine, and isoniazid.
- Drugs causing lupus-like syndrome do not seem to aggravate primary SLE.
- Patients with drug-induced lupus usually present with skin and joint manifestations.
- Although multiple organs are affected, nephritis and central nervous system (CNS) features are not ordinarily present.
- Anti-histone antibodies are characteristic of drug-induced lupus but are not specific for this syndrome; anti-native DNA is almost never detected.
- Clinical manifestations and many laboratory features return to normal after the offending drug is withdrawn.

How useful is the detection of ANAs in the diagnosis of SLE?

ANA antibodies should be positive in any patient with lupus at some point in their life. It is a sensitive test and can aid the diagnosis of SLE. However, their detection very much depends on the specific laboratory and the techniques used, so a false-negative result may occur and should not be taken into account if the clinical suspicion for lupus diagnosis is high. Instead, they should be repeated at a later stage.

What are the patterns of lupus nephritis?

The World Health Organization's morphological classification of lupus nephritis describes five patterns:
- Normal by light, electron, and immunofluorescence microscopy (rare)
- Mesangial lupus glomerulonephritis
- Focal proliferative glomerulonephritis
- Diffuse proliferative glomerulonephritis
- Membranous glomerulonephritis.

Note: None of these patterns is specific for lupus.

How would you manage a patient with SLE?

- Avoidance of sunlight provocation. In Britain, patients should avoid being outside from 11 am to 3 pm from March to September and should wear protective clothing, including hats; patients should holiday in temperate latitudes or during the winter. In addition, sun block creams such as titanium dioxide (rather than barrier cream) are essential.
- Avoid drug provocation: penicillin, sulphonamides.
- Encourage the patient to join the Lupus Society.

- Educate the patient that no therapy is curative and that medical treatment is largely empirical, selected on the basis of specific manifestations:

Disease Manifestation	Treatment
Serological abnormalities and minor cytopenia unaccompanied by symptoms	No treatment
All patients with any disease activity	Antimalarial drugs: hydroxychloroquine, chloroquine
Mild or moderate arthritis, fever, pleuropericarditis	Nonsteroidal antiinflammatory drugs or low-dose prednisolone, azathioprine, or methotrexate if steroid-sparing immunosuppression is needed
Malaise, weight loss, and lymphadenopathy	Low-dose steroids, immunosuppression therapy
High fever, active inflammatory glomerulonephritis, severe thrombocytopenia, severe haemolytic anaemia, and most neurological disturbances	Pulsed methylprednisolone, with or without other immunosuppressive agents (mycophenolate, azathioprine, cyclophosphamide, rituximab)
Rapidly progressive renal disease	Intravenous administration of bolus doses of 1000 mg methylprednisolone
Lupus nephritis with high histological activity score	Immunosuppressive treatment with high-dose steroids
Thromboembolism with antiphospholipid antibody	Long-term anticoagulation

Name some poor prognostic factors for SLE.
Mortality rates in SLE have decreased throughout the last decades; however, they still remain high when compared to non-SLE mortality.

Bad prognostic factors are male patient, hypertension, renal disease, black race, presence of antiphospholipid antibodies, and high disease activity.

What are the common causes of death in SLE?
The most common causes of death are renal failure and intercurrent infections, followed by diffuse CNS and cardiovascular disease.

What do you know about the pathogenesis of SLE?
- *Pathogenic autoantibodies* are the primary cause of tissue damage in patients with lupus, including the following:
  - Anti-double-stranded DNA, anti-nucleosome, and anti-α-actinin antibodies contribute to lupus nephritis (anti-double-stranded DNA antibodies also occur, however, in 23% to 64% of patients with type 1 autoimmune hepatitis, depending on the assay used).
  - Anti-Ro antibodies, anti-La antibodies, or both in pregnancy confer a 1% to 2% risk of fetal heart block.
  - Antibodies against the *N*-methyl-D-aspartate (NMDA) receptor may be important in CNS lupus (NMDA is an excitatory amino acid released by neurons).
  - Anti-Ro and anti-nucleosome antibodies may play a role in cutaneous lupus.
  - Autoantibody-mediated destruction of red cells is important in the haemolytic anaemia that can occur in patients with lupus.

- Anti-platelet antibodies are important in the pathogenesis of thrombocytopenia that can occur in patients with lupus.
- *T lymphocyte help* is critical in the pathogenesis of lupus. The effect on the T cell depends on the interaction between molecules on the surface of the cell with the antigen presented on the surface of the antigen-presenting cell.
- *B cells* acting as antigen-presenting cells also interact with T cells, the costimulation requiring an interaction between CD40 and the CD40 ligand. The interaction stimulates the T cell to produce cytokines, some of which act on the B cell to promote antibody formation, to stimulate cell division, to switch antibody production from immunoglobulin (Ig) M to IgG, and to promote changes in the secreted antibody so that it binds more strongly to the driving antigen. (Note: CD20 and CD22 are present on B cells and interleukin-10 is produced by B cells).
- Plasmacytoid dendritic cells (producing interferon) have been found in the inflamed skin of lupus. They can internalize immune complexes in SLE, which, in turn, triggers the cells to secrete interferon-α through activation of toll-like receptor.

Further Information

Ferdinand von Hebra (1816–1880), from Vienna, described an eruption that occurs 'mainly on the face, on the cheeks and nose in a distribution not dissimilar to a butterfly' in 1845.

Pierre Louis Alphée Cazenave (1795–1877), from Paris, first used the term lupus érythémateux in 1851.

R.R.A. Coombs (1921–2006), Professor of Immunology at Cambridge, is reported to have said 'red blood cells were primarily designed by God as tools for the immunologist and only secondarily as carriers of haemoglobin'.

Sir William Osler (1849–1919) first described the systemic manifestations of SLE under the name exudative erythema between 1895 and 1904.

CHAPTER 74

Small-Vessel ANCA-Associated Vasculitis

Instruction
A patient is brought in by ambulance with acute haemoptysis. Please assess.

Salient Features
HISTORY
- Haemoptysis is a major presentation of anti-neutrophilic cytoplasmic antibody (ANCA)-associated vasculitis (around one-third of cases).
- Patients may become compromised despite an apparently small quantity of blood seen.
- Massive life-threatening haemoptysis may occur with a visible blood loss of more than 100 mL (one-third of a cup).

Ask about:
- Severity, frequency, duration
- Other sites of bleeding-associated dyspnoea
- Associated symptoms that could signify an underlying pathological process (as in this chapter the associated symptoms of vasculitis are described)
- Constitutional symptoms such as fever, malaise, fatigue, and weight loss
- Joint and muscle pains without a particular pattern
- Red gritty eyes
- Neuropathic type pains or paraesthesia without a specific pattern
- Nasal symptoms especially in Wegener's granulomatosis
- Hearing loss in microscopic polyangiitis and Wegener disease can coexist but will not be the main presenting complaint of the patient.

Note: Cough, haemoptysis, wheeze, dyspnoea, and chest pain complicate small-vessel vasculitis when the respiratory system is involved. If the trachea is affected patients can present with stridor and acute dyspnoea.

EXAMINATION
- Vital signs and baseline observations
- Chest examination
- Skin examination for rash, palpable purpura (Fig. 74.1), telangiectasia, splinter haemorrhages
- Ear, nose, and throat examination for nasal crusting, septal perforation, saddle nose deformity
- Neurological examination for peripheral neuropathy or mononeuritis multiplex
- Peripheral vasculature for bruits and diminished pulses
- Lymph node basins for lymphadenopathy in Churg–Strauss disease.

74 — SMALL-VESSEL ANCA-ASSOCIATED VASCULITIS

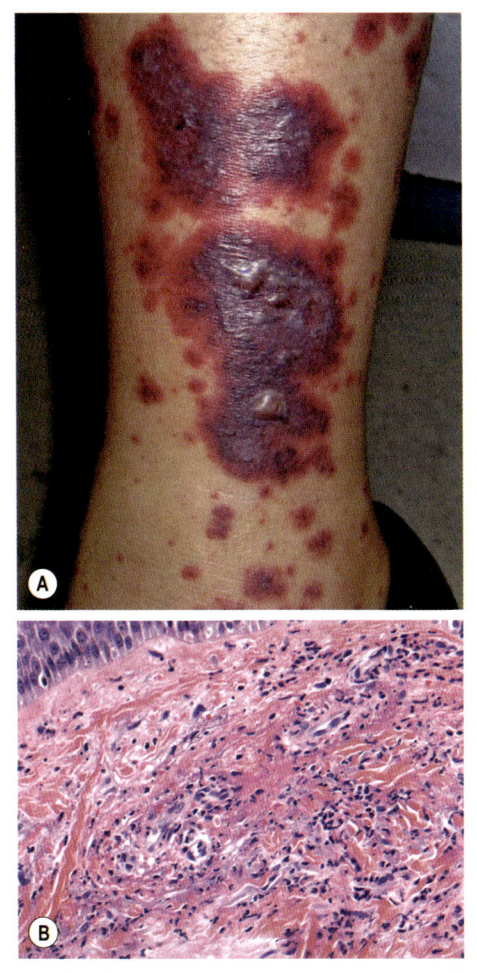

Fig. 74.1 Small-vessel vasculitis **(A, B)**. (A, Courtesy Carlo F. Tomasini, MD; B, Courtesy Christine Ko, MD.)

Proceed as follows:
- Dip the urine.
- Obtain blood for renal function, inflammatory markers, and immunological investigations.

Diagnosis

This young patient has haemoptysis, widespread joint pain, and a rash (lesions). This is caused by Churg Strauss disease, a vasculitis (aetiology). He feels very fatigued and needs to be admitted to hospital to manage his symptoms (functional status).

Questions

How are vasculitides classified dependent on the size of the vessels affected?
Vasculitides are categorized according to the types of vessels affected into three main types—large-vessel vasculitis, medium-vessel vasculitis, small-vessel vasculitis, and variable-vessel vasculitis.

Large-vessel vasculitides are Takayasu arteritis and giant cell arteritis with the affected vessels being involved in the inflammation process being the aorta and its main branches and the temporal artery, respectively.

Medium-vessel vasculitides examples include polyarteritis nodosa and Kawasaki disease.

Small-vessel vasculitides include Wegener syndrome or granulomatosis with polyangiitis, Churg–Strauss syndrome or eosinophilic granulomatosis with polyangiitis, and microscopic polyangiitis, all of which are currently included in the term ANCA-associated vasculitis; and Goodpasture syndrome, IgA vasculitis, cryoglobulinaemic vasculitis, and hypocomplementaemic urticarial vasculitis, all included in the category of immune complex vasculitis of small vessels.

What do you know of the ANCA-associated small-vessel vasculitis?
The three main vasculitides associated with ANCA are Wegener's granulomatosis, microscopic polyangiitis, and Churg–Strauss disease. These vasculitides have been traditionally known by their eponymous syndromes; however, there has been a trend recently to avoid eponymous names and instead use terms that describe the underlying process. These diseases are now known as granulomatosis with polyangiitis, microscopic polyangiitis, and eosinophilic granulomatosis with polyangiitis. All three of them share a common identity; they are associated with ANCAs. The first two also share the same symptomatology whereas Churg–Strauss presentation differs. The fourth small-vessel vasculitis associated with ANCA disease is renal limited vasculitis, and as its name suggests the pathological process is limited to the kidneys.

ANCAs bind to two antigens located in cytoplasmic azurophilic granules of neutrophils: proteinase 3 (PR3) and myeloperoxidase (MPO). Most antibodies against PR3 when binding with their target antigen produce an immunofluorescent pattern called c-ANCA as it is diffuse in the cytoplasm. The antibodies against MPO when binding with their target antigen produce a perinuclear pattern rather than diffuse, named p-ANCA (Fig. 74.2).

Wegener disease, or granulomatosis with polyangiitis, is associated with PR3–ANCA in 80% of cases, 10% have MPO–ANCA and a 10% of patients may not have ANCA detected. In contrast, microscopic polyangiitis is mostly connected with the presence of MPO–ANCA,

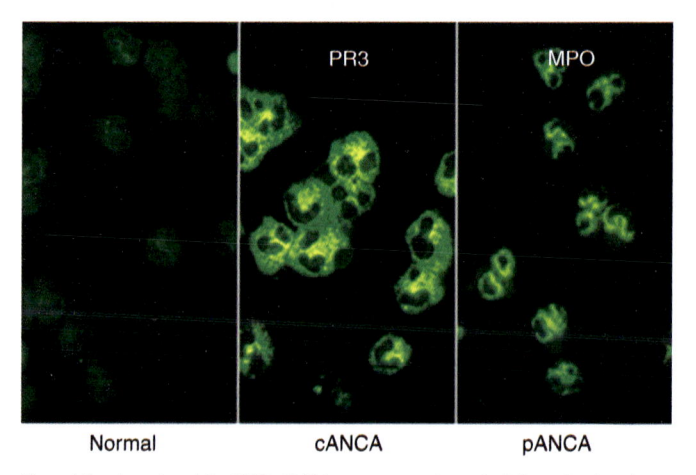

Fig. 74.2 On ethanol-fixed neutrophils, PR3–ANCA causes a characteristic cytoplasmic granular centrally accentuated immunofluorescence pattern, referred to as cANCA. (With permission from Petty, R.E., Laxer, R., Lindsley, C., Wedderburn, L., Fuhlbrigge, R., Mellins, E., 2021. Textbook of Pediatric Rheumatology, eighth edn. Elsevier.)

around 90%. Churg–Strauss disease, or eosinophilic granulomatosis with polyangiitis, is 50% associated with ANCA, of which a 70% is MPO–ANCA.

A negative ANCA does not exclude a diagnosis of vasculitis. As the techniques for immunofluorescence can be very dependent on multiple noncontrolled factors, some patients with ANCA-associated vasculitis can have no detectable ANCA in their blood.

Name some respiratory complications of small-vessel vasculitis.
- Asthma (Churg–Strauss disease)
- Pleural effusion
- Lung nodules
- Interstitial lung disease
- Pulmonary artery stenosis
- Pulmonary embolism
- Diffuse alveolar haemorrhage and haemoptysis.

Name some common medical causes of haemoptysis.
Bronchiectasis, lung malignancy, foreign body, bronchovascular fistula, bronchitis, pneumonia, lung abscess, fungal infections, tuberculosis, vasculitis, pulmonary oedema, pulmonary embolism, coagulopathy.

How would you manage a patient presenting with haemoptysis?
Priority has to be given in determining the severity of the haemoptysis. Massive haemoptysis should be treated as an emergency with immediate resuscitation, possible intubation, and urgent bronchoscopy and imaging. Nonmassive haemoptysis will be evaluated with a thorough history, chest X-ray, and routine blood tests in the first instance. If the chest imaging provides an answer, then treatment is directed towards the underlying pathology. If clinical evaluation and chest X-ray (CXR) have failed to determine an underlying diagnosis, then further work up is warranted. If a clinical suspicion of pulmonary embolism (PE) is raised, then a CT pulmonary angiogram (CTPA) would be the most appropriate next investigation. If the patient has features consistent with possible underlying malignancy, further investigations will depend on initial CT findings. If a patient has clinical signs and CXR consistent with possible bronchiectasis, then high-resolution CT scan in combination with a bronchiectasis noninvasive screen would be indicated.

How would you investigate a patient with small-vessel vasculitis?
- Immunological testing including ANCA, antinuclear antibodies (ANA), anti-glomerular basement membrane antibodies (anti-GBM), complement levels, and cryoglobulins
- Consider HIV screen, hepatitis screen, respiratory virus PCR, blood cultures, and viral serology.
- CT thorax, abdomen, and pelvis to look for respiratory involvement, and exclude underlying occult malignancy.

The confirmation of a small-vessel vasculitis should ideally come from tissue biopsy, and the site will depend on the organs involved (skin, lung, renal biopsy).

SECTION VII

Endocrinology Cases

SECTION OUTLINE

75 Acromegaly
76 Hypopituitarism (Simmonds Disease)
77 Endocrinology Case
78 Graves Disease
79 Orbitopathy
80 Multinodular Goitre
81 Hypothyroidism
82 Hypoparathyroidism
83 Primary Hyperparathyroidism
84 Addison Disease
85 Cushing Syndrome
86 Carcinoid Syndrome
87 Gynaecomastia
88 Falls—Osteoporosis
89 Obesity
90 Type 1 Diabetes
91 Type 2 Diabetes Mellitus
92 Diabetic Foot

CHAPTER 75

Acromegaly

Instruction

You are the medical doctor in the ambulatory medical unit. This 45-year-old patient has presented with chronic headaches. He has noted some changes in his facial characteristics over the last decade and thinks this may be related to his headaches. Please assess the patient and advise on further management.

Salient Features

HISTORY

- Ask the patient for old photographs of themselves for comparison
- Whether the patient has outgrown their wedding ring and shoes
- Hyperhidrosis
- Headaches, visual field defects (depending on the size of the tumour)
- Paraesthesia and symptoms of carpal tunnel syndrome
- Hypertension
- Acral and facial changes
- Oligomenorrhoea/amenorrhoea, galactorrhoea in females (prolactin is coproduced with growth hormone (GH) in approximately 40% of patients with acromegaly)
- Impotence in males
- Shortness of breath (cardiac failure)
- Arthritis (hands, feet, hips, and knees).

EXAMINATION

Hands:
  On shaking hands, there is excessive sweating: moist, doughy, enveloping handshake
  - Large hands with broad palms, spatulate fingers; there is an increase in the 'volume' of the hands (Fig. 75.1)
  - Look for evidence of carpal tunnel syndrome.
Face:
  - Prominent supraorbital ridges
  - Large nose and lips
  - Protrusion of the lower jaw (prognathism): ask the patient to clench his or her teeth and note the malocclusion and splaying of the teeth (i.e. interdental separation).
  - Ask the patient to show his or her tongue and look for macroglossia and for impressions of the teeth on the edges of the tongue.
Proceed by testing:
  - For bitemporal hemianopia and optic atrophy
  - Examine the neck for goitre.
  - Axillae for skin tags (molluscum fibrosum), acanthosis nigricans (black velvety papillomas)
  - Chest for cardiomegaly, gynaecomastia, and galactorrhoea

75 — ACROMEGALY

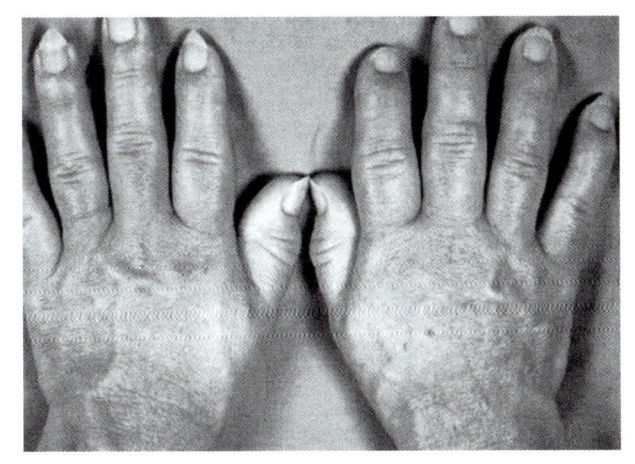

Fig. 75.1 Acromegaly: hands with sausage-shaped fingers. (With permission from Carey, W.D., 2010. Current Clinical Medicine, second edn. Saunders, Philadelphia, PA.)

- Abdomen for hepatosplenomegaly
- Joints for arthropathy, i.e. osteoarthrosis, chondrocalcinosis
- Spine for kyphosis
- Blood pressure for hypertension (present in 15% of cases)
- Tell the examiner that you would like to examine the urine for sugar (impaired glucose tolerance).

Diagnosis

This patient has a protruding lower jaw, splaying of teeth, and large spade-like hands (lesions), which are features of acromegaly caused by a pituitary tumour (aetiology).

Questions

Mention some causes of macroglossia.
- Acromegaly
- Amyloidosis
- Hypothyroidism
- Down syndrome.

How are symptoms of acromegaly explained?
The symptomatology of patients suffering with acromegaly is attributed to:
- metabolic effects of the excess hormone production from the adenoma, GH, and insulin-like growth factor (IGF-1)
- compression symptoms of a macroadenoma, which are symptoms from localized pressure to neighbouring anatomic structures, and symptoms from decreased production of other pituitary hormones.

What are the complications of acromegaly?
- Cardiomegaly and heart failure
- Hypertension

- Impaired glucose tolerance
- Hypopituitarism
- Carpal tunnel syndrome
- Arthritis of the hip, knee, and spine
- Spinal stenosis resulting in cord compression
- Visual field defects
- Increased risk of premalignant polyps and colon cancer: screening colonoscopy should be considered in all patients with GH excess.

What is the initial screening test you would perform for a suspected diagnosis of acromegaly?
The initial investigation for suspected acromegaly is measurement of insulin-like growth factor 1 (IGF-1) in blood. Unlike GH, IGF-1 levels do not vary during the course of the day. If IGF-1 levels in the blood are elevated, then this indicates active acromegaly and further testing is warranted. If IGF-1 levels corrected to the patient's age are low, further investigations are not needed and acromegaly can be excluded. IGF-1 level, and not GH level, is the best blood test for initial screening for acromegaly.

What are the indicators of disease activity?
- Symptoms such as headache, patient requiring increase in size of ring, shoe, or dentures
- Excessive sweating
- Skin tags
- Glycosuria
- Hypertension
- Increased loss of visual fields.

How would you investigate this patient?
- Biochemical tests:
    - Plasma IGF-1 levels (allows assessment of the efficacy of initial therapy and in the post-therapeutic period). Marked elevations establish the diagnosis.
    - When IGF-1 levels are elevated, the diagnosis has to be biochemically confirmed with oral glucose tolerance test with serial GH measurements, before and 2 hours after administration of oral glucose. In normal individuals, a drop in GH is expected after the administration of glucose. In acromegaly, however, GH levels fail to drop in response to glucose.
    - All pituitary axis hormones have to be tested if acromegaly is diagnosed.
    - Routine biochemical profile including calcium levels (to exclude multiple endocrine neoplasia (MEN) type 1 syndrome).

Note: Random GH level measurements are not useful because of pulsatile secretion.

- Once the diagnosis of acromegaly is established biochemically, then localization of the source (adenoma) needs to take place with imaging:
    - Magnetic resonance imaging of the pituitary
    - Chest and abdominal imaging in cases of acromegaly diagnosis with normal brain and pituitary imaging.

Note: Unlike in Cushing disease and prolactinomas, the majority of the patients (~60%) with acromegaly have a macroadenoma.

- Other investigations to assess for complications of acromegaly:
    - Formal perimetry

- Obtain old photographs
- New photographs of face, torso, hands, and the chest
- Electrocardiogram
- Triple stimulation test: if hypopituitarism is suspected.

What therapeutic options are available?
- Neurosurgical intervention, typically transsphenoidal, is the primary therapeutic choice for almost all patients. The goal is complete resection of the adenoma with excision performed for most patients with either microadenoma or macroadenoma. In cases of large macroadenomas that are considered unresectable, surgical debulking can be performed before administering medical therapy.
- Medical therapy is reserved for patients who decline surgical treatment, are poor surgical candidates, or have residual disease after surgical resection. Medical therapy includes:
    - somatostatin analogues (octreotide)
    - dopamine receptor antagonist (cabergolide)
    - pegvisomant, which is a synthetic GH receptor antagonist (the peptide is conjugated (pegylated) to polyethylene glycol to reduce renal clearance and immunogenicity) that lowers IGF-1 in >90% of patients, which is accompanied by clinical benefits (but no effect on tumour).
- Radiation treatment is reserved for failure of medical treatment in patients who cannot have surgery.

Mention four common causes of death in such patients.
- Cardiac failure
- Tumour expansion (mass effect and haemorrhages)
- Effects of hypertension
- Degenerative vascular disease.

Mention other conditions with excess GH secretion.
- MEN type 1: parathyroid hyperplasia, pituitary tumours, and gut tumours
- McCune–Albright syndrome: polyostotic fibrous dysplasia, sexual precocity, and café-au-lait spots
- Carney complex is an autosomal dominant disorder that consists of multicentric tumours in many organs, including myxomas in heart, breast, and testes; pigmented skin lesions; and pigmented nodular hyperplasia.

Further Information

In 1886 Pierre Marie (1853–1940) used the term acromegaly in describing two patients and reviewed eight previously published papers describing patients with presumed acromegaly (Marie, 1886). He also described Charcot–Marie–Tooth disease. In 1887, Minkowski deduced that acromegaly is related to pituitary tumour (Minkowski, 1887).

In 1891, the New Syndenham Society published a translation of Marie's original paper and a review by Souza-Leite of 48 patients (Marie and de Souza-Leite, 1891).

Fuller Albright, Professor of Endocrinology at Massachusetts General Hospital and Harvard Medical School, whose chief interest was calcium metabolism.

CHAPTER 76

Hypopituitarism (Simmonds Disease)

Instruction

This young patient presented to the general medical clinic. She complains of increased fatigue and tiredness and has not had a menstrual cycle for a year, since after giving birth to her first child, who is now 13 months old. Please take a focused history and examination and advise on further management.

Salient Features

HISTORY

- In a male: frequency of shaving, impotence
- In a female: postpartum haemorrhage, amenorrhoea
- History of radiation (e.g. proton-beam radiation): causes hypopituitarism primarily because of its effects on hypothalamic function, whereas high-dose radiation can directly affect the pituitary.

EXAMINATION

- Patient is pale; the skin is soft
- Check for paucity of axillary and pubic hair
- Check for atrophy of the breast (in females)
- Examine the blood pressure for postural hypotension
- Check visual fields: bitemporal hemianopia may be present
- Examine the fundus for optic atrophy
- Tell the examiner that you would like to examine the external genitalia for hypogonadism (small testes).

Diagnosis

This patient has pale soft skin and absence of axillary hair with atrophied breasts (lesion) caused by hypopituitarism (functional status) secondary to postpartum necrosis (aetiology).

Questions

Mention a few causes of hypopituitarism.
- Iatrogenic: from surgical removal of the pituitary or irradiation
- Chromophobe adenoma (particularly in males)
- Postpartum pituitary necrosis (in females): known as Sheehan syndrome
- Hypophysitis, infections, apoplexy, congenital.

Rare causes:
- Craniopharyngioma

76 – HYPOPITUITARISM (SIMMONDS DISEASE)

- Metastatic tumours (breast and lung cancers most likely)
- Granulomas (tuberculosis, sarcoid, haemochromatosis, histiocytosis X).

How would you assess such a patient?
- Full blood count for normochromic normocytic anaemia
- Urea and electrolytes for hyponatraemia
- Measurement of pituitary hormones (adrenocorticotrophic hormone (ACTH), thyroid-stimulating hormone (TSH), luteinizing hormone (LH), growth hormone (GH), prolactin)
- Measurement of target organ secretion: thyroxine (T_4), triiodothyronine (T_3), plasma-free T_4, 8 a.m. serum cortisol, testosterone, oestrogen, and progesterone
- Pituitary stimulation tests:
  - TSH-releasing hormone stimulation tests
  - Tetracosactrin (synacthen) tests
  - Insulin hypoglycaemia test considered the gold standard used to diagnose GH deficiency in adults, using a diagnostic threshold of 3 mg/L
  - LH-releasing hormone tests
- Magnetic resonance imaging (MRI) provides the best imaging of parasellar lesions. The posterior pituitary usually has a high-intensity signal on sagittal MRI that is absent in central diabetes insipidus.
- Assessment of visual fields (formal perimetry).

In what order do the hormone secretions generally fail?
In general, GH, follicle-stimulating hormone, and LH secretions become deficient early, followed by TSH and ACTH. Last of all, antidiuretic hormone secretions diminish and fail.

How would you treat such patients?
The mainstay of therapy is lifetime replacement of deficient end-organ deficiencies (thyroid, adrenal, and gonads).

Does hypopituitarism affect life expectancy?
Even when hormonal replacement therapy (adrenal, gonadal, and thyroid) is carried out in an adequate manner, there is a two-fold risk of death in patients with hypopituitarism. It has been suggested that this is caused by untreated GH deficiency.

What is the Houssay phenomenon?
Houssay showed that diabetes of pancreatectomized dogs improved after hypophysectomy. A diminishing requirement of insulin by diabetics may be a sign of hypopituitarism with diminished secretion of GH and ACTH (and thus corticosteroids). Similarly, diabetes in acromegaly may improve with pituitary surgery or octreotide therapy.

Further Information
Morris Simmonds of Hamburg described this condition in 1914.

Bernado Alberto Houssay (1889–1971), an Argentinian physiologist in Buenos Aires, was awarded the Nobel Prize for his discovery of the part played by the hormone of the anterior pituitary lobe in the metabolism of sugar. The other half of the Nobel Prize was awarded to Carl and Gerty Cori of St. Louis, Missouri, United States, for their discovery of the course of the catalytic conversion of glycogen.

CHAPTER 77

Endocrinology Case

Instruction

Examine the thyroid.
- Test this patient's thyroid status.
- Look at this patient's neck.

Salient Features

EXAMINATION

Introduce yourself to the patient, and while shaking hands, note whether the palms are warm and sweaty.
The neck (Fig. 77.1):
- Look for the jugular venous pulse
- Scars of surgery (often missed by candidates)
- Enlarged cervical lymph nodes
- Goitre.

Palpation:
- Always begin by palpating from behind
- Seat the patient comfortably
- Comment first on exophthalmos
- While palpating the gland, ensure that there is a glass of water to swallow
- Palpate the thyroid and note the following:
  - Size: specify the World Health Organization (WHO) grade (see later)
  - Mobility
  - Texture: simple or nodular (solitary or multiple)
  - Tenderness.
- Pemberton's sign: on raising the arms above the head, patients with retrosternal goitre may develop signs of compression, such as suffusion of the face, syncope, or giddiness
- Palpate cervical lymph nodes
- Feel the carotid arteries
- Palpate for tracheal deviation
- Percuss for retrosternal extension
- Auscultate over the gland for bruit, carotid bruits
- Test sternomastoid function (this muscle may be infiltrated in thyroid malignancy).

Thyroid function:
- Eye signs:
  - Lid lag
  - Exophthalmos
  - Lid retraction (sclera visible above the cornea)
  - Extraocular movements.
- Hands:
  - Pulse for tachycardia or atrial fibrillation

77 — ENDOCRINOLOGY CASE

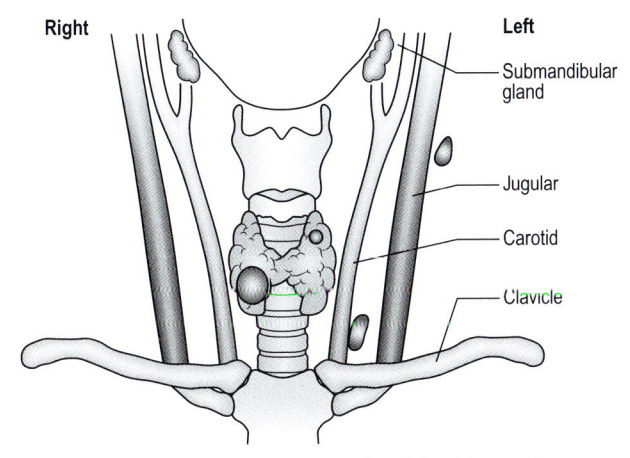

Fig. 77.1 Cervical map helps in communicating anatomic relationships and serves as a reference for follow-up examinations.

- Tremor
- Acropachy or clubbing
- Palmar erythema (thyrotoxicosis)
- Supinator jerks (inverted in hypothyroidism)
- Proximal weakness in the upper arm.
- Skin
  - Look for pretibial myxoedema.
- Elicit the ankle jerks
- If you are permitted to ask questions, enquire about shortness of breath, dysphagia, about iodine-containing medications, and possible exposure to radiation.

Questions

How would you grade the size of the goitre? WHO grading of goitre:
   0: no palpable or visible goitre
   1: palpable goitre (larger than terminal phalanges of examiner's thumbs)
   1A: goitre detectable only on palpation
   1B: goitre palpable and visible with neck extended
   2: goitre visible with neck in normal position
   3: large goitre visible from a distance.

What is the significance of the thyroid bruit?
The thyroid bruit is almost pathognomonic of Graves disease and occurs only rarely in patients with colloid goitres or other thyroid disorders.

Further Information

In 1915, Kendall isolated a crystalline product named thyroxine (Kendall, 1915).
In 1927, Harrington and Barger synthesized thyroxine (Harrington and Barger, 1927).

In 1952, Gross and Pitt-Rivers identified triiodothyronine (Gross and Pitt-Rivers, 1952).

In 1946, HS Pemberton described the sign of the 'submerged' goitre (Pemberton, 1946). Pemberton's manoeuvre is a useful clinical sign for latent superior vena cava syndrome caused by a substernal mass (Anders and Keller, 1997).

CHAPTER 78

Graves Disease

Instruction

This patient presented to the general medical ambulatory care with a history of palpitations and unintentional weight loss. Please take a history, examine the patient, and advise on further management.

Salient Features

- Patient is fidgety and restless.

HISTORY

- Easy irritability, nervousness, insomnia
- Fatigue
- Weight loss with increased appetite
- Frequent defaecation
- Oligomenorrhoea
- Dislike for hot weather, heat intolerance, excessive sweating
- Palpitations, dyspnoea
- Family history of thyroid disease
- Proximal muscle weakness, muscle atrophy, periodic paralysis (particularly in patients of Oriental ethnicity).

EXAMINATION

Hands:
- While shaking hands with the patient, note the warm sweaty palms
- Look for tremor, thyroid acropachy (a hypermetabolic state leading to axial bone destruction; do not confuse it with clubbing, which is usually painless), onycholysis (Plummer's nails), vitiligo, and palmar erythema
- Check pulse for tachycardia or the irregularly irregular pulse of atrial fibrillation.

Eyes:
- Comment on proptosis (after looking at the eyes from behind and above)
- Check for lid lag
- Check for scars of previous tarsorrhaphy.

Neck:
- Mention previous thyroidectomy scar if present
- Examine the neck for goitre and auscultate over the gland.

Chest:
- Gynaecomastia can occur in men as a result of increased oestrogen production
- Examine the cardiovascular system: sinus tachycardia, widened pulse pressure, loud first heart sound, third heart sound, systolic murmur, atrial fibrillation.

Lower limbs:
- Examine the shins for pretibial myxoedema (bilateral pinkish, brown dermal plaques)
- Test for proximal myopathy with hyperreflexia.

Tell the examiner that you would like to check for thyroid-stimulating hormone receptor antibodies (TRAbs): near 100% detection rate in patients with Graves disease.

Diagnosis

This patient has tremor, proptosis, and lid lag (lesions) caused by autoimmune Graves disease (aetiology) and is in fast atrial fibrillation (functional status).

Questions

How would you confirm the diagnosis in this patient?
Serum thyroxine (T_4), serum thyroid-stimulating hormone (TSH; thyrotropin) levels, and thyroid autoantibodies.

What are the causes of hyperthyroidism?
- Primary: Graves disease, toxic nodule, multinodular goitre, Hashimoto's thyroiditis, iodine-induced, excess thyroid hormone replacement, postpartum thyroiditis
- Secondary: pituitary or excess TSH hypersecretion, hydatidiform moles, struma ovarii, factitious.

What are the components of Graves disease?
Hyperthyroidism with goitre, eye changes (see Fig. 79.1), and pretibial myxoedema: they run independent courses.

What happens to radioactive iodine uptake in Graves disease?
Radioactive iodine uptake increases in Graves disease.

Which is the best laboratory test to diagnose hyperthyroidism?
Serum TSH measurement is the single most reliable test to diagnose all common forms of hyperthyroidism, particularly in an outpatient setting. Typically, serum concentrations are <0.1 mIU/L in Graves disease, toxic adenoma, nodular goitre, subacute and lymphocytic (silent, postpartum) thyroiditis, iodine-induced hyperthyroidism, and exogenous thyroid hormone excess. To diagnose hyperthyroidism accurately, TSH assay sensitivity (the lowest reliably measured TSH concentration) must be ≤0.02 mIU/L. Some less-sensitive TSH assays cannot reliably distinguish hyperthyroidism from euthyroidism. Free T_4 and triiodothyronine (T_3) concentrations should also be measured when less sensitive TSH assays are utilized. In rare types of TSH-mediated hyperthyroidism (pituitary adenomas and selective pituitary resistance to thyroid hormone), serum TSH alone will not suffice and again free T_4 and T_3 concentrations should be measured.

Note: Although serum TSH is the best initial diagnostic test, it is not good at assessing response to therapy as it remains suppressed until after patient becomes euthyroid. Clinical assessment and free plasma T_4 are used to monitor response to therapy.

What are the causes of isolated TSH suppression?
- Mild (subclinical) hyperthyroidism
- Recovery from overt hyperthyroidism

- Nonthyroidal illness (which can cause a low serum-free T_4)
- Pregnancy during the first trimester
- Medications such as dopamine and glucocorticoids.

Mention a few causes of hyperthyroidism with reduced iodine uptake.
- Thyroiditis
- Malignancy of the thyroid
- Struma ovarii (ovarian tumour).

What drugs are used in the treatment of thyrotoxicosis?
- Carbimazole
- Methimazole
- Propylthiouracil (PTU).

Note: Carbimazole or methimazole is favoured over PTU because of their simple once-a-day dosing and higher adherence, but PTU is the preferred option in pregnancy due to its lower teratogenic effects.

The medical regimens used clinically to suppress thyroid hormone production are as follows:
- Thionamide alone with regular follow-up and down-titration once euthyroidism has been achieved
- Block and replace therapy: combination of standard (not reducing) dose thionamide with beta-blocker and thyroxine replacement when patient becomes euthyroid.

What are the disadvantages of antithyroid drugs?
- High rates of relapse once treatment is discontinued
- Occasionally complicated by troublesome hypersensitivity reaction and very rarely by life-threatening agranulocytosis and hepatitis.

What are the advantages and disadvantages of radioactive iodine compared with partial thyroidectomy for thyrotoxicosis?

Both radioactive iodine therapy and surgical thyroidectomy are extremely effective and usually result in permanent cure. Patients will require lifelong thyroxine replacement. Thyroid surgery is expensive, inconvenient, and occasionally complicated by injury to surrounding structures in the neck in less skilled hands; it is also complicated by the general risks of anaesthesia. In Graves disease, the indications for surgery include:
- a large goitre
- patient preference
- drug noncompliance
- disease relapse when radioiodine is not available.

Radioactive iodine, although safe and with lower complication rates than surgery, may not be acceptable to patients who are sensitive to the calamities of Chernobyl and Hiroshima. It is also associated with worsening orbitopathy so it is not recommended for patients who have more than mild orbitopathy, unless other treatment options are contraindicated.

What are the contraindications to radioiodine therapy?
- Breastfeeding and pregnancy
- Situations where it is clear that the safety of other persons cannot be guaranteed
- Patients who are incontinent who are unwilling to have a urinary catheter
- Allergy to iodine.

What are the indications for radioiodine therapy in hyperthyroidism?
- Hyperthyroidism in Graves disease with moderate goitre (40–50 g), with no significant eye signs and first presentation
- Toxic multinodular goitre in older persons complicated by heart failure or atrial fibrillation
- Toxic adenoma, usually with mild hyperthyroidism
- Ophthalmopathy with thyroid dysfunction with stable eye disease (Note: radioiodine treatment may exacerbate eye changes in Graves disease and is not recommended in severe Graves ophthalmopathy).
- Ablation therapy in those with severe manifestations such as heart failure, atrial fibrillation, or psychosis.

What advice would you give to patients who are administered radioiodine?
- Depending on the dose, they should avoid journeys on public transport, stay off work, avoid places of entertainment or close contact with other people for up to 12 days, and avoid nonessential close personal contact with children and pregnant women for up to 27 days.
- Patients should be warned that in the first 14 days after administration of therapy, they may experience palpitations or other exacerbations of symptoms, particularly when not euthyroid before treatment.
- The importance of regular follow-up should be emphasized and the need to report the recurrence of thyrotoxic symptoms or the development of hypothyroidism.
- Patients should be informed that atrial fibrillation often reverts to normal rhythm and that digitalis may then be discontinued.
- Patients should be reminded to avoid pregnancy for 4 months after radioiodine therapy.

Does thyrotoxicosis affect the bone?
Yes, chronic thyrotoxicosis is associated with osteoporosis.

If a patient with thyrotoxicosis develops muscle weakness following oral carbohydrate or intravenous dextrose, which condition comes to mind?
Hypokalaemic periodic paralysis, which occurs particularly in Asian men. These attacks may last for 7 to 72 hours.

What is the effect of iodine on thyroid status?
It may cause transient hypothyroidism (Wolff–Chaikoff effect) or hyperthyroidism (Jod–Basedow phenomenon).

What is the prevalence of hyperthyroidism?
The prevalence is 0.2% in the adult population. Mild (subclinical) hyperthyroidism (serum TSH <0.1 mIU/L, free T_4 and T_3 normal) has a prevalence of 0.1% to 6% of the adult population.

What is the role of monitoring thyroid-stimulating antibody in these patients?
Titres for TRAb progressively decrease over 18 months after surgery or an antithyroid drug and ultimately disappears in most patients.

After radioiodine ablation, TRAb levels actually increase during the first year and are less likely to disappear: over a 5-year follow-up, only 60% of patients achieved undetectable levels.

This last observation underscores the importance of TRAb monitoring in pregnant women previously treated with radioiodine who may still harbour TRAb even though they are hypothyroid.

What do you know about the pathogenesis of Graves ophthalmopathy?
It is postulated that the TSH receptor is a target of autoimmunity within the orbit and that its recognition by a circulating TSH-like factor explains the link between hyperthyroidism and Graves ophthalmopathy. A failure of T cells to tolerate the receptor allows autoimmunity to develop against it. The antibodies formed stimulate the TSH receptor located on thyroid follicular epithelial cells, leading to their proliferation and increased production of T_3 and T_4. The antibodies also recognize the TSH receptor on fibroblasts in the orbit and, together with the secreted interferon-γ and tumour necrosis factor, initiate the tissue changes that typically occur in Graves ophthalmopathy.

What is the histopathology in Graves disease?
It is characterized by a nonhomogeneous lymphocytic infiltration with an absence of follicular destruction.

What do you know about amiodarone-induced hyperthyroidism?
Amiodarone, which contains 37% iodine, can induce hyperthyroidism; this disorder is more common in iodine-deficient areas and in patients with nodular goitre and thyroid autoantibodies.

There are two mechanisms by which amiodarone may cause hyperthyroidism: thyroid destruction through an iodine-associated increase in circulating interleukin-6 or an increase in thyroid hormone synthesis. Amiodarone-induced hyperthyroidism sometimes responds to thionamide antithyroid drugs but it may be very resistant to treatment. A combination of potassium perchlorate and carbimazole should be trialed; steroids may be effective, particularly if interleukin-6 concentrations are high, suggesting destructive thyroiditis. In resistant disease, total thyroidectomy should be considered.

Which drug would you prefer in the management of a pregnant woman with thyrotoxicosis?
PTU is preferred for pregnant hyperthyroid women because methimazole and carbimazole may have teratogenic effects.

Further Information
Robert James Graves (1796–1853) was a Dublin physician who described this condition. In 1835, he described three patients and wrote of one patient, 'It was now observed that the eyes assumed a singular appearance for the eyeballs were apparently enlarged, so that when she slept or tried to shut her eyes her lids were incapable of closing, when the eyes were open, the white sclerotic could be seen, to a breadth of several lines all around the cornea' (Graves, 1835). Graves disease is also termed Basedow or Parry disease.

CHAPTER 79

Orbitopathy

Instruction

Examine this patient's face.
Perform a general examination of this patient.

Salient Features

HISTORY

- Obtain a history of thyrotoxicosis.
- Obtain history of smoking; ophthalmopathy is common in cigarette smokers.

EXAMINATION

- Look for prominent eyeballs (Fig. 79.1).
- Look at the patient's eyes from behind and above for proptosis.
- Comment on lid retraction (the sclera above the upper limbus of the cornea will be seen); this is Dalrymple sign (Fig. 79.2).
- Comment on the sclera visible between the lower eyelid and the lower limbus of the cornea (i.e. comment on the exophthalmos). Most patients have bilateral exophthalmos with unilateral prominence.
- Check for lid lag (ask the patient to follow your finger and then move it along the arc of a circle from a point above the patient's head to a point below the nose—the movement of the lid lags behind that of the globe); this is von Graefe sign. Voluntary staring can result in a false lid lag, and the patient must be suitably relaxed before eliciting this sign.
- Check for extraocular movements and comment on the cornea.
- Look for the five important signs of exophthalmos:
  - Eyelid swelling
  - Eyelid redness
  - Conjunctival swelling (chemosis)
  - Conjunctival redness
  - Inflammation of the plica or caruncle, which both lie at the inner corner of the eye medial to the conjunctiva.
- Look for:
  - Signs of thyrotoxicosis: fast pulse rate, tremor, and sweating
  - Goitre (auscultate for a bruit)
  - Postthyroidectomy scar.

Diagnosis

This patient has marked exophthalmos with ophthalmoplegia (lesions) with signs of thyrotoxicosis (functional status) caused by Graves disease (aetiology).

79 — ORBITOPATHY

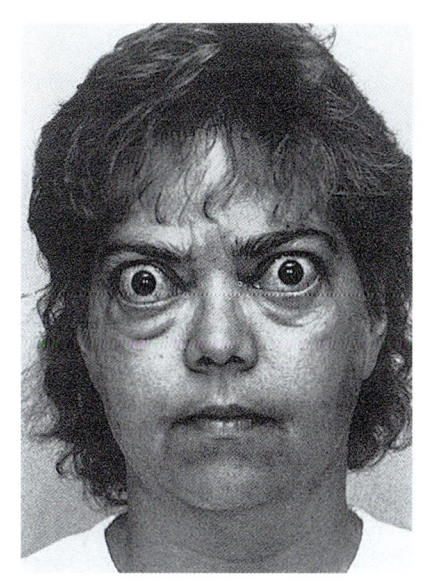

Fig. 79.1 Characteristic signs of Graves orbitopathy: thyroid stare, asymmetry, proptosis, and periorbital oedema. (With permission from Larsen, P.R., Kronenberg, H.M., Melmed, S., 2003. Williams Textbook of Endocrinology, tenth edn. Saunders, Philadelphia, PA.)

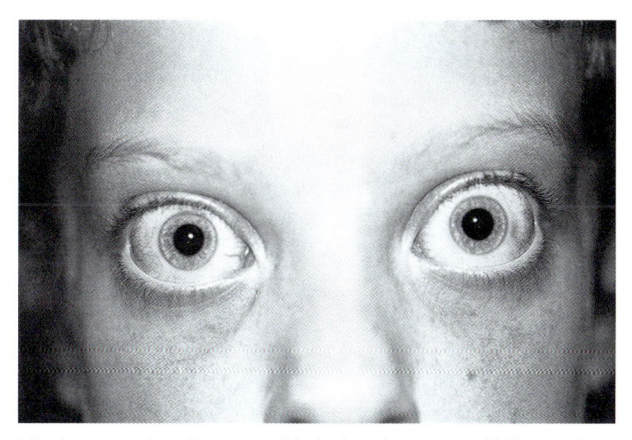

Fig. 79.2 Dalrymple's sign: retraction of upper eyelids in the primary gaze. (With permission from Kanski, J.J. Systemic Diseases and the Eye: Signs and Differential Diagnosis. Mosby, London.)

Questions

What eye signs of thyroid disease do you know?
Werner mnemonic, NO SPECS:
- **N**o signs or symptoms
- **O**nly signs of upper lid retraction and stare, with or without lid lag and exophthalmos
- **S**oft tissue involvement
- **P**roptosis

- **E**xtraocular muscle involvement
- **C**orneal involvement
- **S**ight loss from optic nerve involvement.

How would you investigate this patient?
- History and clinical examination for signs of thyrotoxicosis, thyroid enlargement, and bruit
- Serum thyroxine (T_4), triiodothyronine (T_3), thyroid-stimulating hormone (TSH)
- Thyroid antibodies.

Mention the factors implicated in the phenomenon of lid lag.
- Sympathetic overstimulation, causing overaction of Müller's muscle
- Myopathy of the inferior rectus, causing overaction of superior rectus and levator muscles
- Restrictive myopathy of the levator muscle.

What is euthyroid Graves disease?
The patient will be clinically and biochemically euthyroid but will have manifestations of Graves ophthalmopathy. A TSH-releasing hormone stimulation test will show a flat response curve.

What would you recommend if a patient with unilateral exophthalmos is clinically and biochemically euthyroid?
- Ophthalmological referral
- Ultrasonography of the orbit
- Computed tomography/magnetic resonance scan of the orbit.

How is proptosis quantified?
It is assessed using a Hertel's exophthalmometer. The upper limit of normal is subject to ethnic variation, and usually >20 mm is considered as proptosis.

What are the components of the Clinical Activity Score (CAS) for Graves ophthalmopathy?
The CAS is calculated according to the presence or absence of the characteristics listed. The score ranges from 0 to 7, with 0 to 2 characteristics indicating inactive Graves ophthalmopathy and 3 to 7 characteristics active Graves ophthalmopathy:
- Spontaneous retrobulbar pain
- Pain with eye movement
- Redness of the eyelids
- Redness of the conjunctiva
- Swelling of the eyelids
- Swelling of the caruncle
- Conjunctival oedema (chemosis)
- Increase in proptosis >2 mm over 1 to 3 months
- Decrease in eye movement of > 8 degrees in 1 to 3 months
- Decrease in visual acuity over 1 to 3 months.

The positive predictive value for therapeutic response for a CAS of 3/7 (or 4/10) is 80%, whereas the negative predictive value is 64%. Although the CAS is extremely useful for assessment of activity, its binary scoring makes it much less useful for monitoring change over time. The European Group on Graves' Orbitopathy atlas is one tool for assessment and is freely available at http://www.eugogo.eu.

How would you manage a patient with Graves ophthalmopathy?
The single most important aspect is a close liaison between the physician and the ophthalmologist.

79 — ORBITOPATHY

All patients with orbitopathy, regardless of the severity of the disease, should strongly be advised to stop smoking, all patients should be euthyroid, and all patients should be educated on general measures (artificial tears, dark glasses, elevation of head at night). Further specific treatments depend on the severity:

- Severe disease and visual loss: should be treated immediately with high doses of corticosteroids, and if there is no improvement within 72 to 96 hours, orbital nerve decompression by surgical removal of the floor and medial wall of the orbit is indicated.
- Moderate ophthalmopathy: targeted treatment with course of oral or preferably intravenous steroids. If steroids cannot be tolerated, second-line immunosuppressive agents like rituximab can be used. Symptomatic relief is also needed:
  - Pain and grittiness are treated with methylcellulose eye drops by day and a lubricating eye ointment at night
  - Exposure keratitis may be relieved by lateral tarsorrhaphy surgery of the lower eyelid
  - Diplopia may be relieved by prisms (the Fresnel prism is stuck on to the lens of spectacle) or surgery of the extraocular muscles
  - Static or worsening ophthalmopathy is an indication for steroids, orbital decompression, or orbital irradiation
  - Patients should be advised to stop smoking.
- Mild ophthalmopathy: this can be rectified by cosmetic eyelid surgery. It is important to remember that patients can be distressed by their appearance. During the early acute phase, patients will have considerable symptomatic relief from the following measures:
  - Elevating the head at night
  - Diuretics to reduce oedema
  - Course of selenium for 6 months
  - Tinted glasses for protection from the sun, wind and foreign bodies.

What is the role of radioiodine in thyroid eye disease?

- Since radioiodine treatment carries a substantial risk of exacerbating preexisting thyroid eye disease, it should be avoided as far as possible in patients with active or severe ophthalmopathy, in whom medical therapy with a thionamide drug such as carbimazole is preferable. Radioiodine may be used in patients with mild eye disease, but adjuvant oral corticosteroids should be prescribed.
- Patients without clinical evidence of thyroid disease have a small risk of developing ophthalmopathy and a very low risk of developing severe eye disease. It is prudent to warn all patients of this complication, but the risks do not justify denying most patients the benefits of definitive treatment with radioiodine when indicated. In addition, the risks do not justify the routine use of corticosteroids in patients without ophthalmopathy.
- Smoking, raised serum T_3, and uncorrected hypothyroidism are also factors that can exacerbate thyroid eye disease. Therefore, to reduce the risk of thyroid eye disease, patients should be encouraged to stop smoking, be rendered euthyroid with a thionamide before radioiodine, and be monitored closely to detect and treat early hypothyroidism or persistent hyperthyroidism.

Mention the less important eponyms related to thyroid eye disease.

- Infrequent blinking: Stellwag's sign
- Tremor of closed eyelids: Rosenbach's sign
- Difficulty in everting the upper eyelid: Gifford's sign
- Absence of wrinkling of forehead on sudden upward gaze: Joffroy's sign
- Impaired convergence of the eyes: Möbius' sign
- Weakness of at least one of the extraocular muscles: Ballet's sign

- Paralysis of extraocular muscles: Jendrassik's sign
- Poor fixation on lateral gaze: Suker's sign
- Dilatation of pupil with weak epinephrine solution: Loewi's sign
- Jerky pupillary contraction to consensual light: Cowen's sign
- Increased pigmentation of the margins of eyelids: Jellinek's sign
- Upper lid resistance on downward traction: Grove's sign
- Abnormal fullness of the eyelid: Enroth's sign
- Unequal pupillary dilatation: Knie's sign
- When the eyeball is turned downwards, arrest of the descent of the lid, spasm, and continued descent: Boston's sign.
- When the clinician places his or her hand on a level with the patient's eyes and then lifts it higher, the patient's upper lids spring up more quickly than the eyeball: Kocher's sign.

Further Information

J. Dalrymple (1804–1852), an English ophthalmologist.

Exophthalmos associated with goitre and nonorganic heart disease was first described by the English physician Caleb Hillard Parry (1775–1822) in a paper published posthumously in 1825. He graduated in medicine from Edinburgh and practised in Bath. He described hyperthyroidism before Graves disease.

Robert James Graves (1796–1853), an Irish surgeon trained at Trinity College Dublin was once arrested in Austria on suspicion of being a German spy, such was his aptitude for learning languages.

In 1977, Solomon et al. presented the evidence that three independent autoimmune diseases tended to occur concomitantly in the same euthyroid Graves ophthalmopathy: idiopathic hyperthyroidism, Hashimoto thyroiditis, and Graves ophthalmopathy.

CHAPTER 80

Multinodular Goitre

Instruction

This 70-year-old patient has been suffering from frequent palpitations for a few months and has also noticed a swelling in her neck. Please examine her.

Salient Features

HISTORY

- Stridor: trachea must be narrowed to 20% to 30% for this symptom
- Hoarseness of voice (caused by pressure on recurrent laryngeal nerve); suggests thyroid malignancy
- Acute painful enlargement; suggests bleeding into thyroid nodule
- Suffusion of face when the patient raises the arms above the head, suggests substernal goitre
- Dysphagia
- Deafness: if caused by eighth cranial nerve involvement suggests Pendred syndrome (rare)
- Symptoms of thyroid hyper- or hypofunction
- Family history of thyroid cancer.

EXAMINATION

- Middle-aged or elderly patient
- Multinodular goitre (Fig. 80.1)
- Atrial fibrillation
- Signs of thyrotoxicosis.

Diagnosis

This patient has a multinodular goitre (lesion) and is hyperthyroid with atrial fibrillation (functional status).

Questions

Name a few causes of thyroid goitre.
- Iodine deficiency
- Thyroiditis
- Graves disease
- Multinodular goitre
- Malignancy.

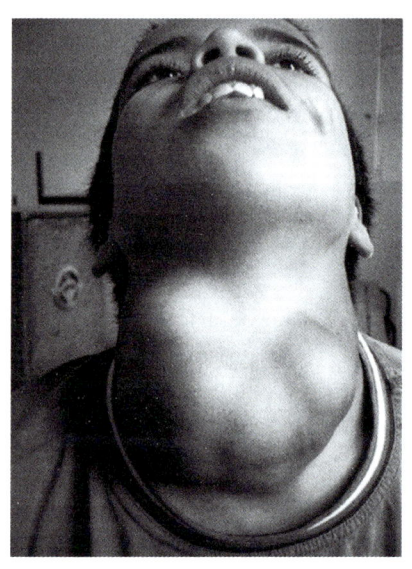

Fig. 80.1 Large nodular goitre. (With permission from Zimmermann, M.B., Jooste, P.L., Pandav, C., 2008. Iodine deficiency disorders. Lancet 372, 1251–1262.)

What is the thyroid status of a patient with goitre?
Patients with goitre can be euthyroid, hyperthyroid, or hypothyroid. The clinical and biochemical status of the patient depends on the underlying cause of the goitre. Multinodular goitre in particular is usually present in older patients and is associated with a hyperthyroid state.

What is the natural history of thyrotoxicosis in nodular goitre?
It is permanent and there are no spontaneous remissions; therefore, antithyroid drugs to decrease thyroid hormone secretion are not appropriate for long-term therapy.

How would you investigate a nodular goitre?
- Serum thyroid-stimulating hormone (TSH) and free thyroxine (T_4) should be measured to identify those with subclinical or overt hyperthyroidism.
- Ultrasonography of the thyroid gland indicates whether goitre is *cystic* or *solid*:
    - If solid, a radioisotope scan is performed to indicate hot or cold nodule
    - If cold nodule is identified, fine-needle aspiration biopsy should follow.
- Patients with features of tracheal compression (inspiratory stridor and dyspnoea) should undergo computed tomography (CT) or magnetic resonance imaging (MRI) of the neck and upper thorax and pulmonary function tests (especially flow volume loop studies). When CT is used, iodinated contrast agents should not be given because of the risk of inducing hyperthyroidism.
- Antibodies against thyroglobulin, anti-thyroid peroxidase antibodies, and TSH receptor antibody should be measured.
- If the patient has a family history of medullary thyroid carcinoma or multiple endocrine neoplasia type 2, the serum calcitonin level should also be checked.

How would you treat a patient with toxic multinodular goitre?
Patients who are clinically hyperthyroid due to toxic multinodular goitre require active treatment:

- Beta-blockers to control thyrotoxicosis
- Formal anticoagulation according to scoring systems in atrial fibrillation to prevent embolic complications
- Radioiodine for hyperthyroidism
- Surgery if the patient declines radioiodine; for large multinodular goitres or malignancy
- In patients <20 years of age, and in the case of a high clinical suspicion for cancer (e.g. follicular neoplasia as diagnosed by fine-needle aspiration and a nonfunctioning nodule revealed on scanning), the patient should be offered hemithyroidectomy regardless of the results of fine-needle aspiration.

What are indications for treatment of patients with nontoxic multinodular goitre?
- Compression of the trachea or oesophagus and venous-outflow obstruction
- Growth of the goitre, especially where there is intrathoracic extension
- Neck discomfort or cosmetic issues.

What are the treatment options available for nontoxic multinodular goitre?
- Surgery is the standard therapy, especially when rapid decompression of vital structures is required. It allows pathological examination of the thyroid. Disadvantages include postoperative tracheal obstruction, recurrent laryngeal nerve injury, hypoparathyroidism, hypothyroidism, and goitre recurrence.
- Thyroxine therapy to shrink goitres is no longer recommended. The disadvantages are that it causes only a small decrease in thyroid volume; long-term efficacy is not known; it causes a decrease in bone mineral density in postmenopausal women; and there are possible cardiac side effects.
- Radioiodine is an alternative to surgery in elderly patients and in those with cardiopulmonary disease. It results in a substantial decrease in thyroid volume and improvement of compressive symptoms in most patients. The disadvantages are that it causes only a gradual decrease in thyroid volume; radiation thyroiditis (usually mild) and radiation-induced thyroid dysfunction (hyperthyroidism in 5%, hypothyroidism in 20%–30%) can occur; and there is a possible risk of radiation-induced cancer.
- Treatment options depend on the nodule:
  - Functioning benign nodule: iodine-131 is generally the therapy of choice independent of concomitant hyperthyroidism.
  - Nonfunctioning cystic nodules: aspiration and ethanol injection therapy may be considered, and ethanol injection or laser therapy if the nodules are solid; patients are followed annually with neck palpation and measurement of the serum TSH, with repeated ultrasonography and fine-needle aspiration if there is evidence of growth of the nodule.

What are the treatment options available for toxic multinodular goitre?
Treatment is always indicated when overt hyperthyroidism is present. In subclinical hyperthyroidism, treatment is advisable in elderly patients and in younger ones who are at risk for cardiac disease or osteoporosis. There are three treatment options:
- Antithyroid drugs are valuable as pretreatment for surgery and before and after radioiodine treatment in elderly patients and those with concurrent health problems. Long-term treatment is recommended only when other therapies cannot be used. The disadvantages are that the treatment is lifelong and there are potential adverse effects such as agranulocytosis.
- Surgery should be considered in large goitres when rapid relief is needed. The other advantage is that it provides tissue for a pathological diagnosis. Disadvantages include surgical mortality and morbidity, hypothyroidism, and persistence or recurrence of hyperthyroidism.

- Radioiodine is an appealing option in the majority of the patients because it is highly effective for reversal of hyperthyroidism. The disadvantages include a gradual diminution of the hyperthyroid state, more than one dose may be necessary, hypothyroidism (<20%), and the theoretical risk of radiation-induced cancer.

How do you differentiate between Graves disease and toxic nodular goitre?

Graves Disease	*Toxic Nodular Goitre*
Younger age group	Older individuals
Diffuse goitre	Nodular enlargement of the gland
Eye signs common	Eye signs rare
Atrial fibrillation uncommon	Atrial fibrillation common (~40% of the patients)
Other autoimmune diseases common	Other autoimmune diseases uncommon

What factors influence the decision to proceed to radiotherapy?
Patient's age, sex, diagnosis, severity of hyperthyroidism, presence of other medical conditions, access to radioiodine, and patient and doctor preference.

CHAPTER 81

Hypothyroidism

Instruction
This patient presents with unintentional weight gain, reduced appetite, and constipation for a few months. Please take a focused history and examine the patient.

Salient Features
HISTORY
- Dryness of skin
- Hair dryness or loss (Fig. 81.1)
- Cold intolerance
- Change in the voice (hoarse, husky)
- Lethargy, undue tiredness
- Constipation
- Moderate weight gain in spite of loss of appetite
- Menstrual irregularity especially menorrhagia
- Infertility
- Depression
- Dementia
- Muscle cramps
- Oedema
- Radioiodine therapy for previous Graves disease (the patient may have associated eye signs of Graves disease)
- Medications and other compounds such as lithium carbonate and iodine-containing compounds (e.g. amiodarone, radiocontrast agents, expectorants containing potassium iodide and kelp)
- Family history of thyroid dysfunction, pernicious anaemia, diabetes mellitus, primary adrenal insufficiency
- Obtain history of hypercholesterolaemia, angina pectoris, and hypertension (remember hypertension occurs in 10% of these patients and disappears with thyroxine replacement).

EXAMINATION
- Coarse, dry skin (look for yellowish tint of carotenaemia: 'peaches and cream' complexion)
- 'Dirty elbows and knees' sign
- Puffy lower eyelids
- Loss of outer third of eyebrows (Queen Anne's sign or sign of Hertoghe)
- Xanthelasma.

Proceed as follows:
- Examine the neck for goitre and the scar of previous thyroidectomy. The typical Hashimoto gland is firm and lobulated.

319

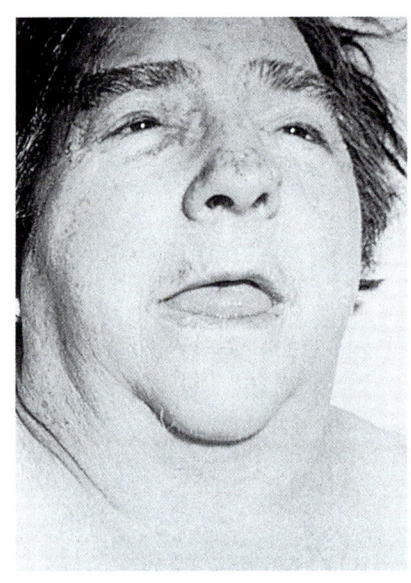

Fig. 81.1 Myxoedema facies: dull, puffy, yellowed skin; coarse, sparse hair; temporal loss of eyebrows; periorbital oedema; prominent tongue. (With permission from Seidel, H.M., Ball, J.W., Dains, J.E., Benedict, G.W., 2004. Mosby's Guide to Physical Examination, fifth edn. Mosby, Philadelphia, PA.)

- Pulse is slow
- Check the ankle jerks, looking for delayed relaxation.

Look for:
- Proximal muscle weakness
- Cerebellar signs
- Carpal tunnel syndrome.

Diagnosis

This patient has delayed ankle jerks, puffy lower eyelids, slow pulse, and hoarse husky voice (lesions), indicating that she has hypothyroidism (functional status); the cause needs to be determined (aetiology).

Questions

How is delayed relaxation best elicited in the ankle?
Get the patient to kneel on a chair with her hands holding the back of the chair and then elicit the jerks on either side.

What are the causes of goitre?
- Idiopathic (majority)
- Hashimoto thyroiditis
- Graves disease
- Iodine deficiency (simple goitre)
- Puberty, pregnancy, subacute thyroiditis, goitrogens (lithium, phenylbutazone).

81 — HYPOTHYROIDISM

What is the thyroid status in Hashimoto disease?
Hypothyroidism (usually).

What do you know of Hashimoto thyroiditis?
Hashimoto thyroiditis is the most common cause of hypothyroidism in iodine-sufficient dietary intake countries. It is an autoimmune disease, where autoantibodies against the thyroid gland (anti-thyroid peroxidase antibodies or anti-TPO and thyroglobulin or TG) cause destruction of the gland and thyroid failure. The main clinical syndrome that Hashimoto manifests is hypothyroidism. However, patients can sometimes be in the initial hyperthyroid phase or be euthyroid for years with presence of antibodies. Patients may or may not have a goitre. Regardless of the clinical syndrome or the presence of a goiter, a chronic thyroiditis with thyroid antibodies is called Hashimoto thyroiditis. Biopsy of the thyroid gland shows lymphocytic infiltration. The treatment is with lifelong thyroid hormonal replacement. However, there are occasions that treatment may be indicated even in euthyroid population (e.g. pregnant women with positive antibodies, elevated thyroid-stimulating hormone (TSH) but normal T4 levels will benefit from treatment with hormone replacement).

What is the single best clinical indicator for hypothyroidism?
Delayed ankle jerks.

What is the best laboratory indicator for hypothyroidism?
Elevated serum TSH. When there is a suspicion of pituitary or hypothalamic disease, the serum-free thyroxine (T_4) should be measured in addition to serum TSH. Serum triiodothyronine (T_3) is a poor indicator of hypothyroid state and should not be used.

What are the laboratory changes in hypothyroidism?
- Hypercholesterolaemia
- Hyponatraemia
- Anaemia
- Elevation of serum creatinine phosphokinase and lactate dehydrogenase
- Hyperprolactinaemia.

What are the causes of isolated TSH elevation?
- Subclinical hypothyroidism (SCH)
- Recovery from hypothyroxinaemia of nonthyroid illnesses
- Medications such as amiodarone or lithium.

What are the causes of isolated TSH suppression?
- Subclinical hyperthyroidism
- Recovery from overt hyperthyroidism
- Nonthyroidal illness, which causes low serum-free T_4
- Pregnancy, during the first trimester
- Medications such as dopamine and glucocorticoids.

How would you investigate a simple goitre?
Estimation of serum T_4, T_3, TSH, and thyroid antibodies (presence of anti-TPOs suggests Hashimoto thyroiditis).

Note: One does not know what free T_4 value is normal for an individual person unless the serum TSH is measured.

What is the cause for delayed relaxation in hypothyroidism?
The exact cause is not known. It is probably caused by decreased muscle metabolism.

How would you manage this patient with hypothyroidism?
Oral T_4 replacement therapy for life. The therapeutic dose varies between 100 and 200 µg/day taken as a single dose. It is taken on an empty stomach (1 hour before or 2–3 hours after food). Dose adjustments are made once in 3 weeks. The dose is adjusted depending on the clinical response and suppression of raised serum TSH. Lack of response to T_4 suggests:
- non-thyroid-related disease
- poor compliance
- underlying psychiatric abnormalities
- presence of pernicious anaemia
- associated autoimmune disease such as Addison disease.

In hypothyroid patients who become pregnant, T_4 requirements go up by ~50% in the first half of pregnancy.

What is the hazard in treating the elderly?
Rapid T_4 replacement may precipitate angina and myocardial infarction. The starting dose in the elderly is 25 to 50 µg/day.

What are the cardiovascular manifestations of hypothyroidism?
- Bradycardia
- Mild hypertension
- Pericarditis and pericardial effusion
- High low-density lipoprotein, low high-density lipoprotein levels, hypercholesterolaemia
- Diminished cardiac output and cardiac failure
- Coronary artery disease
- Electrocardiogram changes: low-voltage T and P waves, prolongation of QT interval.

What are the neurological manifestations of hypothyroidism?
- Delayed deep tendon reflexes (Woltman's sign)
- Carpal tunnel syndrome, peripheral neuropathy
- Myxoedema madness
- Myxoedema coma
- Pseudodementia
- Deafness to high tones (Trotter syndrome)
- In Pendred syndrome, babies are born with a goitre, deafness, and mental retardation
- Cerebellar syndrome
- Hoffmann syndrome (i.e. muscle aches with myotonia in myxoedema). In infants, muscle involvement may result in Kocher–Debré–Sémélaigne syndrome or 'infant Hercules'.

What do you understand by subclinical hypothyroidism?
This is a condition where there is low-normal serum T_4 and there is moderately raised serum TSH (grade 1: 5–10 mIU/L; grade 2: 10.1–20 mIU/L; grade 3: >20 mIU/L). All patients discovered to have subclinical hypothyroidism should have a repeat thyroid function test with the addition of TPOs. Younger patients (<70 years old) with TSH levels more than 10 mIU/L or presence of symptoms should be treated with replacement therapy. All patients started on treatment for subclinical hypothyroidism should have regular clinical and biochemical monitoring, aiming for a TSH within normal range.

What other conditions are associated with Hashimoto thyroiditis?
- Addison disease
- Diabetes mellitus
- Graves disease
- Hypoparathyroidism
- Premature ovarian failure
- Pernicious anaemia
- Rheumatoid arthritis
- Sjögren syndrome
- Ulcerative colitis
- Systemic lupus erythematosus
- Haemolytic anaemia.

What do you understand by the term sick euthyroid syndrome?
In severe acute nonthyroid illness or following surgery, changes in pituitary–thyroid function result in altered thyroid indices, although the patient remains euthyroid. On recovery from the illness, the indices of thyroid function return to normal. The changes in thyroid indices include:
- decrease in extrathyroidal conversion of T_4 to T_3, the active form of thyroid hormone
- decrease in TSH secretion, which causes decreased thyroidal secretion and subsequent decreases in serum T_4 concentrations and further decreases in serum T_3 concentrations—the latter as a result of both decreased secretion of T_4 by the thyroid and diminished availability of T_4 for peripheral conversion to T_3
- decreased production or diminished affinity for thyroidal hormones of one or more major serum thyroid hormone-binding proteins: thyroxine-binding globulin, transthyretin, and albumin. These decreases can result in decreased serum total T_4 levels but not in free T_4 or T_3. Serum concentrations of reverse T_3 (which is inactive) are increased because its deiodination is impaired.

What is the prevalence of hypothyroidism?
The prevalence is 2% of the adult population, whereas mild (subclinical) hypothyroidism is 5% to 17%.

What are the components of Grover disease?
- Hypothyroidism
- Autoimmune alopecia
- Transient acantholytic dermatosis.

Further Information
Laterally truncated eyebrows came to be associated with Anne of Denmark (1574–1619), James I's Queen Consort, likely because a contemporaneous portrait of her by Paul van Somer shows a woman with fair and abbreviated brows (Furdell, 2007). The sign is named after Eugene Hertoghe of Antwerp, a pioneer in thyroid function research.

W.W. Gull (1816–1890), FRS, graduated from Guy's Hospital in London and was created a Baronet when he treated the then Prince of Wales, who had typhoid. He was a good teacher and said that 'Savages explain, science investigates'. In 1873, he described several previously healthy women who acquired clinical features similar to those in cretinism. He coined the term myxoedema to describe a syndrome in five women with coarse features, mental dullness, dry skin, hypothermia, and oedema (Gull, 1873).

Ord in 1878 coined the word myxoedema when, at postmortem, he found extensive deposits of mucin in the skin of the feet (Ord, 1878).

Treatment for hypothyroidism with sheep thyroid extract was first reported by Murray in 1891.

Emil Theodor Kocher (1841–1917), Swiss Professor of Surgery in Berne, was awarded the Nobel Prize in 1909 for his work on the physiology, pathology, and surgery of the thyroid gland. He was the first to excise the thyroid gland for goitre and described myxoedema following thyroidectomy: 'cachexia strumipriva'. His name is associated with Kocher forceps, Kocher's transverse cervical incision for thyroidectomy, Kocher's operation for the wrist, Kocher's oblique right subcostal incision for gallbladder surgery, Kocher manoeuvre for reduction of a dislocated shoulder, and Kocher syndrome describing splenomegaly and lymphadenopathy with thyrotoxicosis.

In 1912, Hashimoto (1881–1934), a Japanese surgeon, described autoimmune thyroiditis in four women with goitres that seemed to have turned into lymphoid tissue (struma lymphomatosa).

Johann Hoffmann (1887–1919), a German neurologist.

In 1914, thyroid hormone was crystallized by Kendall.

In 1927, Harington and Barger reported the synthesis of thyroxine; its initial physiological testing was reported in 1927.

R. Debré and G. Sémélaigne were both French physicians (Debré and Semölaigne, 1935).

In 1948, H.E.W. Roberton, a general practitioner in New Zealand, was the first to recognize postpartum thyroid disease; he successfully treated lassitude and other symptoms of hypothyroidism related to the postpartum period with thyroid extract.

In 1952, triiodothyronine was discovered by Pitt-Rivers and Gross.

In 1956, Roitt and colleagues reported the presence of circulating thyroid autoantibodies in Hashimoto thyroiditis.

In 1963, Condliffe purified thyrotrophin (TSH), and soon thereafter, Odell and Utiger both reported the first immunoassays for human TSH.

In 1970, the endogenous generation of T_3 from T_4 was described by Ingbar, Sterling, and Braverman.

In 1971, Mayberry and Hershman simultaneously described use of TSH immunoassays for diagnosis of hypothyroidism.

CHAPTER 82

Hypoparathyroidism

Instruction

Look at this patient's hands.

Salient Features

HISTORY

- History of thyroid surgery
- Paraesthesia of fingers, toes, and circumoral region
- Muscle cramping, carpopedal spasm, laryngeal stridor, convulsions.

EXAMINATION

- Spasm of the hands: fingers are extended, except at the metacarpophalangeal joints, and the thumb is strongly adducted.

Proceed as follows:
- Look at the feet for spasm.
- Investigate as follows:
  - Tap over the facial nerve (in front of the tragus of the ear): there is contraction of the lips and facial muscles (Chvostek's sign or Chvostek–Weiss sign)
  - Inflate the blood pressure cuff to just above the systolic pressure for 3 min; this will cause the hand to go into spasm: Trousseau's sign
  - Look into the mouth for candidiasis (may be seen in primary hypoparathyroidism) and defective teeth
  - Finger nails may be thin and brittle
  - Check for thyroidectomy scar
  - Look for cataracts.
- Tell the examiner that you would like to perform the following tests:
  - Do a skull radiograph (looking for basal ganglia calcification)
  - Check serum total and ionized calcium, albumin, phosphorus, magnesium, and parathyroid hormone (PTH)
  - Perform electrocardiogram for prolonged QT intervals and T-wave abnormalities
  - Slit-lamp examination for early posterior lenticular cataract formation.

Diagnosis

This patient has carpopedal spasm (lesion) caused by hypoparathyroidism as a complication of thyroidectomy (aetiology).

Questions

How would you manage an acute attack of hypoparathyroid tetany?
- Maintain airway
- Slow intravenous calcium gluconate and oral calcium
- Vitamin D preparations
- Magnesium (if associated hypomagnesaemia)
- Outpatient therapy with calcium carbonate three times daily and calcitriol once or twice daily adjusting the dose to maintain a target level of albumin-corrected serum calcium at the lower end of the normal range (approximately 80–85 mg/L (2.00–2.12 mmol/L)), a 24-hour urinary calcium level of <300 mg, and a calcium–phosphate product <55.

What are the causes of hypoparathyroidism?
- Damage during thyroid or neck surgery
- Idiopathic
- Destruction of the parathyroid gland caused by the following:
  - Radioactive iodine therapy
  - External neck irradiation
  - Haemochromatosis and Wilson's deficiency
  - Metastatic disease from the breast, lung, lymphoproliferative disorder
- Dysembryogenesis (DiGeorge syndrome)
- Polyglandular autoimmune syndrome (type 1), which is also known as autoimmune polyendocrinopathy–candidiasis–ectodermal dystrophy).

How is corrected total calcium calculated?
Albumin-corrected total calcium is calculated as follows:
Corrected calcium (mg/dL) = 0.8(4 − albumin (g/dL)) + Ca (mg/dL).

What is the mechanism of hypocalcaemia?
Hypocalcaemia results from PTH secretion that is inadequate to:
- mobilize calcium from bone
- reabsorb calcium from the distal nephron
- stimulate renal 1α-hydroxylase activity; as a result, insufficient 1,25-dihydroxyvitamin D (1,25-dihydrocholecalciferol) is generated for efficient intestinal absorption of calcium.

What are the biochemical features of hypoparathyroidism?
Typically, it consists of low serum calcium with low serum PTH, high serum phosphate, normal alkaline phosphatase levels, and reduced urine calcium excretion.

> **Note:** Hypomagnesaemia causes resistance to effects of PTH and when severe may decrease PTH release as well. Hypermagnesaemia may also decrease PTH release.

What do you know about pseudohypoparathyroidism?
It is a condition characterized by end-organ resistance to PTH. The biochemistry is similar to that of idiopathic hypoparathyroidism except that patients with pseudohypoparathyroidism have elevated PTH levels that do not respond to injected PTH. These patients are moon-faced, short-statured, and learning disabled and may have short fourth or fifth metacarpals. Patients without hypocalcaemia but who have these phenotypic abnormalities are said to have 'pseudopseudohypoparathyroidism'.

What are the main physiological effects of PTH?
It results in a net increase of ionized calcium in the plasma through:
- increased bone osteoclastic activity, resulting in increased delivery of calcium and phosphorous to the extracellular compartment
- enhanced renal tubular absorption of calcium
- inhibited absorption of phosphate and bicarbonate by the renal tubule
- stimulated synthesis of 1,25-dihydrovitamin D by the kidney.

Further Information

Frantisek Chvostek (1835–1884) was Professor of Medicine in Vienna, Austria.

Nathan Weiss (1851–1883), an Austrian physician.

Armand Trousseau (1801–1867), a Parisian physician, was the first to refer to adrenal insufficiency as Addison disease.

CHAPTER 83

Primary Hyperparathyroidism

Instruction
This patient is referred to the medical admissions unit with nausea and lethargy. Initial blood tests have shown hypercalcaemia. Please examine.

Salient Features

HISTORY
- Gastrointestinal symptoms: nausea, anorexia, constipation
- Neurological symptoms: memory problems, lethargy, cognitive impairment
- Psychiatric symptoms—anxiety, depression
- Abdominal pains—kidney stones can form from hypercalciuria; acute severe hypercalcaemia can also cause acute pancreatitis causing severe nonspecific generalized abdominal pain. If hypercalcaemia is due to hyperparathyroidism accompanied by Zollinger–Ellison syndrome, abdominal pain can be due to acid reflux and peptic ulcer disease.
- Polyuria and polydipsia—chronic hypercalcaemia can give rise to diabetes insipidus.
- Bone pain.

Traditionally a mnemonic has been used to remember the set of symptoms of hypercalcaemia, and that describes all mentioned earlier: 'stones, bones, groans, and psychological moans'.

- Acute severe hypercalcaemia can lead to arrhythmias and palpitations of presyncopal episodes.
- Generalized weakness and fatigue usually coexist especially if the underlying cause is hyperparathyroidism. Other symptoms will depend on the aetiology of hypercalcaemia (respiratory symptoms in sarcoidosis, cachexia and weight loss in malignancy, etc.).

EXAMINATION
- Signs of dehydration can be apparent with postural blood pressure drop, tachycardia, dry mucous membranes, and reduced skin turgor.
- Neurological abnormalities may be the presenting finding from mild generalized weakness to stupor and coma, depending on the onset and level of hypercalcaemia.
- Band keratopathy and corneal calcification can occur from calcium deposits.
- Back tenderness on palpation from vertebral bone fractures
- Dilute urine if renal tubular acidosis with decreased ability in urine concentration is established.
- Cardiac arrhythmias can occur as a result of a short corrected QTc.

Diagnosis
This 65-year-old female presents with fatigue, low mood, and abdominal pain (lesions). This is due to hypercalcaemia which is most likely secondary to a parathyroid adenoma (aetiology).

83 — PRIMARY HYPERPARATHYROIDISM

Questions

How does parathyroid hormone (PTH) increase serum calcium?
PTH, secreted by the parathyroid glands in response to low calcium in plasma, acts on different organs with an end target to increase plasma calcium in the body. It increases osteoclastic activity, calcium absorption in the bowel and reabsorption of calcium in the kidney, synthesis of 1,25 (OH)2-D3, and phosphate excretion.

What are the major causes of hypercalcaemia?
The main causes of hypercalcaemia are excess production of PTH, malignancy, excess calcium intake or vitamin D, several endocrine disorders, and medication. Excessive PTH secretion is seen in primary hyperparathyroidism, which is the commonest cause of hypercalcaemia, and can be due to adenoma (80% of cases), hyperplasia or carcinoma (rare), tertiary hyperparathyroidism and ectopic PTH secretion, or parathyroid hormone-related peptide (PTH-rp). Malignancies that are associated with hypercalcaemia are multiple myeloma, any malignancy with bone metastasis or malignancies that produce PTH-rp, such as squamous cell carcinoma of the lung. Excess calcium intake is seen in the context of milk-alkali syndrome, whereas excess vitamin D can be either iatrogenic or part of underlying lymphoma or granulomatous disease. Other than hyperparathyroidism, other endocrinopathies that can be associated with mild hypercalcaemia are Addison disease and hyperthyroidism. Drugs that can cause hypercalcaemia are most commonly thiazide diuretics. Rare causes of hypercalcaemia are chronic immobility and familiar hypocalciuric hypercalcaemia.

Name some familiar syndromes that primary hyperparathyroidism can be part of.
Primary hyperparathyroidism can be part of multiple endocrine neoplasia 1 (MEN1), also known as the '3 P' MEN or Wermer syndrome. MEN1 comprises parathyroid adenoma, enteropancreatic tumour, and anterior pituitary adenoma. The mnemonic of 3Ps derives from the initials of parathyroid, pancreas, and pituitary.

Primary hyperparathyroidism can also be part of multiple endocrine neoplasia 2 A (MEN2A), together with medullary thyroid carcinoma and pheochromocytoma.

What are the biochemical consequences of primary hyperparathyroidism?
The most common finding of primary hyperparathyroidism is incidental and asymptomatic hypercalcaemia in the biochemical profile of a patient. Excess parathyroid hormone can also cause hypophosphataemia, hypomagnesaemia, and hyperuricaemia. Patients may have metabolic acidosis with extremely high levels of PTH. Renal failure and a normocytic anaemia of chronic disease are rarely seen probably reflecting an element of bone marrow failure.

Can the underlying cause of hypercalcaemia be suspected from the presenting symptoms?
The underlying cause of hypercalcaemia is usually evident from the history and clinical examination of the patient before any investigation takes place. An acute symptomatic presentation with severe hypercalcaemia is most commonly associated with an underlying malignancy. Careful history taking will reveal constitutional symptoms including weight loss, sweats, or fever. Clinical examination may reveal pallor, cachexia, and specific symptoms that may direct the astute clinician towards a primary source.

In contrast, chronic mild hypercalcaemia would mostly be associated with primary hyperparathyroidism. Although patients present incidentally and are usually asymptomatic, the history will reveal symptoms and signs of coexistent hypertension, heart disease, and renal problems that are associated with the hyperparathyroidism. Family history may be significant for either hyperparathyroidism or an inherited syndrome. Obviously, the existence of symptoms suggesting a MEN syndrome, such as multiple peptic ulcers difficult to treat, will point towards primary hyperparathyroidism.

Tertiary hyperparathyroidism affects patients with end-stage renal failure on renal replacement therapy or patients with sarcoidosis. Bone pain is an important symptom for suspecting metastatic bone disease as, although commonly described as one of the main symptoms of hypercalcaemia, in the current era with frequent biochemical tests, bone pain is rarely a presenting symptoms of hypercalcaemia in general.

Detailed diet and drug history is essential, as it is not uncommon for the hypercalcaemia to be iatrogenic.

How is hypercalcaemia treated?
Mild and asymptomatic hypercalcaemia usually does not need any specific treatment. Patients should be advised of the importance of hydration and drugs that can cause or contribute to hypercalcaemia should be withdrawn. Severe hypercalcaemia (corrected calcium to albumin in blood >3 mmol/L) and symptomatic hypercalcaemia will need treatment in the acute setting with fluid resuscitation and rehydration, with additional treatment in specific cases or nonresponding cases. Intravenous normal saline for the first 24 to 48 hours should be initiated and, if calcium fails to respond to hydration, treatment is with intravenous bisphosphonate. Denosumab is an alternative option to bisphosphonate in patients with severe kidney failure or with underlying malignancy, or a third line option if hypercalcaemia does not respond to bisphosphonates. Certain conditions will require disease-specific treatment such as hypercalcaemia secondary to sarcoid or lymphoma which will respond to steroids.

What do you know of familiar hypocalciuric hypercalcaemia?
It is a rare inherited disorder where there is increased renal reabsorption of calcium despite persistent hypercalcaemia. It is inherited in an autosomal dominant way and it can be diagnosed by calculating the creatinine to calcium ration in blood and urine. The mutation is on the long arm of chromosome 3 encoding for the calcium-ion-sensing G protein-coupled receptor in kidney and parathyroid tissue. The mutation can be detected by genetic analysis. The condition is usually benign and only causes mild hypercalcaemia.

CHAPTER 84

Addison Disease

Instruction

This patient presented with weakness, loss of appetite, and weight loss. Please take a focused history, examine the patient, and advise on further management and investigations.

Salient Features

HISTORY

- Dizziness, syncope
- Skin pigmentation (ask if the patient has been sitting in the sun)
- Ask questions regarding fatigue, weakness, apathy, anorexia, nausea, vomiting, weight loss, and abdominal pain.
- Depression.

EXAMINATION

- The striking abnormality is hyperpigmentation.

Proceed as follows:
- Examine for hyperpigmentation, typically localized to palmar creases and knuckles:
    - Hand: compare the creases with your own
    - Mouth and lips for pigmentation
    - Areas not usually covered by clothing, nipples, areas irritated by belts, straps, collars, or rings
    - Look for vitiligo.
- Tell the examiner that you would like to investigate as follows:
    - blood pressure, in particular for postural hypotension
    - looking for sparse axillary and pubic hair
    - abdomen for adrenal scar (if the scar is pigmented, think of Nelson syndrome and examine field defects).
- If you suspect Addison disease, tell the examiner that you would like to do a short synacthen test.

Diagnosis

This patient has postural hypotension, marked hyperpigmentation, and sparse axillary hair (lesion) caused by autoimmune Addison disease (aetiology). The patient has marked hypoadrenalism (functional status).

Questions

What is the size of the heart in Addison deficiency?
The heart is small.

331

Mention some causes of hyperpigmentation.
- Suntan
- Ethnic background
- Uraemia
- Haemochromatosis
- Primary biliary cirrhosis
- Ectopic adrenocorticotrophic hormone (ACTH)
- Porphyria cutanea tarda
- Nelson syndrome
- Malabsorption syndromes.

Mention some causes of primary adrenal insufficiency.
- Idiopathic—autoimmune (80%)
- Tuberculosis
- Metastasis
- HIV infection
- Waterhouse–Friderichsen syndrome (haemorrhagic adrenal infarction caused by septicaemia).

Which conditions may be associated with Addison disease?
- Graves disease
- Hashimoto thyroiditis
- Primary ovarian failure
- Pernicious anaemia
- Autoimmune polyglandular syndromes (APS).

What are the components of Schmidt syndrome?
Autoimmune adrenal insufficiency, autoimmune hypothyroidism, and type 1 diabetes. It is part of the polyglandular autoimmune syndrome type II.

What do you know about polyglandular syndromes?
They are autoimmune in nature and are of three main types:
1. chronic mucocutaneous candidiasis, hypoparathyroidism, and Addison disease
2. Addison disease, insulin-dependent diabetes, and thyroid disease (hyperthyroidism or hypothyroidism); this syndrome is also known as 'autoimmune polyendocrinopathy–candidiasis–ectodermal dysplasia'.
3. Also known as Carpenter disease, this is identical to APS 2 but without Addison disease. It is sometimes referred to as APS type 2b.

In rare cases where there is evidence of diverse polyglandular endocrinopathies that do not satisfy the criteria of APS 1–3, patients are labelled with APS 4, a diagnosis of exclusion.

What are the features of Allgrove syndrome?
Adrenal insensitivity to ACTH (resulting in cortisol deficiency), achalasia, alacrima, and neurological disease.

How would you investigate this patient?
- Full blood count (for lymphocytosis, eosinophilia)
- Electrolytes (for hyponatraemia, hyperkalaemia, hyperchloraemic acidosis, hypercalcaemia)
- Blood glucose, looking for hypoglycaemia
- ACTH and cortisol levels: in Addison disease, the 9 a.m. ACTH is elevated (>300 ng/L).

- Dynamic cortisol test: Short synacthen test is performed if 9 a.m. cortisol has not excluded the disease. Synthetic ACTH is administered and serial measurements of corticotropin (ACTH) and cortisol take place before and at half and one hour after the administration; low cortisol with high ACTH measurements are found in primary adrenal insufficiency, whereas low cortisol and low ACTH measurements are found in secondary or tertiary adrenal insufficiency.
- Serum renin and aldosterone levels: increased plasma renin with low aldosterone levels are found in primary adrenal insufficiency.
- Adrenal autoantibodies: 21-hydroxylase autoantibodies are elevated in 80%.
- Chest radiography
- Plain radiograph of the abdomen may show adrenal calcification.
- Computed tomography scan of the abdomen to review the adrenals for calcification, haemorrhage, hyperplasia, or masses.

How would you manage this patient if the underlying aetiology is autoimmune?
- Immediate treatment of adrenal failure with replacement steroids; hydrocortisone in three daily divided doses
- Fludrocortisone 0.025 to 0.15 mg daily; adjust dose depending on postural hypotension
- Give steroid card and Medic Alert bracelet
- Stress the importance of regular therapy and increase the dose in the event of stress such as dental extraction or urinary tract infection. It is also important to tell the patient that this therapy is lifelong and that an ampoule of hydrocortisone should be kept at home.
- Follow up every 6 months.
- Double the steroid during concurrent illnesses that impose stress (e.g. infections).
- Treat adrenal crisis with high-dose hydrocortisone and fluid resuscitation.

Note: In Addisonian crisis, intravenous fluids and hydrocortisone should be administered (after drawing a blood sample for cortisol determination).

Further Information

Thomas Addison (1793–1860) qualified from Edinburgh and worked at Guy's Hospital, London. He wrote 'The constitutional and local effects of the disease of the suprarenal capsules'. He was one of the three 'Giants of Guy's Hospital' and all three studied in Edinburgh. The others were Richard Bright (1789–1858) and Thomas Hodgkin (1798–1866).

Armand Trousseau in Paris labelled the disease 'maladie d'Addison'. Addison also first described morphoea. The original description of the disease was reported in the following paper: Addison, T., 1855. Disease of the suprarenal capsules. London Med. Gaz. 43, 517.

John F. Kennedy, past president of the United States, reportedly had Addison disease and was on replacement corticosteroid therapy.

CHAPTER 85

Cushing Syndrome

Instruction

This young patient was recently diagnosed with resistant hypertension. She also reports weight gain that she finds difficult to control with diet, and weakness of her legs and arms. Please assess the patient with focused history and examination and advise on further investigations.

Salient Features

HISTORY

- History of steroid therapy
- Central weight gain
- Hirsutism
- Easy bruising
- Acne
- Weakness of muscle
- Menstrual disturbance
- Loss of libido
- Depression, sleep disturbances
- Back pain as a result of spinal osteoporosis.

EXAMINATION

- Look for moon-like facies (Fig. 85.1), acne, hirsutism, and plethora (from telangiectasia).
- Examine the following:
    - The mouth for oral thrush
    - The interscapular area for 'buffalo hump'
    - Increased fat pads and bulge above the supraclavicular fossae (more specific for Cushing syndrome)
    - The abdomen for thinning of skin and purple striae (also seen over the shoulders and thighs): said to be present on almost all patients
    - The limbs for bruising, wasting of the limbs, weakness of the muscles of the shoulders and hips: get the patient to squat (proximal myopathy).
- Ask the patient whether he or she has back pain and then examine the spine, looking for evidence of osteoporosis and collapse of vertebra, kyphoscoliosis.
- Measure the blood pressure.
- Tell the examiner you would like to:
    - test the urine for glucose
    - check visual fields (for pituitary tumour)
    - examine the fundus for optic atrophy, papilloedema, signs of hypertensive or diabetic retinopathy.

85 — CUSHING SYNDROME

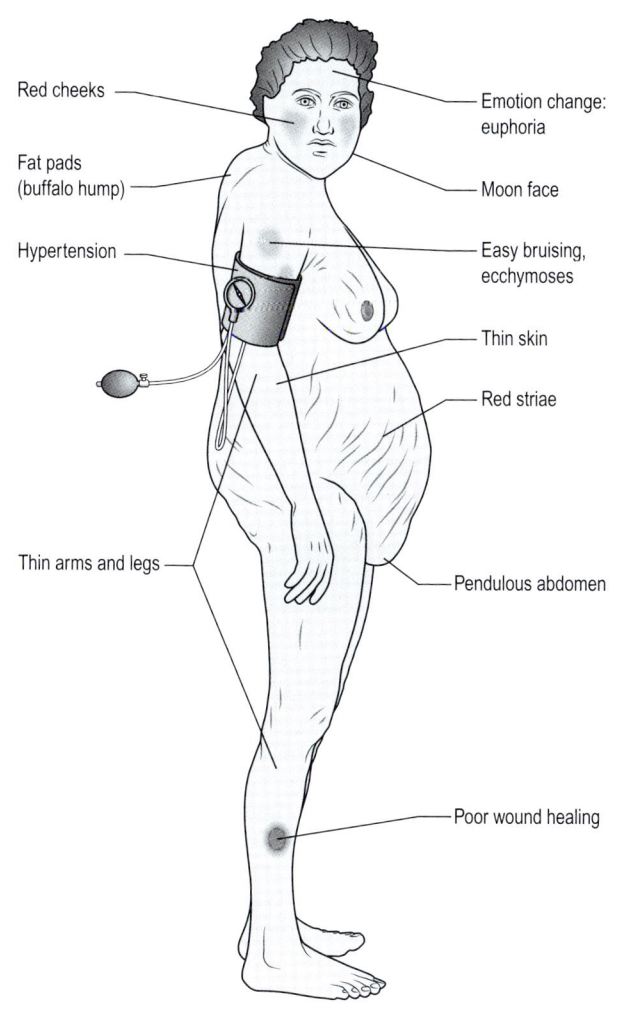

Fig. 85.1 Typical findings in Cushing syndrome.

- Comment on signs of asthma, rheumatoid arthritis, systemic lupus erythematosus, pulmonary fibrosis (conditions that are treated with long-term steroids).

Note: Hirsutism is not common in Cushing syndrome caused by exogenous steroids because they suppress adrenal androgen secretion.

Diagnosis

This patient has moon-like facies, acne, and supraclavicular pads of fat (lesions), which are features of Cushing syndrome caused by long-term steroid therapy (aetiology) for asthma. The patient is now steroid dependent and is disabled by proximal myopathy and kyphoscoliosis because of osteoporosis (functional status).

Questions

Mention some causes of Cushing syndrome.
- Steroid use
- Pituitary adenoma (Cushing disease)
- Adrenal adenoma
- Adrenal carcinoma
- Ectopic adrenocorticotrophic hormone (ACTH) (usually by small-cell carcinoma of the lung): the presence of hyperpigmentation or hypokalaemic alkalosis suggests that the Cushing syndrome results from ectopic ACTH secretion.

What is the difference between Cushing disease and Cushing syndrome?
Cushing disease is increased production by the adrenals secondary to excess pituitary ACTH, whereas Cushing syndrome is caused by excess steroid from any cause.

How would you investigate such a patient?
Tests to confirm the diagnosis of hypercortisolism:
- Urinary free cortisol 24-hour collection: this is the most direct and reliable practical index of cortisol secretion. The reason is that plasma concentrations of ACTH and cortisol fall and rise episodically, in normal subjects, in Cushing syndrome and in ectopic ACTH syndrome.
- Measurement of midnight salivary cortisol levels
- Overnight dexamethasone test
- Plasma cortisol.

Tests to determine the site of hormone production:
- Measure plasma ACTH to decide whether the Cushing syndrome is ACTH dependent (20% of cases) or due to primary adrenal pathology (80% of cases).
- If ACTH-independent Cushing syndrome is suspected, adrenal imaging should follow.
- In ACTH-dependent disease, high-dose dexamethasone test will help with localization: low-dose dexamethasone fails to suppress ACTH in Cushing disease and other causes of Cushing syndrome, whereas high-dose dexamethasone (2 mg every 6 hours for 2 days) suppresses at least 50% of urinary steroid secretion in Cushing disease but not other causes of Cushing syndrome (we describe Cushing disease as 'hard of hearing' but 'not completely deaf' as in all other causes of Cushing syndrome. Cushing disease may not respond to a whisper (the low-dose dexamethasone test), but if we 'shout' (high-dose dexamethasone test) it will respond—while other forms of Cushing syndrome are completely deaf, they will not respond to a whisper or a shout). If initial screening has confirmed Cushing syndrome with either low-dose dexamethasone test or 24-hour urinary cortisol, then high-dose dexamethasone test will help localize disease to the pituitary.
- Cushing disease responds to corticotrophin-releasing hormone (CRH) stimulation test.
- Perform chest radiography for carcinoma of the bronchus.
- Perform plain radiograph of the abdomen for adrenal calcification.
- Perform ultrasonography of the abdomen for adrenal tumours.
- If Cushing disease is suspected:
    - Plasma ACTH: >10 pg/mL (2 pmol/L) suggests ACTH dependency; a level below 5 pg/mL (1 pmol/L) suggests an adrenal source.
    - Pituitary magnetic resonance imaging (MRI) with gadolinium enhancement: MRI can identify pituitary tumours approximately 60% of the time once ACTH dependency is established.
    - Bilateral measurement of ACTH in the inferior petrosal sinus: Cushing disease is the most likely diagnosis if the sinus-to-peripheral-vein ratio of plasma ACTH is at least

85 — CUSHING SYNDROME

2:1 before or at least 3:1 after injection of ACTH-releasing hormone (CRH) during sampling from the inferior petrosal sinus.
- Inferior petrosal sinus sampling is used to distinguish primary and ectopic sources of ACTH when the source of the ACTH is not obvious based on clinical circumstances, biochemical evaluation, and imaging studies.

How would you manage Cushing syndrome?
- Cushing disease: transsphenoidal microadenomectomy, pituitary irradiation, total bilateral adrenalectomy
- Adrenal tumour: surgical resection, mitotane therapy, resection of recurrent tumour
- Ectopic ACTH: surgical resection of tumour
- Taper corticosteroid therapy.

What is pseudo-Cushing syndrome?
In chronic alcoholism and patients with depression, there may be increased urinary excretion of steroids, absent diurnal variation of plasma steroids, and a positive overnight dexamethasone test. All these investigations return to normal on discontinuation of alcohol or improvement of emotional status.

What do you know about Nelson syndrome?
It is a syndrome that occurs after bilateral adrenalectomy and is characterized by rapidly growing pituitary adenoma, very high ACTH levels, and hyperpigmentation. As the incidence may be as high as 50%, patients with Cushing disease who have undergone adrenalectomy should be followed by regular plasma ACTH levels and imaging for pituitary tumours.

Further Information

Harvey Williams Cushing (1869–1939) was Professor of Surgery at Harvard. He was awarded the Pulitzer Prize for his biography of Osler (Cushing, 1932).

CHAPTER 86

Carcinoid Syndrome

Instruction

This patient presented to the general medical clinic with persistent diarrhoea and recurrent 'troublesome flushing sensations', which she describes as multiple episodes of purplish discolouration of her face associated with a burning sensation. Please assess and advise on further investigations.

Salient Features

HISTORY

- Confirm a history of chronic intermittent diarrhoea.
- Flushing attacks, which may be associated with increased lacrimation and periorbital oedema. Flushing may be provoked by eating, exertion, excitement, or ethanol.
- Wheeze (caused by bronchoconstriction during flushing attacks).

EXAMINATION

- Flushed face ('fire-engine' face)
- Telangiectasia.

Proceed as follows:

- Listen to the chest for wheeze (bronchial carcinoid).
- Listen to the heart (right-sided murmurs in intestinal, gastric, hepatic, and ovarian carcinoid, left-sided murmurs in bronchial carcinoid).
- Look for hepatomegaly (nodular and firm from metastases, may be pulsatile from tricuspid regurgitation).

Diagnosis

This patient has facial flushing and tricuspid regurgitation (lesion) caused by carcinoid syndrome (aetiology) and is in cardiac failure (functional status).

> **Note:** Carcinoid tumours are referred to as neuroendocrine tumours (NETs). NETs include a wide spectrum of neoplasms and clinical behaviours depending on their site of origin, hormonal production, and differentiation.

Questions

What are the cardiac lesions seen in metastatic carcinoid from the liver?

- Right-sided valvular lesions including tricuspid stenosis or regurgitation, and pulmonary stenosis or regurgitation. Bronchial carcinoids metastasize to the left side of the heart.
- Endocardial fibrosis.

86 — CARCINOID SYNDROME

Serotonin is related to the progression of carcinoid heart disease, and the risk of progressive heart disease is higher in patients who receive chemotherapy than in those who do not.

Name some causes of flushing.
- Phaeochromocytoma
- Systemic mastocytosis
- VIPoma
- Drug induced
- Menopause.

What are the types of gastric NETs?
There are three types:
- Type I is associated with chronic atrophic gastritis.
- Type II develops in patients with combined multiple endocrine neoplasia type 1 and the Zollinger–Ellison syndrome. (The multiple endocrine neoplasia type 1 gene locus may be involved in type II gastric carcinoid tumours).
- Type III is sporadic.

Hypergastrinaemia has an important role in the development of types I and II.

How is the diagnosis confirmed?
- Raised urinary levels of 5-HIAA (hydroxyindoleacetic acid; Fig. 86.1)
- Plasma and platelet serotonin levels.

How are these tumours treated?
- Emergency treatment includes prednisolone.

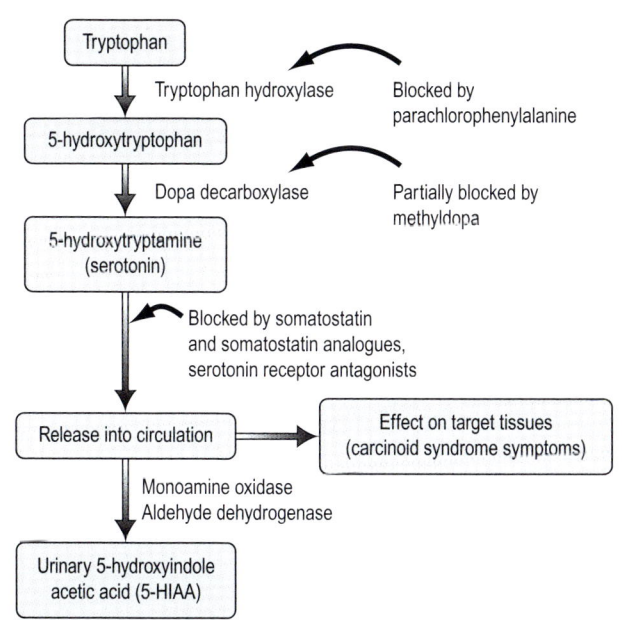

Fig. 86.1 Typical biochemical carcinoid pathway.

- Octreotide (a somatostatin analogue) is associated with a significant reduction in 5-HIAA concentration. NET cells express somatostatin receptors on their surface. Octreotide binds into the receptors and inhibits the release of the hormones by the cells.
- Surgery is useful for localized carcinoid.
- Hepatic resection of metastasis or hepatic artery embolization in unresectable metastasis
- Antidiarrhoeal agents for symptom control in severe diarrhoea
- Chemotherapy in advanced disease (fluorouracil, streptozocin, dacarbazine)
- Interferon-α and tryptophan hydroxylase inhibitors may be useful in those who do not respond to surgery and octreotide treatment.

Further Information

Carcinoid was described in 1888 by Lubarsch, the term Karznoid, or carcinoma-like, was introduced by Oberndorfer in 1907 when he described a midgut tumour that was morphologically distinct and less aggressive in behaviour than intestinal adenocarcinoma.

Erspamer succeeded in demonstrating serotonin (5-HT) in the enterochromaffin cells, and in 1953, Lembeck was able to extract 5-HT from a carcinoid tumour.

In 1914, Gosset and Mason suggested that carcinoid tumours arose from the enterochromaffin cells of the gastrointestinal tract.

CHAPTER 87

Gynaecomastia

Instruction
This patient presents to the general medical clinic complaining of excess breast tissue. Please take a focused history and examine the patient and advise on further management.

Salient Features
HISTORY
- Take a drug history: oestrogens, digoxin, spironolactone, cimetidine, diazepam, alkylating agents, methyldopa, clomiphene
- Ask the patient whether it is painful.

EXAMINATION
- Unilateral or bilateral enlargement of the breasts in a male patient.

Proceed as follows:
- Palpate to confirm the presence of glandular tissue (before palpation ask the patient to lie flat on his back with his hands clasped beneath his head). Using the separated thumb and forefinger, slowly bring the fingers together from either side of the breast. In patients with true gynaecomastia, a rubbery or firm mound of tissue that is concentric with the nipple–areolar complex is felt, whereas in patients with pseudogynaecomastia, no such disc of tissue is felt.
- Tell the examiner that you would like to look for stigmata of cirrhosis.

Diagnosis
This patient has gynaecomastia (lesion) caused by spironolactone therapy (aetiology), which is cosmetically distressing to the patient (functional status).

Questions
Mention the physiological causes of gynaecomastia.
- Newborn
- Adolescence
- Ageing.

Mention a few pathological causes.
- Chronic liver disease
- Thyrotoxicosis
- Klinefelter syndrome
- Viral orchitis

- Renal failure
- Neoplasms (bronchogenic carcinoma, testicular carcinoma, hepatoma)
- Bulbospinal muscular atrophy or Kennedy syndrome (a defect in the androgen receptor alters function of motor neurons; 50% of patients have gynaecomastia)
- Drugs associated with gynaecomastia include:
  - antimicrobials: isoniazid, ketoconazole, metronidazole, miconazole
  - cardiovascular drugs: atenolol, captopril, digoxin, enalapril, methyldopa, nifedipine, spironolactone, verapamil
  - antiulcer drugs: cimetidine, ranitidine, omeprazole
  - psychoactive drugs: diazepam, tricyclic antidepressants
  - anticancer drugs: imatinib (used in treatment of chronic myeloid leukaemia), bicalutamide.

How would you investigate such a patient?

Bilateral nontender gynaecomastia with an obvious cause elicited by the patient's history does not require further investigations. However, in unilateral gynaecomastia, painful and tender gynaecomastia, further tests may be needed to exclude a tumour.

- Mammogram to assess the breast tissue
- Plasma β-human chorionic gonadotrophin: detectable levels implicate a testicular tumour or lung or liver neoplasm
- Plasma testosterone and luteinizing hormone in the diagnosis of hypogonadism
- Serum oestradiol (usually normal)
- Other: serum prolactin, serum thyroxine, and thyroid-stimulating hormone, and chromosomal analysis for Klinefelter syndrome.

What are the causes of a feminizing state?

The pathophysiological process of gynaecomastia involves an imbalance between free oestrogen and free androgen actions in the breast tissue. Multiple processes can alter the pathways of oestrogen and androgen production and action, resulting in gynaecomastia from an enhanced oestrogen effect or a diminished androgen effect at the target-tissue level. Causes include:

- absolute increase in oestrogen formation by tumours
- increased availability of oestrogen precursors, e.g. as a result of cirrhosis
- increased extraglandular oestrogen synthesis
- relative increase in ratio of oestrogen to androgen, e.g. as a result of testicular failure
- drugs (estradiol and estrone, displaced by some drugs, resulting in an increase in free oestrogen).

How would you manage the patient?

- Acute florid stage of gynaecomastia: tamoxifen, 20 mg/day for up to 3 months, may be useful.
- When gynaecomastia has not regressed by 1 year or in patients who present with long-standing gynaecomastia who are troubled by their appearance, surgical removal of the breast glandular tissue and subareolar fat can be done for cosmetic reasons.
- Asymptomatic patients not bothered by the gynaecomastia without a suggestive history or physical examination, a more minimalist evaluation (i.e. measurements of testosterone and luteinizing hormone levels, although even the use of these tests may not be warranted): weight reduction.

Further Information

Ancient Egyptian sculptures and paintings suggest that the pharaoh Tutankhamun (1357–1339 BCE) had gynaecomastia.

CHAPTER 88

Falls—Osteoporosis

Instruction
This elderly man has recently sustained a Colles fracture. Please take a history of how he sustained the injury and perform a focused examination.

Salient Features
HISTORY
- Circumstances of the fall, including location, time, activity
- Whether it was provoked by cough, micturition, eating, or prolonged standing
- If it occurred when turning or bending over
- Preceding symptoms to suggest a postural or cardiovascular cause: dizziness, palpitations, chest pain
- Loss of consciousness (up to one-third of older people who lose consciousness will not recall this. A witness may be able to describe if there was pallor or cyanosis or seizure activity and the duration and recovery time)
- Injuries
- Previous falls and fractures: whether there is a pattern
- History of gait or balance problems, neurological deficit, incontinence, cardiac history, visual impairment, diabetes
- Medications, including antihypertensives, anticholinergics, antipsychotics, sedatives, opiates, antidepressants, hypoglycaemics. Polypharmacy (>5 medications) is an independent risk factor for falls.
- Detailed social history, including mobility aids used, trip hazards in the home
- History of alcohol or drug use
- Do they drive?—relevant if syncope is suspected.

EXAMINATION
- Check function: ask the person to stand, walk 5 to 10 metres, turn around, and sit down to assess gait, use of walking aids and footwear, turning speed, and balance
- Cardiovascular examination for pulse rate and rhythm, lying and standing blood pressure (BP), and presence of cardiac murmurs
- Neurological examination, particularly the lower limbs, looking for evidence of stroke, Parkinson disease, peripheral neuropathy, foot drop, cerebellar signs, and proprioception problems
- Examine the feet and joints
- Check vision
- Check cognition
- Consider Dix–Hallpike test if there are symptoms of vertigo.

Diagnosis

This elderly man sustained a fall caused by postural hypotension (aetiology), exacerbated by peripheral neuropathy, poor vision, and polypharmacy. This has resulted in a fracture and he needs assistance mobilizing and with personal care (functional status).

Questions

How would you investigate someone who is falling?
- Blood tests to exclude contributory factors including anaemia, hypoglycaemia, dehydration, infection, vitamin B_{12} deficiency, vitamin D deficiency
- Electrocardiogram can be carried out, looking for evidence of arrhythmia or previous cardiac disease
- Lying and standing BP: should be done with the person rested flat for at least 5 min, checked immediately on standing, and after 3 min of standing. Note the lowest recorded BP and presence of any symptoms. Postural hypotension is defined as a drop in systolic BP of greater than 20 mm Hg or a drop in diastolic BP of greater than 10 mm Hg shortly after standing.
- Further investigation of syncope includes tilt table test and carotid sinus massage.

How would you treat someone with recurrent falls?
Multifactorial interventions have the best evidence for both community-based and in-hospital falls. These include the following:
- Treat underlying acute cause: medical illness, delirium
- Treat postural hypotension
- Medication review, aim to reduce polypharmacy and reduce or stop medications associated with falls
- Ensure appropriate footwear
- Git and balance training by a physiotherapist; may include using a mobility aid
- Environmental assessment by an occupational therapist: looking at trip hazards, assistance for dressing, toileting; appropriate lighting
- Consider pendant alarms or pullcord in rooms if the person has fallen
- Those with cognitive impairment who need assistance mobilizing may benefit from bed or chair sensors to alert carers they are attempting to mobilize on their own and need help or have fallen.

How common are falls?
Some 30% of people over 65 years of age fall at least once a year, increasing to 50% of people over 80 years old.

What is the relationship between vitamin D and falls?
Vitamin D deficiency is associated with proximal myopathy and impairment of the neuromuscular junction, which may result in falls. Vitamin D therapy is associated with a 14% reduction in falls, but has no effect on fracture reduction.

Combined vitamin D and calcium supplementation has been shown to reduce falls in people in residential care, again with no effect on fractures.

Who should be assessed for bone protection?
All people with a fragility fracture (a fracture from a fall from standing height or lower), commonly occurring in the spine, hip, wrist, humerus, or pelvis, should be assessed for bone protection medications, including bisphosphonates.

Those who have not fractured but are at high risk should be considered for primary prevention of fragility fractures, e.g. those on long-term steroids and those with rheumatoid arthritis. There are various tools available to help assess risk. In the United Kingdom, FRAX and Q-fracture are widely used.

What is the role of falls clinics?
These are multispecialty clinics aiming to provide multiinterventions to reduce falls and fall-related harm.
- Investigate recurrent or unexplained falls
- Review polypharmacy
- Holistic assessments include gait and balance, vision, continence, cognition, and environment, aiming to optimize all where possible
- Review osteoporosis risk
- Instigate or refer for strength and balance training programmes (home based or group).

What is osteoporosis management?
Lifestyle modifications:
- Exercise—exercise is proven to have a positive effect on bone mineral density and reduce fracture risk
- Maintain a normal BMI
- Smoking cessation—smoking is associated with reduction in bone mineral density
- Alcohol consumption in moderation
- Diet rich in calcium and vitamin D.

Medications:
- Oral bisphosphonates for a maximum of 5 to 10 years from diagnosis
- Intravenous bisphosphonates for a maximum of 3 to 5 years
- Denosumab can be used as first line treatment or in patients who cannot tolerate bisphosphonates. However, there is lack of evidence of long-term benefit, more adverse effects, and an association with increased risk of vertebral fractures on discontinuation, needing bisphosphonate infusion upon stopping
- Hormone replacement therapy in young postmenopausal women
- Anabolic agents for male patients or severe osteoporosis.

CHAPTER 89

Obesity

Instruction

This patient presents to the general medical clinic complaining of weight gain. After multiple unsuccessful attempts to lose weight with diet and exercise, he decided to ask for medical advice regarding weight loss. Please examine the patient and advise on further management.

Salient Features

HISTORY

- Family history of obesity (parental obesity more than doubles the risk of adult obesity among both obese and nonobese children under 10 years of age)
- History of sleep apnoea, snoring, and insomnia
- History of hypertension, diabetes, hyperlipidaemia, cardiovascular disease
- Gastrooesophageal reflux
- History of gallstones (cholesterol gallstones more prevalent in obesity)
- History of endometrial cancer in women (two to three times more common in obese than in lean women)
- History of breast cancer (risk increases with body mass index [BMI] in postmenopausal women)
- Cancer of gallbladder and biliary system (obese women have a higher incidence)
- Cancer of colon, rectum, prostate, and renal cell (higher in obese men)
- Medication history: antipsychotics, antidepressants, corticosteroids, oral contraceptives, beta-blockers, oral hypoglycaemic agents, insulin, anticonvulsants, antihistamines, pizotifen
- Onset and duration of weight gain
- Attempts to lose weight, methods used, success rates, and duration of any weight loss
- Diet pattern and eating behaviours
- Patient's determination, motivation, and willingness to change lifestyle
- Medical history of endocrine problems (thyroid disease, polycystic ovarian syndrome, Cushing syndrome)
- Social and lifestyle history, including physical activity levels, alcohol, and smoking
- Explore reasons behind desired weight loss, as it may affect the overall management and treatment success.

EXAMINATION

- The patient has excessive adipose tissue.

Proceed as follows:
- Measure the height and body weight to determine BMI
- Measure waist circumference
- Check blood pressure (the prevalence of hypertension is approximately three times higher in the obese)

- Examine the joints to exclude osteoarthrosis
- Examine the skin for intertrigo in redundant folds of skin (fungal infections of skin are also common).

Tell the examiner that you would like to:
- Perform fasting glucose and oral glucose tolerance test (the prevalence of diabetes is three times higher in overweight than in nonoverweight persons)
- Check serum lipids (these patients often have an adverse pattern of plasma lipoproteins that generally improve with weight loss)
- Conduct endocrine tests and fasting insulin, liver function tests, and renal function tests
- Assess pulmonary function (sleep apnoea)
- Exclude secondary causes (hypothyroidism, Cushing syndrome, polycystic ovarian syndrome)
- Obtain a history of eating disorders.

Diagnosis

This patient has gross obesity (lesion) of genetic origin, complicated by hypertension and osteoarthrosis.

Questions

Does obesity have a genetic origin?
Obesity is a multifactorial disease, with genetic predisposition being one of the different risk factors of its development. There are many identified genes connected with obesity, some of which are responsible for a syndromic phenotype that obesity is part of and some are contributing factors to obesity developing. There are more than 90 genes identified to date that can play a role in obesity development. The *ob* gene is an adipocyte-specific gene that encodes leptin, a protein that regulates body weight. Animals with mutations in *ob* are obese and lose weight when given leptin. In humans, serum leptin concentrations correlate with the percentage of body fat, suggesting that obese people may be insensitive to endogenous leptin (leptin resistance). A variant of the fat mass and obesity (FTO) gene is proved to be associated with obesity and subsequently type 2 diabetes. Congenital deficiencies of specific genes like proprotein convertase subtilisin/kexin type 1 or melanocortin-4 receptor are associated with early onset obesity. Despite the identification of multiple genes that can directly cause obesity, contribute to obesity, or are associated with obesity syndromes, routine genetic testing is not recommended and has no role in clinical practice as yet.

What is the BMI?
It is a measure used to determine the presence of excessive adipose tissue and is calculated by dividing the body weight in kilograms by the height in metres squared. The normal range of BMI is from 20 to 25 kg/m^2.

What is morbid obesity?
It is relative weight greater than 200% (or BMI >40) and is associated with a 10-fold increase in mortality rate.

Mention some adverse health consequences of obesity.
Persons who are obese have a greater risk for diabetes mellitus, stroke, dyslipidaemia, coronary artery disease, premature mortality, hypertension, thromboembolism, gallstones, reflux oesophagitis, liver disease, sleep apnoea, kidney disease, osteoarthritis, pregnancy complications, polycythaemia, and cancer of the colon, rectum, prostate, uterus, breast, and ovary. The risk of death from all

causes is increased. Higher maternal weight before pregnancy increases the risk of late fetal death, although it protects against delivery of a small-for-gestational age infant.

How common is obesity?
Obesity is becoming increasingly common all over the world. About one-third of adults ≥20 years of age are now obese in the developed world. Obesity rates significantly increased in the last decade and according to the World Health Organization there were around 1.9 billion overweight adults worldwide.

What patterns of obesity correlate with premature coronary artery disease?
Central obesity (abdomen and flank) and when there is excessive visceral fat within the abdominal cavity rather than subcutaneous fat around the abdomen.

How would you manage such patients?
Approach is based on BMI and comorbidities such as cardiovascular disease (Fig. 89.1):
- Multidisciplinary approach to weight loss: hypocaloric diets, exercise, social support. Individualized targets should be set for patients to decide the best approach to weight loss. For instance, lifestyle modifications with diet control without the use of medications is ideal for patients who would benefit from losing 5% to 10% of their body weight, whereas individuals who need more weight loss than 10% of their starting weight will need a combination of therapies including medical and/or surgical management. Risk stratification of patients depending on their overall weight and risk of complications will also play an important role in the choice of treatment.
- Activity can be incorporated into everyday life or be part of a supervised exercise programme. Although individualized to each patient's targets, as general advice to prevent obesity, patients need 45 to 60 min of moderate-intensity activity daily, and more than that is advised for patients who have lost weight in order to prevent regain.
- Diets that are encouraged are hypocaloric and nutritionally balanced ones; a 600-kcal deficit diet or reduced-fat intake diet, combined with expert support and regular follow-up, is encouraged, as their results are sustainable.

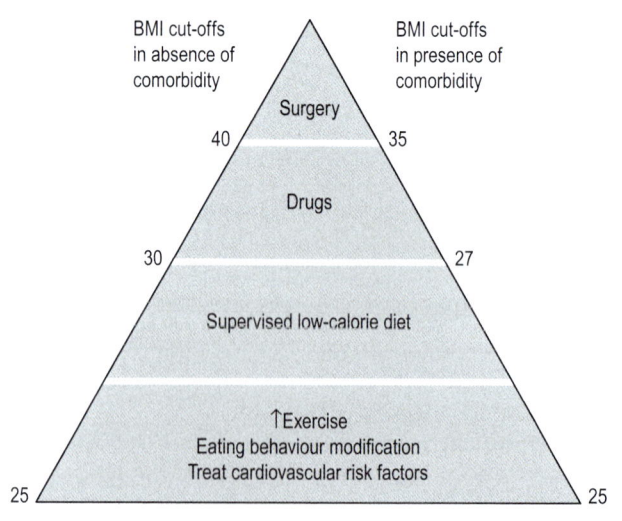

Fig. 89.1 Therapeutic options for obesity with increasing body mass index (BMI) and comorbidity.

- Behaviour modification and social support are needed for every patient regardless of the treatment options chosen for each patient.
- Medical therapy: orlistat partially inhibits absorption of dietary fat (binds to pancreatic lipase in the gastrointestinal tract). Side effects include oily spotting, flatus with discharge, and faecal urgency. The National Institute for Health and Clinical Excellence (NICE) recommends the prescription of orlistat in patients with a BMI of more than 30 kg/m^2 or a BMI more than 28 kg/m^2 with associated risk factors. Treatment should be continued if the patient has managed to lose more than 5% of their body weight in 3 months' time. Rimonabant (a selective blocker of the cannabinoid receptor CB1) and sibutramine (serotonin–norepinephrine reuptake inhibitor that reduces appetite) have shown to result in 5% weight loss when compared with placebo. Liraglutide is another pharmacological therapy for treating obesity, even in nondiabetic population, given in patients who have a BMI of more than 35 kg/m^2 and who have nondiabetic hyperglycaemia and cardiovascular risk factors alongside with obesity
- Surgery: bariatric surgery is reserved for patients who have a BMI more than 40 kg/m^2 (or more than 35 kg/m^2 associated with developed risks related to obesity like diabetes type 2), where all other treatments have failed despite intensive management, and the patient is fit for anaesthetic and can commit to long-term follow-up postoperatively. It is also the treatment of choice in those with BMI more than 50 kg/m^2. Different techniques have been used and they all fall under the umbrella of bariatric surgery:
    - Adjustable gastric banding and vertical (sleeve) gastrectomy
    - Roux-en-Y gastric bypass: a procedure that combines restriction and malabsorption and is considered by many to be the gold standard because of its high level of effectiveness and its durability.
    - Biliopancreatic diversion procedures: commonly performed with a duodenal switch in which a short, distal, common-channel length of small intestine severely limits caloric absorption; the procedure also includes a sleeve gastrectomy.

Note: Jejuno-ileal bypass is rarely used.

What are the mechanisms of obesity?
The pathophysiology of obesity is complex and poorly understood, but it includes genetic, behavioural, psychological, and other factors:
- Insensitivity to leptin, presumably in the hypothalamus
- Neuropeptide Y-induced hyperphagia
- Deficiency of production or action of anorexigenic hypothalamic neuropeptides
- Increased secretion of insulin and glucocorticoid.

Mutation in the gene for the nuclear receptor peroxisome proliferator-activated receptor-γ accelerates differentiation of adipocytes and may cause obesity. The thiazolidinedione class of antidiabetic drugs acts at this point.

Mention some syndromes where obesity is a prominent feature.
Cushing syndrome, Laurence–Moon syndrome, Alström syndrome, Prader–Willi syndrome.

What is the link between obesity and diabetes?
Fat cells release free fatty acids and tumour necrosis factor-α, which cause insulin resistance, and leptin, which causes insulin sensitivity. A protein called resistin that is secreted by fat cells also causes insulin resistance. The antidiabetic group of drugs, the thiazolidinediones, reduce insulin resistance by suppressing the expression of resistin by the fat cells.

Which is the best type of diet for weight loss?
There are a variety of diet types and methods, most claiming results, but the facts so far from literature review are that:
- There are only a few types of diets that have proven health benefits (Mediterranean diet)
- The composition of macronutrients in the diet does not play an important role in weight loss
- Fashionable and popular diets like intermittent fasting, or ketonic diets have not been shown to be effective in any studies published to date.
- The most important diet in losing weight is a hypocaloric diet with a variety of micronutrients.

CHAPTER 90

Type 1 Diabetes

Instruction

This 45-year-old female with known type 1 diabetes presents with reflux, bloating, and bowel habit disturbance. Please examine her.

Salient Features

HISTORY

- Duration and onset of original diabetes diagnosis
- Symptoms relating to hyperglycaemia: polyuria, polydipsia, dry mouth, blurred vision
- Episodes of hypoglycaemia and symptoms:
  - Frequency
  - Pattern
  - Warning signs
  - Hypoglycaemia awareness.
- Complications of diabetes:
  - Coronary artery disease
  - Peripheral vascular disease (exercise, activity, intermittent claudication, previous vascular surgery, cold peripheries)
  - Cerebrovascular disease (previous stroke or transient ischaemic attack)
  - Peripheral neuropathy (particularly sensory symptoms in extremities)
  - Renal disease (previous urine dipstick results, renal function)
  - Retinal disease (problems with vision, routine check-ups with retinal screening history of laser treatment)
  - Foot ulcers (known ulcers, routine checks by chiropodist or podiatrist, previous admissions for antibiotics or surgery)
  - Autonomic dysfunction.
- Previous admissions to hospital related to diabetes control
- Comorbidities and risk factors:
  - Cardiovascular disease
  - Hypertension
  - Hyperlipidaemia
  - Smoking and excessive alcohol
  - Other autoimmune conditions like thyroid disease, coeliac disease, pernicious anaemia.

EXAMINATION

- Visual acuity and fundoscopy
- Cardiovascular examination, including blood pressure specifically to look for orthostatic hypotension
- Abdominal inspection to check injection sites and examination of the gastrointestinal tract

351

- Peripheral neurological examination for peripheral neuropathy
- Foot examination for foot disease and signs of arteriopathy
- Inspection of diabetic control records if patient using continuous glucose or flash glucose monitoring.

Diagnosis

This patient has features of diabetic autonomic neuropathy (DAN) (lesion) caused by poorly controlled type 1 diabetes (aetiology). Their mobility is currently limited due to postural hypotension and they are only able to eat small quantities of food due to gastroparesis (functional status).

Questions

What is the underlying pathology in the development of type 1 diabetes?
Progressive destruction of beta cells in the islets of Langerhans of the pancreas. Type 1A diabetes is autoimmune mediated and immune markers can be tested for in affected individuals. It is increasingly clear that T-cell immunity as well as humoral autoimmunity is important in the development of type 1A diabetes. Less common is type 1B diabetes which is characterized by loss of insulin expression but no evidence of autoimmunity.

What immune markers are associated with type 1 diabetes?
- Islet cell antibodies (ICA) and antibodies to glutamic acid decarboxylase 65 (anti-GAD65) are the commonest markers though a range of other antibodies may also be found in type 1A diabetes.
- Other autoantigens include insulinoma-associated protein 2 and zinc transporter ZnT8.

What do you understand by the term 'epitope spreading'?
As autoimmunity in type 1A diabetes progresses from the activation stage to chronic disease, the number of autoantigens targeted by the host immune system increases. This phenomenon is termed epitope spreading. It is likely this that tips the patient into overt diabetes as the pace of islet cell destruction increases and the critical mass of islet cell function is reached such that insulin production no longer keeps up with demand.

Do you know of any genetic markers that are associated with type 1 diabetes?
There are many such markers which have variable influence on the development of type 1 diabetes. Major susceptibility genes are in the human leukocyte antigen (HLA) region of chromosome 6 with the highest risk conferred to those with DR3/DR4 heterozygosity. The risk of developing type 1 diabetes can be calculated with some accuracy depending on genetic markers and the presence of a first degree relative with type 1 diabetes with the most at risk individuals carrying a one in four chance of developing type diabetes.

What do you understand by the term latent autoimmune diabetes in adults?
This group of patients have varying degrees of autoimmunity associated with diabetes development and a variable body mass index. They are often misdiagnosed as having type 2 diabetes but respond poorly to oral diabetic drugs and need insulin early on in their illness. Measuring high levels of anti-GAD65 or ICA in younger thinner patients with a positive family history of autoimmunity who have had a suboptimal response to oral medication allows clinicians to reach the diagnosis and start appropriate insulin therapy at an earlier stage.

How would you manage type 1 diabetes in adulthood?

Type 1 diabetes is best managed by a combination of dietary optimization and insulin therapy, so called intensive diabetes therapy. Aggressive use of insulin achieves the best glycaemic control and thereby reduces the risk of long-term complications of diabetes. Patient education is the key to making intensive diabetes therapy work as it is the patient who will need to be exercise caution in dietary choices, estimate carbohydrate content of meals, regularly measure glucose levels, and administer appropriate doses of insulin. Traditionally total daily dose of insulin at initiation will be 0.2 to 0.5 units per kg per day, although insulin requirements often rise with time. Approximately half of this should be in the form of a long-acting bolus insulin given once or twice daily, with the rest delivered as fast-acting insulin at or around mealtimes. The exact dosing of fast-acting insulin will depend on premeal glucose levels and the type of meal the patient will consume.

What do you know about diabetic autonomic dysfunction?

DAN is a common complication of poorly controlled diabetes. It can manifest in many ways but is most commonly seen in the cardiovascular, gastrointestinal, and genitourinary systems. Cardiovascular DAN often presents with resting tachycardia, exercise intolerance, orthostatic hypotension, and postural tachycardia. The diagnosis of postural tachycardia syndrome (POTS) should not be given to patients with diabetes. It is thought that the increased cardiac mortality associated with diabetes is in part explained by a reduced perception of cardiac ischaemia and higher incidence of silent cardiac events. Gastroenterological DAN presents with gastroesophageal reflux due to autonomic dysfunction affecting the lower oesophageal sphincter, gastroparesis, and chronic diarrhoea. Treatment is supportive with better glycaemic control being the best way of preventing progressive symptoms. Sadly, once gastroparesis has evolved it does not improve even with tighter diabetic control. Genitourinary DAN presents as bladder dysfunction.

What other autoimmune diseases do you know of that are associated with type 1 diabetes?

The most common concurrent autoimmune conditions affecting patients with type 1 diabetes are autoimmune thyroid disease and coeliac disease, with both conditions affecting approximately 5% of type 1 diabetics. The risk appears to be related to shared alleles for disease expression such as HLA subtypes DR3 and DR4. These conditions should be screened for at the time of diagnosis of type 1 diabetes. Rarer associated autoimmune conditions include type 2 autoimmune polyglandular syndrome, Addison disease (autoimmune adrenalitis), autoimmune gastritis, and IPEX (Immune dysregulation, Polyendocrinopathy, Enteropathy, X-linked).

Further Information

Many well-known people from all walks of life manage type 1 diabetes, amongst them Sharon Stone (Hollywood actress).

The word diabetes comes from the Ancient Greek for siphon thought to describe the large quantities of urine produced by sufferers.

CHAPTER 91

Type 2 Diabetes Mellitus

Instruction

This patient, who is known to suffer from type 2 diabetes, has presented to the general medical clinic for a routine review. She also complains of some recent visual problems. Please take a history and examine the patient.

Salient Features

HISTORY

- Patient's age
- Time of diagnosis of diabetes and duration of diabetes
- Presenting symptoms on diagnosis and current symptoms of hyperglycaemia
  - Routine screening and biochemical diagnosis
  - Symptomatic presentation with polyuria and polydipsia.
- Episodes of hypoglycaemia and symptoms
  - Frequency
  - Pattern
  - Warning symptoms
  - Hypoglycaemia awareness.
- Complications of diabetes
  - Coronary artery disease
  - Peripheral vascular disease (exercise, activity, intermittent claudication, previous vascular surgery, cold peripheries)
  - Cerebrovascular disease (previous stroke or transient ischaemic attack)
  - Peripheral neuropathy (particularly sensory symptoms in extremities)
  - Renal disease (previous urine dipstick results, renal function)
  - Retinal disease (problems with vision, routine check-ups with the optician, history of laser treatment)
  - Foot ulcers (known ulcers, routine checks by chiropodist or podiatrist, previous admissions for antibiotics or surgery)
  - Previous admissions to hospital related to diabetes control.
- Other cardiovascular risk factors
  - Hypertension
  - Smoking
  - Hyperlipidaemia.
- Medication history
  - Oral diabetes medication
  - Insulin
  - Primary cardiovascular prevention medications
  - Medication for diabetic nephropathy
  - Other drug history for other medical conditions.

- Other medical history
- Social history
  - Disability issues
  - Diet
  - Lifestyle.
- Compliance with treatment
- Knowledge of diabetes.

EXAMINATION

- Visual acuity and fundoscopy
- Cardiovascular examination, including blood pressure
- Abdominal inspection if on insulin to check injection sites
- Peripheral neurological examination for peripheral neuropathy
- Foot examination for foot disease and signs of arteriopathy.

Diagnosis

This patient has evidence of proliferative diabetic retinopathy (lesion) previously treated with laser, and peripheral sensory neuropathy in his feet. This is due to type 2 diabetes (aetiology), which is poorly controlled. He needs an urgent referral to the ophthalmology team for his visual problem, but in general, a multidisciplinary approach of diabetes management is needed together with patient education.

Questions

What are the diagnostic criteria for type 2 diabetes?
Diabetes is diagnosed if a patient is symptomatic (polyuria, polydipsia) and:
- fasting plasma glucose is more than or equal to 7 mmol/L or
- random plasma glucose is more than 11 mmol/L or
- 2-hour plasma glucose post oral glucose tolerance test is more than 11 mmol/L.

If the patient is not symptomatic, then the previous criteria have to be demonstrated on two separate occasions for the diagnosis of diabetes to be established.

What is the role of HbA1c in diagnosing type 2 diabetes?
An HbA1c of 48 mmol/mol is recommended as the cut-off point for diagnosing diabetes, but a value of less than 48 mmol/mol does not exclude diabetes diagnosed using glucose tests, as there are not enough data for recommendations to be made for levels lower than 48 mmol/mol. In asymptomatic patients with HbA1c more than 48 mmol/mol, levels should be repeated. If the second sample is <48 mmol/mol, the patient should be treated as at high risk of diabetes and the test should be repeated in 6 months or sooner if symptoms develop.

Name some conditions for which HbA1c cannot be used for the diagnosis of diabetes.
- Children and pregnancy
- Haemoglobinopathies and haemolytic anaemias
- Recent pancreatic surgery
- Medication use (steroids, antipsychotics)
- Acutely unwell patients
- Suspicion of type 1 diabetes.

What are the drug treatment recommendations for type 2 diabetes in nonpregnant women according to the National Institute for Health and Clinical Excellence?

Antihypertensives:
- Blood pressure should be adequately controlled with a blood pressure target lower than that of the general population (130/80 mm Hg in patients with evidence of end-organ damage); first-line treatment is an angiotensin-converting enzyme inhibitor unless contraindicated
- Second-line treatment is the addition of calcium channel blocker or thiazide diuretic or a combination of the two if target blood pressure is not achieved with dual antihypertensive therapy.

Secondary prevention medications:
- Antiplatelet therapy is not offered routinely to all diabetic patients.
- Statin therapy is not offered for primary prevention to all diabetic patients with type 2 diabetes. Instead, the QRISK2 assessment tool is used to identify people with increased 10-year cardiovascular risk who would benefit from primary prevention: in patients with type 2 diabetes, statins are offered to patients for primary prevention if the 10-year risk is more than 10% or if renal disease has developed.

Oral diabetes medications:
- First-line treatment: First-line treatment is standard release metformin; when metformin is introduced, the dose should be gradually titrated within a couple of weeks to avoid gastrointestinal side effects associated with treatment. If these occur, modified-release metformin can be substituted. Metformin should be reduced if estimated glomerular filtration rate (eGFR) falls below 45 mL/min/1.73 m^2 and stopped when eGFR falls below 30 mL/min/1.73 m^2.
- First intensification: If metformin is not sufficient to achieve targets and HbA1c rises above 58 mmol/mol, treatment should be escalated with the addition of a second oral diabetes drug depending on the patient's comorbidities and preferences:
    - Sulfonylurea (SU)
    - Pioglitazone
    - Dipeptidyl-peptidase-4 inhibitor (DPP-4)
    - Sodium-glucose transport protein 2 (SGLT2) inhibitor.
- Second intensification: If dual therapy does not achieve targets and HbA1c rises above 58 mmol/mol, then triple therapy should be considered with a combination of any of the first intensification medication options, depending on the individual patient's characteristics:
    - Metformin, DPP-4, and SU
    - Metformin, pioglitazone, and SU
    - Metformin, pioglitazone, and SGLT2 inhibitor
    - Metformin, SU, and SGLT2 inhibitor
    - Alternatively, insulin can be started at this stage.
- Glucagon-like peptide (GLP)-1 mimetics: If triple therapy is not sufficient to achieve targets or not tolerated then the combination of metformin, SU, and GLP-1 mimetic can be considered for patients who:
    - have a body mass index (BMI) of ≥35 kg/m^2 with obesity-related problems *or*
    - have a BMI <35 kg/m^2 but insulin could affect their occupation circumstances significantly or weight loss would benefit obesity-related comorbidities.

Treatment with GLP-1 mimetic therapy should only be continued if a beneficial metabolic response has been achieved at 6-month review, defined as a reduction of HbA1c by 11 mmol/mol and more than 3% of weight loss.

When starting insulin for type 2 diabetes:
- Metformin should be continued unless contraindicated
- Other oral therapies other than metformin should be reviewed

- Neutral protamine hagedorn (NPH) insulin is recommended
- Combination of NPH with short-acting insulin can be used especially if HbA1c is high (more than 75 mmol/mol)
- Detemir and glargine are alternatives to NPH for certain groups of patients (carer needed to administer insulin, recurrent hypoglycaemia, NPH needed twice daily with oral hypoglycaemic)
- Patients on NPH or biphasic insulin should be monitored for the need for short-acting insulin before meals.

How often should diabetic control be checked?
Diabetes control should be monitored with HbA1c measurements. HbA1c should be measured 3-monthly until it is stable on a particular treatment regimen and 6-monthly thereafter if the blood sugar levels are stable. HbA1c target levels should be 48 mmol/mol, unless they are on antidiabetic medication that can cause hypoglycaemia, where the target should be set higher, at 53 mmol/mol. Treatment of diabetes needs to be escalated if HbA1c levels are higher than 58 mmol/mol.

What is the recommendation regarding self-monitoring for type 2 diabetes?
Routine self-monitoring is not needed unless under specific circumstances (insulin treatment, driver, hypoglycaemia episodes, steroid treatment, pregnant or planning pregnancy).

What do you know about flash glucose monitoring?
Since 2017, patients with type 2 diabetes requiring insulin have been able to monitor their body glucose levels with a wearable device that can be placed on to skin. This measures the glucose content of interstitial fluid and allows the patient to better understand their diabetic control and self manage insulin dosage. Currently there is one product on the market—the Freestyle Libre device.

CHAPTER 92

Diabetic Foot

Instruction
Examine this patient's legs and feet.

NEUROPATHIC FOOT

Salient Features

HISTORY
- Pain (usually painless neuropathy, but may be painful)
- Blistering (usually caused by an ill-fitting shoe)
- Previous history of foot ulcers
- History of diabetes.

EXAMINATION
- Dry, warm, and pink with palpable pulses
- Impaired deep tendon reflexes
- Reduced pinprick, light touch, and vibration sensation
- Ulcers usually painless and on plantar surface.

ISCHAEMIC FOOT

Salient Features

HISTORY
- Pain (usually painful)
- Rest pain and claudication
- History of diabetes.

EXAMINATION
- Skin is shiny and atrophic with sparse hair
- The foot is cold to touch
- Peripheral pulses are absent (calcified arteries may make pulse examination less reliable)
- Ulcers are usually painful and present on the heels and toes
- Check all peripheral pulses.

NEUROPATHIC AND ISCHAEMIC FOOT PRESENTING TOGETHER

EXAMINATION
- Ulcer on the foot with callosities at pressure points
- Loss of the arch of foot

- Stocking distribution of sensory loss of all modalities
- Loss of dorsalis pedis and/or posterior tibial pulsations.

Proceed as follows:
- Tell the examiner that you would like to:
  - Check the urine for sugar
  - Perform a simple neurologic examination of the lower extremities using a 10-g monofilament to test sensation.

Note: When asked to examine the feet, remember that the evaluation should include assessment of:
- degree of neuropathy (clinically)
- severity of ischaemia (clinically, Doppler, computed tomography angiography)
- bone deformity (clinically, radiograph, magnetic resonance imaging (MRI))
- infection (local swab, blood culture, radiograph, MRI).

The common conditions affecting the feet are diabetes and atherosclerosis. Pay particular attention to the pulses and the skin.

Diagnosis

This patient has features of both an ischaemic and neuropathic foot (lesion), which is caused by diabetes mellitus (aetiology); walking is limited by the plantar ulcer (functional status).

QUESTIONS

What are the types of diabetic foot?
- Neuropathic foot (Fig. 92.1)
- Ischaemic foot (Fig. 92.2).

Note: Features of both types often occur together.

What is the pathophysiology of the ischaemic foot?
Occlusive vascular disease involving both microangiopathy and atherosclerosis of large- and medium-sized arteries.

Mention a few conditions in which neuropathic ulcers are seen.
- Progressive sensory neuropathy
- Tabes dorsalis
- Leprosy
- Amyloidosis
- Porphyria.

How would you manage this patient?
- Patient education: avoid tobacco smoking, inspect the feet daily for blisters, no walking barefoot, avoid tight shoes, and avoid cutting toenails straight across. 'The patient should be advised to take care of their foot as well as their face'.
- Radiograph of the foot
- Antibiotics
- Removal of necrotic tissue

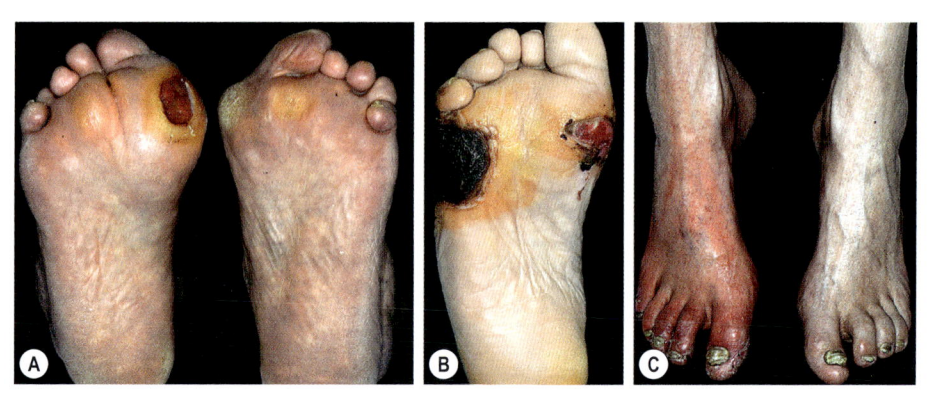

Fig. 92.1 The various presentation of diabetic foot ulcers. **(A)** Classical neuropathic diabetic foot ulceration on the right foot with peri ulcer callus overgrowth over the bony prominence of first MTPJ. Note the forefoot deformities on both feet and preulcerative lesions on the left plantar foot. **(B)** Lateral neuroischemic diabetic foot ulceration. Noted limited foot deformity and extensive lateral necrosis. **(C)** Ischemic features in a young individual with longstanding type 1 diabetes. Note the ischemic rubor and areas of early dry gangrene over dorsal second toe. The individual did not report significant rest pain and ignored early symptoms and signs. MTPJ, metatarsophalangeal joint. (With permission from Vas, P.R.J., Kavarthapu, V., 2022. Management of diabetic foot disease. In: Tavakoli, M. (ed.), Diabetic Neuropathy, first edn. Elsevier, 235–258.)

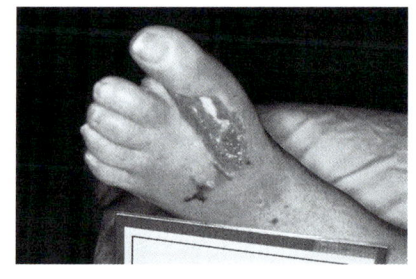

Fig. 92.2 Ischaemic diabetic foot: exposed tendon at the base of a left foot wound. (With permission from Auerbach, P.S., 2007. Wilderness Medicine, fifth edn. Mosby, St Louis, PA.)

- Removal of weight bearing and friction from ulcerated areas; use of appropriate footwear such as moulded insoles or plaster cast, instant total contact cast, or crutches to avoid weight bearing
- Control of hyperglycaemia
- Chiropody
- Surgical opinion and arteriography if reconstructive vascular surgery or angioplasty is considered. When irreversible arterial insufficiency occurs, it is often quicker and more humane for the patient to undergo early major amputation rather than be subjected to a series of debilitating conservative procedures.
- Hyperbaric oxygen, platelet-derived growth factor, and tissue-engineered skin; intermittent negative pressure applied to a wound to stimulate cellular proliferation; electrical stimulation and hydrotherapy.

How would you monitor a diabetic patient at annual review?
- Eyes: visual acuity, fundoscopy
- Sensory system: touch, pinprick, and vibration sense

- Deep tendon reflexes
- Cardiovascular system: blood pressure, peripheral pulses
- Biochemistry: urine and blood sugar, albumin, HbA1c, creatinine.

What is the importance of the Neuropathy Disability Score?

The Neuropathy Disability Score is based on impairment of sensation. A score (for *both* feet) of ≥6 is predictive of foot ulceration. The annual risk of ulceration is 1.1% if the score is <6 and 6.3% if it is ≥6. A maximum of 5 points can be scored for each foot:
- Vibration threshold (apply 128-Hz tuning fork to apex of great toe):
    - Normal (can distinguish between presence and absence of vibration) 0
    - Abnormal: 1.
- Temperature (to dorsum of foot, apply a tuning fork placed in a beaker of ice water or warm water):
    - Normal (can distinguish between hot and cold): 0
    - Abnormal: 1.
- Pinprick (apply pin proximal to great toenail to barely depress skin):
    - Normal (can distinguish sharpness or lack of sharpness): 0
    - Abnormal: 1.
- Achilles reflex
    - Present: 0
    - Present with reinforcement: 1
    - Absent: 2.

What do you know about measurement of cutaneous pressure perception?

Semmes–Weinstein monofilaments assess sensory perception. Individuals with normal feet can usually feel the 4.17 monofilament (~1 g linear pressure). Patients who cannot feel the 5.07 monofilament (~10 g of linear pressure) before it buckles are considered to have lost protective sensation. A seven-fold increase in the risk of ulceration has been reported in patients insensitive to the 5.07 monofilament. However, up to 10% of persons who feel the monofilament before it buckles may still have cutaneous breakdown.

SECTION VIII

Eye Cases for Internal Medicine

SECTION OUTLINE

93 The Eye Case
94 Age-Related Macular Degeneration
95 Cataracts
96 Cholesterol Embolus in the Fundus
97 Diabetic Retinopathy
98 Hypertensive Retinopathy
99 Optic Atrophy
100 Osteogenesis Imperfecta
101 Papilloedema
102 Retinal Detachment
103 Retinal Vein Occlusion
104 Retinitis Pigmentosa
105 Subhyaloid Haemorrhage
106 Vitreous Opacities

CHAPTER 93

The Eye Case

Instruction

Examine this patient's eyes.

Examination of the Eye

EXAMINATION

- Tell the patient, 'Look straight ahead with your right (R) or left (L) eye while I look into your L/R eye'. (The candidate need not remove his or her spectacles while the fundus is being examined.) The candidate should use his or her own R/L eye to examine the patient's R/L eye.
- Look at the eye from a distance of at least 50 cm and check for the red reflex. The presence of a red reflex indicates that the media in front of the retina is transparent and that the retina is firmly in apposition with the underlying choroid. Red reflex may be absent when there is a lens opacity, vitreous haemorrhage, or retinal detachment.
- Look systematically at the following:
  - The optic discs (comment on the colour, contour, cup, and lamina cribrosa)
  - The macula (one- or two-disc diameters away from and a little below the temporal margin of the optic disc); it appears darker than the surrounding retina, and in young individuals has a central yellow point called the fovea centralis (Fig. 93.1)
  - The nasal and temporal halves of the fundus
  - The retinal vessels (remember that the retinal artery has four main branches and the normal ratio of the artery to the vein is 2:3); assess the transparency of the vessels (the arteries usually have a shiny central reflex stripe), the presence of pressure effects such as arteriovenous (AV) nicking, the presence of focal narrowing of arteries, as well as the tortuosity of the venule.

> **Note**:
> - Lesions in the fundus are measured using the disc diameter as the reference size
> - Elevation of any lesion is measured by noting the difference between lens powers that focus clearly on the top of the lesion and an adjacent normal area of the fundus. Elevation of 3-dioptres lens changes is approximately equal to 1 mm in actual elevation.

Clinicopathologic Correlations of Retinal Haemorrhages and Exudates

The location of the haemorrhage within the retina determines its appearance by ophthalmoscopy. The retinal nerve fibre layer is oriented parallel to the internal limiting membrane.

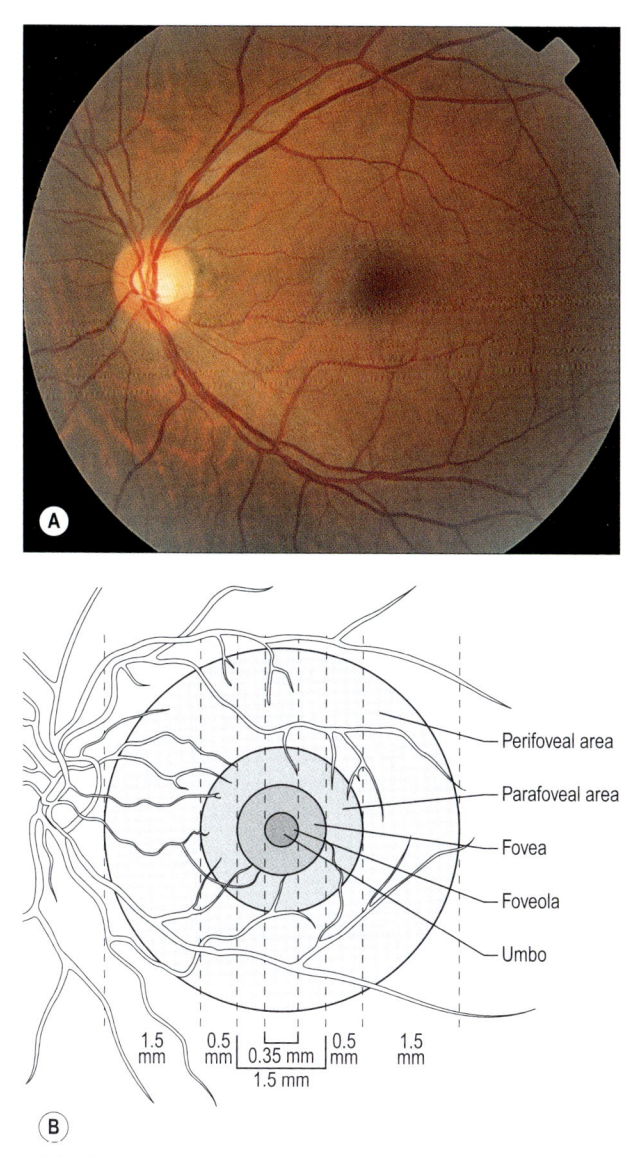

Fig. 93.1 (A) Normal fundus with macula encompassed by major vascular arcades. **(B)** The components, from centre to periphery, of the macula. (With permission from Yanoff, M., Duker, J.S., 2008. Ophthalmology, third edn. Mosby, Philadelphia, PA.)

Haemorrhages here appear to be flame shaped. The deeper retinal layers are oriented perpendicular to the internal limiting membrane and haemorrhages here appear as 'dots'.

Exudates from leaky retinal vessels accumulate in the outer plexiform layer.

CHAPTER 94

Age-Related Macular Degeneration

Instruction
Look at this patient's fundus.

Salient Features
HISTORY
- Visual loss often detected when one eye is covered for testing visual acuity
- Loss of ability to read, recognize faces, or drive a car; however, patients have enough peripheral vision to walk unaided
- Decrease in visual acuity (severe loss suggests choroidal neovascularization)
- Metamorphopsia (distortion of the shape of objects in view)
- Paracentral scotoma
- Variable visual loss from atrophy of a large area of retinal pigment epithelium involving the fovea
- Family history
- History of smoking
- High blood pressure (increases risk of choroidal neovascularization).

EXAMINATION
- Drüsen
- Disruption of pigment of the retinal pigment epithelium into small areas of hypopigmentation and hyperpigmentation (Fig. 94.1)
- Choroidal neovascularization.

Proceed as follows:
- Comment on the white walking aid by the bedside, which indicates the patient is registered blind
- Check visual acuity and visual field (in most patients, there is loss of central vision and maintenance of peripheral vision). Patients with only drüsen typically require additional magnification of text and more intense light to read small print text.
- Tell the examiner you would like to use an Amsler grid to confirm your diagnosis.

Remember: Age-related macular degeneration (AMD) is now the commonest cause of registrable blindness in the United Kingdom.

Diagnosis
This patient has senile macular degeneration (aetiology) and is registered blind, as evidenced by the white walking aid (functional status).

94—AGE-RELATED MACULAR DEGENERATION

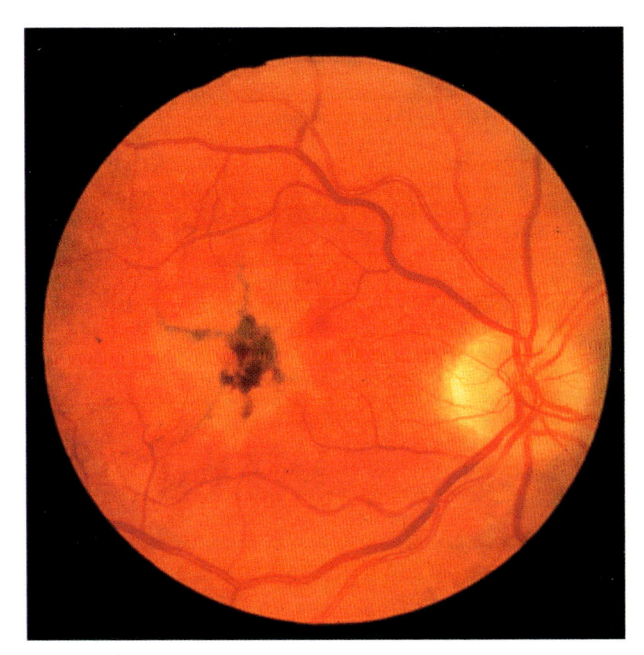

Fig. 94.1 Macular degeneration.

Questions

What are drüsen?
Drüsen are pale yellow spots that occur individually or in clusters throughout the macula (Fig. 94.2). Nearly all individuals over 50 years of age have at least one small drüsen ($\leq 63\,\mu m$) in one or both eyes. They consist of amorphous material accumulated between the Bruch membrane and pigment epithelium. Although the exact origin is not known, it is believed that drüsen occur from accumulation of lipofuscin and other cellular debris derived from cells of the retinal pigment epithelium that are compromised by age and other factors. Only eyes with large drüsen ($>63\,\mu m$) are at increased risk for senile macular degeneration. The clinical hallmark and usually the first clinical finding of AMD is the presence of drüsen. In most cases of AMD, drüsen are present bilaterally.

What are the types of AMD?
There are two types:
  Dry AMD: Findings include subretinal drüsen and pigment epithelial clumping, geographical atrophy of the retinal pigment epithelium, and pigment epithelial detachments. It is responsible for approximately 10% of AMD related blindness.
  Wet AMD: This is characterized by neovascularization from the choroidal and less commonly the retinal circulations into the subretinal space. Leak from these vessels allows fluid and blood to accumulate in this space. Although wet AMD accounts for only around 15% of AMD, it causes 80% of AMD related blindness (Fig. 94.3).

What do you know about neovascularization in these patients?
It leads to substantial visual loss as choroidal vessels proliferate across the Bruch membrane under the retinal pigment epithelium and, in some cases, continue their extension into the

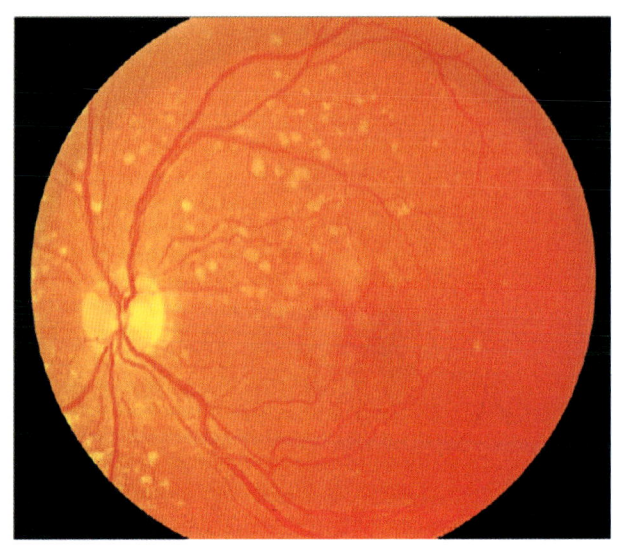

Fig. 94.2 Intermediate age-related macular degeneration with large drüsen. (With permission from Coleman, H.R., Chan, C.-C., Ferris, F.L., Chew, E.Y., 2008. Age-related macular degeneration. Lancet 372, 1835–1845.)

subretinal space. Substantial leakage from these neovascular membranes can lead to retinal detachment. The most devastating consequence is haemorrhage, which resolves forming a disciform scar.

What are the risk factors for choroidal neovascularization in the other eye of a patient with disorder in one eye?
- Large drüsen (>63 µm)
- Drüsen number >5
- Focal hyperpigmentation of the retinal pigment epithelium.

What investigations are performed to detect choroidal neovascularization?
- Rapid-sequence fluorescein angiography
- Retinal angiography using indocyanine green and infrared photography
- Optical coherence tomography (OCT) provides high-resolution images of the retina in cross section, allowing early and sensitive diagnosis.

What are the risk factors for macular degeneration?
- Elderly
- Genetic factors
- A history of smoking within the past 20 years
- White race
- Obesity
- High dietary intake of vegetable fat
- Aspirin use
- Low dietary intake of antioxidants and zinc
- Complement factor H, Y402H variant
- *LOC387715/ARMS2*, A69S variant.

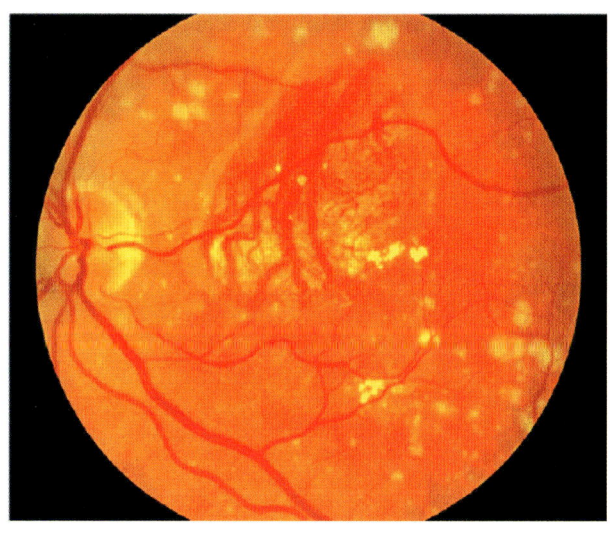

Fig. 94.3 Geographic atrophy involving the centre of the fovea, with sharply demarcated loss of normal retinal pigment epithelial cells and evidence of deeper, larger choroidal vessels. (With permission from Coleman, H.R., Chan, C.-C., Ferris, F.L., Chew, E.Y., 2008. Age-related macular degeneration. Lancet 372, 1835–1845.)

What is the treatment for dry AMD?
Smoking cessation is essential; for patients with dry macular degeneration, it is proven that smoking exacerbates the progression of the disease to wet stage. Antioxidants have shown to be beneficial, and supplements with high doses of vitamin A, C, zinc, omega-3 fatty acids, zeaxanthin, and lutein are used with proof that they can reduce the risk of developing advanced AMD in those at least at moderate risk.

What are the treatment options for advanced disease?
- When visual loss is severe, low-vision devices, such as electronic video magnifiers and spectacle-mounted telescopes, as well as low-vision rehabilitation services are available. The options available are vascular endothelial growth factor (VEGF) inhibitors injected intravitreously, inhibitor-like medications, photodynamic therapy, laser treatment, intravitreous surgery, or a combination of the aforementioned.
- Ranibizumab is a monoclonal antibody that inhibits all forms of VEGF. When ranibizumab is injected into the vitreous, it has stabilized loss of vision and, in some cases, improved vision in individuals with neovascular AMD.
- Bevacizumab, a monoclonal antibody to VEGF used intravenously as an anticancer agent, is also increasingly being used off-label as intravitreal therapy for neovascular AMD.
- Aflibercept and brolucizumab have recently been approved in the United States for wet AMD.
- Photodynamic therapy to reduce angiogenesis involves the use of an intravenously administered light-sensitive dye, verteporfin (Visudyne, Novartis), that preferentially concentrates in new blood vessels and is activated with the use of a 689-nm laser beam focused over the macula. It causes localized choroidal neovascular thrombosis through a nonthermal chemotoxic reaction.
- Some surgical techniques have been trialled of which the most effective to date is subretinal injection of tissue plasminogen activator (tPA).
- Radiation therapy has not been proven to have a good therapeutic profile so far.

What are the lifestyle modifications that a patient should be encouraged to make in order to prevent the disease as primary prevention?
Eating healthy with plenty of fish, fruit, and vegetables is encouraged as there are numerous studies so far that have proven the benefits of it. Antioxidants reduce the free radicals produced during light absorption and hence prevent cellular damage; however, they have not shown to have any role in primary prevention. Regular exercise has been proven to reduce the risk of the disease developing, but the best lifestyle modification one can do to prevent the disease is smoking cessation.

What is the difference between krypton and argon laser photocoagulation?
The krypton red photocoagulator is useful to treat when the neovascularization is closer than 200 μm but not under the fovea because of its ability to spare the inner retina by its virtual lack of absorption by haemoglobin (unlike the argon laser). The conventional argon laser has blue and green wavelengths. The green wavelength is absorbed by haemoglobin and may damage the retina, while the blue wavelength is absorbed by the macular xanthophyll and results in foveal damage.

Argon laser photocoagulation therapy was once the most common therapy for neovascular AMD. It is now used only occasionally to treat choroidal neovascularization that extends by >200 μm from the centre of the macula, since this therapy can create a large retinal scar, which is itself associated with permanent visual loss.

Mention some drugs that can cause maculopathy.
Chloroquine, thioridazine, chlorpromazine.

CHAPTER 95

Cataracts

Instruction
Examine this patient's eyes.

Salient Features
HISTORY
- Drug history (steroids, chloroquine, phenothiazines, chlorambucil, busulfan)
- History of gradual deterioration of vision
- History of diabetes
- Inquiry about smoking and alcohol consumption as both cigarette smoking and heavy alcohol consumption increase the risk of cataract formation
- History of sun exposure
- History is important even in age-related nuclear cataract as it explains about 50% variation in the severity of disease.

EXAMINATION
- Bilateral cataracts (shine light obliquely across the lens; Fig. 95.1, see also Fig. 97.3H)
- Patients will sometimes report an increase in near sightedness before the visual disturbance attributed to cataract is evident.

Proceed as follows:
- Tell the examiner that you would like to check the urine for sugar.

Diagnosis
This patient has premature bilateral cataracts (lesion) caused by diabetes mellitus (aetiology) and has had a gradual deterioration of vision (functional status).

Questions
Mention a few causes of cataracts.
- Common causes:
  - Old age (look for arcus senilis). The Framingham Study reported that 13% of people aged 65 to 74 years and about 40% of those over the age of 75 years had cataracts.
  - Diabetes mellitus. Nonenzymatic glycosylation of lens protein is twice as high in diabetic patients as in age-matched controls and may contribute to the premature occurrence of cataracts.
- Uncommon causes:
  - Trauma
  - Metabolic: Cushing syndrome, Wilson disease (stellate cataracts), galactosaemia

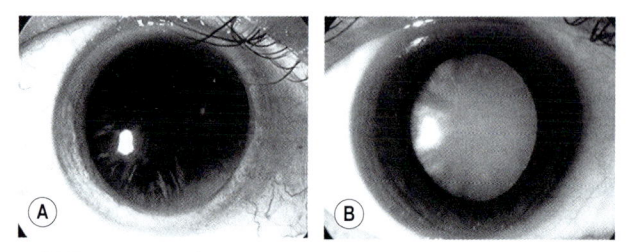

Fig. 95.1 Cataracts. **(A)** Early cataract. **(B)** White mature cataract. (With permission from Kumar, P., Clark, M. 2005. Clinical Medicine, sixth edn. Saunders, Edinburgh.)

- Chromosomal disorders: myotonic dystrophy, Turner syndrome
- Congenital infections (rubella or cytomegalovirus)
- Drugs (see earlier)
- Dermatological disorders: atopic dermatitis, ichthyosis
- Radiation: infrared (glassblower's cataract), X-ray, microwave radiation.

How are cataracts treated?
Cataract extraction can be performed by removing the lens nucleus and cortex from within the lens capsule (extracapsular) with placement of a hard prosthetic plastic lens. Multifocal intraocular lens implants in some instances have reduced the need for both reading and distance spectacles. Lens extraction improves vision in 95% of instances. In the remaining cases, prior retinal disease or postoperative complications such as haemorrhage, glaucoma, infection, or retinal detachment may be the cause. Phacoemulsification involves disruption of the native lens with ultrasound waves, which is then removed through a small incision, and replaced with a soft flexible lens. There are data suggesting that there is substantial benefit from bilateral cataract eye surgery in that it improves visual functioning.

How is early cataract detected using direct ophthalmoscopy?
Examination of the red reflex with +4 dioptres at approximately 20 cm from the patient will reveal a black opacity in the lens against the reddish hue of the reflex. If this opacity appears to move down on upward gaze, it is located in the posterior half of the lens, but if it appears to move up, then it is located in the anterior half of the lens.

Is the use of inhaled steroids associated with cataracts?
The use of inhaled steroids is associated with nuclear and posterior subcapsular cataracts.

Are there any ways to prevent cataract formation?
Although there is no proven prevention, certain interventions are associated with a reduced risk of developing cataracts. The importance of a healthy diet, especially one rich in the B vitamins riboflavin and B_{12}, is well known, as is smoking cessation.

However, large studies have not provided any evidence that vitamin E, selenium, or lutein with zeaxanthin have any positive impact on development of cataracts.

CHAPTER 96

Cholesterol Embolus in the Fundus

Instruction
Examine this patient's fundus.

Salient Features
HISTORY
- Severe, acute, and painless diminution or loss of vision
- History of atherosclerosis
- Risk factors of atherosclerosis: family history, diabetes, hypertension, ischaemic heart disease, peripheral vascular disease, cerebrovascular disease.

EXAMINATION
- Presence of a cholesterol embolus (Hollenhorst plaques) (Fig. 96.1) in one of the branches of the retinal artery.

Proceed as follows:
- Look for a cherry-red spot at the fovea (the ischaemic retina at the posterior pole becomes milky white and swollen, and the choroid is seen through the fovea as a cherry-red spot) (Fig. 96.2).
- Tell the examiner that you would like to check for visual field defects.

Remember: Retinal artery occlusion results in infarction of the inner two-thirds of the retina, reflex vasoconstriction of the retinal arterial tree, and stasis in the retinal capillaries.

Diagnosis
This patient has a cholesterol embolus in one of the branches of the retinal artery (lesion) caused by underlying atherosclerotic disease (aetiology).

Questions

What are the complications of such an embolus?
Retinal artery occlusion causing field defects or loss of vision.

Where is the likely origin of this embolus?
The most likely origin is an atherosclerotic plaque in the carotid circulation which is reported to be associated with carotid stenting.

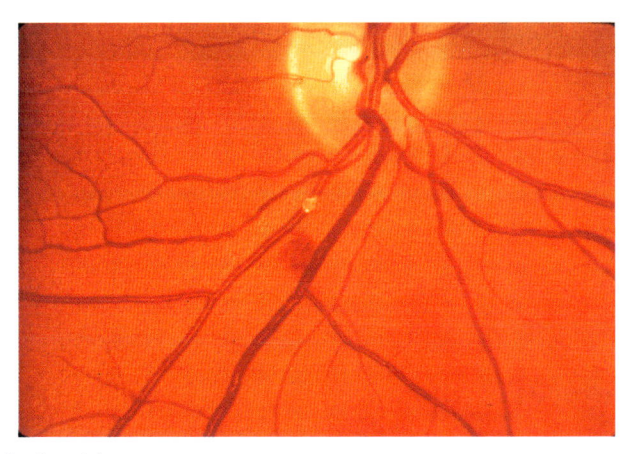

Fig. 96.1 Cholesterol crystal.

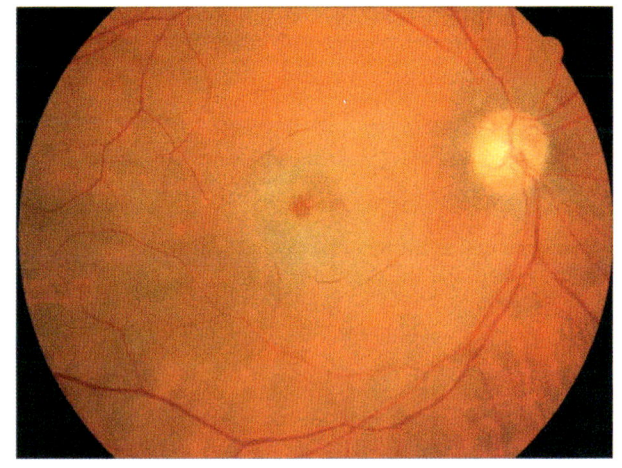

Fig. 96.2 Central retinal artery occlusion. (With permission from Wong, T., Mitchell, P., 2007. The eye in hypertension. Lancet 369, 425–435.)

What are the causes of retinal arterial occlusion?
- Commonest cause: emboli arising from the major arteries supplying the head or from the left side of the heart; embolic particles consist of platelet clumps, cholesterol crystals, or Hollenhorst plaques and others (mixed thrombus, calcific or septic material from cardiac valves, fat, myxoma, talc in intravenous drug abusers, or silicone in those who receive injections for cosmetic purposes).
- Other causes:
    - Temporal arteritis
    - Collagen vascular diseases
    - Increased orbital pressure, e.g. retrobulbar haemorrhage, Graves exophthalmos
    - Sickle cell disease
    - Acute arteriolar spasm caused by intranasal cocaine
    - Syphilis.

What do you understand by the term amaurosis?
Amaurosis means blindness from any cause.

What do you understand by the term amblyopia?
Amblyopia means that impaired vision is not caused by refractive error or ocular disease.

What do you understand by the term amaurosis fugax?
Amaurosis fugax is a retinal artery transient ischaemic attack that manifests with a painless, unilateral loss of vision that usually lasts a few minutes.

How would you manage this patient?
- Aspirin
- Ophthalmology opinion
- Ultrasonography of the carotid arteries
- Advise the patient to stop smoking
- Control of hypertension
- Carotid angiography with a view to performing carotid endarterectomy.

What is the effect of cholesterol crystals?
Cholesterol crystals rarely cause significant obstruction to the retinal arterioles.

What manoeuvre would you use to make the cholesterol crystals more apparent?
Mild lateral pressure on the globe may make the presence of unobtrusive crystals clearly visible when the retinal arteries pulsate.

How would you manage an acute occlusion of the retinal artery?
- Lie the patient in a supine position to ensure adequate circulation.
- Intermittent ocular massage is applied for 15 min to dislodge the emboli, lower intraocular pressure, and improve circulation.
- Intravenous acetazolamide to lower intraocular pressure
- Inhalation of a mixture of 5% carbon dioxide and 95% oxygen
- Anterior chamber paracentesis.

If the investigation of a patient with amaurosis fugax comes up with no evidence of carotid artery disease, embolism, or other recognized causes of the disorder, then the diagnosis by exclusion should be vasospasm. In such cases, a calcium channel blocker should be tried.

CHAPTER 97

Diabetic Retinopathy

Instruction

Examine the fundus in these patients.
- You will be expected to comment on whether it is background (Fig. 97.1) or proliferative (Fig. 97.2) retinopathy.
- You may have a clue about the underlying diabetes either from a diabetic chart or from the presence of diabetic fruit juices at the bedside. If you inspect their hands, you will see pinpricks on the nondominant hand from glucose monitoring.

PATIENT 1
Salient Features
HISTORY

- Gradual or acute loss of vision
- History of floaters
- History of diabetes, hypertension
- Ask about renal disease (renal–retinal syndrome of diabetes).

EXAMINATION

- Background retinopathy, caused by microvascular leakage into the retina
- Microaneurysms, usually seen in the posterior pole temporal to the fovea
- Dot and blot haemorrhages (Fig. 97.3B)
- Hard exudates (Fig. 97.3C)
- Cotton-wool spots (Fig. 97.3D).

Diagnosis

This patient has dot and blot haemorrhages and cotton-wool spots (lesions), probably caused by diabetic retinopathy (aetiology), and good visual acuity (functional status).

Questions

What symptoms will this patient have?
The patient will be asymptomatic as the macula is spared.

How would you manage such a patient?
- Treat diabetes and associated hypertension
- Conduct annual fundal examination
- No targeted treatment is required at this stage, unless there is macular oedema.

97 — DIABETIC RETINOPATHY

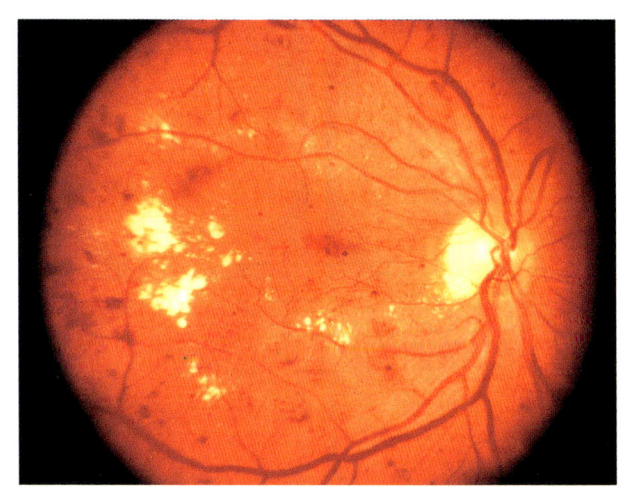

Fig. 97.1 Background retinopathy.

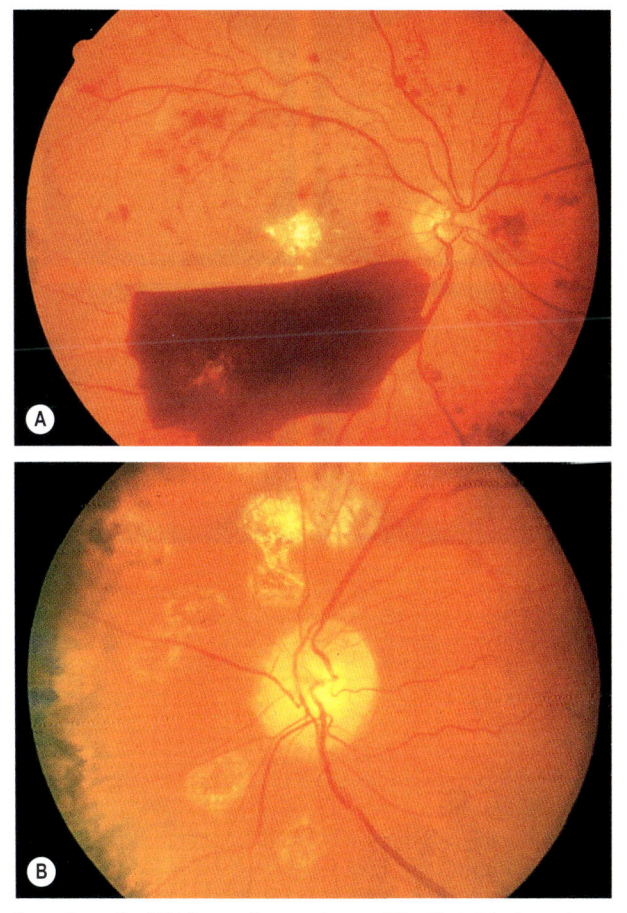

Fig. 97.2 Proliferative retinopathy. **(A)** Vitreous haemorrhages; **(B)** retinal detachment.

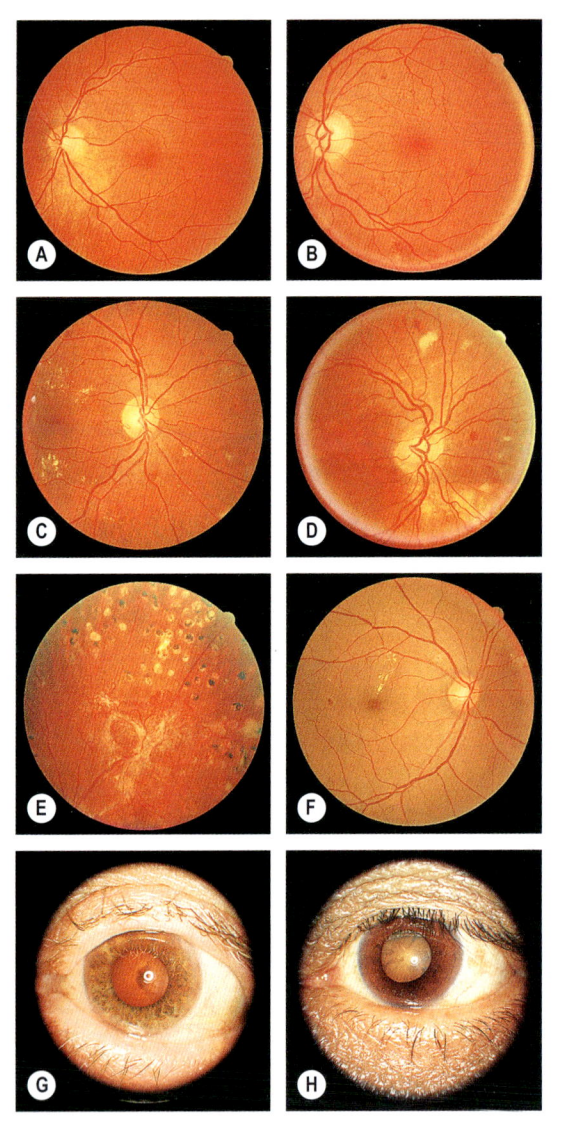

Fig. 97.3 Diabetic eye disease. **(A)** Normal macula and optic disc. **(B)** Early background retinopathy, dot and blot haemorrhages. **(C)** Early background retinopathy, plus hard exudates. **(D)** Preproliferative retinopathy, with multiple cotton-wool spots. **(E)** Proliferative retinopathy, with hallmark frond-like new vesicles. **(F)** Exudative maculopathy, with exudates within a disc-width of the macula. Central **(G)** and cortical **(H)** cataracts seen against the red reflex of the ophthalmoscope. (With permission from Kumar, P., Clark, M. 2005. Clinical Medicine, sixth edn. Saunders, Edinburgh.)

- In selected cases with very severe changes and high risk of progression, laser photocoagulation may be considered.

The Early Treatment of Diabetic Retinopathy Study has established that early peripheral (panretinal) argon laser photocoagulation is not indicated for mild to moderate nonproliferative retinopathy.

PATIENT 2
Salient Features
EXAMINATION
- Signs of background retinopathy with hard exudates or oedema of the macula.

Diagnosis
This patient has diabetic maculopathy, caused by the oedema and/or the hard exudates.

Questions
What symptoms may this patient have?
There will be a gradual impairment of central vision, such as difficulty in reading small print or seeing road signs.

PATIENT 3
Salient Features
EXAMINATION
- Cotton-wool spots
- Venous dilatation, beading, looping, or sausage-like segmentation
- Arteriolar narrowing
- Haemorrhages: large dark blots
- Intraretinal microvascular abnormalities.

Diagnosis
This patient has severe nonproliferative retinopathy.

Questions
What symptoms may this patient have?
Asymptomatic if the macula is spared.

How would you manage this patient?
Semiurgent referral to the ophthalmologist for close follow-up to enable early detection and treatment of proliferative retinopathy.

PATIENT 4
Salient Features
EXAMINATION
- Neovascularization around the disc or away from the disc; in early stages, the vessels are bare and flat and easily missed. In later stages, they are elevated and may be associated with a white fibrous component.
- Presence of laser burns (in treated cases).

Diagnosis

This patient has proliferative retinopathy caused by retinal hypoxia, usually seen in insulin-dependent diabetic retinopathy.

Questions

What symptoms may this patient have?
Asymptomatic in the absence of complications.

How would you manage this patient?
Urgent referral to an ophthalmologist for laser treatment and anti-VEGF injections.

How is diabetic retinopathy classified?
Diabetic retinopathy can be nonproliferative or proliferative, depending on whether neovascularization has taken place or not.
- In nonproliferative retinopathy, new-vessel formation has not taken place, but the characteristic changes are haemorrhages, microaneurysms, venous beading, soft exudates, and intraretinal microvascular abnormalities. It is subclassified into mild, moderate, severe, and very severe, depending on the extent of these changes within the retinal map.
- In proliferative diabetic retinopathy, new vessels are formed. In severe proliferative diabetic retinopathy, the retina may be detached.

What are the complications of proliferative retinopathy?
- Vitreous haemorrhage
- Traction retinal detachment
- Rubeosis irides
- Rubeotic glaucoma: some of these patients can have partial restoration of vision by microsurgery called pars plana vitrectomy.

What are the signs of macular oedema?
Macular oedema includes any of the following signs:
- Retinal thickening at or within 500 μm of the centre of the macula (Fig. 97.3F)
- Retinal thickening of one-disc area or larger, in any part of the retina, which is within the one-disc diameter from the centre of the macula
- Hard exudates at or within 500 μm of the centre of the macula
- Optical coherence tomography (OCT) has vastly increased the sensitivity of diagnosis and has allowed many more cases to be managed earlier on in the natural history of the condition.

How will you manage the patient with macular oedema?
Nonurgent referral to an ophthalmologist for photocoagulation, which will stabilize (seldom improve) visual acuity in 50% of patients. The ability to alter the course of visual loss in diabetic macular oedema favourably is a major advance, but patients must be cautioned that the most likely result of treatment is stabilization, not improvement, of visual acuity.

What is the principal mechanism of visual loss in nonproliferative retinopathy?
The principal mechanism of visual loss in nonproliferative retinopathy is through macular oedema, which results from focal vascular leakage from microaneurysms in the macular capillaries, as well

as from diffuse vascular leakage. With time, areas of leakage progress to macular thickening associated with hard exudates or cystoid changes.

What are the different types of clinical presentation of nonproliferative retinopathy?
Patients may present with no visual symptoms, paracentral scotomata, or various degrees of central visual loss. Consequently, the diagnosis and management of macular oedema depend crucially on the determination of macular thickening by fundus examination. Ophthalmoscopy detects intraretinal haemorrhages and hard exudates but does not detect substantial retinal thickening. A critical evaluation of retinal thickening requires stereoscopic examination of the retina by slit-lamp biomicroscopy with lens for retinal visualization, stereoscopic fundus photography, and OCT.

What is the relationship between the duration of diabetes and retinopathy?
There is a close relationship: in patients diagnosed to have diabetes before the age of 30 years, the incidence of retinopathy is about 50% after 10 years and 90% after 30 years. It is unusual for retinopathy to develop within 5 years of onset of diabetes; however, 5% of patients with type 2 diabetes have background retinopathy at presentation. Sight-threatening retinopathy can be expected to develop in 50% of patients with type 1 diabetes and 30% of those with type 2; these patients will need intervention to reduce the risk of vision loss. Diabetic blindness can be reduced or prevented without preventing retinopathy. Systematic screening for diabetic retinopathy and preventive laser treatment for those who develop macular oedema or proliferative retinopathy reduce the rate of blindness to about 0.5% in the diabetic population, irrespective of the prevalence of retinopathy.

What associated systemic conditions worsen diabetic retinopathy?
- Pregnancy
- Hypertension
- Anaemia
- Renal failure.

What is the relationship between diabetic control and retinopathy?
The Diabetes Control and Complications Trial compared intensive treatment for blood glucose control with conventional treatment in patients with and without retinopathy at baseline who were followed for a mean of 6.5 years. Intensive treatment had profound benefits in both subgroups and was associated with a reduction in the incidence of both the development of new retinopathy and the risk of progression of existing retinopathy.

What is the relationship between diabetic retinopathy and pregnancy?
Retinopathy can progress rapidly in pregnant patients with preexisting diabetes; careful and more frequent evaluation is indicated during and after pregnancy, until a year postpartum. Gestational diabetes is not associated with retinopathy, so regular evaluation is not indicated in this group of patients.

How often would you screen diabetic patients for retinopathy?
- Type 2 diabetics: annually
- Type 1 diabetics:
  - Newly diagnosed: no screening for the first 5 years
  - 5 to 10 years from initial diagnosis: annually
  - >10 years after initial diagnosis: every 6 months.

What is the earliest sign of retinal change in diabetes?
An increase in capillary permeability, evidenced by the leakage of dye into the vitreous humour after fluorescein injection, is the earliest sign.

What do you know about the role of growth factors in the formation of new vessels in proliferative retinopathy?
In response to constant hyperglycaemia, oxidative stress, loss of endothelial integrity, and subsequent hypoxia, growth factors are produced by the retinal cells. Growth factors that have been found in diabetic retinas and have been proved to be implicated in the development of new vessels are insulin growth factor-1, fibroblast growth factor, platelet-derived growth factor, and vascular endothelial growth factor. These growth factors, in turn, promote neovascularization. Vascular endothelial growth inhibitors have been produced and are currently used in combination with laser treatment for cases of diabetic proliferative retinopathy.

What do you know about photocoagulation?
Photocoagulation is a technique whereby several thousand lesions are produced over a 2-week therapy period with lasers. Panretinal photocoagulation reduces the risk of severe visual loss (50% in patients with severe diabetic retinopathy). The laser is used to ablate a portion of the retina and does not directly cauterize the neovascularization. It is believed that the regression of neovascularization results from the destruction of ischaemic and hypoxic retina, thus reducing angiogenic factors. Photocoagulation decreases the incidence of haemorrhage or scarring in proliferative retinopathy. Photocoagulation is also useful in the treatment of microaneurysms, haemorrhages, and oedema. Some loss of peripheral vision may be inevitable with this technique. Photocoagulation reduces the risk of visual loss in patients with proliferative retinopathy.

What surgical technique may be used for a nonresolving vitreous haemorrhage and retinal detachment?
Pars plana vitrectomy may be used and is recommended for severe proliferative diabetic retinopathy when it is unresponsive to panretinal photocoagulation, is associated with severe vitreous haemorrhage, or is associated with traction on the macula. However, it is often complicated by retinal tears, retinal detachment, glaucoma, infection, cataracts, and loss of the eye.

CHAPTER 98

Hypertensive Retinopathy

Instruction
Examine this 53-year-old man's eyes, including fundoscopy.

Salient Features
HISTORY
- Usually no ocular symptoms
- History of hypertension.

EXAMINATION
- Arteriovenous nipping (Figs 98.1A and 98.2B)
- Arteriolar narrowing
- Macular star (Fig. 98.2D)
- Flame-shaped and blot haemorrhages (Figs 98.1B and 98.2C)
- Cotton-wool exudates (Figs 98.1B and 98.2C)
- Papilloedema may or may not be present (Fig. 98.2D).

Tell the examiner that you would like to:
- check the blood pressure (BP).
- auscultate for bruits.
- examine the urine for proteinuria.
- examine the cardiovascular system for heart failure and obtain a 12-lead electrocardiogram (ECG) for signs of left heart strain or ischaemia.

Diagnosis
This patient has flame-shaped haemorrhages with a macular star (lesions) caused by hypertension (aetiology).

Questions
How would you grade hypertensive retinopathy?
Keith–Wagener–Barker classification
This combines the clinical findings of hypertension and atherosclerosis:
- Stage I: arteriolar narrowing
- Stage II: irregular calibre of arterioles
- Stage III: cotton-wool exudates; flame and blot haemorrhages, retinal oedema
- Stage IV: papilloedema.

383

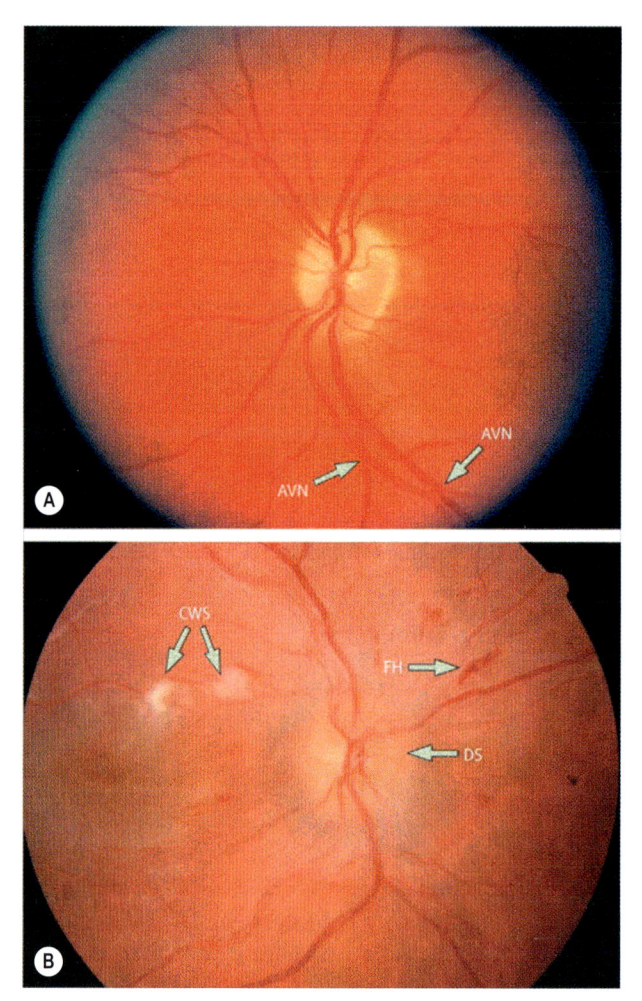

Fig. 98.1 (A) Mild retinopathy in an eye with ischaemic optic neuropathy. **(B)** Severe hypertensive retinopathy. *AVN*, Arteriovenous nipping; *CWS*, cotton-wool spots; *DS*, swelling of the optic disc; *FH*, flame-shaped retina haemorrhage. (With permission from Wong, T., Mitchell, P. 2007. The eye in hypertension. Lancet 369, 425–435.)

Mitchell and Wong have since simplified this system to the following:
- Grade 1: Mild retinopathy. Arteriolar narrowing (generalized and focal), atrioventricular nicking, and/or arteriolar wall opacity
- Grade 2: Moderate retinopathy. Haemorrhage, microaneurysm, cotton-wool spot, and/or hard exudate
- Grade 3: Malignant retinopathy. Moderate retinopathy plus optic disc swelling.

Scheie classification

This separates the clinical findings of hypertension and atherosclerosis (Fig. 98.2).
- Hypertension:
  - Grade 0: no changes
  - Grade 1: barely detectable arteriolar narrowing
  - Grade 2: obvious arteriolar narrowing with focal irregularities

98 — HYPERTENSIVE RETINOPATHY

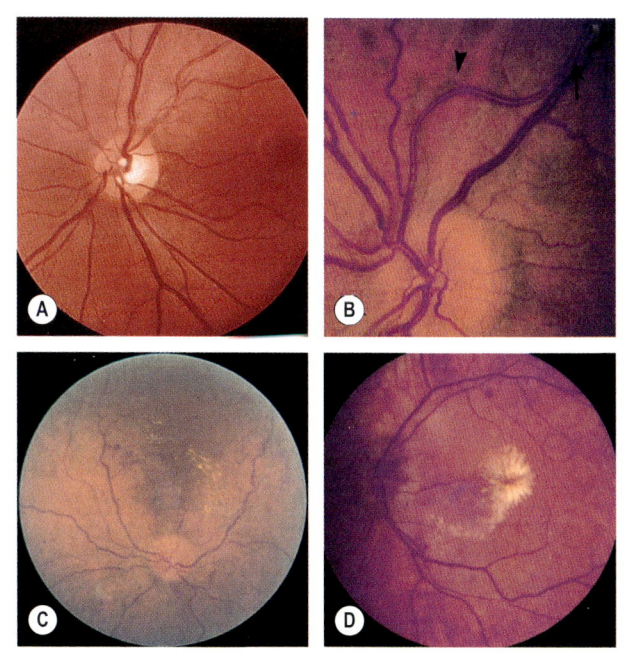

Fig. 98.2 **(A)** Grade 1: early and minor changes include increased tortuosity of a retinal vessel and increased reflectiveness (silver wiring) of a retinal artery (at 1 o'clock in this view). **(B)** Grade 2: increased tortuosity and silver wiring (arrowhead) plus 'nipping' of the venules at arteriovenous crossings (arrow). **(C)** Grade 3: as grade 2 plus flame-shaped retinal haemorrhages and soft 'cotton-wool' exudates. **(D)** Grade 4: swelling of the optic disc (papilloedema), retinal oedema, and hard exudates around the fovea, producing a typical 'macular star'. (With permission from Forbes, C.D., Jackson, W.F. 2003. Color Atlas and Text of Clinical Medicine, third edn. Mosby, London.)

- Grade 3: grade 2 plus retinal haemorrhages and/or exudates
- Grade 4: grade 3 plus papilloedema.
- Arteriolar sclerosis:
    - Grade 0: normal
    - Grade 1: barely detectable light reflex changes
    - Grade 2: obvious increased light reflex changes
    - Grade 3: copper-wire arterioles
    - Grade 4: silver-wire arterioles.

What is the significance of retinal arteriolar narrowing in normotensive individuals?
Retinal arteriolar narrowing might also be used to predict subsequent development of hypertension in individuals initially classified as normotensive.

Mention some causes of cotton-wool spots.
- HIV infection
- Anaemias
- Infective endocarditis
- Leukaemias
- Diabetic retinopathy.

What is the relationship between morbidity and hypertensive retinopathy?
Neurological link
- In a 3-year population-based cohort study of atherosclerosis risk, incident stroke events were more common in participants with signs of hypertensive retinopathy than in participants without retinopathy. When controlled for BP, diabetes, lipids, and other risk factors, moderate signs of hypertensive retinopathy (cotton-wool spots, retinal haemorrhages, and microaneurysms) were associated with a two- to four-fold higher risk of incident stroke. Weaker associations between signs of mild hypertensive retinopathy and risk of stroke were also present.
- Hypertensive retinopathy is also reported to be associated with cognitive decline, cerebral white-matter lesions identified by cerebral magnetic resonance imaging, lacunar infarctions, cerebral atrophy, and stroke mortality.

Cardiovascular link
- Studies of the association between hypertensive retinopathy signs and heart disease have produced inconsistent results. However, hypertensive retinopathy has been linked with coronary artery stenosis and with incident coronary heart disease events. A large study revealed that individuals with retinal microaneurysms and haemorrhages were twice as likely to die of a cardiovascular event compared to those without these signs.
- Some investigators suggest that moderate hypertensive retinopathy could be used to predict incident congestive heart failure, even in individuals without a history of myocardial infarction.

Other links
- Retinopathy signs are also associated with indicators of target organ damage, such as microalbuminuria, renal impairment, and left ventricular hypertrophy.

What are Elschnig spots?
They are black flecks surrounded by yellow or red halos and occur in advanced hypertensive retinopathy. They are caused by focal occlusion of the choroidal capillaries, which leads to necrosis and atrophy of retinal pigment epithelium. Acutely, these spots are punctate tan-white lesions that leak on fluorescein angiography through breakdown in the blood–brain barrier.

Further Information

Anton Elschnig (1863–1939) was an Austrian ophthalmologist.

Marcus Gunn first described hypertensive retinopathy in the 19th century in a series of patients with hypertension and renal disease (Gunn, 1892).

In 1939, Keith, Wagner, and Barker showed that the signs of retinopathy were predictive of death in patients with hypertension (Keith, Wagener and Barker, 1939).

CHAPTER 99

Optic Atrophy

Instruction
Examine this patient's eyes.
Examine this patient's fundus.

Salient Features
HISTORY
- Visual loss: onset of symptoms depends on underlying aetiology
- History of multiple sclerosis
- History of glaucoma
- Optic nerve tumour
- Vitamin B_{12} deficiency
- Paget disease
- Exposure to toxins: lead, methanol, arsenic.

EXAMINATION
- Pale disc with sharp margins (Fig. 99.1)
- Intact consensual light reflex but impaired direct light reflex: Marcus Gunn pupillary response (seen in asymmetrical involvement of the two eyes)
- Central scotoma on testing of visual fields.

Proceed as follows:
- Tell the examiner that you would like to look for cerebellar signs (remember that multiple sclerosis is the commonest cause of optic atrophy).

Diagnosis
This patient has primary optic atrophy (lesion) caused by multiple sclerosis (aetiology). I would like to check the visual fields for central scotoma (functional status).

Questions
What is the differential diagnosis?
- Demyelinating disorders (multiple sclerosis)
- Optic nerve compression by tumour or aneurysm
- Glaucoma
- Toxins: methanol, tobacco, lead, arsenical poisoning
- Ischaemia, including central retinal artery occlusion in thromboembolism, temporal arteritis, idiopathic acute ischaemic optic neuropathy, syphilis

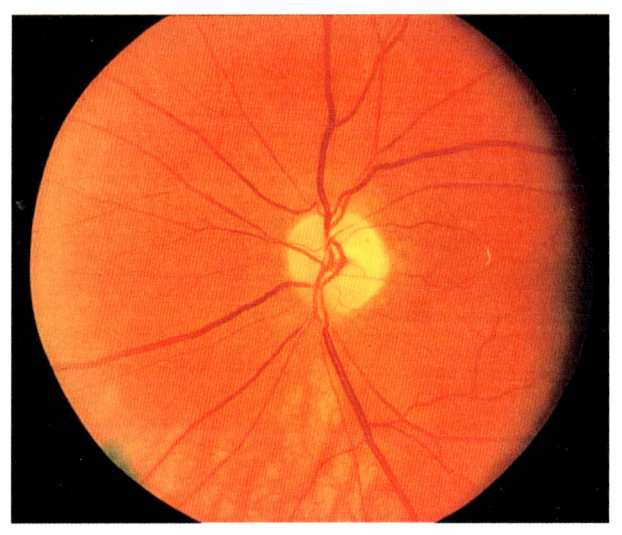

Fig. 99.1 Optic atrophy.

- Hereditary disorders: Friedreich ataxia, Leber optic atrophy (sex linked, seen in young males)
- Paget disease
- Vitamin B_{12} deficiency
- Secondary to retinitis pigmentosa.

What is the difference between primary and secondary optic atrophy?

Primary	*Secondary*
White and flat with clear-cut edges	Greyish-white, edges indistinct
Visible lamina cribrosa	Cup filled and lamina cribrosa not visible
Arteries and veins normal	Arteries thinner than normal, veins may be dilated
Capillaries decreased in number	Capillaries decreased in number (fewer than seven): Kestenbaum sign

What is consecutive optic atrophy?
Consecutive optic atrophy is a controversial term and is best avoided. Some use it as an equivalent or alternative for what has been described earlier as secondary optic atrophy, but others use the term to indicate an atrophy complicating retinitis or, rarely, Tay–Sachs disease or retinitis pigmentosa.

What is glaucomatous optic atrophy?
Glaucomatous optic atrophy denotes loss of disc substance, referred to as increased cupping.

How would you investigate a patient with optic neuropathy?
- Full blood count, erythrocyte sedimentation rate
- Blood glucose
- Serology for syphilis

- Serum vitamin B_{12} and B_1
- Skull radiograph of pituitary fossa, optic foramina and sinuses, or computed tomography scan of the brain and orbit
- Optical coherence tomography
- Electrocardiogram
- Pattern-stimulated visual evoked responses
- Electroretinography.

Further Information

R. Marcus Gunn (1850–1909), a Scottish ophthalmologist who worked at Moorfields Eye Hospital, London.
T. von Leber (1840–1917), Professor of Ophthalmology at the University of Heidelberg, Germany.
W. Tay (1843–1927), a British ophthalmologist, Moorfields Eye Hospital, London.
B.P. Sachs (1858–1944), a German neuropsychiatrist who worked in New York. He described this condition independent of Tay.

CHAPTER 100

Osteogenesis Imperfecta

Instruction
Look at this patient's eyes.

Salient Features
HISTORY
- Ask about previous fractures.
- Ask whether or not the condition runs in the family.

EXAMINATION
- Blue sclera
- Look for the following signs:
  - Hearing loss as a result of otosclerosis
  - Signs of old fractures
  - Defective dentine formation in the teeth
  - Kyphosis and scoliosis (Fig. 100.1)
  - Joint hypermobility
  - Herniae
  - Aortic regurgitation.

Diagnosis
This patient has blue sclera with abnormalities of the skeleton and teeth (lesions) caused by osteogenesis imperfecta tarda (aetiology) and uses a wheelchair (functional status).

Questions

Why is the sclera blue?
Because the choroid pigment is visible.

Mention other conditions in which the sclera is blue.
- Marfan syndrome
- Ehlers–Danlos syndrome.

What is the inheritance pattern?
Usually autosomal dominant although it may be autosomal recessive. The gene defects are in the two genes *COL1A1* or *COL1A2* that encode the procollagen chains of type I collagen. Mutant type I collagen results from autosomal dominant osteogenesis imperfecta. Mutations affecting either of two components of the collagen prolyl 3-hydroxylation complex (cartilage-associated

100 — OSTEOGENESIS IMPERFECTA

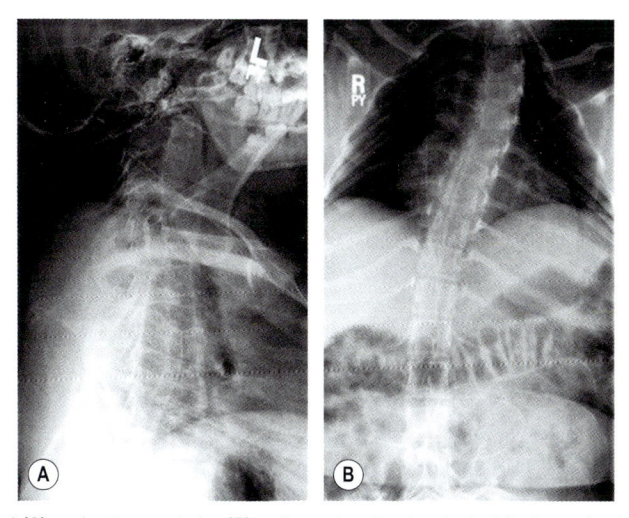

Fig. 100.1 Lateral **(A)** and anteroposterior **(B)** radiographs showing typical findings of osteogenesis imperfecta: diffuse osteopenia, scoliosis, compression of several cervical vertebral bodies, and a focal kyphosis at the midcervical level. (With permission from Song, D., Maher, C.O., 2007. Spinal disorders associated with skeletal dysplasias and syndromes. Neurosurg. Clin. North Am. 18, 499–514.)

protein and prolyl 3-hydroxylase 1) cause the autosomal recessive form with rhizomelia (shortening of proximal segments of upper and lower limbs) and delayed collagen folding.

What is the characteristic pathology?
The most characteristic pathology is a primary reduction in bone matrix with secondary mineralization.

What are the clinical types?
The Sillence classification is into four types (I–IV):
  I. Nearly normal stature, imperfect dentition, blue sclera, fractures of variable number, and minimal deformity
  II. Usually fetuses die in utero or shortly after birth; multiple fractures of ribs and long bones with little mineralization of calvarium and pulmonary hypertension.
  III. (Osteogenesis imperfecta congenita, fetal type): stature markedly diminished as a result of multiple fractures and deformity of long bones in utero; blue sclera, imperfect dentition, and hearing loss
  IV. (Osteogenesis imperfecta tarda): stature usually reduced, bone deformity and fractures common; sclera bluish to normal; imperfect dentition; may or may not have loss of hearing.

How would you manage this patient?
- Genetic counselling
- Calcium, vitamin D
- Bisphosphonates may improve bone density and growth in children.
- Bone marrow transplantation to correct mesenchymal defect in children.

CHAPTER 101

Papilloedema

Instruction
Examine this patient's fundus.

Salient Features
HISTORY
- Headache (positional, worsening headache on lying flat, diurnal pattern of headache with the headache being worse in the morning)
- Transient visual disturbances
- Diplopia (from associated sixth cranial nerve palsy, presenting as binocular horizontal diplopia)
- History of hypertension, brain tumour
- History of ingestion of steroids, hypervitaminosis A (causes of benign intracranial hypertension).

EXAMINATION
- There is swelling of the optic disc (look for haemorrhages and soft exudates; Fig. 101.1).

> **Note:** Common causes are:
> - intracranial space-occupying lesion
> - hypertensive retinopathy
> - idiopathic intracranial hypertension.

Diagnosis
This patient has bilateral papilloedema (lesion) and I would like to investigate for an intracranial space-occupying lesion (aetiology).

Questions

What do you understand by the term papilloedema?
Papilloedema is the swelling of the nerve head as seen on ophthalmoscopy secondary to raised intracranial pressure. The colour of the optic disc becomes redder, approximating to that of the rest of the retina; its contour becomes blurred and the cup and cribrosa are filled in.

What is the first manifestation of papilloedema?
The earliest manifestation of papilloedema is the engorgement of the veins.

101 – PAPILLOEDEMA

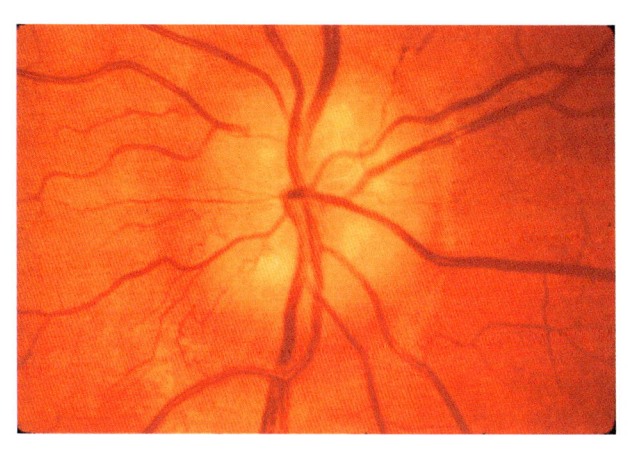

Fig. 101.1 Papilloedema.

What is the nature of the field defect in papilloedema?
Papilloedema is always associated with enlargement of the blind spot, with a consequent diminution of visual fields and gradual loss of visual acuity, but a fair degree of acuity may remain until papilloedema is marked.

Mention a few causes of papilloedema.
- Idiopathic intracranial hypertension (pseudotumour cerebri)
- Raised intracranial pressure resulting from one of the following conditions:
    - Impaired circulation of the cerebrospinal fluid (CSF) in aqueduct stenosis
    - Meningitis
    - Obstructive hydrocephalus
    - Intracranial mechanical pathology (space-occupying lesions, haemorrhage, haematoma, abscess).
- Cerebral oedema:
    - Following head injury
    - Following cerebral anoxia.
- Metabolic causes that can cause diffuse cerebral oedema:
    - Carbon dioxide retention
    - Steroid withdrawal
    - Thyroid eye disease
    - Vitamin A intoxication
    - Lead poisoning.
- Increased protein in the CSF in:
    - Guillain–Barré syndrome
    - Spinal cord tumours
    - Any spinal block.
- Haematological and circulatory disorders and venous outflow obstruction:
    - Central retinal vein thrombosis
    - Sinus venous thrombosis
    - Superior vena cava obstruction
    - Polycythaemia vera
    - Multiple myeloma
    - Macroglobulinaemia.

Mention a few conditions that simulate papilloedema.
- Deep optic cup:
  - Nasal edge appears heaped up.
  - Vessels plunge into the optic cup.
  - Temporal edge is quite normal.
- Medullated nerve fibres: seen on the disc or even on the retina. The appearance is typically flared and on focusing will reveal fibres traversing the area. Field defects are the result of the retinal vessels being obscured. Since these are present from birth, the patient is unaware of the defect.
- Bergmeister papilla: whitish elevation of the centre of the disc with venous and arterial sheathing. It is common and seen at all ages. There is an equal sex and racial incidence.
- Pseudopapilloedema: congenitally elevated discs secondary to hyaloid tissue (Drüsen) or hyperopia.

> **Note:** Elevation or swelling on the optic disc occurs in the following conditions:
> - Papilloedema
> - Papillitis
> - Drüsen
> - Infiltration of the nerve head by malignant cells.

What do you know about Foster Kennedy syndrome?
Unilateral papilloedema with or without 'secondary' optic atrophy on the other side suggests a tumour of the opposite side on the olfactory lobe or orbital surface of the frontal lobe or of the pituitary body.

What do you understand by the term papillitis?
Papillitis is inflammation of the anterior portion of the optic nerve, commonly associated with inflammation of the retina. The fundoscopic findings can resemble papilloedema, as the optic nerve is swollen and congested, with or without haemorrhages. Causes can be viral infections, autoimmune diseases, and vasculitides.

How do you differentiate papillitis from papilloedema?

Papillitis	*Papilloedema*
Usually unilateral	Usually bilateral
Visual acuity is considerably reduced in relation to the degree of swelling of the disc	Visual acuity only slightly reduced until late stages
Visual field defect is usually central, particularly for red and green	Peripheral constriction or enlargement of the blind spot
Eye movements may be painful	Eye movements are never painful

> **Note:** A Marcus Gunn pupil is one that shows better constriction to an indirect response than to direct light. An example is decreased constriction of both pupils when a light is shone into the left eye, indicating a relative afferent pupillary defect.

What investigations does a patient with bilateral papilloedema warrant?
Any patient presenting with new onset bilateral papilloedema of unknown aetiology should have urgent brain imaging in the form of computed tomography (CT) or magnetic resonance imaging (MRI), with sequences that help identify potential sinus venous obstruction (venogram).

If neuroimaging does not reveal the cause of the papilloedema, then lumbar puncture should take place on an urgent basis to estimate the opening CSF pressure and send CSF for further analysis, and proceed to therapeutic drainage of CSF fluid if indicated. All patients found to have papilloedema will need a detailed evaluation by an ophthalmologist and formal visual field testing.

What are the stages of papilloedema?
- Stage I: increase in venous calibre and tortuosity
- Stage II: optic cup becomes pinker and less distinct, the vessels seeming to disappear suddenly on the surface of the disc
- Stage III: blurring of the discs on the nasal side (in many normal discs, the nasal edge is less distinct and one of the most frequent false-positive signs is questionable blurring of the nasal disc margins)
- Stage IV: the whole disc becomes suffused and slightly elevated. The margins may disappear and the vessels seem to emerge from a mushy swelling. The optic cup is filled and there are haemorrhages around the disc.

What are the diagnostic criteria for diagnosis of idiopathic intracranial hypertension?
- Unimpaired consciousness
- Clinical features and signs of increased intracranial pressure
- No localizing neurological signs (except sixth cranial nerve palsy)
- Opening pressure of CSF during lumbar puncture is >250 mmH$_2$O and CSF is of normal composition.
- Normal ventricles and normal study on CT or MRI
- No other apparent cause for raised intracranial pressure.

What treatment options are available for pseudotumour cerebri?
Treatment of idiopathic intracranial hypertension aims at relieving the symptoms and, most importantly, preventing permanent visual loss.
- General measures: weight loss, avoid medications that can raise intracranial pressure
- Drugs: carbonic anhydrase inhibitors, diuretics
- Serial lumbar punctures, lumboperitoneal shunt
- Optic nerve sheath fenestration, subtemporal decompression.

Further Information

Foster Kennedy (1884–1952) was born in Belfast. He was Professor of Neurology at Cornell University. He described his syndrome in 1923.

CHAPTER 102

Retinal Detachment

Instruction
Examine this patient's eye.

Salient Features
HISTORY
- Patient complaints of a dark curtain progressing across the visual field
- Floaters, flashes
- History of diabetes, hypertension
- History of kidney disease (diabetic renal-retinal syndrome).

EXAMINATION
- The retina has lost its pink colour and appears grey and opaque.
- When the collection of subretinal fluid is large, the retina shows ballooning detachment with numerous folds (Fig. 102.1).
- Examine visual acuity and visual fields.

Proceed as follows:
- Tell the examiner that you would like to:
  - check urine for sugar
  - check the blood pressure.
- Comment on any walking aid for the registered blind.

Diagnosis
This patient has neovascularization and retinal detachment (lesion) caused by underlying diabetes mellitus (aetiology). She has a walking aid for the registered blind (functional status).

Questions

What is the pathology of retinal detachment?
It is a separation within the retina between the photoreceptors and the retinal pigment epithelium, characterized by collection of fluid or blood in this potential space.

What are the types of retinal detachment?
Rhegmatogenous retinal detachment. This is defined as the presence of a hole or break in the retina that allows fluid from the vitreous cavity to enter the subretinal space. It usually occurs spontaneously in those who have a predisposition to it following trauma to the eye or after intraocular surgery. Most of these patients develop symptoms. A break in the peripheral retina is associated with a sudden burst of flashing lights or sparks, which may be followed by small floaters or spots

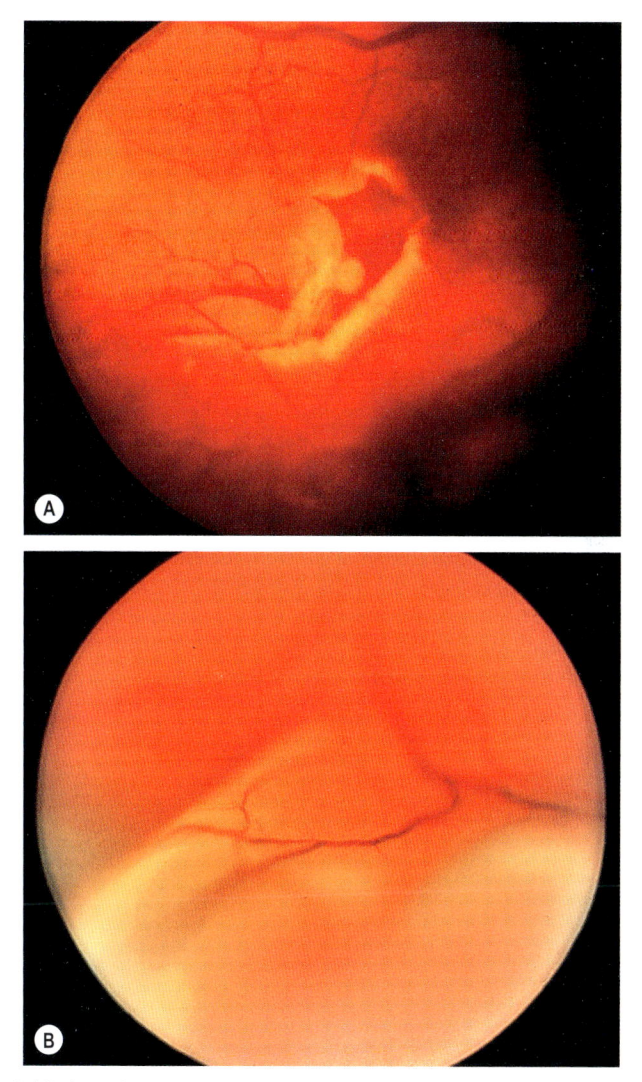

Fig. 102.1 Retinal detachment.

in the field of vision. When the retina detaches, the patient perceives a dark curtain progressing across the visual field, and when the fovea detaches, central vision is abruptly diminished. Small detachments can be treated with retinopexy, either with laser or cryotherapy. Larger detachments require pneumatic retinopexy or a scleral buckling procedure.

Traction retinal detachment. This occurs when the intact retina is forcibly elevated by contracting membranes on the surface of the retina or by vitreous traction on areas of retinal neovascularization. Causes include diabetes, intraocular foreign body, perforating eye injuries, and loss of vitreous humour following cataract surgery. These retinal detachments are difficult to treat and pars plana vitrectomy is the only option.

Secondary retinal detachments. This occurs secondary to systemic disorders, including hypertension, toxaemia of pregnancy, chronic glomerulonephritis, retinal venous occlusive disease, and retinal vasculitis. Treatment is directed towards the underlying cause as these detachments are not amenable to scleral buckling surgery.

What surgical procedures are available for retinal detachment?
The four principal methods for reattachment of the retina are scleral buckling, vitrectomy, pneumatic retinopexy, and cryoretinopexy:
- *Scleral buckling* is an extraocular approach that indents the eye wall to restore contact with the detached retina. All retinal breaks are localized and adhesions between the choroid and retina are performed around the break with diathermy or a cryoprobe. After draining the subretinal fluid, the detached portion of the retina is indented towards the vitreous cavity by a scleral implant or explant. This pushes the retina towards the vitreous humour, causing closure of the retinal break (by the buckled sclera and choroid) and release of traction on the vitreous humour.
- *Pars plena vitrectomy* is an intraocular approach that relieves traction by removing the vitreous humour attached to the retinal breaks, permitting reapproximation to the retinal pigment epithelium, where the breaks are permanently closed with retinopexy.
- *Pneumatic retinopexy* closes retinal breaks using a small bubble of pure sulphur hexafluoride or perfluoropropane injected intravitreally; this allows the retinal pigment epithelium pump to reattach the retina. Gradual elution of gas from the eye coupled with permanent closure of the break by retinopexy leaves the retina reattached.
- *Laser retinopexy or cryoretinopexy* uses heat or cold to spot weld the detached retina back in place. These methods are only suitable for small breaks and small rhegmatogenous detachments, and further surgery is sometimes needed if these procedures are ineffective.

CHAPTER 103

Retinal Vein Occlusion

Instruction
Examine this patient's eyes and perform fundoscopy.

Salient Features
HISTORY

- Age: In the general population, central retinal vein occlusion has an incidence of 0.5%, and branch retinal vein occlusion, an incidence of 1.8% of adults. This incidence increases with age so that patients above the age of 80 have an incidence of 4.6%.
- Branched retinal vein occlusion: decreased vision and floaters suggest vitreal haemorrhage
- Central retinal vein occlusion: loss or decreased vision, headache (associated increase in intraocular pressure), floaters
- History of hypertension, diabetes, glaucoma, blood coagulation disorders, systemic inflammatory disorders, or hyperlipidaemia.

EXAMINATION
Patient 1
Central retinal vein occlusion (Fig. 103.1), the occlusion is behind the cribriform plate:
- Multiple retinal and preretinal haemorrhages surround the optic nerve head; there is marked dilatation and tortuosity of the veins, hyperaemia, or oedema of the nerve head and soft exudates: 'blood and thunder' appearance.
- Visual acuity is only slightly reduced.

Patient 2
Branch vein occlusion (Fig. 103.2), the occlusion is in front of the cribriform plate:
- Occlusion occurs just distal to the arteriovenous crossing and haemorrhages can be seen surrounding the occluded vein; the superior temporal vein is most commonly involved.
- May cause a quadrantic field defect.

For both patients, proceed as follows:
Tell the examiner that you would like to check for the following conditions:
- Diabetes (glycosuria on urine dipstick)
- Hypertension (participants with hypertension were five times more likely to have a branch retinal vein occlusion than those without hypertension)
- Chronic simple glaucoma
- Systemic inflammatory disorders: polyarteritis nodosa, sarcoidosis, Wegener granulomatosis, Goodpasture syndrome, Behçet disease
- Coagulation disorders: Wäldenstroms macroglobulinaemia, myelofibrosis, multiple myeloma, hyperhomocysteinaemia, anticardiolipin antibodies, protein S and C deficiencies, activated protein C resistance, and factor V Leiden mutation.

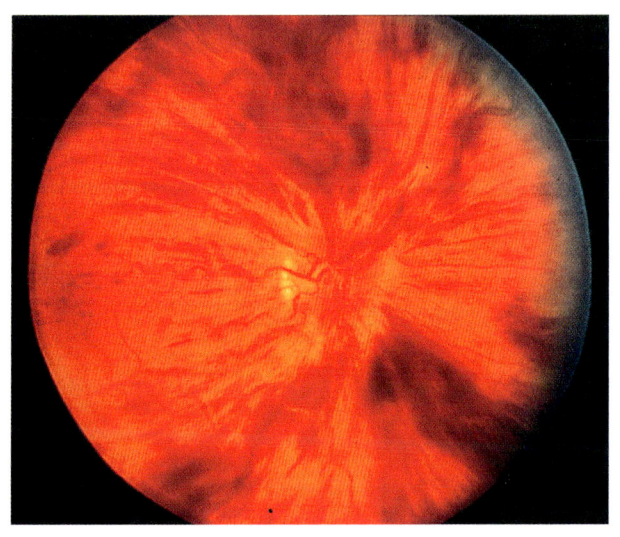

Fig. 103.1 Central retinal vein thrombosis.

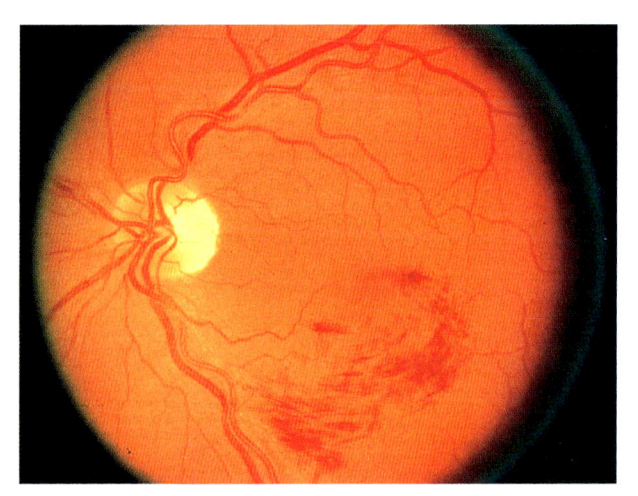

Fig. 103.2 Branch retinal vein thrombosis.

Diagnosis

Patient 1 has multiple retinal haemorrhages (lesions) caused by central retinal vein occlusion with underlying diabetes mellitus (aetiology).

Patient 2 has branch vein occlusion (lesion). (**Note:** Visual prognosis is good if the haemorrhages do not extend to the macula with accompanying macular oedema.)

Questions

What are the usual sites of occlusion in branch retinal vein occlusion?
- At arteriovenous crossings, causing classic quadrantic or small macular occlusions
- Along the main veins, as in diabetes mellitus

- At the edges of the optic disc, resulting in occlusion of the hemisphere
- Peripherally, as in sickle cell disease.

What are the vascular responses to retinal vein occlusion?
- Dilatation of retinal capillaries
- Abnormal vascular permeability
- Retinal capillary closure.

What is the prognosis in branch retinal vein occlusion?
It varies from complete resolution with no residual visual deficits to a progressive deterioration resulting in permanent loss of vision.

What is the clinical course in central retinal vein occlusion?
- In mild cases, there is minimal dilatation of veins and haemorrhages with little or no oedema of the macula and no visual deficit
- In severe instances, the vision may deteriorate to hand motions, with extensively deep and superficial haemorrhages with stagnation of blood in the markedly dilated veins and several cotton-wool spots.

What are the complications of central retinal vein occlusion?
These include macular oedema, neovascularization of the retina, rubeosis iridis (usually visible by 1 month), and rubeotic glaucoma (usually by 3 months). Ophthalmic follow-up is needed to diagnose and prevent the two main complications of retinal vein occlusion: neovascularization and macular oedema.

How would you manage such eyes?
- Treat the underlying condition
- Fluorescein angiography to determine areas of retinal ischaemia
- Optical coherence tomography to assess macular oedema
- Macular oedema is increasingly treated with newer antivascular endothelial growth factor agents like ranibizumab, aflibercept, and bevacizumab. Other treatments include intravitreal dexamethasone implant as well as the more established technique of laser photocoagulation. These biological agents are repeatedly used to prevent the onset of ocular neovascularization
- Prompt referral and follow-up by the ophthalmologist as secondary neovascularization and deteriorating visual acuity are common complications. Panretinal photocoagulation prevents the dreaded complications of neovascular glaucoma.

Randomized clinical trials have demonstrated that prophylactic panretinal laser treatment does not prevent neovascularization in ischaemic vein occlusions and that laser treatment can be withheld unless the patient develops evidence of ocular neovascularization.

What is the role of arteriovenous crossing sheathotomy?
Arteriovenous crossing sheathotomy is commonly used as an adjuvant to pars plana vitrectomy. Branch retinal vein occlusion typically occurs at arteriovenous crossings, where the artery and vein share a common adventitial sheath. Cutting the sheath around the vessels and physically separating them where they cross should improve blood flow through the vein.

Further Information
J.G. Waldenström (1906–1996), Professor of Medicine, Uppsala University, Sweden.

CHAPTER 104

Retinitis Pigmentosa

Instruction
Examine this patient's fundus.
Examine this patient's eyes.

Salient Features
HISTORY
- Family history of blindness (can be autosomal recessive, which is more severe, or autosomal dominant, which is more benign)
- Decreased nocturnal vision
- Altered colour vision
- Loss of peripheral vision
- Blurry vision.

EXAMINATION
- Peripheral retina shows perivascular 'bone spicule pigmentation' and arteriolar narrowing (Fig. 104.1). The retinal veins (never the arteries) often have a sheath of pigmentation for part of their course. The pigment spots that lie near the retinal veins are seen to be anterior to them, and so they hide the course of the vessel. (In this respect, they differ from the pigment around the spots of choroidal atrophy, in which the retinal vessels can be traced over the spots.)
- Optic disc is pale.
- Check for maculopathy, which is atrophic or cystoid.

Proceed as follows:
- Look for polydactyly in the hands and feet (Laurence–Moon syndrome)
- Comment on the white walking aid (if any) used by the registered blind
- Tell the examiner that you would like to check visual fields.

Diagnosis
This patient is obese, has polydactyly and retinitis pigmentosa (lesion) caused by Laurence–Moon syndrome (aetiology), and is registered blind (functional status).

Questions
What is the prognosis in retinitis pigmentosa?
Most patients are registered blind by the age of 40 years, with central field <20 degrees in diameter. Almost all patients lose central vision by the seventh decade.

104 – RETINITIS PIGMENTOSA

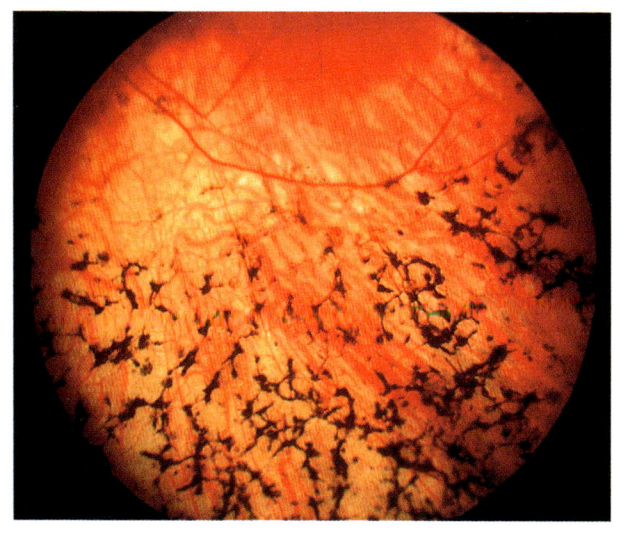

Fig. 104.1 Retinitis pigmentosa.

What do you know about retinitis pigmentosa?
Retinitis pigmentosa is a slow degenerative disease of the retina. It occurs in both eyes, begins in early childhood, and often results in the loss of sight by middle or advanced age. The degeneration primarily affects the rods and cones, in particular the rods. Rods mediate achromatic vision in starlight or moonlight, whereas cones are important for colour vision and fine acuity in daylight.

How may retinitis pigmentosa present?
It may present with defective vision at dusk (night blindness), which may occur several years before the pigment is visible in the retina.

Mention a few systemic disorders associated with retinitis pigmentosa.
- *Laurence–Moon syndrome*, which is a recessively inherited disorder characterized by mental disability, polydactyly, syndactyly, hypogonadism, obesity, and renal disease (structural abnormalities such as calyceal cysts or calyceal clubbing and blunting)
- *Bassen–Kornzweig syndrome* (abetalipoproteinaemia), characterized by fat malabsorption, abetalipoproteinaemia, acanthocytosis, and spinocerebellar ataxia
- *Refsum disease* (phytanic acid storage disease), an autosomal recessive disorder characterized by hypertrophic peripheral neuropathy, deafness, ichthyosis, cerebellar ataxia, raised cerebrospinal fluid protein levels in the absence of pleocytosis
- *Kearns–Sayre syndrome*, a triad of retinitis pigmentosa, progressive external ophthalmoplegia, and heart block
- *Usher disease*, a recessively inherited disorder characterized by congenital, nonprogressive, sensorineural deafness
- *Friedreich ataxia*.

What do you know about the genetics of retinitis pigmentosa?
Mutations in more than 70 genes linked to retinitis pigmentosa have been described. These genes account for only about 60% of all patients; the remainder have defects in as yet unidentified genes. The most common genes involved are:
- *RHO* gene for rhodopsin, which leads to about 25% of dominant retinitis pigmentosa

- *USH2A*, which might cause about 20% of recessive disease (including many with Usher syndrome type II)
- *RPGR*, which accounts for about 70% of X-linked retinitis pigmentosa.

Which ocular conditions are associated with retinitis pigmentosa?
- Open-angle glaucoma
- Posterior subcapsular cataracts
- Myopia
- Keratoconus.

What is secondary retinitis pigmentosa?
Secondary retinitis pigmentosa is a sequela to inflammatory retinitis. It is often ophthalmoscopically indistinguishable from the primary condition; the electroretinographic and electro-oculographic responses are slightly subnormal unless the condition is far advanced. (In the primary type, the electroretinograph and electro-oculograph responses are markedly subnormal.)

What is retinitis pigmentosa sine pigmento?
A variety of retinitis pigmentosa but without visible pigmentation of the retina.

What is inverse retinitis pigmentosa?
Bone corpuscles are visible in the perifoveal area, whereas the retinal periphery is normal.

How would you manage this patient?
- Refer for genetic counselling.
- Suggest impaired vision training and aids for daily living.
- Consider a diet rich in vitamin A and marine omega-3-fatty acids.
- Gene therapy (Luxturna) for patients with biallelic *RPE65* mutation associated retinal dystrophy.

Further Information

J.Z. Laurence (1830–1874), an English ophthalmologist.
R.C. Moon (1844–1914), a US ophthalmologist.
F.A. Bassen (b. 1903), physician, and A.L. Kornzweig (b. 1900), ophthalmologist, Mount Sinai Hospital, New York.
S. Refsum, a Norwegian physician.

CHAPTER 105

Subhyaloid Haemorrhage

Instruction

Examine this patient's fundus.

Salient Features

HISTORY

- Sudden, painless loss of vision
- Sudden appearance of floaters and black spots with or without flashing lights
- History of stroke (subarachnoid haemorrhage)
- History of diabetes, retinal tears, vitreous detachment, retinal vein occlusion
- History of trauma.

EXAMINATION

- A large, solitary subhyaloid haemorrhage (there may be no fluid level if the patient is lying flat) (Fig. 105.1)
- There may be associated retinal haemorrhage.
- Mild papilloedema in 20%
- Comment on any obvious hemiplegia.

Note: When the subhyaloid (preretinal) haemorrhage extends into the vitreous humour, it is called Terson syndrome (Fig. 105.2).

Diagnosis

This hemiplegic patient has a subhyaloid haemorrhage (lesion) caused by subarachnoid haemorrhage (aetiology).

Questions

What is the commonest cause of subhyaloid haemorrhage?
Subarachnoid haemorrhage.

What are the other causes of haemorrhage into the vitreous humour?
- Local injury
- Blood diseases
- Hypertension
- Diabetes
- Idiopathic.

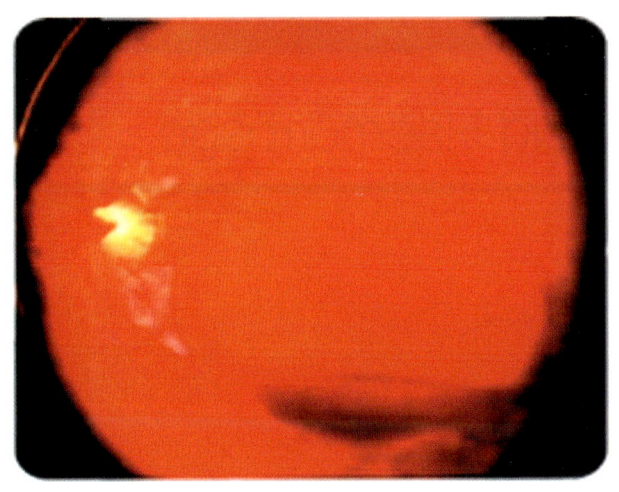

Fig. 105.1 Funduscopic photograph of a subhyaloid haemorrhage. (With permission from Field, T.S., Heran, M.K., 2010. Teaching NeuroImages: middle cerebral artery aneurysm rupture presenting as pure acute subdural hematoma. Neurology. 74, e13.)

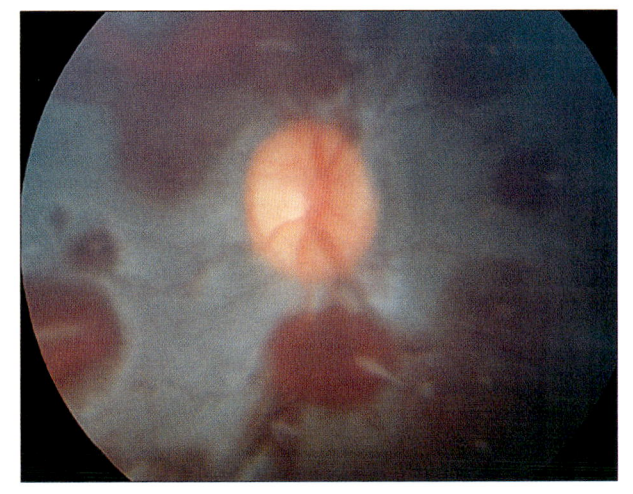

Fig. 105.2 Terson syndrome. (With permission from Yanoff, M., Duker, J.S., 2008. Ophthalmology, third edn. Mosby, Philadelphia, PA.)

Mention some causes of neck stiffness.
- Subarachnoid haemorrhage
- Meningitis
- Posterior fossa tumours
- Local neck pathology, such as cervical spondylosis.

What is the cause of subarachnoid haemorrhage?
- Aneurysms are the cause of subarachnoid haemorrhage in 85% of cases. Intracranial aneurysms are not congenital, as was once believed, but develop in the course of life

- The best estimate of the frequency of aneurysms for an average adult without specific risk factors is 2.3% (95% confidence interval, 1.7–3.1); this proportion increases with age.
- Saccular aneurysms arise at sites of arterial branching, usually at the base of the brain, either on the circle of Willis itself or at a nearby branching point.
- Most intracranial aneurysms will never rupture. The rupture risk increases with the size of aneurysm, but paradoxically, most ruptured aneurysms are small (<1 cm); the explanation is that 90% of all aneurysms are small and even though only a small fraction of these rupture, this total outnumbers the greater fraction of the large aneurysms that rupture. The case fatality after aneurysmal haemorrhage is 50%; one in eight patients with subarachnoid haemorrhage dies outside the hospital.

What are causes of deterioration in a patient with subarachnoid haemorrhage?
- Rebleed
- Cerebral infarction as a result of reflex vasospasm of cerebral vessels (hence the rationale for using nimodipine)
- Secondary hydrocephalus.

How would you investigate such a patient?
Computed tomography head scan; if this rules out intracranial hypertension, then a lumbar puncture to diagnose minor leaks.

What is the management of subarachnoid haemorrhage?
- Rebleeding: occlusion of the aneurysm. Endovascular obliteration by means of platinum spirals (coiling) is the preferred mode of treatment, but some patients require a direct neurosurgical approach (clipping).
- Cerebral ischaemia: the risk is reduced with oral nimodipine and probably by maintaining circulatory volume.
- Hydrocephalus might cause gradual obtundation in the first few hours or days; it can be treated by lumbar puncture or ventricular drainage, dependent on the site of obstruction.

What are the indications of vitrectomy in Terson syndrome?
- Retinal detachment with vitreous haemorrhage
- Nonclearing vitreous haemorrhage in the patient who is monocular
- Subfoveal haemorrhage
- Late complications of intraocular haemorrhage, such as epiretinal membrane formation (macular pucker)
- Occupational necessity for rapidly cleared vision.

CHAPTER 106

Vitreous Opacities

Instruction
Examine this patient's fundus.

Salient Features
HISTORY
- History of diplopia (monocular diplopia)
- Floaters
- History of diabetes, hypertension.

EXAMINATION
- Small white opacities are present in front of the retinal vessels.
- The patient may complain of diplopia (monocular diplopia).
- Tell the examiner that you would like to:
  - test for monocular diplopia
  - check urine for sugar
  - check the blood pressure.

Diagnosis
This patient has vitreous opacities (lesions) with monocular diplopia (functional status) and has underlying diabetes mellitus (aetiology).

Questions
What are the causes of vitreous opacities?
- Blood: diabetes, retinal vein occlusion, trauma, subarachnoid haemorrhage, sickle cell retinopathy
- Cholesterolosis bulbi: where free-floating, highly refractile crystals are seen in liquified vitreous humour in patients with severe intraocular disease.
- Asteroid hyalitis (Benson disease): where whitish yellow solid bodies containing calcium palmitate and stearate are suspended in normal vitreous. Prognosis for vision good
- Synchysis scintillans: gold or yellowish-white particles made up of cholesterol located in the vitreous humour; they settle to the bottom of the eye through gravity. Associated with previous trauma or surgery to the eye
- Other: retinoblastoma, primary amyloidosis.

What are the other causes of monocular diplopia?
- Opacities in the lens
- Corneal opacities
- Retinal detachment.

SECTION IX

Dermatology Cases for Internal Medicine

SECTION OUTLINE

107 Acanthosis Nigricans
108 Acne Vulgaris
109 Alopecia Areata
110 Arterial Leg Ulcer
111 Arteriovenous Fistula
112 Atopic Dermatitis—Eczema
113 Bullous Eruption
114 Mycosis Fungoides (Cutaneous T-Cell Lymphoma)
115 Dermatitis Herpetiformis
116 Eruptive Xanthomata
117 Erythema Ab Igne
118 Erythema Multiforme
119 Erythema Nodosum
120 Fungal Nail Disease
121 Hairy Leukoplakia
122 Henoch–Schönlein Purpura
123 Hereditary Haemorrhagic Telangiectasia (Osler–Weber–Rendu Syndrome)
124 Herpes Simplex
125 Herpes Zoster Syndrome (Shingles)
126 Ichthyosis
127 Lichen Planus
128 Lichen Simplex
129 Lipodystrophy

130 Lupus Pernio
131 Maculopapular Rash
132 Malignant Melanoma
133 Molluscum Contagiosum
134 Nail Changes
135 Necrobiosis Lipoidica
136 Neurofibromatosis
137 Onycholysis
138 Palmar Xanthomata
139 Peutz–Jeghers Syndrome
140 Phlebitis Migrans
141 Pretibial Myxoedema
142 Pseudoxanthoma Elasticum
143 Psoriasis
144 Purpura
145 Pyoderma Gangrenosum
146 Raynaud's Phenomenon
147 Rosacea
148 Seborrhoeic Dermatitis
149 Sturge–Weber Syndrome (Encephalotrigeminal Angiomatosis)
150 Tuberous Sclerosis (Bourneville or Pringle Disease)
151 Urticaria
152 Urticaria Pigmentosa
153 Venous Ulcer
154 Vitiligo
155 Xanthelasma
156 Xanthomata

CHAPTER **107**

Acanthosis Nigricans

Instruction
Perform a general examination.

Salient Features

HISTORY
- Age
- Carcinoma of the stomach or other neoplasms (in 80% the cancer is abdominal and in 60% the cancer is in the stomach): symptoms of weight loss, asthenia and decreased appetite, diabetes mellitus type II, obesity, polycystic ovarian syndrome (insulin-resistant states)
- Other endocrinopathies: acromegaly, Cushing disease, hypothyroidism, hyperthyroidism
- Family history of similar lesions (hereditary benign)
- Drug history (steroids, insulin, hormonal treatments).

EXAMINATION
- Black, velvety overgrowth seen in the axillae, neck, umbilicus, nipples, groins, or facial skin
- Acrochordons or skin tags may accompany acanthosis nigricans and occur in similar areas.

Proceed as follows:
- Look for the following signs:
  - Tripe palms (roughness of the palmar and plantar skin; usually associated with internal malignancy)
  - Filiform growths around the face and mouth and over the tongue (when mouth and tongue are involved it is highly suggestive of an underlying neoplasm).
- Tell the examiner that you would like to investigate for:
  - underlying malignancy, in particular adenocarcinoma of the stomach
  - for endocrine disorders (diabetes, Cushing syndrome, acromegaly).
- Comment on the patient's body mass index if appropriate.

Diagnosis
This patient has a velvety black overgrowth in the axillae (lesion) and I would like to exclude an underlying adenocarcinoma, particularly of the stomach (aetiology).

Questions

What are the types of acanthosis nigricans?
(1) Benign, (2) obesity associated, (3) hereditary, (4) malignant, (5) medication induced, (6) syndromic, and (7) mixed type.

What is the histology of acanthosis nigricans?
- Undulating epidermis with numerous sharp peaks and valleys
- Variable amount of hyperplasia, hyperkeratosis, and slight pigmentation of the basal cell layer (but no melanocytic hyperplasia).

With which conditions is acanthosis nigricans associated?
- Benign conditions:
  - Diabetes, associated with marked insulin resistance
  - Cushing syndrome
  - Acromegaly
  - Polycystic ovarian syndrome
  - Obesity: nearly 75% of these patients develop acanthosis nigricans.
- Malignant conditions (caused by abnormal production of epidermal growth factors):
  - Adenocarcinomas (usually stomach, gastrointestinal tract, and uterus; less commonly lung, ovary, breast, and prostate)
  - Lymphoma (rarely).

Name some characteristics of malignant acanthosis nigricans.
Acanthosis nigricans when associated with internal malignancy can have very rapid progression of skin lesions, the patient is not obese, or has no reason to have insulin resistant state, and up to half of cases are associated with mucosal involvement with lesions in the mouth or lips. It usually occurs in older adults and other paraneoplastic cutaneous manifestations may be present.

What is the relationship between the course of the skin lesion and the underlying malignancy?
Acanthosis nigricans may precede the neoplasm by >5 years. In about two-thirds of cases, the course parallels that of the tumour, including remission with cure.

Mention some cutaneous manifestations of visceral malignancy.
- Dermatomyositis (in individuals >40 years of age, the prevalence of internal malignancy particularly lung and breast cancer is increased)
- Migratory thrombophlebitis
- Ichthyosis (when acquired suggests gastrointestinal leiomyosarcoma, lymphoma, multiple myeloma)
- Paget disease of the nipple
- Tylosis or palmar hyperkeratosis (suggests oesophageal cancer)
- Leser–Trélat sign, which is the sudden appearance of multiple seborrheic keratosis and suggests underlying cancer in the elderly
- Necrotic migratory erythema suggests tumours of the alpha cells of the pancreas, which secrete glucagon.
- Bazex syndrome or acrokeratosis paraneoplastica suggests malignancy of the upper respiratory tract, particularly squamous cell carcinomas of the mouth, pharynx, larynx, oesophagus, and bronchus.
- Lymphomatoid papulosis is cutaneous lymphoid infiltration associated with T-cell lymphomas or Hodgkin disease.

What is the therapy for acanthosis nigricans?
Acanthosis nigricans related to an underlying cause can subside if the underlying cause is treated. Success has been reported with laser therapy.

Note: Acanthosis is hyperplasia of the stratum spinosum of the epidermis.

CHAPTER 108

Acne Vulgaris

Instruction
Look at this patient.

Salient Features
HISTORY
- Steroid
- Isoniazid
- Occupational exposure to oils (oil-induced acne).

EXAMINATION
- Comedones or blackheads (Fig. 108.1), caused by plugging of hair follicles by keratin, which are hallmarks of acne
- Generally found over the chin, face, neck, chest, upper back, and upper arms (areas which have the most and the largest sebaceous glands)
- Whiteheads (i.e. distended sebaceous glands without a pore)
- Cysts (larger, deeper masses of retained sebum)
- Greasy skin
- There may be associated scarring: ice-pick scars.

Remember: Acne vulgaris is a multifactorial disease affecting the pilosebaceous follicle and characterized by open and closed comedones, papules, pustules, nodules, and scars.

Diagnosis
This patient has blackheads on the face with greasy skin (lesions), which is acne vulgaris caused by *Propionibacterium acnes* (aetiology).

Questions

What do you know about the pathogenesis of acne?
Follicular keratinization, seborrhoea, and colonization of the pilosebaceous unit with *P. acnes* are central to the development of these lesions. Genetic and hormonal factors also play a role, possibly by optimizing the follicular environment suitable for the growth of *P. acnes* or by influencing the inflammatory response and thus the nature of these lesions.

How is the severity of acne graded?
Lesions can be inflammatory or noninflammatory and are graded by severity (Fig. 108.2):
- Mild disease: open and closed comedones and some papules and pustules

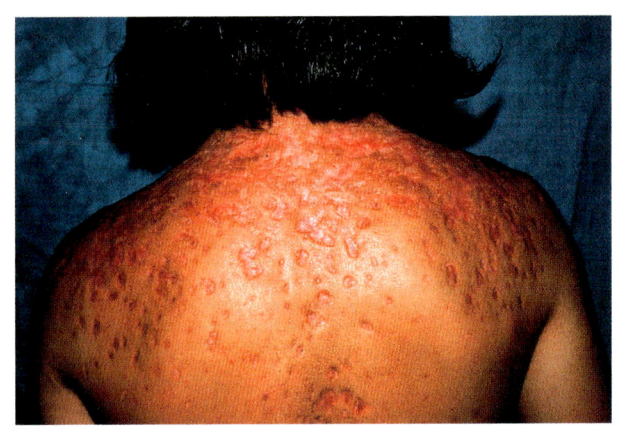

Fig. 108.1 Acne vulgaris.

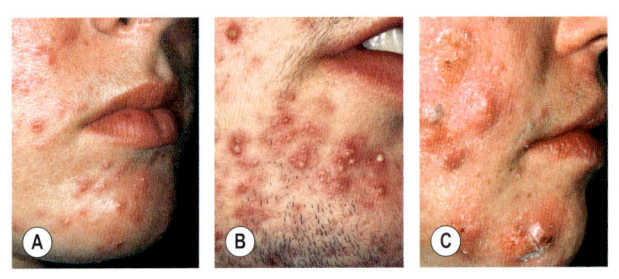

Fig. 108.2 Acne classification. **(A)** Mild, open, and closed comedones and some papules/pustules. **(B)** Moderate, many papules/pustules plus some nodules. **(C)** Severe, with multiple papules/pustules and nodules, leading to scarring. (With permission from Habif, T.P., 2009. Clinical Dermatology, fifth edn. Mosby, Philadelphia, PA.)

- Moderate: more frequent papules and pustules with mild scarring
- Severe disease: all of the previous plus nodular abscesses; leads to more extensive scarring, which may be keloidal in some instances.

What factors may exacerbate acne?
- Cosmetics, oils
- Clothing (turtlenecks, bra straps, sports helmets)
- Trauma
- Excessive sweating.

How would you manage acne?
The aims of treatment are to prevent scarring, limit the disease duration, and reduce the impact of the psychological stress, which may affect over half of sufferers:
- Wash affected parts with soap not more than twice a day.
- Avoid steaming: saunas, Turkish baths.
- Dietary restriction has no role in therapy.
- Reduce *P. acnes* proliferation:
    - Topical therapy: sulfur, benzyl peroxide, retinoic acid, azelaic acid, tetracycline
    - Systemic therapy: tetracycline.

- Reduce sebum overproduction with systemic agents: isotretinoin.
- Reduce inflammation:
  - Systemic agents: corticosteroids, isotretinoin
  - Topical agents: metronidazole, intralesional steroids.
- Reduce abnormal desquamation of follicular epithelium:
  - Systemic agents: isotretinoin, antibiotics by indirect effect
  - Topical agents: tretinoin (most effective), salicylic acid, adapalene, tazarotene, isotretinoin, antibiotics.
- Physical or surgical methods: comedo extraction, dermabrasion, chemical peeling, laser resurfacing, pulsed-dye laser treatment, and punch grafts
- Maintenance therapy with topical retinoids.

What is and how do you treat acne fulminans?

It is a rare but severe variant seen exclusively in adolescent boys. It is caused by an immune complex reaction to *P. acnes*. The lesions eventually become necrotic and form haemorrhagic crusts, causing disfigurement and scarring. There may be associated systemic features such as fever, malaise, arthralgia, arthritis, and vasculitis. Osteolytic bone lesions can arise. Inpatient treatment with systemic steroids is necessary. Recent panel expert recommendation includes use of systemic steroids, followed by delayed addition of oral isotretinoin.

What do you know about acne conglobata?

It is seen in tall White males with cystic skin lesions and multiple abscess formation. It rarely regresses.

CHAPTER 109

Alopecia Areata

Instruction
Examine this patient's scalp.

Salient Features

HISTORY
- Young adult (75% of patients are below the age of 40 years)
- History of atopy
- Ask whether there is a family history (25%).
- Ask the patient whether there are any local symptoms and if the hair loss is cosmetically unacceptable.

EXAMINATION
- Well-defined patch of hair loss (Fig. 109.1); short, fractured, exclamation-point hairs may be seen at periphery.
- Regrowing hair in the patch appears as a fine, depigmented downy growth.

Proceed as follows:
- Look for patches of hair loss over the eyebrows and beard area.
- Examine the nails for fine pitting, transverse lines, dystrophy, fragmentation (anonychorrhexis), and ridging and 20-nail dystrophy (roughened nail surface and brittle free nail edge) (Fig. 109.2).
- Tell the examiner that you would like to:
  - look for atopy
  - look for other autoimmune conditions including vitiligo (see later).

Diagnosis
This patient has alopecia areata (lesion), which is suspected to be of autoimmune origin (aetiology).

Questions

What are the signs of disease activity?
At the advancing edge, broken hairs that look like exclamation marks indicate active disease. These are very short hairs, tapering and becoming depigmented as the scalp is approached. Plucking reveals such hair to be in the telogen phase.

Mention some associated disorders.
- Autoimmune conditions (vitiligo, thyrotoxicosis, Addison disease, pernicious anaemia)
- Down syndrome
- Hypogammaglobulinaemia.

109—ALOPECIA AREATA

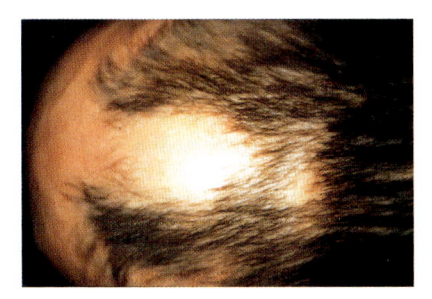

Fig. 109.1 Alopecia areata.

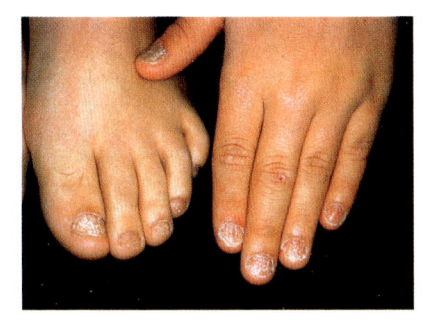

Fig. 109.2 Nail dystrophy.

What is the difference between alopecia totalism and alopecia universalis?
Both of these conditions can occur in alopecia areata. Alopecia totalis is the loss of all scalp hair and alopecia universalis is the loss of hair from all body sites.

Is alopecia areata associated with scarring?
No.

Mention the causes of hair loss associated with scarring.
Discoid lupus erythematosus, lichen planus.

What is the treatment for alopecia areata?
- Steroids (both topical and intralesional)
- Psoralen plus ultraviolet A (PUVA), but alopecia often returns after discontinuation of PUVA
- Topical minoxidil
- Topical immunotherapy: dinitrochlorobenzene, squared acid dibutylester, and diphencyprone have been used for contact sensitization.

Cessation of treatment may be associated with recurrent hair loss.

Mention some causes of drug-induced alopecia.
Anticoagulants, retinoids, vitamin A, antithyroid drugs, oral contraceptives, anticancer drugs (invariably reversible).

What do you understand by the term trichotillomania?
It is the self-inflicted pulling out of one's own hair and can be differentiated from alopecia areata as the hair loss is irregular and there is always growing hair, since these cannot be pulled out until they are long enough. These patches are unilateral and are usually on the same side as the patient's dominant hand. The patient may be unaware of this habit.

What do you know about the growth of the hair follicle?
Each follicle has cyclical growth controlled by a constitutional 'time clock'. It has three phases of growth (anagen), with >90% of hair in this phase, a short involutional phase (catagen), and a resting (telogen) phase. The anagen phase is 3 to 5 years, catagen is 2 to 3 weeks, and the telogen phase is 2 to 4 months. Anagen hairs are anchored deeply into the subcutaneous fat and cannot be pulled out easily. Each hair shaft may persist on the scalp for 3 to 7 years before falling out and being replaced by a new hair. Compared with anagen hair, telogen hair is located higher in the skin and can be pulled out relatively easily. Hair found on the pillow and hairbrush is telogen hair and can be recognized by the fact that the club is depigmented as well as expanded; anagen hair obtained by traction is fully melanized.

How much hair is usually lost by a normal person?
About 70 to 100 hairs/day. The human scalp contains about 100,000 follicles, 5% to 10% are in telogen at any time, i.e. 5000 to 10,000. As telogen lasts for about 100 days, the number of telogen hairs pushed out each day is 70 to 100.

What is telogen effluvium?
It is a transitory (about 2–4 months) increase in the number of hairs in the resting (telogen) phase of the hair growth cycle. There is a sudden increase in shedding of hairs, with white bulbs about 3 to 5 months after a period of stress. The amount of hair loss exceeds 150/day. It is associated with high fever, stress, crash dieting, malnutrition, surgery, termination of pregnancy, or oral contraceptives. The prognosis is good.

What do you know about male pattern baldness?
On the scalps of men who have a predisposition for this pattern of baldness, androgens cause a switch from terminal to vellus or vellus-like follicles and a reduction in the duration of anagen. In these individuals, androgen receptors and 5α-reductase activity (converts testosterone to 5-dihydrotestosterone) are greater in frontal hair follicles than occipital follicles; higher activities of aromatase (involved in conversion of testosterone to oestradiol) are found in occipital follicles. This is one explanation for frontal baldness in men. Finasteride, a 5α-reductase inhibitor that does not affect the androgen receptor, results in some regrowth of hair in about 70% of men after 2 years of continuous use. If treatment is successful, the drug is continued indefinitely because the balding process continues when it is stopped.

What do you understand by the term trichorrhexis nodosa?
It is the fracture of the hair shaft and is common in Black patients who straighten their hair. Usually, the hair regrows healthily if gentle hair care practices are adopted.

CHAPTER 110

Arterial Leg Ulcer

Instruction

Look at this patient's leg.

Salient Features

HISTORY

- Intermittent claudication
- History of underlying cardiovascular or cerebrovascular disease
- Cardiovascular risk factors (smoking, hypertension, diabetes)
- Pain in the distal foot when the patient is supine ('rest pain' syndrome)
- Impotence
- Absence of bleeding from the ulcer
- History of precipitating trauma or underlying deformity.

EXAMINATION

- Tender, punched-out ulcers on the leg (usually away from the ankle region) (Fig. 110.1)
- Ulcer usually in the plantar surface over the heads of first and fifth metatarsals (uncommon on the dorsum of the foot because the pressure is less sustained and perfusion is better)
- Cold atrophic skin
- Loss of hair
- Thickened nails
- Peripheral pulses diminished or not palpable (in patients with diabetes and in chronic renal failure, the arteries may be calcified, making the results of pulse examination less reliable)
- Pallor on elevation
- Redness of foot on lowering the leg (dependent rubor)
- Sluggish filling of toe capillaries.

Diagnosis

This patient has an arterial ulcer (lesion) caused by vascular insufficiency, as evidenced by the absence of popliteal pulses (aetiology).

Remember: An ankle–brachial index of <0.6 suggests arterial compromise.

Questions

What bedside tests can be performed to aid with the diagnosis of arterial ulcers?
- Capillary refill time of the toes—prolonged more than 2 s

419

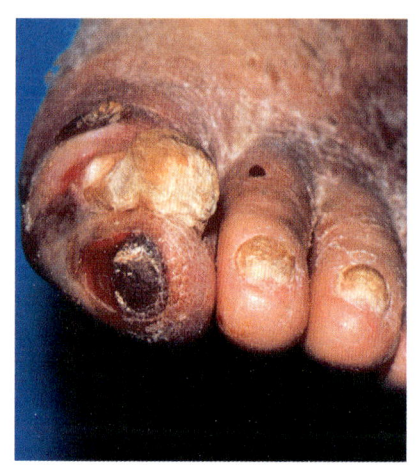

Fig. 110.1 Circumscribed necrotic arterial ulcer. (With permission from Libby, P., Bonow, R.O., Mann, D.L., Zipes D.P., 2007. Braunwald's Heart Disease, eighth edn. Saunders, Philadelphia, PA.)

- Measuring ankle brachial pressure index—decreased ratio less than 0.9
- Buerger test—positive test when the foot becomes pale when elevated and erythematous when lowered below the patient's level.

How would you investigate such a patient?
- Radiographs may show calcification of the arteries of the leg
- Perform Doppler ultrasonography to define the severity of arterial involvement
- Measure segmental limb pressures
- Pulse–volume waveform and transcutaneous oxygen are particularly useful in evaluating perfusion of the diabetic foot because they are not affected by vessel calcification
- Arteriography shows narrowing and stenosis of the leg arteries.

How would you manage arterial ulcers?
- General: stop smoking; control diabetes, obesity, and hypertension
- Limbs: should be kept warm (but avoid local heat)
- Feet: see a chiropodist and apply foot care, use appropriate footwear
- Exercise regularly to promote development of anastomotic collateral vessels
- Low-dose aspirin
- Surgery: balloon dilatation may be used for local iliac or femoral stenoses and aortoiliac bypass; amputation when complicated by gangrene
- Flow-limiting arterial lesions should be evaluated and reconstructed or bypassed: prosthetic vascular grafts or autologous vein grafts may be used.

Mention other causes of leg ulcers.
- Venous ulcers
- Neuropathic: diabetes mellitus, leprosy
- Vasculitis: rheumatoid arthritis, systemic lupus erythematosus, pyoderma gangrenosum

- Haematological disorders: sickle cell anaemia, spherocytosis
- Neoplastic: basal cell carcinoma, Kaposi sarcoma
- Trauma or artefact
- Infection: postcellulitis, fungal.

CHAPTER 111

Arteriovenous Fistula

Instruction
Look at this patient's arms.

Salient Features
HISTORY
- History of haemodialysis and artificial arteriovenous fistula.

EXAMINATION
- Hypertrophy of the affected arm
- Prominent, dilated, tortuous veins (arteriovenous fistula; Fig. 111.1)
- Continuous thrill over the fistula; listen for continuous bruit
- Collapsing pulse; increased pulse pressure indicating hyperdynamic circulation.

Proceed as follows:
- Elicit Branham's sign: slowing of the pulse on occluding the feeding vessel of the fistula
- If the fistula is in the upper limb, then perform Allen's test: the radial and ulnar arteries are occluded at the wrist and the hand is exercised; the arteries are then released one at a time to establish which is the dominant feeding vessel
- Look for signs of chronic renal failure
- Palpate and auscultate the arteriovenous fistula for bruits.

Note: An arteriovenous fistula is a *direct subcutaneous anastomosis of an artery and vein without prosthetic material* and is the preferred means of vascular access for haemodialysis.

Diagnosis
This patient has an arteriovenous fistula (lesion) that has been surgically created (aetiology) for haemodialysis and is functioning well.

Questions
How would you manage a patient with an arteriovenous fistula?
- Clinical examination
- Doppler ultrasonography
- Intraaccess flow monitoring
- Angiography
- Referral to a vascular surgeon if problems arise.

111 — ARTERIOVENOUS FISTULA

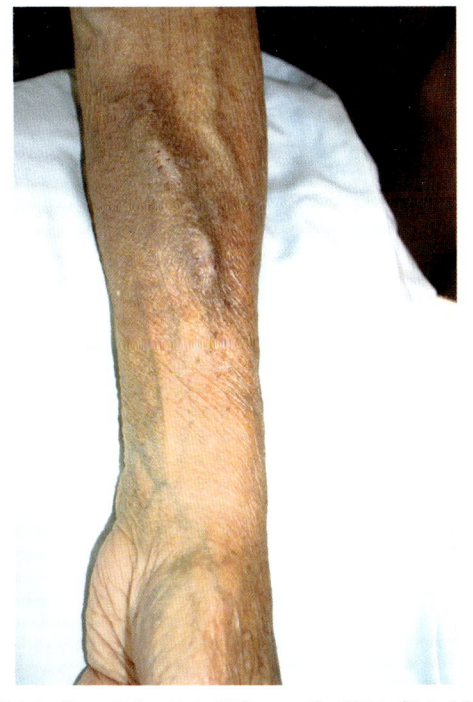

Fig. 111.1 Arteriovenous fistula. (From Talley, N.J., O'Connor, S., 2014. Clinical Examination: A Systematic Guide to Physical Diagnosis, seventh edn. Elsevier, Chatswood, NSW.)

Why are fistulae preferred to prosthetic grafts?
Fistulae have a far lower risk of failure and a reduced requirement for revision compared with prosthetic grafts. They are associated with lower morbidity and mortality compared to grafts. In addition, they are patent for longer periods.

What are the alternatives when a fistula cannot be formed in a patient requiring long-term haemodialysis?
Placement of synthetic grafts subcutaneously or of a long central line into a great vein.

Name some potential complications of arteriovenous fistula placement.
- Bleeding
- Stenosis
- Thrombosis
- Aneurysm
- Infection
- Failure.

What is the leading cause of failure of a prosthetic arteriovenous haemodialysis-access graft?
The leading cause of failure of a prosthetic arteriovenous haemodialysis-access graft is venous anastomotic stenosis. Balloon angioplasty, the first-line therapy, has a tendency to lead to subsequent recoil and restenosis. Percutaneous revision of venous anastomotic stenosis in patients with

a prosthetic haemodialysis graft is improved with the use of an expanded polytetrafluoroethylene endovascular stent graft, which appears to provide longer-term and superior patency and freedom from repeat interventions than standard balloon angioplasty.

Further Information

H.H. Branham, an American surgeon in the 19th century.

E.V. Allen (1900–1961), Professor of Medicine at the Mayo Clinic, Rochester, Minnesota, introduced coumarin anticoagulants into clinical practice and edited one of the first comprehensive textbooks on peripheral vascular disease.

CHAPTER 112

Atopic Dermatitis — Eczema

Instruction
Look at this patient's skin.

Salient Features
HISTORY
- Pruritus: this is an important symptom because it affects the quality of life.
- Tell the examiner that you would like to know whether there is a personal or family history of atopy (asthma, allergic rhinitis, atopic dermatitis) or food allergy.

EXAMINATION
- Scratch marks
- Hyperpigmented or hypopigmented lichenified lesions in flexures (including face, neck, upper trunk, wrists, hand, in the antecubital and popliteal folds) (Fig. 112.1).

Diagnosis
This patient has atopic dermatitis (lesion), which is caused by atopy as supported by a history of asthma (aetiology); it is causing the patient severe itching (functional status).

Questions
What are the stages (and patterns) of atopic dermatitis?
There are three age-related stages, which are separated by remission.
> *Infantile stage (up to 2 years of age).* Red, scaly, itchy crusted rash on both cheeks and extensors of the extremities. The napkin area is generally spared. Eczema of the scalp may also be seen.
> *Childhood stage (2–12 years of age).* There is population (rather than exudation) in the flexural areas, including neck, cubital fossa, popliteal fossa, and volar aspect of wrists and ankles. The plaques show both excoriation and lichenification.
> *Adults (puberty onwards).* The face is commonly involved and there is lichenification of flexures including wrists, hands, fingers, ankles, toes and feet, head and neck.

What are the criteria for diagnosis?
Hanifin and Rajka's major criteria require three or more of the following:
- Pruritus
- Typical morphology and distribution: flexural lichenification in adults, facial, or extensor involvement in children
- Chronic or chronically relapsing dermatitis
- Family or personal history of atopy (asthma, allergic rhinitis, atopic dermatitis).

425

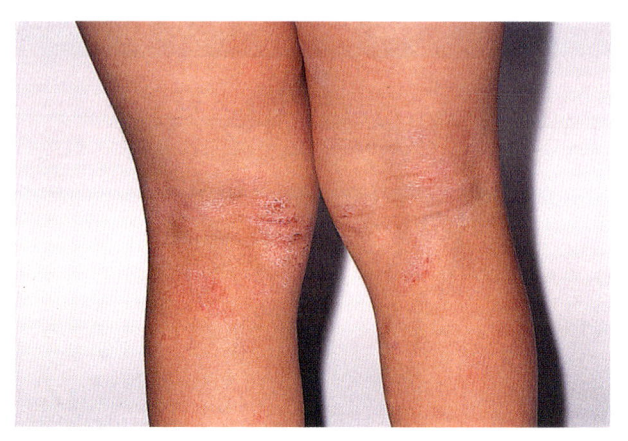

Fig. 112.1 Flexural atopic dermatitis. (With permission from Kumar, P., Clark, M., 2005. Clinical Medicine, sixth edn. Saunders, Edinburgh.)

Many of the minor criteria are under dispute and include ichthyosis, nipple eczema, food intolerance, keratoconus, subcapsular anterior cataracts, cheilitis, pityriasis alba, and anterior neck folds. Fissuring below the auricles of the ear and diffuse scaling of the scalp may be seen in severe disease.

How would you treat such patients?
- Foods (typically dairy products, peanuts, eggs, and wheat) that cause itching should be avoided
- The patient should be instructed about skin care, including avoiding frequent baths and scratchy fabrics and regular use of emollients
- Adequate cutaneous hydration
- Treatment of infected skin
- Antihistamines to control itching
- Corticosteroid lotion, cream, or ointment: topical steroids are first-line drug therapy
- Phototherapy with psoralen plus ultraviolet A in those unresponsive to topical treatment
- Severe recalcitrant disease: ciclosporin, azathioprine, tacrolimus, mycophenolate mofetil, pimecrolimus, Grenz-rays
- Investigational treatment: phosphodiesterase inhibitors, interleukin-2, and thymopentin.

What are the potential complications of atopic dermatitis?
- Staphylococcal superinfection; a deficiency in the expression of antimicrobial peptides may account for the susceptibility of patients with atopic dermatitis to skin infection with *Staphylococcus aureus*
- Eczema herpeticum.

What do you know about the natural history of atopic dermatitis?
- Nonatopic dermatitis is the first manifestation of atopic dermatitis (as a result of genetically determined epidermal barrier dysfunction and the effect of environmental factors)
- Sensitization occurs subsequently (because of the genetic predisposition for immunoglobulin E (IgE)-mediated sensitization). This phenomenon is favoured by *S. aureus* enterotoxin products

- Tissue damage and the release of structural proteins occur finally (from scratching), which triggers an IgE response in patients with atopic dermatitis. This sensitization to self-proteins can be the result of the homology of allergen-derived epitopes and human proteins in the context of molecular mimicry.

What is known about the genetic aspects of atopic dermatitis?
Atopic dermatitis is a complex genetic disease that emerges in the context of two major groups of genes:
- Genes encoding epidermal or other epithelial structural proteins
- Genes encoding major elements of the immune system.

What are the proposed mechanisms of atopic dermatitis?
One mechanism proposes that the primary defect resides in an immunologic disturbance that causes IgE-mediated sensitization, with epithelial barrier dysfunction as a consequence of local inflammation.

Another proposal is that an intrinsic defect in the epithelial cells leads to the barrier dysfunction and that the immunologic aspects are epiphenomena.

CHAPTER 113

Bullous Eruption

Instruction
Look at this patient.

Salient Features
HISTORY
- Onset and blisters
- History of mucosal involvement (mouth ulcers)
- Drug history: thiols (e.g. benzylpenicillin), angiotensin-converting enzyme inhibitors, aspirin, nonsteroidal antiinflammatory drugs, rifampin, levodopa, phenobarbital, interferon, propranolol, nifedipine.

EXAMINATION
- Bullous eruption (Fig. 113.1)
- Crusts or superficial erosions (these suggest a preceding fluid-filled lesion).

Proceed as follows:
- Comment on the distribution: knee, thighs, forearms, and umbilicus in the elderly (pemphigoid)
- Look in the mouth for ulceration; if the blisters break easily leaving denuded skin, it is more likely to be pemphigus
- Tell the examiner that a biopsy of the skin is essential to confirm the diagnosis.

Diagnosis
This patient has a bullous eruption (lesion) caused by sulphonamides (aetiology); it is widespread with involvement of mucous membranes and mild dehydration (functional status).

Questions

What do you understand by the term bulla?
It is a circumscribed elevation of the skin, larger than 0.5 cm and containing fluid.

How would you confirm the diagnosis?
A biopsy of a fresh blister (<12 hours old) with a portion of perilesional skin for histology and immunofluorescent studies.

113 — BULLOUS ERUPTION

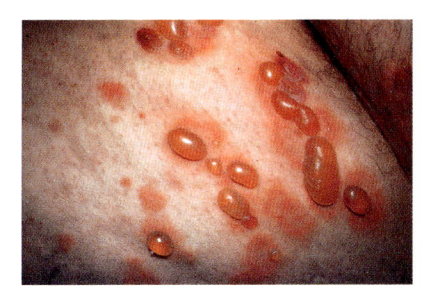

Fig. 113.1 Bullous eruption.

Mention a few blistering conditions.
- Common: friction, insect bites, drugs, burns, impetigo, contact dermatitis
- Uncommon:
    - Autoimmune bullous diseases (pemphigoid, pemphigus vulgaris, dermatitis herpetiformis, immunoglobulin A (IgA)-mediated diseases, bullous erythema multiforme, epidermolysis bullosa acquisita)
    - Porphyria cutanea tarda
    - Paraneoplastic pemphigus.

How would you manage a patient with pemphigus vulgaris?
Barrier nursing, antibiotics, intravenous fluids, large doses of systemic steroids, usually with immunosuppressive drugs (azathioprine, cyclophosphamide, methotrexate, infliximab), which act as steroid-sparing agents. Other drugs used include dapsone, nicotinamide, gold, and ciclosporin.

What are the forms of pemphigus?
There are two main forms; both occur commonly in middle age:
- Pemphigus vulgaris and its variant pemphigus vegetans; the vulgaris form begins in the mouth in over 50% of cases.
- Pemphigus foliaceus and its variant pemphigus erythematosus, which are more superficially blistering conditions; the foliaceus form may be drug induced (e.g. penicillamine toxicity) or is associated with autoimmune disease.

What are the characteristics of pemphigus vulgaris?
Pemphigus vulgaris is characterized by bullae in the epidermis. It is often preceded by bullae in the mucous membranes. Superficial separation of the skin after pressure, trauma, or on rubbing the thumb laterally on the surface of uninvolved skin may cause easy separation of the epidermis (Nikolsky's sign), indicating acantholysis. Biopsy shows disruption of epidermal intercellular connections (acanthocytolysis). Immunofluorescence shows intercellular deposition of IgG in the epidermis.

What are the characteristics of bullous pemphigoid?
It is a relatively benign condition with remissions and exacerbations. Characteristically, tense blisters are present in nonmucosal surfaces such as flexural areas and trunk, typically in the elderly. The blisters are tense and do not rupture easily. The bullae are subepidermal and rich in eosinophils; immunoelectron microscopy shows deposits of IgG and complement 3 (C3) in the lamina lucida of the basement membrane. It has a chronic course marked by exacerbation and remission.

Although clinical findings often lead to a correct diagnosis, positive histopathological studies represent the usual diagnostic standard, particularly direct immunofluorescence studies of perilesional skin demonstrating deposition of C3 and Igs (IgG) in a linear pattern at the epidermal basement membrane.

Therapy involves systemic glucocorticoids and/or immunosuppressives such as azathioprine, methotrexate, mycophenolate mofetil, rituximab, and intravenous Ig.

What do you know about the pathogenesis of pemphigus?

In pemphigus vulgaris, autoantibodies are directed against desmoglein 3 on the surface of the keratinocytes. In pemphigus foliaceus, the antibodies are directed against desmoglein 1 on keratinocytes in the subcorneal region. The desmogleins are desmosomal glycoproteins in the cadherin family of cell adhesion molecules. There is strong evidence that the endemic form of pemphigus foliaceus is initiated by an environmental vector, whose antigens mimic those of desmoglein. The quantitative levels of desmoglein 1 or 3 are used to guide treatment because changes in antibody titre correlate with disease activity: disappearance of the antibody from the serum often precedes clinical remission.

How would you manage generalized forms of autoimmune bullous disease?

- Systemic steroid therapy is usually chosen first to treat patients with generalized forms of any autoimmune bullous disease except those mediated by IgA. Very potent topical steroids can be used effectively, although in extensive disease, use is limited due to side effects and practical implications.
- Other immunosuppressive drugs: many patients with moderate to severe pemphigus, bullous pemphigoid, cicatricial pemphigoid, or epidermolysis bullosa acquisita require a second immunosuppressive drug (such as azathioprine or cyclophosphamide), either for its corticosteroid-sparing effect or to achieve complete remission. The specific choice is a matter of personal experience, concern over the relative toxic effects, and possible contraindications. Some patients have been treated successfully with prednisolone and ciclosporin, but the latter alone is not beneficial. Low-dose methotrexate plus prednisolone may benefit patients with pemphigus or bullous pemphigoid.
- Azathioprine is usually used as a steroid-sparing agent. Alternatives include methotrexate, intravenous chlorambucil, cyclophosphamide, and mycophenolate mofetil
- Dapsone and related drugs: dapsone is the drug of choice for patients with dermatitis herpetiformis or linear IgA dermatosis who are not allergic to sulphonamides. It inhibits the chemotaxis of neutrophils, reducing their accumulation in the upper dermis and thus diminishing tissue inflammation. The response is rapid, with most lesions resolving within 48 to 72 hours. Alternatives to dapsone include sulfapyridine, sulfoxone sodium, and sulfamethoxypyridazine. Dapsone is effective as monotherapy in only a minority of patients with bullous pemphigoid.
- Chrysotherapy: systemic gold is rarely used as an alternative or adjunct to prednisone therapy in patients with pemphigus because it is efficacious in only a subgroup of patients and carries the potential risk of side effects on prolonged administration.
- Intravenous Ig therapy, intravenous rituximab, is usually reserved for patients with recalcitrant disease.
- Plasmapheresis is used in patients with severe pemphigus unresponsive to conventional therapy and high titres of pemphigus autoantibodies. Plasmapheresis may also be beneficial in patients with bullous pemphigoid even in the absence of detectable autoantibodies, although its mechanism of action in such patients is not known.
- Gluten-free diets are advised in dermatitis herpetiformis.
- Other therapies: extracorporeal absorption of antibodies for pemphigus, combination tetracycline and nicotinamide in bullous pemphigoid, colchicine in IgA dermatosis.

What do you know about herpes gestationis?
It is a self-limiting disease with the initial appearance of bullae in the periumbilical region, trunk, and extremities, usually in the fifth or sixth month of pregnancy. Pruritus is typically severe. It may recur in subsequent pregnancies. Menses and oestrogen are known to precipitate flare-ups. The blisters are eosinophil-rich and subepidermal, with C3 in the basement membrane and serum complement-fixing Ig antibody. Corticosteroids, usually systemic, are the treatment of choice.

Further Information

P.V. Nikolsky (1858–1940), Professor of Dermatology, first in Warsaw and later in Rostov.
Pemphigus (from the Greek *pemphix*, meaning blister or bubble).

CHAPTER 114

Mycosis Fungoides (Cutaneous T-Cell Lymphoma)

Instruction
Look at this patient's skin.

Salient Features
HISTORY
- Age (usually fifth and seventh decade)
- Pruritus.

EXAMINATION
- Itchy, brownish-red plaques on the hips, buttocks, and interscapular region (Fig. 114.1)

Proceed as follows:
- Tell the examiner that it may also involve the lymph nodes and viscera.

Diagnosis
This patient has itchy brownish-red plaques with lymph node involvement (lesions), indicating mycosis fungoides (aetiology).

Questions

What is the classification of cutaneous T-cell lymphoma and where is mycosis fungoides in this classification?
Cutaneous T-cell lymphoma is divided into two types, depending on the clinical behaviour of the disease: indolent and aggressive. The first type, slow-growing lymphomas, include mycosis fungoides, mycosis fungoides variants, primary cutaneous acral CD8+ lymphoma, EBV+ mucocutaneous ulcer, primary cutaneous CD30+ lymphoproliferative disorders, primary cutaneous CD4+ T-cell lymphoproliferative disorder, and subcutaneous panniculitis-like T-cell lymphoma, of which mycosis fungoides is the commonest.

How would you confirm the diagnosis?
Skin biopsy to detect *Pautrier's microabscesses*, atypical cells in the nests in the epidermis, atypical mononuclear cell infiltrates, large hyperchromic cells with irregular nuclei—the 'mycosis cells'. The hallmark of mycosis fungoides is the identification of the *Sézary–Lautner cells*. These are 'T' helper cells (CD4 positive) that characteristically form band-like aggregates within the superficial dermis and invade the dermis as single cells and small clusters (Pautrier microabscesses).

114—MYCOSIS FUNGOIDES (CUTANEOUS T-CELL LYMPHOMA)

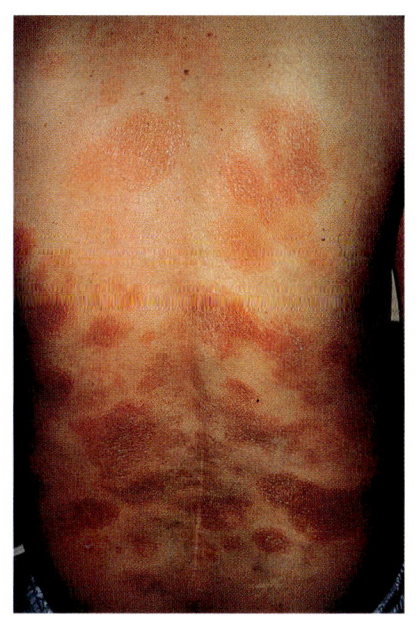

Fig. 114.1 Patch-stage mycosis fungoides: itchy, brownish-red plaques.

What is the prognosis?
Very slow progression of skin lesions with eventual tumour formation and systemic dissemination of lymphoma. In most patients, this process takes several weeks.

What is the differential diagnosis?
Psoriasis.

How would you treat this patient?
Treatment is palliative with steroids, chemotherapeutic agents, and electron-beam therapy.

What are the stages of cutaneous T-cell lymphoma?
- Stage I: eczematoid or psoriasiform erythematous lesions
- Stage II: infiltrated plaques
- Stage III: nodules (Fig. 114.2), ulcers, tumours
- Stage IV: lymph node involvement with or without systemic dissemination.

Prognosis is good for early mycosis fungoides.

Staging is by a tumour/node/metastases/blood system or by the World Health Organization indolent versus aggressive clinical behaviour system.

What are the treatment options for mycosis fungoides?
- Various superficial treatments: topical steroids and chemotherapeutic agents (mechlorethamine and carmustine), psoralen plus ultraviolet A, and electron-beam radiotherapy improve skin disease, the choice of which depends on the staging of the disease
- Systemic therapies are offered to patients with extensive disease (brentuximab vedotin, mogamulizumab, vorinostat, methotrexate, interferons).

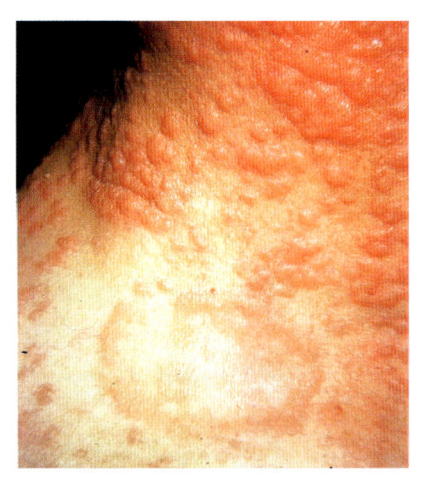

Fig. 114.2 Mycosis fungoides. Tumour stage III with nodules.

Have you heard of Sézary syndrome?
It is a rare leukaemic, erythrodermic variant of cutaneous T-cell lymphoma characterized by lymphadenopathy and large mononuclear cells (*Sézary cells*) in the skin and blood. It belongs on the aggressive arm of cutaneous T-cell lymphoma and clinically affects the skin of the entire body, which becomes erythematous, thick, scaly, and itchy. It is often resistant to traditional treatment and has a poor prognosis, with a median survival between 2 and 4 years from diagnosis.

Further Information
Jean Louis M. Alibert, a French dermatologist, first described this condition in 1806.
A. Sézary (1880–1956), a French dermatologist.

CHAPTER 115

Dermatitis Herpetiformis

Instruction
Look at this patient's skin. She has a history of chronic diarrhoea.

Salient Features

HISTORY
- History of diarrhoea
- History of gluten intolerance (although these patients rarely have gross malabsorption)
- Ask the patient whether the rash itches.

EXAMINATION
- Dry, itchy vesicles and urticarial plaques (Fig. 115.1) occurring bilaterally and symmetrically over the extensor surfaces, elbows, knees, posterior neck, back, and buttocks.

Proceed as follows:
Look for similar lesions on the scalp, face, neck, shoulders, buttocks, knees, and calves.

Diagnosis

This patient has itchy vesicles on the elbows (lesion) caused by dermatitis herpetiformis (aetiology).

Questions

From which other itchy skin disorder should dermatitis herpetiformis be differentiated?
Scabies.

What conditions can be associated with dermatitis herpetiformis?
- Gluten-sensitive enteropathy (frequent, asymptomatic)
- Autoimmune thyroid disease (especially hypothyroidism)
- Type 1 diabetes
- Pernicious anaemia
- Lymphoma (especially gastrointestinal).

How would you investigate such a patient?
- Skin biopsy: fibrin and neutrophils accumulate selectively at the *tips of dermal papillae*, forming small microabscesses. Subepidermal vesicles have a neutrophilic infiltrate. Immunofluorescence demonstrates granular dermal papillary immunoglobulin A (IgA) deposits
- Serology: circulating antiendomysial antibodies, antitissue transglutaminase antibodies
- Jejunal biopsy is not required, but if performed, it consists of patchy abnormality showing subtotal villous atrophy with increased lymphocyte infiltration in the epithelium.

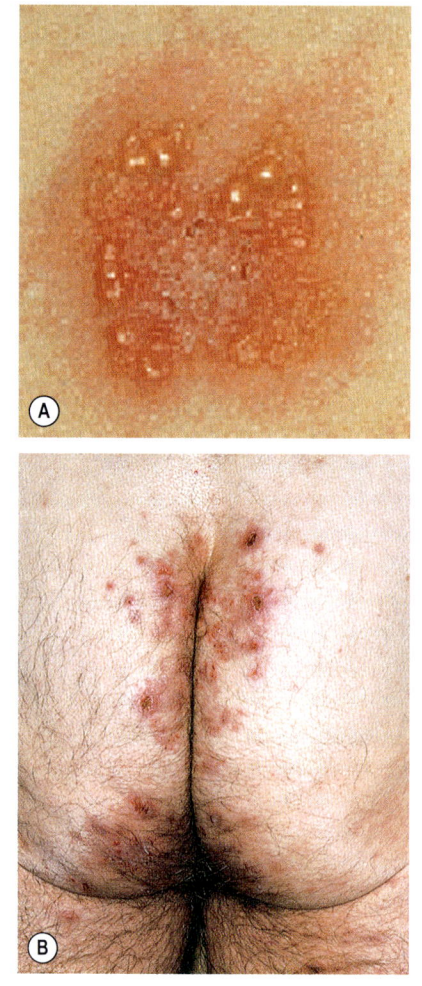

Fig. 115.1 Dermatitis herpetiformis. **(A)** Pruritic, urticarial papules, and small blisters. **(B)** Occurrence in the lumbosacral area. (With permission from Habif, T.P., 2009. Clinical Dermatology, fifth edn. Mosby, Philadelphia, PA.)

How would you treat such a patient?
- Gluten restriction
- Dapsone or sulfapyridine: neither drug should be given to a patient with glucose-6-phosphate dehydrogenase deficiency. Treatment is lifelong; there is usually a rapid relapse if the drug is stopped.

In which foods is gluten found?
Wheat, barley, and rye (rice and maize are permitted in these patients).

What do you know about gluten?
Gluten is the protein component that persists following the removal of water and starch from defatted flour. Gliadin is a class of protein found in the gluten fraction of flour. There are four gliadin fractions (α, β, γ, and ω). α-Gliadin is injurious to the small intestinal mucosa, although there

is some disagreement about the toxicity of other peptides. Patients with dermatitis herpetiformis develop IgA and IgG antibodies to gliadin and reticulin (the latter a component of the anchoring fibrils that tether the epidermal basement membrane to the upper dermis).

What are the benefits of a gluten-free diet?
It gradually improves skin lesions, improves any associated manifestations of malabsorptive enteropathy, and may reduce the late risk of intestinal lymphoma. It also normalizes histological abnormalities.

Further Information

Dermatitis herpetiformis was first described in 1884 by L.A. Duhring (1845–1913), Professor of Diseases of the Skin at the University of Pennsylvania. He studied dermatology in Paris, London, and Vienna and wrote the first American textbook of dermatology. Others believe that dermatitis herpetiformis was first described by F. von Hebra, who also wrote a textbook of dermatology.

Samuel J. Gee (1839–1911) of St Bartholomew's Hospital, London, provided the first thorough description of coeliac sprue in 1888 (Gee, 1888).

Dutch paediatrician W.K. Dicke astutely observed that wheat and rye were harmful in children with this disease (Dicke, 1950).

CHAPTER 116

Eruptive Xanthomata

Instruction

Examine this patient's skin.
This patient with uncontrolled diabetes has developed a profuse eruption; what are these lesions?

Salient Features

HISTORY

- Duration and treatment of diabetes
- History of hyperlipidaemia
- Rash: duration, onset, and evolution and associated symptoms such as itching.

EXAMINATION

- Multiple, itchy, red-yellow vesicles or nodules seen over extensor surfaces, i.e. buttocks, back, knees, and elbows (Fig. 116.1).

Proceed as follows:
Tell the examiner that you would like to:
- examine the fundus for lipaemia retinalis
- check the urine for sugar
- do a lipid profile (remember that eruptive xanthomata signify triglyceridaemia).

Diagnosis

This patient has eruptive xanthomata (lesion) caused by hypertriglyceridaemia (aetiology).

Questions

In which conditions are eruptive xanthomata seen?
- Type IV hyperlipidaemia
- Familial hypertriglyceridaemia
- Lipoprotein lipase deficiency
- Apolipoprotein CII deficiency
- Type I hyperlipidaemia: chylomicronaemia
- Type V hyperlipidaemia: increased levels of triglycerides and chylomicrons.

Mention some other causes of hypertriglyceridaemia.
- Primary hypertriglyceridaemia (usually >5.0 mg/L): familial hypertriglyceridaemia, familial combined hyperlipidaemia

438

116 – ERUPTIVE XANTHOMATA

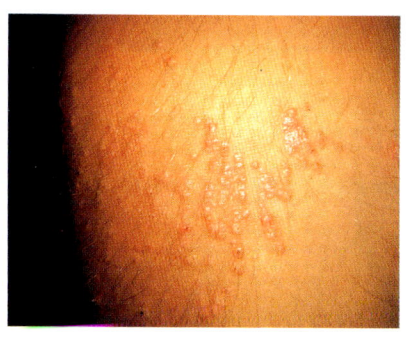

Fig. 116.1 Eruptive xanthomata.

- Secondary hypertriglyceridaemia: diet, obesity, excess alcohol intake, diabetes mellitus, hypothyroidism, uraemia, dysproteinaemias, drugs (beta-blockers, oral contraceptives, and oestrogens, retinoids).

What is the relationship between hypertriglyceridaemia and coronary artery disease?
Triglycerides are an independent risk factor for coronary artery disease irrespective of low-density lipoprotein (LDL) cholesterol. For every increase in serum triglyceride of 890 mg/L, the risk increases by ~30% in men and ~75% in women.

What are the particular risks for patients with serum triglycerides markedly raised (>10.0 mg/L)?
They are more susceptible to acute pancreatitis and hyperchylomicronaemia.

How would you manage a patient with raised levels of serum triglycerides?
- Diet: restrict dietary fat, decrease intake of alcohol and simple sugars
- Weight loss if the patient is overweight
- Exercise
- Discontinuation of drugs, e.g. beta-blockers
- Control secondary causes
- Niacin, gemfibrozil, or omega-3 fatty acids may be used to treat elevated triglycerides (>5.0 mg/L) regardless of LDL or high-density lipoprotein cholesterol.

CHAPTER 117

Erythema Ab Igne

Instruction
Examine this patient's legs.
Examine this patient's abdomen.

Salient Features
HISTORY
- Ask the patient whether she exposed the affected area to heat.

EXAMINATION
- Reticular erythematous or pigmented rash, usually on the forelegs (or abdomen), known as 'Granny's tartan'.

Proceed as follows:
- Look for features of hypothyroidism (pulse, ankle jerks).
- Tell the examiner that you would like to measure thyroxine and thyroid-stimulating hormone levels.

> **Note:** Erythema ab igne used to be seen in people who sat in front of open fires to warm up. Nowadays, with the use of central heating, it is not commonly seen. However, it is still seen from the use of hot water bottles, heated car seats, and electric blankets.

Diagnosis
This patient has a reticular pigmented rash (lesion) on the abdomen caused by local heat from a hot-water bottle (aetiology).

Questions

What do you know about erythema ab igne?
It is dusky discolouration of the skin that is associated with repeated exposure to heat. Typically, the heat is not painful (<45°C) and does not burn the skin but produces a net-like reticulated pigmentation. It is usually found on the front of the lower legs of the elderly who sit in front of open fireplaces (Fig. 117.1) and/or on the abdomen or back of patients with chronic conditions who seek relief of pain by the long-term application of hot-water bottles or heating pads (Fig. 117.2).

How may erythema ab igne be complicated?
Epitheliomas may develop in keratoses, which form in later stages of this condition.

117—ERYTHEMA AB IGNE

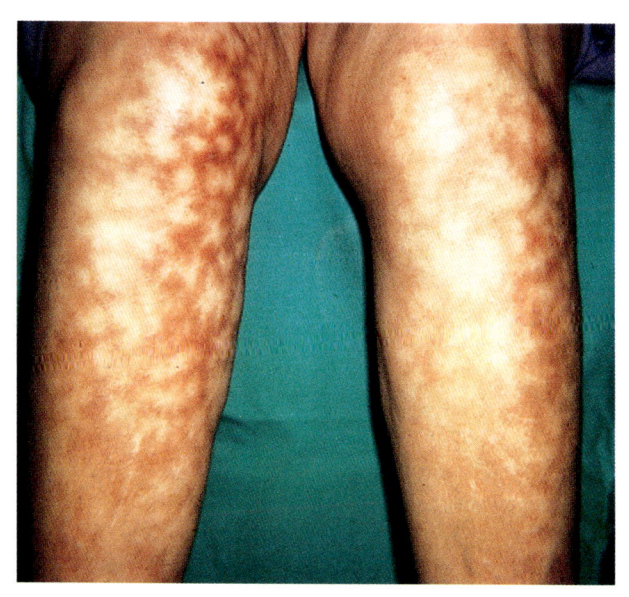

Fig. 117.1 Erythema ab igne.

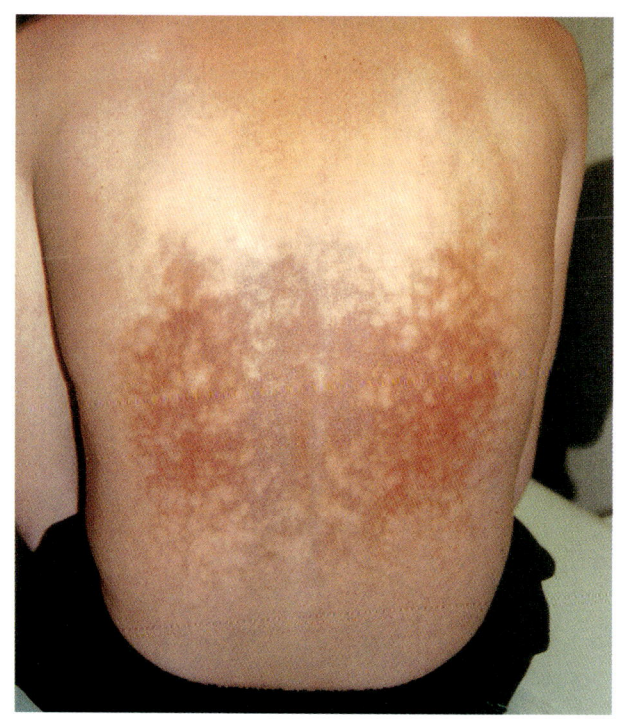

Fig. 117.2 Erythema ab igne produced by applying a heating pad to a painful back. (With permission from Townsend, C.M., Jr., Beauchamp, R.D., Evers, B.M., Mattox, K.L., 2007. Sabiston Textbook of Surgery, eighteenth edn. Saunders, Philadelphia, PA.)

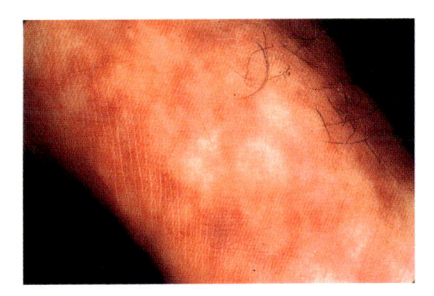

Fig. 117.3 Livedo reticularis.

What other reticulated rashes do you know?
- Livedo reticularis (Fig. 117.3), seen in the following conditions:
  - Polyarteritis nodosa
  - Systemic lupus erythematosus
  - Occult malignant neoplasm
  - Atherosclerotic microemboli to the skin
  - Physiological in young women (it is most apparent on the thighs of young females playing outdoor sports on a cold day)
- Cutaneous marmorata seen in children.

Mention some skin abnormalities related to heat or cold.
- Erythema ab igne
- Livedo reticularis (as a result of cold in young women)
- Raynaud's phenomenon
- Chilblains.

CHAPTER 118

Erythema Multiforme

Instruction
Perform a general examination.

Salient Features

HISTORY
- History of preceding sore throat or cold
- Low-grade fever
- Drug history: barbiturates, sulphonamides, phenytoin, penicillins
- Blister-like skin rash with intense itching
- Mouth ulcers: mucosal involvement suggests Stevens–Johnson syndrome
- History of recurrent episodes: suggests herpes simplex infection.

EXAMINATION
- Target-shaped lesions (Fig. 118.1), usually over the palms, soles, and skin. A classic target lesion consists of three concentric zones of colour change: typically, there is a central, dark, purple area or blister surrounded by a pale, oedematous round zone; this, in turn, is surrounded by a peripheral rim of erythema
- Pleomorphic eruption with macules, papules, and bullae.

Proceed as follows:
- Look at the mucous membranes of the mouth (cutaneous and mucosal lips, gingival sulcus, sides of tongue), nares, and conjunctiva (Stevens–Johnson syndrome)
- Tell the examiner that you would like to examine the external genitalia for ulcers.

Note: Erythema multiforme is a cell-mediated hypersensitivity reaction to many different immunological insults, including drugs and infectious agents such as viruses (most notably herpes simplex). In its so-called 'minor' form, it is manifested by heterogeneous cutaneous eruption, at times bullous.

Diagnosis
This patient has target-shaped lesions (lesion) caused by sulphonamides (aetiology), which usually resolve on discontinuing the drug (functional status).

Questions

What is the underlying aetiology?
- Infections (herpes simplex, mycoplasma, streptococcal)
- Drug hypersensitivity (sulphonamides, penicillin, barbiturates, salicylates, antimalarials)

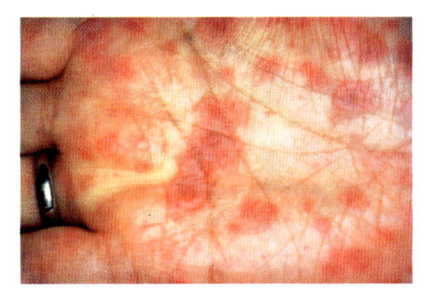

Fig. 118.1 Erythema multiforme with 'target' or 'iris' lesions.

- Collagen vascular disorder (systemic lupus erythematosus, dermatomyositis, periarteritis nodosa)
- Malignancy (carcinomas and lymphomas)
- Multiple myeloma
- Idiopathic: in 50%, no cause may be found.

How would you investigate this patient?
- Viral titres, in particular for herpes simplex type 1
- Complement fixation test for mycoplasma
- Antistreptolysin O titres.

If the previous ones are negative:
- Serum antibodies
- Protein electrophoresis, urine for Bence-Jones protein.

What is the histology of erythema multiforme?
Early lesions. Superficial perivascular lymphocytic infiltrate with oedema of the dermis, accompanied by degeneration and necrosis of keratinocytes and margination of lymphocytes at the dermoepidermal junction

Late lesions. Upward migration of lymphocytes into the epidermis; discrete and confluent portions of the epidermis necrose, resulting in blister formation and, subsequently, erosions (as a result of sloughing of the epidermis)

Target lesions. Characterized by central necrosis surrounded by perivenular inflammation.

What do you understand by Stevens–Johnson syndrome?
Stevens–Johnson syndrome, also referred to as erythema multiforme major, is characterized by fever and mucous membrane involvement (usually oral cavity, eye and genital) in addition to the eruptions of erythema multiforme.

How would you manage a patient with erythema multiforme and Stevens–Johnson syndrome?
Erythema multiforme is a self-limiting condition and treatment is not required, but Stevens–Johnson syndrome may be fatal:
- Symptomatic treatment with antipyretics, intravenous fluids, and antibiotics
- Systemic corticosteroids, although the role of steroids is controversial
- Other immunosuppressive drugs used in recurrent erythema multiforme and Stevens–Johnson syndrome: levamisole, azathioprine, dapsone, thalidomide, high-dose intravenous immunoglobulin, and ciclosporin
- Aciclovir recommended by some authors as a therapeutic trial in any patient with severe recurrent erythema multiforme if suspected herpetic infection is causing the rash

- Antibiotic treatment for *Mycoplasma pneumoniae*, if this is the cause of the disease
- Other therapeutic options:
  - Localized care including use of antibiotic creams, ointments, sterile dressing, special beds containing beads, amnion dressings on denuded skin
  - Ophthalmological care including use of artificial tears and topical vitamin A
  - Extensive denudation of the skin is best treated in a burns unit.

Further Information

F.C. Johnson (1894–1934) and A.M. Stevens (1884–1945), both American paediatricians, described this condition in 1922 (Stevens and Johnson, 1922).

H. Bence-Jones (1814–1873), English physician, St George's Hospital, London

CHAPTER 119

Erythema Nodosum

Instruction
Look at this patient's shins.

Salient Features
HISTORY
Elicit a history of:
- fever, malaise, generalized symptoms
- painful nodules
- arthralgia
- conjunctivitis
- sore throat (β-haemolytic streptococcal infection)
- drugs (sulphonamides, penicillins, oral contraceptives)
- gastrointestinal symptoms (*Yersinia enterocolitica* infections, inflammatory bowel disease)
- infections (tuberculosis, leprosy, coccidioidomycosis, histoplasmosis)
- sarcoidosis.

> **Remember:**
> - About half the cases are idiopathic.
> - Lesions can be less intense in coloration, like large pink hives.
> - Lesions appear in crops; consequently, there may be lesions in different stages of evolution.

EXAMINATION
- Poorly defined, exquisitely tender, erythematous nodules (which are better felt than seen) (Fig. 119.1).

Diagnosis
This patient has tender erythema nodosum (lesions) on the shins caused by the use of oral contraceptives (aetiology).

Questions
How can a definitive diagnosis be obtained?
With a deep wedge biopsy of the tissue.

119—ERYTHEMA NODOSUM

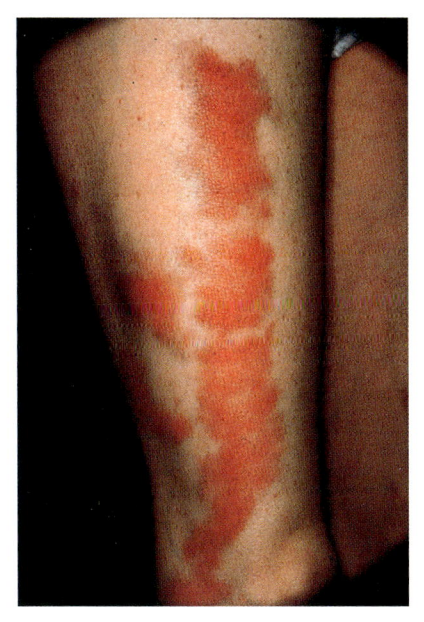

Fig. 119.1 Erythema nodosum lesions.

What is the histology?
Erythema nodosum is a panniculitis, which is an inflammatory reaction in the subcutaneous fat:
- In early lesions, there is widening of the connective tissue septa owing to oedema, fibrin exudation, and infiltration by neutrophils.
- Later, there is infiltration by lymphocytes, histiocytes, multinucleated giant cells, and occasionally eosinophils, associated with septal fibrosis.

Note: Vasculitis is absent.

Mention some examples of panniculitis.
- Erythema induratum (associated vasculitis)
- Weber–Christian disease (relapsing febrile nodular panniculitis)
- Factitial panniculitis.

How would you treat these patients?
Local: hot or cold compresses
Systemic: nonsteroidal antiinflammatory drugs, saturated solution of potassium iodide, corticosteroid therapy, salicylates. Treatment of underlying cause is important.
If lesions are associated with limb oedema, elevation and compression stockings are advised.

Further Information

F.P. Weber (1863–1962), a British physician who graduated from St Bartholomew's Hospital, London, and was a keen collector of coins and vases. He was an alpinist, like his father, Sir H.D. Weber (1823–1918), who described Weber syndrome.

Henry A. Christian (1876–1951), Professor of Medicine and the first Physician-in-Chief of the Peter Bent Brigham Hospital. He also described histiocytosis X (Hand–Schüller–Christian disease).

CHAPTER 120

Fungal Nail Disease

Instruction

Look at this patient's toenails.

Salient Features

HISTORY

- Embarrassment from a cosmetic perspective
- Mechanical problems (uneven nails getting snagged in clothing, etc.)
- History of diabetes.

EXAMINATION

- Nails are white, green, or, occasionally, black when the infection is superficial or proximal (Fig. 120.1A,B)
- When the infection is distal, there may be onycholysis (Fig. 120.1C,D).

Proceed as follows:

- Look at the toenails: thickened, yellow, or white nail with scaling under the elevated distal free edge of the nail plate.
- Tell the examiner that you would like to look for underlying immunodeficiency states such as HIV and circulatory disorders (Raynaud syndrome).

Diagnosis

This patient has fungal nail disease (lesion), which is usually caused by *Trichophyton* or *Candida* (aetiology), and it is cosmetically unacceptable to the patient (functional status).

Questions

What do you understand by the term onychomycosis?
It refers to a fungal infection of nails. Diagnostic criteria include the following:

- Clinical primary criteria:
  - White/yellow or orange/brown patches or streaks
- Clinical secondary criteria:
  - Onycholysis
  - Subungual hyperkeratosis/debris
  - Nail-plate thickening.

Note: Tinea pedis often occurs concomitantly with pedal onychomycosis, and tinea manuum, with infected fingernails.

120 — FUNGAL NAIL DISEASE

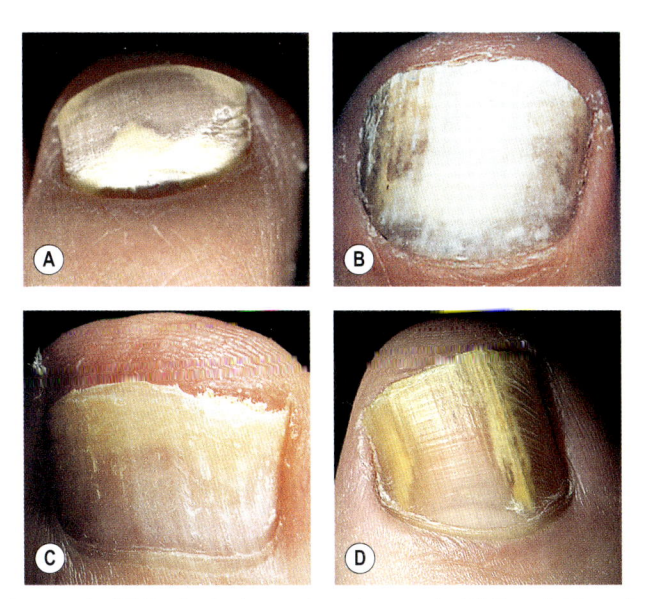

Fig. 120.1 Onychomycosis. **(A)** Proximal subungual onychomycosis. **(B)** Superficial onychomycosis with a dry, white, powdery surface that can be easily scraped away. **(C)** Distal onychomycosis: early changes. **(D)** Distal onychomycosis: late changes where the infection has progressed along a linear channel. (With permission from Habif, T.P., 2009. Clinical Dermatology, fifth edn. Mosby, Philadelphia, PA.)

- Laboratory criteria:
    - Positive microscopic evidence
    - Positive culture of dermatophyte.

What are the different causative organisms?
- Dermatophytes (ringworm, tinea unguium): *Trichophyton rubrum* and *Trichophyton interdigitale* (toenails are more commonly affected than fingernails). *T. rubrum* infection is associated with distal or lateral involvement of the nail plate that spreads proximally, eventually affecting the whole nail; this may be associated with proximal subungual nail dystrophy associated with separation of the nail from the bed. *T. interdigitale* infection, characteristically seen in patients with AIDS, produces superficial white onychomycosis with crumbly white areas on the nail surface
- Yeasts: *Candida albicans* and *Candida parapsilosis* (fingernails are more commonly affected than toenails)
- Nondermatophytes (moulds): *Fusarium, Scopulariopsis brevicaulis* (toenails are more commonly affected than fingernails).

Does the clinical picture vary according to the nature of the infecting organism?
Yes, as follows:
- Dermatophytes: distal or lateral nail involvement spreading proximally, proximal subungual dystrophy, superficial white dystrophy, white or yellow thickened nails, crumbling of nail plate, adjacent web or skin involvement may be present.
- *Candida*: chronic paronychia, shiny red bolstered nailfold, almost exclusively affects finger nailfolds, loss of cuticle, pus exuding from under nailfold, usually proximal nail involvement, distal nail dystrophy (associated with circulatory disorders), total dystrophic onychomycosis, nails white, green or occasionally black

- Nondermatophyte: superficial white onychomycosis, solitary nail involvement; colour of the nail may be influenced by the nature of the infecting mould (e.g. the nails are white with *Fusarium*; white, yellow, brown, or green with *S. brevicaulis*).

What are the patterns of fungal nail involvement?
- Distal lateral subungual onychomycosis
- Superficial white onychomycosis
- Proximal white subungual onychomycosis
- Total dystrophic onychomycosis (i.e. all the previous three sites are affected).

Is laboratory diagnosis essential before starting treatment?
Yes, for the following reasons:
- Antifungal treatment is prolonged and the causative organism may be nonfungal.
- To identify contacts of the patient
- To exclude mixed infection
- To optimize treatment as certain fungi are less responsive to treatment.

What are the poor prognosis factors?
- Areas of nail involvement >50%
- Significant lateral disease
- Subungual hyperkeratosis >2 mm
- White/yellow or orange/brown streaks in the nail
- Total dystrophic onychomycosis (with matrix involvement)
- Nonresponsive organisms (e.g. *Scytalidium* mould)
- Immunosuppression
- Diminished peripheral circulation.

Mention some nonfungal nail infections.
Bacterial nail infection, e.g. *Pseudomonas aeruginosa* (green or blackish discoloration of the nails) and *Staphylococcus aureus* (causes acute paronychia or whitlow).

How are specimens obtained for mycological diagnosis?
Scrapings are taken with a blunt scalpel as proximally as possible in the nail:
- In distal and lateral onychomycosis, specimens are taken from the proximal part of the diseased portion of the nail and subungual material
- In superficial white onychomycosis, the scrapings are taken from the diseased nail surface
- In proximal white mycosis, the scrapings are taken from the nail surface.

In the laboratory, 20% to 30% potassium hydroxide is added to part of the specimen to macerate nail keratin before direct microscopy and the rest of the specimen is inoculated on different media.

What is the recommended treatment for onychomycosis?
- Dermatophyte infections: Localized distal nail disease: tioconazole with undecylenic acid paint, amorolfine paint weekly and 40% urea paste for dissolution
- Proximal or extensive nail disease: terbinafine, itraconazole, fluconazole, griseofulvin, and amorolfine nail paint. Data have suggested that terbinafine is the treatment of choice for onychomycosis
- Candidal infections:
  - Chronic paronychia (localized): imidazole creams or paints, nystatin ointment, terbinafine cream; insufficient evidence on the effects of topical antifungal agents in people with frequently infected toenails

- Distal infection: tioconazole with undecylenic acid paint, amorolfine nail paint
- Severe infection or severe chronic paronychia: itraconazole.
- Nondermatophyte (mould) onychomycosis:
  - Localized disease: tioconazole with undecylenic acid paint, amorolfine paint weekly, 40% urea paste for dissolution or even avulsion of the nail
  - Persistent disease: itraconazole.

Mention some fungal infections that do not respond to oral treatment.
Scopulariopsis, Scytalidium, Fusarium, and *Acremonium* spp.

What is the definition of cure in fungal nail infections?
Cure in fungal nail infections is defined by the absence of clinical signs or the presence of negative nail culture and/or microscopy results with one or more of the following minor clinical signs:
- minimal distal subungual hyperkeratosis
- nail-plate thickening.

Persistent onychomycosis is suggested at the end of the observation period by:
- white/yellow or orange/brown streaks or patches in or beneath the nail plate
- lateral onycholysis with subungual debris.

Although nail appearance will usually continue to improve after therapy is stopped, the nails may have a persistent abnormal appearance even where therapy has been effective.

CHAPTER 121

Hairy Leukoplakia

Instruction
Look at this patient's tongue.

Salient Features

HISTORY
- Patients are usually asymptomatic
- Patients may complain of pain or voice changes
- Tell the examiner that you would like to know whether the patient is immunocompromised (caused by HIV or immunosuppressive treatment particularly in kidney transplant recipients).

EXAMINATION
- Shaggy, hairy, white lesions on the lateral margins of the tongue (remember that it does not affect the vaginal or anal mucosa) (Fig. 121.1).

Note: Oral hairy leukoplakia may be difficult to distinguish from oral candidiasis, but, in contrast to oral candidiasis, it does not rub off, does not respond to antifungal therapy, and may change its appearance daily.

Diagnosis
This patient has whitish hairy lesions on the lateral edges of the tongue (lesions), which is oral hairy leukoplakia caused by the Epstein–Barr virus (aetiology).

Questions

What is the cause of this lesion?
Hairy leukoplakia is caused by the Epstein–Barr virus. The risk of developing the condition is much higher in patients with HIV infection and smokers.

What are the histological features of this condition?
- Hyperkeratosis
- Hyperplasia and ballooning of prickle cells (acanthosis)
- Depletion of Langerhans cells.

Why is the tongue dark coloured?
The dark colour is secondary to porphyrin pigment deposition by bacterial metabolism.

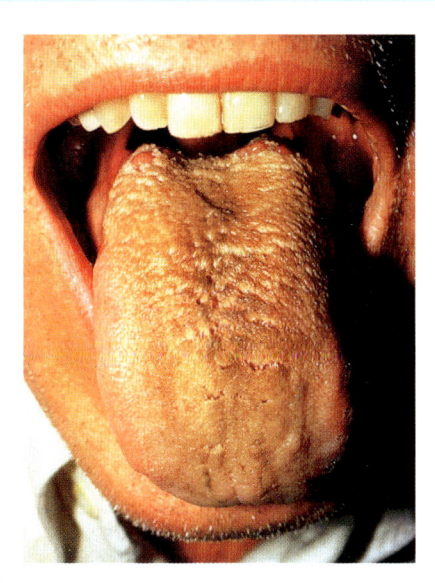

Fig. 121.1 Hairy leukoplakia.

How would you treat this condition?
Treatment is seldom indicated, but ganciclovir or aciclovir may be helpful if the patient has discomfort. Also, podophyllin and retinoin have been used. Secondary candida infection can be treated with antifungals.

Further Information
P. Langerhans (1847–1888), German pathologist and dermatologist.
Oral 'hairy' leukoplakia was initially reported in the Lancet in 1984 (Greenspan et al., 1984).

CHAPTER 122

Henoch–Schönlein Purpura

Instruction
Look at this patient's legs.

Salient Features
HISTORY
Ask the patient about the following:
- The rash: its onset and evolution
- Recent upper respiratory tract infection, fever
- Joint pains (knees and ankles are commonly involved)
- Abdominal pain
- Recent drug ingestion.

EXAMINATION
- Purpuric rash over the legs (Fig. 122.1) and buttocks.

Remember: Palpable purpura implies an inflammatory process, most classically cutaneous small cell vasculitis.

Proceed as follows:
- Tell the examiner that you would like to examine the rest of the body—including arms, body, scalp, and behind the ears—for distribution of rash.
- Examine the mouth to confirm or rule out involvement of mucous membranes.
- Tell the examiner that you would like to examine the urine for haematuria.

Diagnosis
This patient has purpuric rash over the legs and buttocks with renal involvement (lesions) caused by Henoch–Schönlein purpura (aetiology). I would like to know his 24-hour urine output and levels of urea and electrolytes to determine renal function (functional status).

Questions

What do you know about Henoch–Schönlein purpura?
Henoch–Schönlein or anaphylactoid purpura is a distinct, self-limiting small-vessel vasculitis that occurs in children and young adults, with a peak incidence in the first two decades of life. It is a disorder characterized by nonthrombocytopenic purpura, arthralgia, abdominal pain, and glomerular nephritis. It is the result of circulating immunoglobulin (Ig) A-containing immune complexes. It usually lasts between 1 and 6 weeks and subsides without sequelae if renal involvement is mild.

122 — HENOCH–SCHÖNLEIN PURPURA

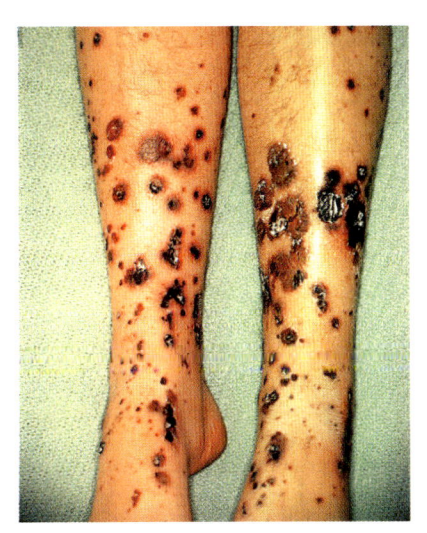

Fig. 122.1 Henoch–Schönlein purpura: palpable purpuric lesions.

The presence of IgG indicates a worse prognosis. Adults are more likely to develop renal involvement. In biopsy specimens obtained from the skin of patients with Henoch–Schönlein purpura, the dermal vessels frequently contain IgA deposits.

What investigations would you like to do?
- Examine the urine for haematuria and proteinuria to determine renal involvement.
- Skin biopsy to detect arteriolar and capillary vasculitis. This is often not necessary in children
- Throat swab is often positive for beta-haemolytic streptococcus, a common precipitant.
- If diagnostic uncertainty, antinuclear factor or venereal disease research laboratory test may be useful.

What is the differential diagnosis?
- Drug-induced purpura
- Systemic lupus erythematosus
- Gonococcal arthralgia
- Keratoderma blenorrhagicum
- Secondary syphilis.

How would you classify vasculitis clinically?
- Purpuric disorders: Henoch–Schönlein purpura, leukocytic vasculitis
- Microscopic polyarteritis: polyarteritis nodosa
- Aortic type: Takayasu disease, polyarteritis nodosa (in the latter, the subclavian artery is spared)
- Pulmonary type: Wegener's granulomatosis, Churg–Strauss syndrome.

How would you treat this patient?
- First line: rest, reduced activity, and leg elevation
- First-line oral therapy: antihistamines and nonsteroidal antiinflammatory drugs
- Second-line therapy: colchicine, dapsone
- Chronic or severe disease may require systemic immunosuppressants.

Patients with IgA nephropathy with protein excretion >500 mg/day should be treated with an angiotensin-converting enzyme inhibitor and/or an angiotensin receptor blocker. Patients with IgA nephropathy, increased urinary protein excretion (1.0–3.5 g daily), and plasma creatinine concentrations of ≤133 μmol/L (≤15 mg/L) may benefit from a 6-month course of steroid treatment. Steroids, plasma exchange, immunoglobulins, and cytotoxic agents have all been used in complicated cases, but the role of immunotherapy in IgA nephropathy remains controversial, with limited benefits but increased adverse effects. A recent randomized controlled trial using rituximab also had disappointing results.

What is the prognosis of immunoglobulin A nephropathy?
IgA nephropathy tends to progress slowly, and only about half the patients develop end-stage renal disease within 25 years. Factors that predict an accelerated course are persistent proteinuria, persistent microscopic haematuria, elevated serum creatinine at the time of diagnosis, poorly controlled hypertension, and extensive glomerulosclerosis or interstitial fibrosis on renal biopsy.

What is the difference between primary immunoglobulin A nephropathy and Henoch–Schönlein purpura?
IgA nephropathy (or Berger disease) was first described by Berger and Hinglais as recently as 1968 and is now generally accepted to be the most common form of primary glomerulonephritis. There are two conditions that should be distinguished from primary IgA nephropathy: Henoch–Schönlein purpura and thin glomerular basement membrane disease. Thin glomerular basement membrane disease is a common condition that occurs more often in female patients and has a benign clinical course in that end-stage renal disease does not develop. Its diagnosis is established by electron microscopy, where glomerular capillary loops can be shown to have diffusely attenuated basement membranes.

What are the other cutaneous manifestations of immune complex-mediated small vasculitis?
Vesicles, pustules, superficial ulcerations, urticaria, splinter haemorrhages, hyperpigmentation (Fig. 122.2).

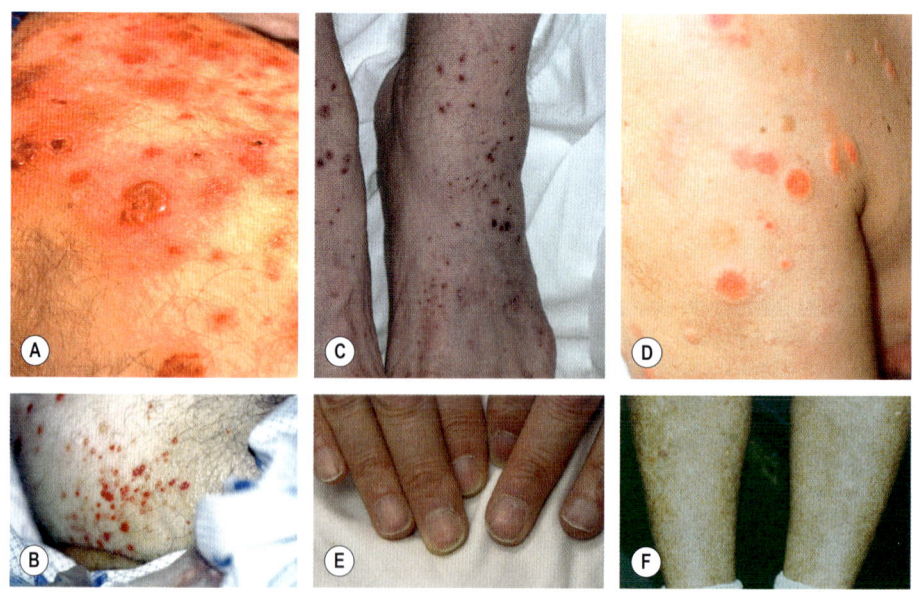

Fig. 122.2 Immune complex-mediated small vessel vasculitis. **(A)** Vesicles. **(B)** Pustules. **(C)** Superficial ulcerations. **(D)** Urticaria. **(E)** Splinter haemorrhages. **(F)** Hyperpigmentation. (With permission from Firestein, G.S., Budd, R.C., Harris Jr., E.D., et al., 2008. Kelley's Textbook of Rheumatology, eighth edn. Saunders, Philadelphia, PA.)

What are the different types of immune complex-mediated vasculitis?
- Henoch–Schönlein purpura
- Cutaneous leukocytoclastic angiitis
- Mixed cryoglobulinaemia
- Connective tissue disease/rheumatoid vasculitis.

Further Information

This disorder was first reported in the English literature by Willan in 1808.

Eduard Heinrich Henoch (1820–1910) qualified in Berlin, where he ran the neurology department; he studied under Schönlein and eventually became a paediatrician. In 1874, he reported the coexistence of purpura and gastrointestinal haemorrhage.

Johannes Lucas Schönlein (1793–1864) was initially Professor of Medicine in Würzburg, but because of his liberal views, he was dismissed; he eventually became Professor of Medicine, first in Zurich and then in Berlin. In 1837, he reported the coexistence of purpura and arthritis.

CHAPTER 123

Hereditary Haemorrhagic Telangiectasia (Osler–Weber–Rendu Syndrome)

Instruction

Examine the patient's face and obtain a relevant history.
Perform a general examination.
Look at this patient's face.

Salient Features

HISTORY

- Does it run in the family (autosomal dominant)?
- Is there a history of gastrointestinal (GI) bleeding?
- Is there a history of epistaxis?
- Is there a history of repeated blood transfusions?
- Is there a history of dyspnoea, fatigue, cyanosis, or polycythaemia (pulmonary arteriovenous malformations)?
- Is there a history of headaches, subarachnoid haemorrhage (cerebral arteriovenous malformations)?

EXAMINATION

- Punctiform lesions and dilated small vessels present on the face, in particular around the mouth (Fig. 123.1)
- The patient may be pale as a result of iron-deficiency anaemia.

Proceed as follows:
- Look into the patient's mouth and inspect the tongue and palate for telangiectasia
- Examine the nail beds, arms, and trunk for telangiectasia
- Examine the chest for bruits (pulmonary arteriovenous malformations with a predilection for lower lobes)
- Look for signs of cardiac failure caused by left-to-right shunting and hepatic bruits (both from hepatic arteriovenous malformations).

Diagnosis

This patient has multiple telangiectasia around the mouth and on the tongue and lips (lesion), probably hereditary in nature (aetiology). The patient is severely anaemic, probably as a result of upper GI bleeding, and is currently receiving a blood transfusion (functional status).

123 – HEREDITARY HAEMORRHAGIC TELANGIECTASIA (OSLER–WEBER–RENDU SYNDROME)

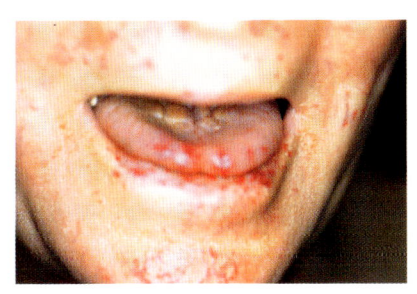

Fig. 123.1 Hereditary haemorrhagic telangiectasia. Lesions are commonly on or close to mucous membranes. Lesions may occur anywhere on the body, such as on the fingers. The lesions are dilated capillaries, and they blanch if pressure is applied with a glass slide. (With permission from Forbes, C.D., Jackson, W.F., 2003. Color Atlas and Text of Clinical Medicine, third edn. Mosby, London.)

Questions

What do you understand by the term telangiectasia?

Telangiectasia is a cluster of dilated capillaries and venules. The lesions blanch if pressure is applied with a glass slide. The word derives from the Greek words *angio* and *ectasia*; *angio* = vessel and *ectasia* = stretched or dilated. In hereditary haemorrhagic telangiectasia (HHT), the telangiectasias consist of focal dilatations of postcapillary venules. Lesions are commonly on or close to mucous membranes but may occur anywhere on the body, such as on the fingers.

Mention a few conditions in which telangiectasia are seen.

- Face:
    - Those who work outdoors in a temperate or cold climate (e.g. farmers)
    - Mitral stenosis
    - Myxoedema
    - Transitory phenomenon during pregnancy.
- Other sites:
    - Secondary to irradiation
    - Scleroderma (CREST syndrome)
    - Dermatomyositis
    - Systemic lupus erythematosus
    - Acne rosacea
    - Lupus pernio
    - Polycythaemia
    - Necrobiosis lipoidica diabeticorum.

What do you know about the genetics of hereditary telangiectasia?

Mutations have been identified in multiple genes, which include those encoding proteins expressed on vascular endothelial cells and involved in signalling by members of the transforming growth factor-β superfamily: endoglin-β (chromosome 9q3) and activin receptor–like kinase 1. Interestingly, heterozygote endoglin knockout mice develop a phenotype similar to that of humans who are heterozygous for a null mutation in the gene for endoglin-β. These heterozygous mice develop nosebleeds and cutaneous telangiectasia, and curiously, the ears are more commonly affected than in human beings. In patients with this condition and juvenile polyposis, there may be mutations in one gene—the *MADH4* gene (also known as *SMAD4*). Pulmonary hypertension in association with HHT can involve mutations in *ALK1*.

What do you know about the pathology of the condition?

Skin:
- The small telangiectasias are focal dilatations of postcapillary venules with prominent stress fibres in the pericytes along the luminal border.
- In fully developed telangiectasia, there is marked dilatation of the venules, which are also convoluted. They extend along the entire dermis, with excessive layers of smooth muscle devoid of elastic fibres. These often are directly connected to dilated arterioles.
- Mononuclear cells, predominantly lymphocytes, accumulate in the perivascular space.

Lungs, liver, and brain:
- Arteriovenous malformations lack capillaries and consist of direct connections between arteries and veins.

What are the clinical criteria for diagnosing hereditary haemorrhagic telangiectasia?

Curacao criteria using Shovlin's 'suggestive findings':
- Recurrent epistaxis
- Telangiectasia at a site other than in the nasal mucosa
- Evidence of autosomal dominant inheritance
- Visceral involvement.

The HHT diagnosis is definite if three criteria are present. A diagnosis of HHT cannot be established in patients with only two criteria but should be recorded as possible or suspected to maintain a high index of clinical suspicion. If fewer than two criteria are present, HHT is unlikely, although children of affected individuals should be considered at risk in view of age-related penetration in this disorder.

What are the complications of hereditary telangiectasia?

- Epistaxis (usually begins by the age of 10 years and by 21 years of age in most; it becomes more severe in later decades in about two-thirds of affected patients)
- GI haemorrhage (usually does not manifest until the fifth or sixth decade). Arteriovenous malformations, angiodysplasias, and telangiectasias are present in the stomach, duodenum, small bowel, colon, and liver.
- Symptomatic liver involvement: the typical clinical presentations include high-output heart failure, portal hypertension, and biliary disease
- Iron-deficiency anaemia
- Haemoptysis, cyanosis, clubbing, cerebral abscess, and embolic stroke from the pulmonary arteriovenous malformations
- Headache and subarachnoid haemorrhage
- High-output cardiac failure is almost always associated with shunts from the hepatic artery to the hepatic veins.

How would you manage such patients?

- Anaemia: ferrous sulfate, multiple blood transfusions
- Epistaxis: local treatments to prevent epistaxis (local ointments and saline spray), ear, nose, and throat invasive therapies (laser therapy, cauterization), emergency interventions (nasal packing)
- Cutaneous telangiectasia: cosmetic therapy with topical agents, laser ablation
- Pulmonary arteriovenous malformations: radiological embolization, surgical resection, or ligation of arterial supply
- GI telangiectasia: blood transfusions, endoscopic ablation, embolization
- Brain and spinal cord arteriovenous malformations: embolization, neurosurgery, stereotactic surgery

- Hormonal therapy can be used
- Anti-vascular endothelial growth factor antibody, bevacizumab.

Further Information

This condition was described by H.J.L.M. Rendu, a French physician, in 1896, by Sir William Osler in 1901, and by F. Parkes Weber, a London physician, in 1936.

Prof. Claire Shovlin is a Professor in NHLI Cardiovascular Sciences and Honorary Consultant in Respiratory Medicine for Imperial College Healthcare NHS Trust (Hammersmith Hospital campus) whose research focuses on gene identification of this condition.

CHAPTER 124

Herpes Simplex

Instruction

Look at this patient's mouth.

Salient Features

HISTORY

- Pain, itching, burning lasting several hours
- Vesicles
- Sore mouth
- Fever
- Gum swelling
- Mouth ulcers.

EXAMINATION

- Small vesicles with an erythematous base on the lips and around the mouth (Fig. 124.1)
- Look for:
  - vesicles in the mouth (gingiva, tongue, soft and hard palate) and pharynx
  - tender anterior cervical lymph nodes.

Diagnosis

This patient has small vesicles around the mouth (lesion) from herpes simplex (aetiology), which is causing severe itching (functional status).

Questions

What usually causes a 'cold sore'?
Skin manifestations include vesicular lesions on an erythematous base. Only 10% to 30% of new infections are symptomatic.
   Herpes simplex virus (HSV) type 1 causes an asymptomatic gingivostomatitis in children.
   In adults, there may be severe stomatitis with mouth ulcers, local lymph node enlargement, and systemic features.

What do you know about herpes simplex virus type 2?
HSV-2 causes a genital infection called vulvovaginitis. Women with genital herpes should have cervical screening as a link is suspected with carcinoma of the cervix.

124 — HERPES SIMPLEX

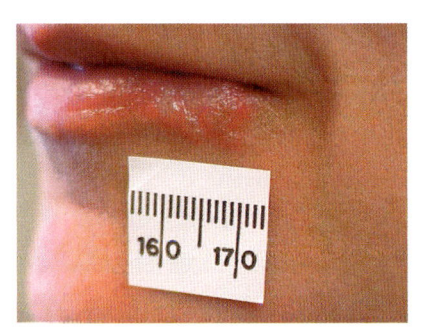

Fig. 124.1 Clustered intact vesicles at the skin–vermilion junction. (With permission from DeLee, J.C., Drez Jr., D., Miller, M.D., 2009. DeLee and Drez's Orthopaedic Sports Medicine, third edn. Saunders, 2009, Philadelphia, PA.)

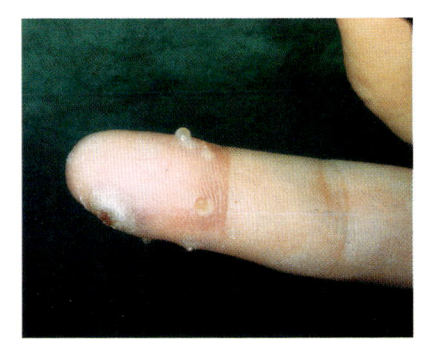

Fig. 124.2 Herpetic whitlow.

What are the complications of herpes infections?
- Erythema multiforme
- Disseminated infection in the immunocompromised individual
- Herpes keratitis, scarring, and visual impairment
- Herpes simplex encephalitis (propensity for the temporal lobe)
- Herpetic whitlow (infection of the finger) (Fig. 124.2)
- Herpes gladiatorum (infection of the skin, described among wrestlers)
- Visceral infections, especially in viraemia in HIV (oesophagitis, pneumonitis, hepatitis)
- Neonatal HSV infection (neonates <6 weeks of age); usually visceral and/or central nervous system (CNS) infection
- CNS complications: aseptic meningitis, sacral radiculopathy, transverse myelitis, and benign recurrent lymphocytic meningitis (Mollaret meningitis).

After initial infection, what causes recurrence of the lesions?
- Local trauma
- Systemic infections
- Emotional and physical stress.

How would you confirm your clinical diagnosis?
- Diagnosis is usually a clinical one
- If there is any clinical doubt, a viral swab can be taken for polymerase chain reaction (PCR) and cultures.

How would you treat lesions of herpes simplex?
Aciclovir cream applied locally.

In a patient suspected of herpes encephalitis, which test allows early detection?
PCR of the cerebrospinal fluid to detect HSV DNA.

What do you know about the pathogenesis of herpes simplex mucocutaneous infections?
In the initial infection, HSV enters through breaks in the skin or mucosa; it then attaches to and enters epithelial cells to replicate. It is taken up by free sensory nerve endings found at the dermis, and the nucleocapsid containing the viral genome is transported by retrograde axonal flow to the nucleus in the sensory ganglion.

After recovery from the initial infection, the virus remains latent in the sensory ganglion for the life of the host. Periodically, the virus reactivates from the latent state and travels back down the sensory nerves to the skin or mucosal surface.

Viral shedding from mucosal surfaces occurs from lesions (clinical reactivation) but can occur with very mild or no symptoms (subclinical reactivation). Shedding leads to transmission to other sexual partners, and in some cases, HSV can be transmitted from mother to infant at delivery.

CHAPTER 125

Herpes Zoster Syndrome (Shingles)

Instruction
Look at this patient.

Salient Features
HISTORY
- Pain across a dermatome (pain can precede the rash for a few days or even weeks. It is the most commonly presenting symptom and affects around 70%–75% of the patients with herpes zoster)
- History of chickenpox
- Systemic symptoms (fever, malaise, general aches, and headache in around 20% of cases)
- Presence of an underlying immunocompromised state
- Herpes zoster rash.

EXAMINATION
- Vesicular rash along a dermatome (usually affects thoracic and lumbar dermatomes). If the ophthalmic branch of the trigeminal nerve is involved, then it can present as herpes ophthalmicus (Fig. 125.1) with clinically serious complications
- Enlargement of a draining lymph node.

Remember: The virus affects both the posterior horn of the spinal cord and the skin supplied by sensory fibres that pass through the diseased root ganglion (Fig. 125.2).

Diagnosis
This patient has a vesicular rash along the sixth thoracic dermatome (lesion) caused by herpes zoster (aetiology) and has severe local pain (functional status).

Questions

Can you describe the rash of herpes zoster?
Depending on the timing of the examination, different types of rash can be seen. Initially, there are erythematous papules across a dermatome distribution. These turn into vesicles and bullae and, subsequently, pustules.

How does this condition present?
Pain in the distribution of the dermatome; malaise; fever, followed a few days later by a rash in the same distribution as the pain.

465

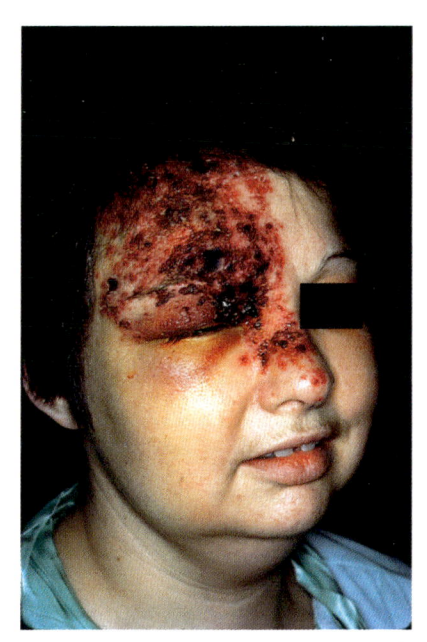

Fig. 125.1 Vesicular rash and pain in the ophthalmic branch of the trigeminal nerve.

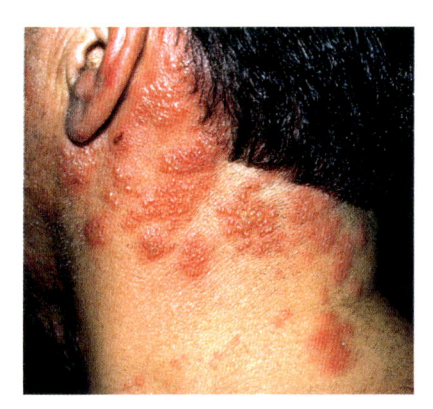

Fig. 125.2 Rash in skin supplied by sensory fibres of the nerve.

Which nerve is affected when the lesions are present on the tip of the nose?
The ophthalmic division of the trigeminal nerve.

How is shingles transmitted?
The transmission is mainly through direct contact with the herpetic rash, and the lesions are infective until they crust. However, airborne transmission has also been reported. Herpes zoster is only infectious to patients who do not have immunity to VZV virus (have not had chickenpox in the past or the vaccination against the virus). Varicella zoster can be transmitted vertically in utero and perinatally.

How would you confirm the diagnosis?
The diagnosis is mainly clinical. Laboratory tests that can be used in specific cases are polymerase chain reaction, direct fluorescent antibody testing, and Tzanck smear test from the lesion. The Tzanck smear demonstrates a multinucleated giant cell and viral inclusions when material scraped from the floor of a vesicle is stained with the Wright stain. The Tzanck test can be positive in infections with any herpes virus and is not specific to varicella zoster virus.

How would you manage such a patient?
- Pain relief, including gabapentin, pregabalin, lidocaine patch, topical capsaicin, and amitriptyline in severe cases
- Antiviral therapy (aciclovir, valaciclovir, or famciclovir) results in faster healing, lessening of acute pain, and reduced incidence and intensity of postherpetic neuralgia, only if prescribed early during the course of the disease (within 1–5 days of onset).

What is the role of vaccination?
There is waning cell-mediated immunity to the virus in the elderly. Therefore, vaccination in patients >60 years reduces the incidence of herpes zoster by 50% and lessens the severity and chance of complications. Apart from usage preexposure, the vaccination for varicella zoster virus has a role when given postexposure in susceptible adults; if given early after exposure, it can both prevent infection and reduce the potential severity in patients who become ill.

What are the complications of herpes zoster?
- Corneal ulcerations
- Phrenic nerve palsy
- Meningoencephalitis, acute retinal necrosis, myelitis, Guillain–Barré syndrome
- Ramsay Hunt syndrome (herpes reactivation within the geniculate ganglion; facial pain, ear pain, vesicles in the auditory canal)
- Postherpetic neuralgia
- Disseminated zoster including pneumonia
- Herpes zoster ophthalmicus (herpes in the trigeminal ganglion)
- Superadded bacterial skin infections.

What are the features of herpes zoster in patients with human immunodeficiency virus infection?
It may be unidermatomal and uneventful. However, it may be multidermatomal, disseminated recurrent, or chronically persistent. Disseminated herpes zoster can be either limited to the skin or involve internal organs, causing multiorgan failure and life-threatening syndromes. These patients are also at increased risk of developing the herpes zoster–related complications described earlier.

Further Information
J. Ramsay Hunt (1874–1937), an American neurologist.
Shingles, from the Latin *cingulum* or 'girdle'.

CHAPTER 126

Ichthyosis

Instruction

Examine this patient's skin.
Perform a general examination on this patient.

Salient Features

HISTORY

- Take a family history of the disorder.
- Ask for weight loss, night sweats, fevers, other systemic features (underlying malignancy).
- Ask for symptoms of hypothyroidism.

EXAMINATION

- Rough, dry skin with fish-like scales (Fig. 126.1).

Proceed as follows:
- Examine the palms for dry skin and hyperkeratotic creases.

Note: Although ichthyosis is said not to be more frequent in HIV/AIDS, it may be more severe when associated with this condition.

Diagnosis

This patient has rough, dry skin with fish-like scales (lesion) caused by ichthyosis (aetiology), which causes severe itching (functional status).

Questions

What do you know about ichthyosis?
Ichthyosis is a disorder of keratinization characterized by the development of dry, rectangular scales. It can be classified as inherited, metabolic, or malignant.
- Inherited ichthyosis:
  - *Inherited ichthyosis* is present from birth or childhood and may be apparent only in winter.
  - *Ichthyosis vulgaris* (Fig. 126.2A) is autosomal dominant and present from childhood. It has white, translucent, quadrangular scales on the extensor aspects of the arms and legs, sparing flexural areas, and is associated with atopy.
  - *X-linked ichthyosis* (Fig. 126.2B) is present from birth. It occurs all over the trunk with large, brown, quadrangular scales that may encroach on the antecubital and popliteal fossae; it is associated with corneal opacities. Affected individuals have a deficiency of steroid sulfatase, an enzyme important for the removal of proadhesive cholesterol sulfate

126 — ICHTHYOSIS

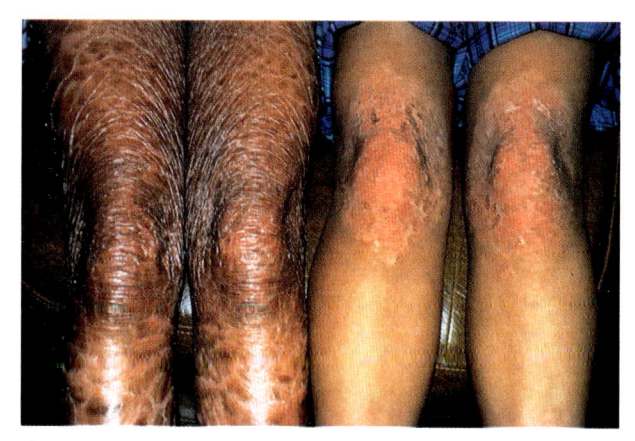

Fig. 126.1 Ichthyosis.

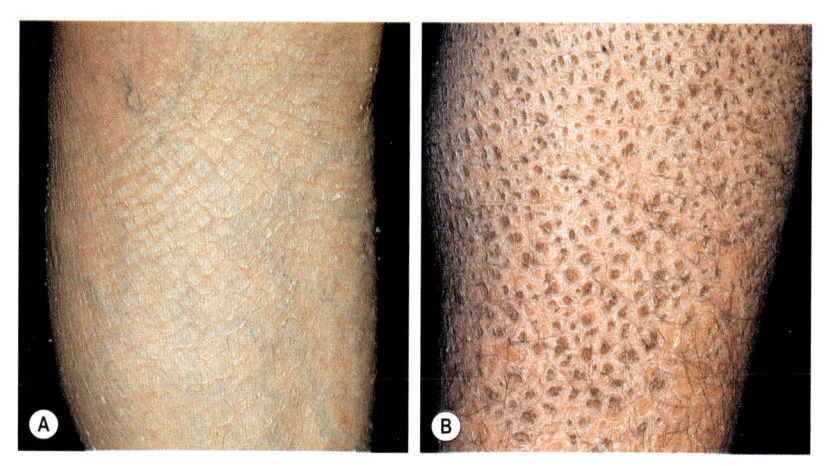

Fig. 126.2 Inherited ichthyosis. **(A)** Dominant ichthyosis vulgaris. **(B)** X-linked ichthyosis vulgaris. (With permission from Habif, T.P., 2009. Clinical Dermatology, fifth edn. Mosby, Philadelphia, PA.)

secreted into the intercellular spaces. The desquamation process is impaired by the accumulation of cholesterol sulfate, which results in persistent cell-to-cell adhesion within the stratum corneum.
- *Lamellar ichthyosis* is autosomal recessive and present from birth. It is seen over the body, palms, and soles and is associated with ectropion.
- *Epidermolytic hyperkeratosis* is autosomal dominant and present from birth. There is predominant flexural involvement.

Note: Filaggrin is a key protein involved in skin barrier function. Mutations in the gene for filaggrin have been reported in patients with ichthyosis.

- **Metabolic ichthyosis:** Refsum disease: a metabolic disorder of lipid metabolism
- **Malignancy:** Hodgkin disease, multiple myeloma, breast cancer.

How would you manage such patients?
Regular use of emollients and moisturizing creams. Creams containing urea are useful. Bathing in salt water can be useful. Treatment of superadded infections with antibiotics orally.

Further Information
S. Refsum, a Norwegian physician.

CHAPTER 127

Lichen Planus

Instruction

Look at this patient's skin.

Salient Features

HISTORY

- Age
- Itching
- Medication and occupational history for drug-induced lichen planus: thiazides, beta-blockers, angiotensin-converting enzyme inhibitors, gold, chloroquine, methyldopa, quinine, proton pump inhibitors
- Hepatitis C infection.

EXAMINATION

- Papular, purplish, flat-topped eruption with fine white streaks in a lace-like pattern (Wickham striae) (Fig. 127.1) over the anterior wrists and forearms, sacral region, ankles, legs, and penis
- Involvement of the skin is characterized by the '4Ps': purple, polygonal, pruritic papules.

Proceed as follows:
- Look into the mouth (buccal mucosa, tongue, gum, or lips) for a lace-like pattern of white lines and papules (Fig. 127.2). (Remember that oral lichen planus must be differentiated from leukoplakia.)
- Examine the scalp for cicatricial alopecia.
- Examine the nails for longitudinal ridging, pterygium formation from the cuticle (Fig. 127.3), 20-nail dystrophy (roughened nail surface and brittle free nail edge), and total nail loss.
- Comment on eruptions that present along linear scratch marks (Koebner's phenomenon).
- Comment on the residual hyperpigmented macules that lichen planus leaves in their wake.

Note: The three cardinal features of lichen planus are the typical skin lesions, histopathological features of T-cell infiltration of the dermis in a band pattern, and immunoglobulin and complement immunofluorescence at the dermal–epidermal junction.

Diagnosis

This patient has violaceous, flat-topped eruptions (lesion) caused by lichen planus (aetiology), with several scratch marks indicating moderately severe pruritus (functional status).

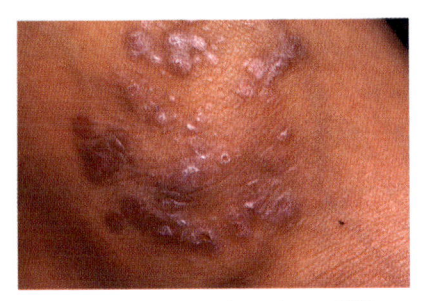

Fig. 127.1 Flat-topped, purple polygonal papules of lichen planus. (With permission from Kliegman, R.M., Behrman, R.E., Jenson, H.B., Stanton, B.F., 2007. Nelson Textbook of Pediatrics, 18th edn. Saunders, Philadelphia, PA.)

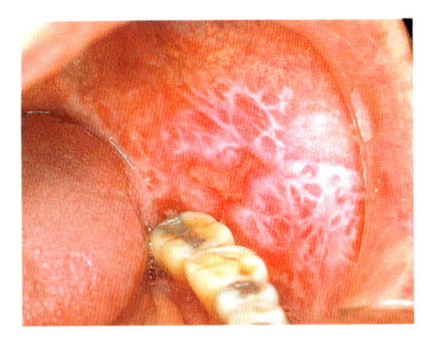

Fig. 127.2 Lace-like keratoses, erythema, and ulceration of the buccal mucosa. (With permission from Goldman, L., Ausiello, D.A., 2007. Cecil Textbook of Medicine, 23rd edn. Saunders, Philadelphia, PA.)

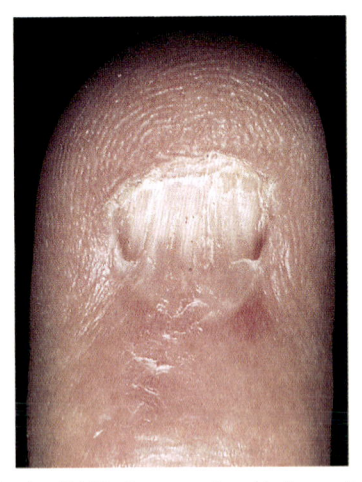

Fig. 127.3 Adhesion of the proximal nailfold to the scarred matrix throws the nail plate into folds, pterygium. (With permission from Habif, T.P., 2009. Clinical Dermatology, fifth edn. Mosby, Philadelphia, PA.)

127—LICHEN PLANUS

Questions

Mention a few conditions that present as white lesions in the mouth.
- Leukoplakia
- Candidiasis
- Aphthous stomatitis
- Squamous papilloma
- Verruca vulgaris
- Secondary syphilis.

Mention a few conditions in which ulcers can be found in the mouth.
- Erosive lichen planus
- Pemphigus vulgaris
- Recurrent aphthous ulcers
- Behçet disease (also known as Adamantiades–Behçet disease)
- Stevens–Johnson syndrome
- Recurrent herpes simplex.

What is the prognosis in lichen planus?
Lichen planus is a benign condition that lasts for months to years. It may be recurrent. Oral lesions may be persistent.

How would you manage these lesions?
- Local measures: high-potency topical steroid creams or intralesional steroids
- Oral corticosteroids
- Phototherapy
- Retinoids
- Antihistamines for symptomatic control of pruritus.

Further Information

L.F. Wickham (1860–1913), a French dermatologist.
H. Koebner (1838–1904), a German dermatologist.

CHAPTER 128

Lichen Simplex

Instruction
Look at this patient's skin.

Salient Features
HISTORY
- Itching (self-perpetuating itch–scratch cycle).

EXAMINATION
- Several scratch marks (from pruritus)
- Well-circumscribed plaque with lichenified or dry, thickened, leathery skin (Fig. 128.1)
- Look for similar plaques in common areas, including the posterior nuchal region, wrists, perineum, dorsum of the feet, or ankles (Fig. 128.2).

Diagnosis
This patient has lichen simplex (lesion), which is caused by chronic itching and scratching (aetiology) and is cosmetically disturbing to the patient.

Questions

How would you treat such a patient?
- Break the scratch–itch–scratch cycle by administering antipruritic agents
- Topical steroids (under occlusion or intralesional injection) may be used
- The area should be protected
- The patient should be made aware of when he or she is scratching.

What is the prognosis?
The disease tends to remit during treatment; however, it may recur or develop at another site.

What is the classification of itch?
Twycross classification of itch is based on peripheral and central origins of itch:
- *Pruritoceptive itch* is itch that originates in the skin from inflammation, dryness, or other skin damage and is transmitted by nerve C-fibres, e.g. itch caused by reactions to insect bite, scabies, urticaria.
- *Neuropathic itch* is itch that arises because of disease located at any point along the afferent pathway, e.g. post–herpes zoster neuropathy, the itch occasionally associated with multiple sclerosis and brain tumours.

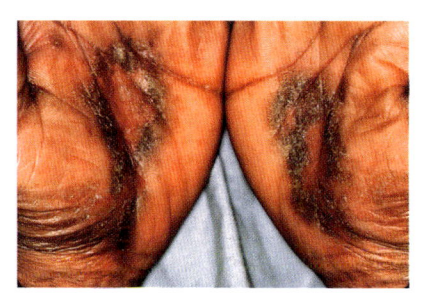

Fig. 128.1 Lichen simplex chronicus.

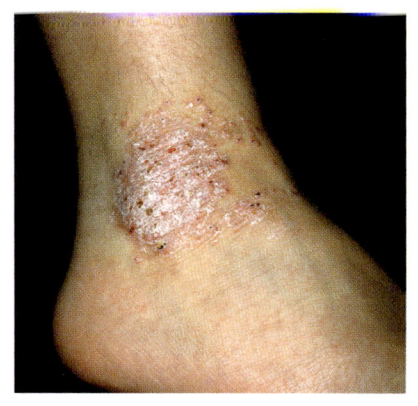

Fig. 128.2 Lichen simplex chronicus. (With permission from Habif, T.P., 2009. Clinical Dermatology, fifth edn. Mosby, Philadelphia, PA.)

- *Neurogenic itch* is itch that originates centrally but without evidence of neural pathology, e.g. itch of cholestasis, which is the result of the action of opioid neuropeptides on opioid μ-receptors.
- *Psychogenic itch*, as in the delusional state of parasitophobia.

Often one type of itch can coexist with another, for example in the itch of atopic eczema, neurogenic as well as pruritoceptive itches seem to arise in the same patient.

Which spinal tracts conduct itch and pain information?

Information on itch and pain is conveyed centrally in two separate systems that both use the lateral spinothalamic tract.

CHAPTER 129

Lipodystrophy

Instruction
Look at this patient.

Salient Features
HISTORY
- Ask whether the patient is taking insulin for diabetes.
- Is there a history of renal disease (mesangiocapillary glomerulonephritis)?
- Ask if there is a history of HIV and whether the patient is receiving antiretroviral agents.
- Ask for family history.

EXAMINATION
- Atrophy of the subcutaneous fat leading to disfiguring excavations and depressed areas (Figs 129.1 and 129.2).

Diagnosis
This patient has atrophy of subcutaneous fat or lipodystrophy (lesion) caused by local injection of subcutaneous insulin (aetiology).

Questions

With which conditions is lipodystrophy associated?
- Membranoproliferative glomerulonephritis
- Diabetes, insulin resistance, hypercholesterolaemia
- Viral infections
- Autoimmune conditions
- Chronic relapsing panniculitis
- Patients with human immunodeficiency virus (HIV) infection on antiretroviral treatment.

What is the mechanism of acquired lipodystrophy?
It results from an immune reaction. It is thought that, after exposure, antibodies develop against adipocyte membranes, which results in loss of subcutaneous fat and lipodystrophy.

Can lipodystrophy occur with insulin injections?
It used to be more common before the introduction of purified insulin, as a consequence of insulin being deposited repeatedly in the same location. It can still rarely occur with purified insulins, but rotation of the injection sites should prevent this complication.

129 — LIPODYSTROPHY

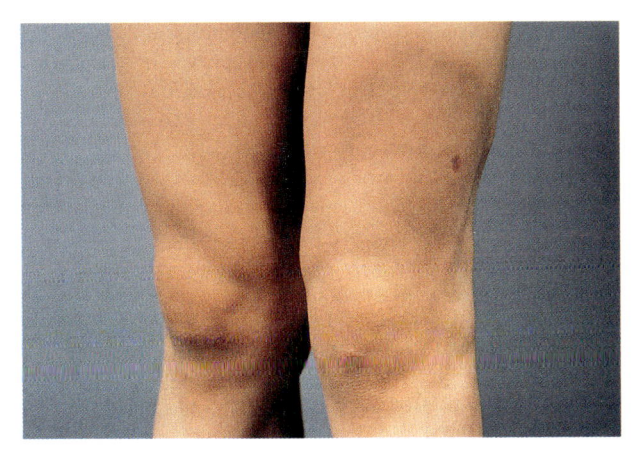

Fig. 129.1 Lipodystrophy.

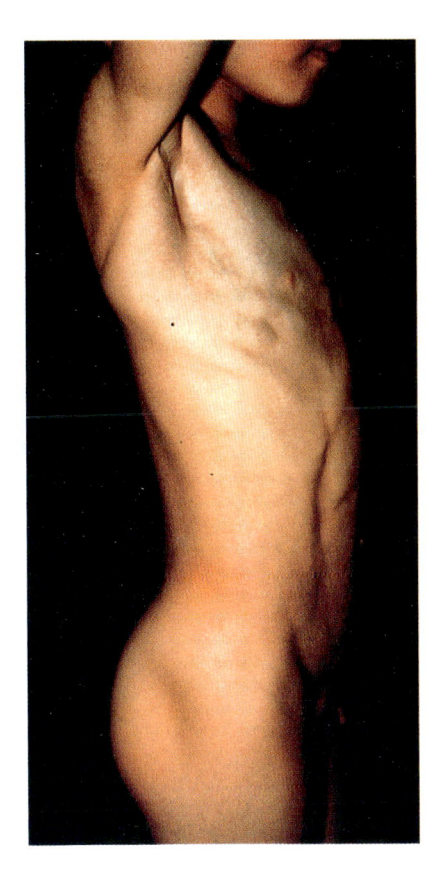

Fig. 129.2 Lipoatrophy.

What is relationship between lipodystrophy and human immunodeficiency virus?
Patients infected with HIV-1 receiving antiretroviral therapy have been reported to have abnormal fat distribution, including (a) lipodystrophy or loss of subcutaneous fat and (b) central or visceral fat accumulation. Typically, these patients have wasting of face and limbs along with adipose tissue accumulations in the abdomen and back of the neck, the latter giving a 'buffalo hump' appearance. It was initially considered only to be caused by HIV-1 protease inhibitors, but subsequently, this has not been substantiated. It has also been associated with nucleoside reverse transcriptase inhibitors, via mitochondrial toxicity and interference with lipid metabolism. Stavudine-based regimens have a higher cumulative prevalence of lipodystrophy than regimens based on zidovudine, abacavir, or tenofovir. Regimens based on nelfinavir are associated with more rapid fat loss than efavirenz. In general, thymidine-based nucleoside analogues have been most associated with lipodystrophy and protease inhibitor drugs most associated with the metabolic syndrome. Leptin deficiency contributes to the insulin resistance and other metabolic abnormalities associated with severe lipodystrophy. Leptin therapy improves glycaemic control and triglyceride levels in patients with lipodystrophy and leptin deficiency.

What are genes implicated in familial lipoatrophy?
- Familial partial lipodystrophy of the Dunnigan variety (FPL2). LMNA genes encoding lamins A and C
- The other inherited forms of lipodystrophy are much rarer and involve mutations in peroxisome-proliferator–activated receptor-γ (PPARG), PLIN1, AKT2 and CIDEC genes.

Further Information

The 1923 Nobel Prize in Medicine was awarded for the discovery of insulin to a Canadian surgeon, Sir Fredrick G. Banting (1891–1941), and a Scottish physiologist, John J.R. Macleod (1876–1935), working in Toronto. Banting shared his monetary prize with Charles Best, whereas Macleod shared his prize with J.J. Collip (the latter purified insulin to the point that it could be used in humans). Macleod corrected Banting's deficiencies on carbohydrate metabolism and provided him with laboratory support including the services of a graduate student in physiology, Charles Best. Macleod was from Aberdeen.

CHAPTER 130

Lupus Pernio

Instruction

Look at this patient's face.

Salient Features

HISTORY

- Shortness of breath, cough, chest discomfort
- Fatigue, weight loss, malaise, anorexia
- History of therapy with interferon-α (particularly in patients with hepatitis C; interferon-α increases interferon-γ and interleukin-2, thus promoting granuloma formation).

EXAMINATION

- Reddish blue or violaceous plaques on the nose (Fig. 130.1), cheeks, ears, and fingers, with telangiectasia over and around the plaques (Fig. 130.2).

Proceed as follows:
- Tell the examiner that you would like to examine the patient's eyes and respiratory system and you would like to obtain a chest X-ray to look for pulmonary sarcoidosis and an electrocardiogram to rule out heart block or arrhythmias.

Diagnosis

This patient has violaceous plaques on his face (lesion), which look like lupus pernio, a form of cutaneous sarcoidosis (aetiology).

Questions

What is the differential diagnosis of such a lesion?
- Rhinophyma
- Lupus vulgaris
- Leprosy.

Name some cutaneous manifestations of sarcoid.
- Erythema nodosum
- Papular sarcoid
- Nodular sarcoidosis
- Scar infiltration
- Lupus pernio
- Sarcoid plaques of limbs, shoulders, buttocks, and thighs
- Ulcers, atrophic lesions, and subcutaneous sarcoidosis.

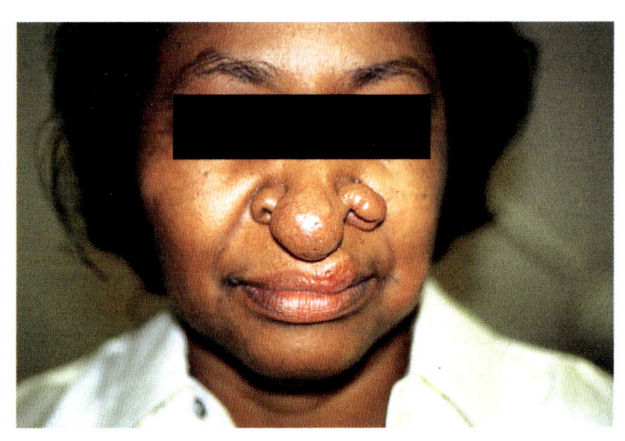

Fig. 130.1 Nodular sarcoidosis with lupus pernio plaques on the nose.

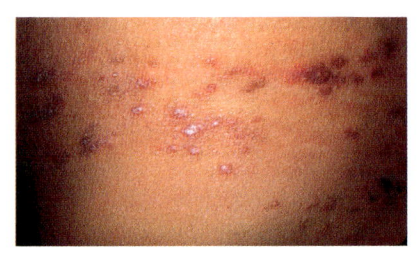

Fig. 130.2 Telangiectasia over and around the plaques.

How may sarcoid present?
- Asymptomatic (incidental diagnosis from imaging)
- Respiratory symptoms (dyspnoea, chest pain, cough)
- Generalized symptoms (weight loss, malaise, low-grade fever)
- Skin lesions (erythema nodosum)
- Symptoms of hypercalcaemia.

How would you investigate such a patient?
- Routine blood tests: leukopenia, eosinophilia, raised inflammatory markers, hypercalcaemia
- Chest radiography and high-resolution computed tomography. Four stages of sarcoidosis are defined depending on radiographic findings, although these stages do not indicate chronology of disease:
  - I: bilateral hilar adenopathy alone
  - II: both hilar adenopathy and lung parenchymal involvement
  - III: parenchymal involvement alone
  - IV: pulmonary fibrosis (usually upper lobe).
- Slit-lamp examination of the eyes
- Kviem's test is of no clinical use
- Mantoux test or interferon assay to search for tuberculosis
- Serum angiotensin-converting enzyme levels: raised in 40% to 80% with active disease, although this finding is neither sensitive nor specific enough to have diagnostic significance

- Lung function tests: usually restrictive changes with decreased lung volumes and diffusing capacity; occasionally airflow obstruction
- Bronchoalveolar lavage: usually characterized by an increase in lymphocytes and a high CD4:CD8 T-cell ratio
- Histological confirmation by the presence of noncaseating granulomas with typical manifestations (fibrotic response develops over time) in biopsy of lung (transbronchial), lymph node, skin, liver, gums, or minor salivary glands
- Radiotracker tests (Gallium 67) can be used if diagnosis is uncertain and biopsy is technically difficult.
- Electrocardiogram (ECG) to rule out arrhythmias and heart block.

What are the treatment options for sarcoidosis?
Asymptomatic patients with pulmonary sarcoidosis with no extrapulmonary features, normal calcium, and no affected pulmonary function can be observed with regular follow-up in the respiratory clinic. All other patients should be treated with oral steroids. Refractory cases can be treated with methotrexate, azathioprine, leflunomide, or mycophenolate. The overall prognosis is good.

What is the treatment of cutaneous sarcoid?
Monthly intralesional triamcinolone injections, topical and systemic steroids, hydroxychloroquine, allopurinol, thalidomide, and tranilast.

What are the specific indications for systemic steroids in sarcoidosis?
- Progressive deterioration in lung function or symptomatic pulmonary fibrosis
- Extrapulmonary manifestations (central nervous system involvement, hypercalcaemia, severe ocular disease, hepatitis, cutaneous lesions).

What are the ocular manifestations of sarcoidosis?
- Anterior uveitis, seen in about 5% of all cases and either acute or chronic: mutton fat keratic precipitates, iris nodules
- Retinal vasculitis, neovascularization
- Vitreous opacities
- Choroidal granulomata
- Optic nerve granuloma.

What is Löfgren syndrome?
Erythema nodosum, hilar adenopathy, and polyarthralgia in a patient with sarcoidosis. It is associated with good prognosis, with spontaneous remission without the need of steroids.

What is the source of the raised serum angiotensin-converting enzyme in sarcoidosis?
It is derived from the cell membranes of epithelioid cells in the sarcoid granuloma and its synthesis is controlled by epithelioid cells.

What is Blau syndrome?
It is a multisystem granulomatous disorder of the skin, eyes, and joints that resembles childhood sarcoidosis; it was described by Edward Blau, a Wisconsin paediatrician.

Is there any relationship between viral infections and sarcoid?
Variant human herpes virus type 8 DNA sequences have been found in sarcoid tissue. Also, mycobacteria-like 16 S ribosomal RNAs are more frequently found in sarcoid tissue, but this does not indicate infection by a particular mycobacterial species.

What is the cardinal feature in the pathogenesis?
The cardinal feature of sarcoidosis is the presence of CD4 T cells that interact with antigen-presenting cells to initiate the formation and maintenance of granulomata.

What are the diagnostic features of cardiac sarcoidosis?
- *Histologic diagnosis group*: cardiac sarcoidosis is confirmed when histologic analysis of operative or endomyocardial biopsy specimens demonstrates epithelioid granuloma without caseating granuloma.
- *Clinical diagnosis group*: in patients with a histologic diagnosis of extracardiac sarcoidosis, cardiac sarcoidosis is suspected when item (a) and one or more of items (b) to (e) are present:
    (a) ECG: complete right bundle branch block, left axis deviation, atrioventricular block, ventricular tachycardia, premature ventricular contraction or abnormal Q or ST-T change
    (b) Abnormal wall motion, regional wall thinning, or dilatation of the left ventricle (LV)
    (c) Myocardial scintigraphy: perfusion defect detected by thallium-201 or abnormal accumulation of gallium-67 or technetium-99m
    (d) Abnormal intracardiac pressure: low cardiac output, abnormal wall motion, or depressed ejection fraction of the LV
    (e) Interstitial fibrosis or cellular infiltration over moderate grade, even if the findings are nonspecific.

Further Information

M.A. Kviem (b. 1892), a Norwegian pathologist.

C. Mantoux (1877–1947), a French physician from Cannes, who showed that his intradermal test was more sensitive than the older Pirquet subcutaneous tests using tuberculin.

Norwegian dermatologist Caesar P.M. Boeck (1845–1917) from Olso, Norway, coined the term to describe skin nodules characterized by compact, sharply defined foci of 'epithelioid cells with large pale nuclei and also a few giant cells'. Thinking this resembled sarcoma, he called the condition 'multiple benign sarcoid of the skin'.

S. Löfgren (1910-1978), a Swedish physician.

CHAPTER 131

Maculopapular Rash

Instruction

Look at this patient.

Salient Features

HISTORY

- Ask if the rash is itchy.
- Ask where the rash started and ask the patient to describe its evolution.
- Take a drug history (e.g. penicillin, cephalosporins, allopurinol, nonsteroidal antiinflammatory drugs); include over-the-counter and herbal therapies.
- Ask if there is a history of fever (viral exanthems).
- Determine if there is mucosal involvement.
- Ask if there is a history of allergies.

EXAMINATION

- Reddish, blotchy maculopapular rash over the trunk (check the chest, back, and axillae) and limbs (Fig. 131.1).

Proceed as follows:
- Palpate the surface of the rash to confirm your inspection findings.
- Check the mucous membranes of the mouth.
- Examine for lymph nodes (glandular fever): some examiners may expect you to examine the lymph nodes as a part of the general examination. If the lymph nodes are palpable, then examine all groups (cervical, supraclavicular, axillary, and inguinal).

Note: Avoid waffling descriptions such as 'skin rash'.

Diagnosis

This patient has a maculopapular rash (lesion) caused by penicillin ingestion (aetiology), which usually resolves on discontinuing the drug (functional status).

Questions

What is your differential diagnosis?
- Drug-induced rash
- Glandular fever (rash seen in only 3% of patients with infectious mononucleosis but approaches 100% when these patients take amoxicillin).
- Viral exanthems (measles, rubella).

483

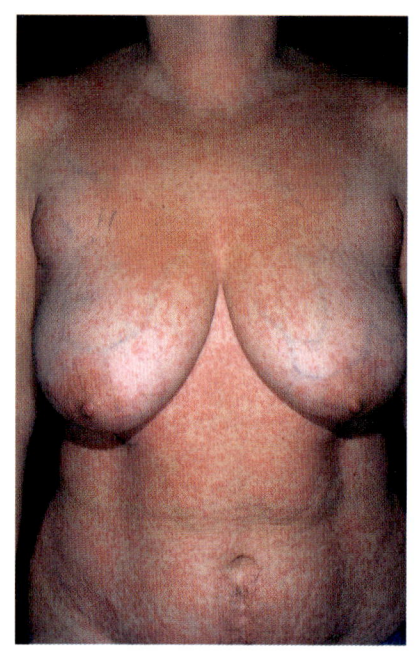

Fig. 131.1 Drug eruption (ampicillin): asymmetric, confluent maculopapular eruption. (With permission from Habif, T.P., 2009. Clinical Dermatology, fifth edn. Mosby, Philadelphia, PA.)

What is your differential diagnosis when the rash is associated with lymphadenopathy?
- Glandular fever
- Lymphoproliferative disorders such as Hodgkin disease
- HIV infection.

CHAPTER 132

Malignant Melanoma

Instruction
Look at this skin lesion.

Salient Features
HISTORY
- Age
- Family history (a patient with a dysplastic naevus with two relatives having malignant melanoma has a 300 times increased chance of having a malignant melanoma).
- Ask the patient:
  - has the mole changed in colour?
  - does the mole itch?
  - has it changed in shape/morphology?
  - does your skin have freckles or tendency to freckling?
  - how many moles does your skin have?
  - how many times in your life have you had bad sunburn (with peeling of your skin)?
- Remember MacKie's four independent risk factors for melanoma: freckles, moles (Fig. 132.1), atypical naevi (Fig. 132.2), and a history of severe sunburn.

EXAMINATION
- Irregular and asymmetrical, with a fuzzy border where the pigment appears to be leaking into the surrounding skin (Fig. 132.3). (The American Cancer Society mnemonic to suspect malignancy in a mole is ABCDE: **a**symmetry, **b**order irregular, **c**olour variegation and **d**iameter >6 mm, **e**levated lesions are more suspicious.)

Proceed as follows:
- Comment if the mole stands out from the patient's other moles.
- Comment if bleeding and ulceration are present (these are ominous signs).
- Examine regional lymph nodes and the liver (for metastatic spread).

Diagnosis
This patient has a malignant melanoma (lesion) as evidenced by its irregular border. Urgent biopsy and histological examination must be performed to exclude or confirm the diagnosis.

Questions

How would you describe a melanotic lesion?
There are different systems to use to aid the description and clinical identification of a potentially sinister lesion, one of which is the ABCDE description.

485

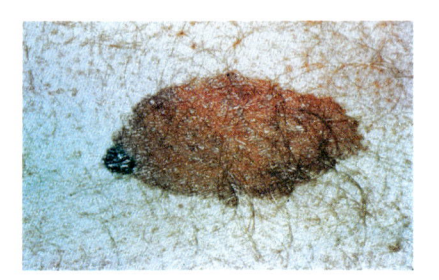

Fig. 132.1 Mole.

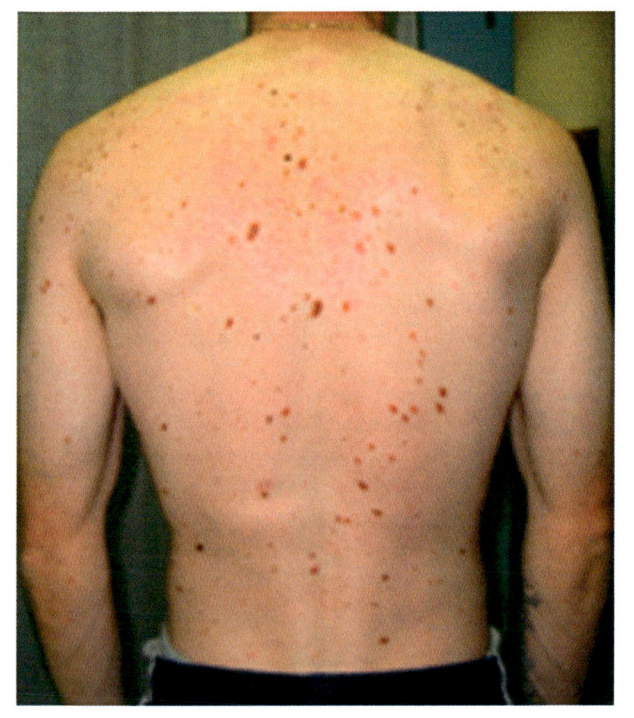

Fig. 132.2 The back of an individual with multiple atypical naevi.

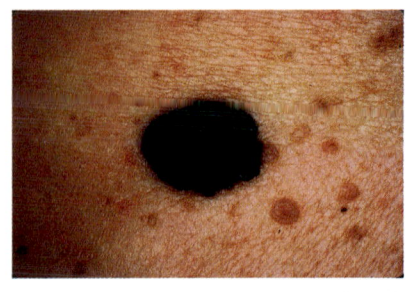

Fig. 132.3 Mole with pigment that appears to be leaking into surrounding skin.

Using the ABCDE description of melanoma, a suspicious lesion has the following characteristics:
- Asymmetry
- Border irregularity
- Colour variation
- Diameter more than 6 mm
- Evolving (changing in appearance or becoming larger).

What are the different types of malignant melanoma?
Depending on the clinical picture and histological findings, these include:
- superficially spreading malignant melanoma
- nodular malignant melanoma
- acral lentiginous melanomas (arising on the palms, soles, and nail beds)
- malignant melanoma on mucous membranes
- lentigo maligna melanoma (arising in lentigines in older individuals)
- amelanotic (nonpigmented) melanoma
- miscellaneous: melanoma arising from blue naevi, congenital, and giant naevocytic naevi.

What is the commonest type of melanoma?
The superficial spreading melanoma.

Name some risk factors for developing superficial spreading melanoma.
- Age
- Family history of melanoma
- Previous diagnosis of melanoma
- Previous basal or squamous cell carcinoma
- Multiple naevi
- Skin type and sunlight exposure/sunburns.

What are the patterns of growth of malignant melanoma?
- Radial growth: where the growth is horizontal within the epidermis and superficial dermal layers (e.g. lentigo maligna, acral/mucosal lentiginous, superficial spreading types). During this stage of growth, the tumour does not have the capacity to metastasize.
- Vertical growth: occurs with time, and the melanoma grows downward into the deeper dermal layers as an expansile mass lacking cellular maturation; this correlates with the emergence of a clone of cells with metastatic potential. The nature and extent of this vertical growth phase determine the biological behaviour of malignant melanoma

What is the treatment of such lesions?
Surgery remains the mainstay of treatment, and the extent of surgery depends on the thickness of the primary melanoma:
- Excision: following histological examination, the area is usually reexcised with margins dictated by the thickness of the tumour.
- Elective lymph node dissection is controversial; in general, it is indicated only in melanomas of intermediate thickness with one draining chain of lymph nodes.
- Adjuvant immunotherapy may be beneficial in selected patients.

What do you understand of the term Breslow thickness produced in a pathology report of an excised melanoma?
- It refers to the vertical thickness of the lesion excised from the superficial ulcer to the deepest end of the tumour, and it is a predictor of general outcome, as the thicker the lesion,

the more chances for metastasis. (Thin melanomas (<0.76 mm) approach 100% cure rate, whereas only 20%–30% survive for 5 years if the lesion has a depth of >1.6 mm.)

Name some other prognostic factors in melanoma except for tumour thickness.
- Level of invasion (deeper Clark levels are associated with greater chance of metastasis)
- Gender of the patient (female patients have a better prognosis)
- Anatomical location: melanomas in the TANS areas (thorax, upper arms, neck, and scalp) show a higher relative risk
- Specific mutations are associated with greater risk (mutation in the mitogen-activated protein kinase pathway carries a worse prognosis).

What are melanoma-associated genes?
Loss of CDKN2A alleles are observed in invasive melanoma. Other inherited forms of melanoma may be related to CDK4 mutations.

Further Information
Rona MacKie is contemporary Professor of Dermatology at the University of Glasgow.

CHAPTER 133

Molluscum Contagiosum

Instruction
Look at these skin lesions.

Salient Features
HISTORY
- Ask the patient whether there are similar lesions elsewhere.
- Ask for social history (travel history, towel, or bath share).
- Look for other areas affected.
- History of immunosuppression.

EXAMINATION
- Multiple rounded, dome-shaped, waxy papules that are 2 to 5 mm in diameter and contain central umbilication with a caseous plug (Fig. 133.1).
- The common sites are face, hands, lower abdomen, and genitals.

Proceed as follows:
- Tell the examiner that you would like to investigate for an underlying HIV infection.

Diagnosis
This patient has molluscum contagiosum (lesion), which is of viral aetiology; you would like to rule out an underlying HIV infection as the lesions are extensive and widely distributed on the face, neck, and other parts of the body.

Questions
How do these lesions spread?
- Direct body-to-body contact
- Indirect contact (towel share)
- Sexual contact
- Autoinoculation by scratching.

What is the histology of these lesions?
Microscopically, they show cup-like verrucous epidermal hyperplasia. Large inclusion bodies called 'molluscum bodies' are present in the cells of the stratum corneum and granulosum. These bodies are also seen in the curd-like material that can be expressed from the central umbilication. Numerous virions are present within the molluscum bodies.

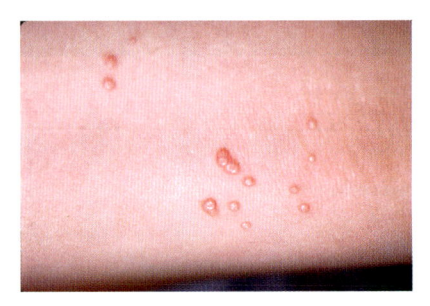

Fig. 133.1 Molluscum contagiosum. Multiple raised nodules, with areas of confluent lesions. (With permission from Rakel, D., 2007. Textbook of Family Medicine, seventh edn. Saunders, Philadelphia, PA.)

What is the aetiology of these lesions?
It is caused by a pox virus that is characteristically brick shaped and has a central dumb-bell-shaped DNA core.

How are these lesions treated?
- Cryotherapy (applications of liquid nitrogen to freeze the lesions)
- Curettage (scraping the lesion with a curette)
- Topical agents applied by physicians or patients (podophyllotoxin, antiseptics, salicylates, cantharidine).

Note: In children, these lesions tend to resolve spontaneously.

CHAPTER 134

Nail Changes

Instruction

Look at this person's fingernails.

Salient Features

- Disorders of the nail bed:
    - Terry's nail (Fig. 134.1): brownish-red distal transverse band; occurs normally in the elderly, also seen in cirrhosis and congestive cardiac failure
    - Lindsay's half-and-half nail (Fig. 134.2): distal brown band occupying about 25% to 50% of the nail bed and seen in chronic renal failure
    - Muehrcke's nail: pale transverse bands resulting from oedema of the nail bed; seen in hypoalbuminaemia
    - Onycholysis (see Fig.137.1).
- Disorders of the lunula:
    - Blue lunula: in Wilson disease, the normally white lunula becomes blue; the lunula has the largest area in the fingers closest to the thumb; in the elderly, it becomes smaller or absent.
- Disorders of the nail plate:
    - Clubbing
    - Leukonychia (Fig. 134.3): whitish discoloration, which may be diffuse (liver disease, congenital, fungal), punctate, or linear (Mees' lines (Fig. 134.4) seen in arsenical poisoning) or vasculitic
    - Koilonychia (spoon-shaped nails) seen in iron-deficiency anaemia, thyrotoxicosis
    - Onychogryphosis: hypertrophy and thickening of the nail
    - Onychomycosis: dystrophy, destruction of the nail caused by fungal or yeast infections
    - Pitting: seen in psoriasis, alopecia areata
    - Pterygium formation: growth of the cuticle onto the nail plate
    - Longitudinal brown streaks: junctional naevi seen in Black patients
    - Beau's lines (Fig. 134.5): transverse depression occurring in severe systemic illness; it allows estimation of the date of the illness (normal nail grows at the rate of 0.1 mm/day and it takes approximately 3 to 4 months for the nail plate to grow out completely).
- Disorders of the nailfold:
    - Nailfold telangiectasia: seen in dermatomyositis, scleroderma, collagen vascular disease
    - Paronychia: may be acute or chronic and includes the swelling and inflammation of the proximal or lateral nailfolds.

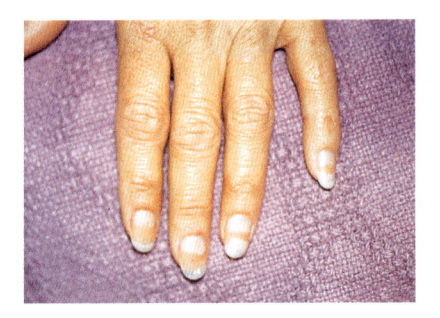

Fig. 134.1 Terry's nail.

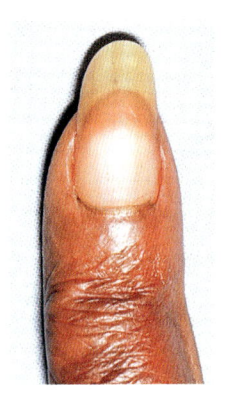

Fig. 134.2 Lindsay's half-and-half nail.

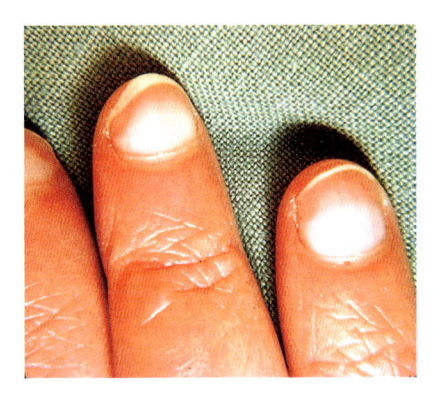

Fig. 134.3 Leukonychia.

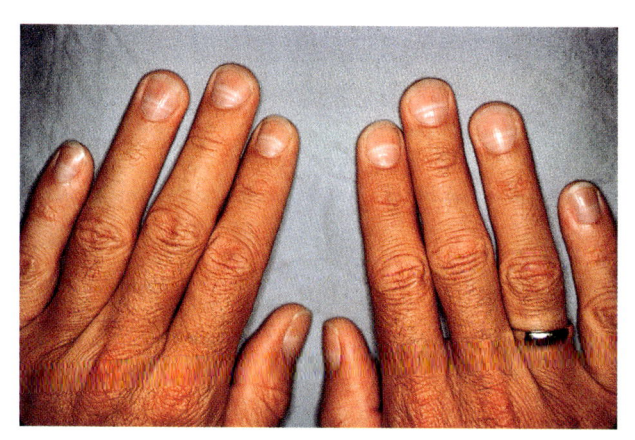

Fig. 134.4 Mees' lines.

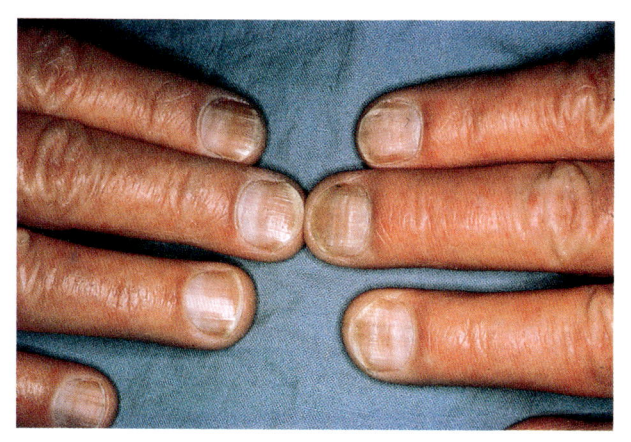

Fig. 134.5 Beau's lines.

- Disorder of the hyponychium:
  - Koenen subungual angiofibromas seen in tuberous sclerosis
  - Warts.

Note: The hyponychium is the most distal region of the nail bed and marks the transition to normal skin.

CHAPTER 135

Necrobiosis Lipoidica

Instruction

Look at this patient's legs.

Salient Features

HISTORY

- History of diabetes (previously the disease was thought to be exclusively related to diabetes).
- History of other autoimmune condition (thyroid disease, coeliac disease)
- Age and gender.

EXAMINATION

- Usually seen in females (two to four times more frequently than in men)
- Sharply demarcated oval plaques seen on the shin (Fig. 135.1), arms, or back
- The plaques have a shiny surface with yellow waxy atrophic centres and brownish red margins with surrounding telangiectasia.

Proceed as follows:
- Tell the examiner that you would like to check the urine for sugar.

Diagnosis

This patient has plaques with yellow waxy centres on the shins (lesions), likely to be necrobiosis lipoidica (aetiology), and there are clinical signs consistent with insulin use.

Remember: In necrobiosis lipoidica, the shins, ankles, and feet are typically affected, although 15% of patients may have lesions elsewhere.

Questions

What is the histology of these lesions?
Microscopy studies have shown that it is a disorder of collagen degeneration characterized by a granulomatous response (surrounded by epithelioid and giant cells), thickening of the walls of blood vessels, and fat deposition. The duration of the lesion can alter its histology; earlier lesions are richer in inflammatory cells, whereas older lesions are more atrophic and fibrotic.

What may complicate it?
Ulceration of the plaque.

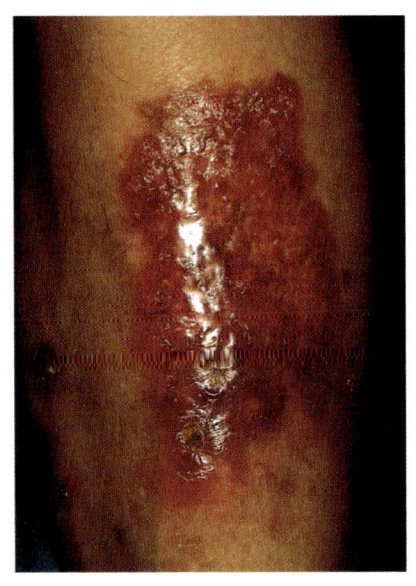

Fig. 135.1 Necrobiosis lipoidica diabeticorum. Well-demarcated, waxy erythematous plaques with prominent telangiectasias.

What treatment is available for such lesions?
- Topical steroids, or intralesional steroid injections
- Topical tacrolimus
- Phototherapy
- Hyperbaric oxygen.

Flare-ups are frequent. No treatment is completely effective.

What other skin lesions are usually seen on the shins?
- Erythema nodosum
- Pretibial myxoedema
- Diabetic dermopathy
- Erythema ab igne
- Livedo reticularis.

Name some other skin lesions that are seen in diabetes.
- Granuloma annulare
- Chronic pyogenic infections and carbuncles (indicating poor control)
- Eruptive xanthomata (from hypertriglyceridaemia associated with poor glycaemic control)
- Xanthelasmata
- Lipoatrophy and lipohypertrophy
- Leg ulcers and gangrene
- Acanthosis nigricans
- Diabetic dermopathy
- Peripheral anhidrosis (from autonomic neuropathy)
- Vulval candidiasis.

CHAPTER 136

Neurofibromatosis

Instruction

Examine this patient's skin.

Salient Features

HISTORY

- Presents in childhood with cutaneous features including café-au-lait spots, axillary freckles, and neurofibromas
- Obtain history of learning disabilities (about half the patients with neurofibroma 1 are affected).
- Childhood leukaemia: the risk of malignant myeloid disorders, particularly juvenile myelomonocytic leukaemia and the monosomy 7 syndrome (a childhood variant of myeloid dysplasia), is 200 to 500 times the normal risk.

EXAMINATION

- Check for multiple neurofibroma and café-au-lait spots (brown macules, >2.5 cm diameter and more than five lesions)
- Examine the axilla for freckles.
- Check visual acuity and fundus for retinal tumour (neurofibromatosis (NF); Fig. 136.1).
- Check hearing and corneal sensation for acoustic neuroma.
- Check the iris for Lisch nodules (often apparent only by slit-lamp examination). The incidence of Lisch nodules in type 1 increases with age (at the age of 5 years, only 22% have Lisch nodules, whereas at the age of 20 years, 100% have them). Therefore, older individuals who do not have Lisch nodules are unlikely to have type 1 NF (Fig. 136.2).
- Check the spine for kyphoscoliosis.
- Tell the examiner that you would like to check the blood pressure (for renal artery stenosis or phaeochromocytoma).

The triad for NF—neurofibroma, café-au-lait spots, and Lisch nodules—allows identification of virtually all patients with NF type 1.

Diagnosis

This patient has multiple café-au-lait spots and neurofibromas (lesion) caused by type 1 NF (von Recklinghausen disease) (aetiology), which are cosmetically disfiguring (functional status).

136 — NEUROFIBROMATOSIS

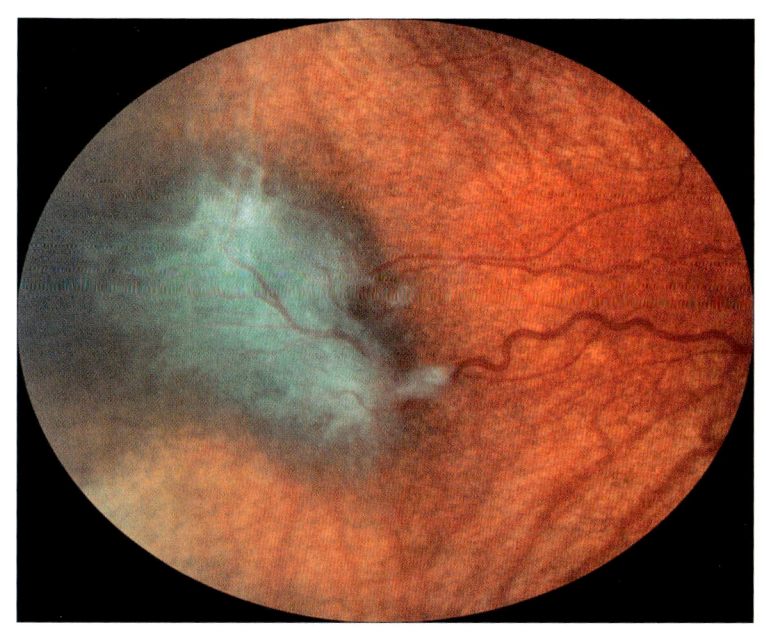

Fig. 136.1 Peripheral combined hamartoma of retina (From Yanoff, M., Duker, J., 2009. Ophthalmology, fifth edn. Elsevier.)

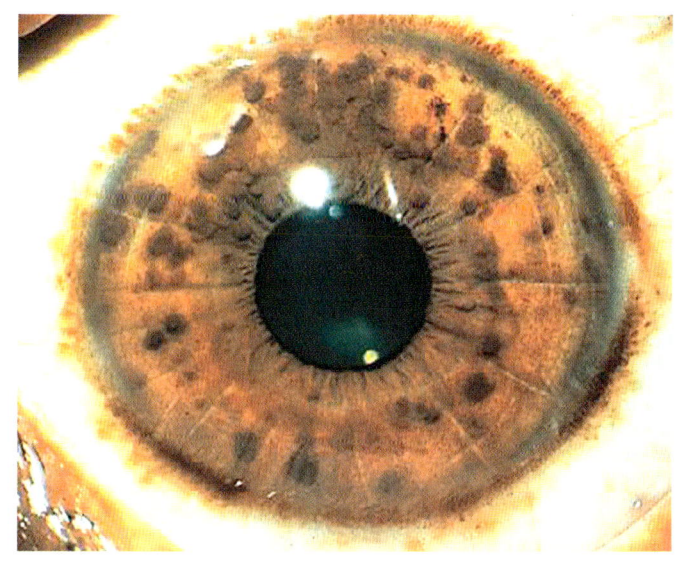

Fig. 136.2 Pigmented hamartomas of the iris (Lisch nodules). (From Zitelli, B.J., McIntire, S.C., Nowalk, A.J. (Eds.), 2012. Atlas of Pediatric Physical Diagnosis. Elsevier, Philadelphia.)

Questions

What are the criteria for neurofibromatosis type 1 (von Recklinghausen disease)?
NF type 1 may be diagnosed when two or more of the following are present:
- Six or more café-au-lait spots, the greatest diameter of which is >5 mm in prepubertal patients and >15 mm in postpubertal patients
- Two or more neurofibromas or one plexiform neurofibroma. Plexiform neurofibroma is considered by some to be a defining lesion of neurofibroma type 1.
- Freckling in the axilla or inguinal region (Crowe's sign)
- Retinal hamartoma
- Two or more Lisch nodules (iris hamartoma)
- A distinctive osseous lesion such as sphenoid dysplasia or thinning of long bone cortex with or without pseudarthroses
- A parent, sibling, or child with NF or a heterozygous pathogenic NF1 variant with a variant allele fraction of 50% in apparently normal tissue.

What are the diagnostic criteria for Legius syndrome?
Legius syndrome is an NF1-like disease but without the neurofibromata. The criteria are six or more café-au-lait macules bilaterally distributed and no other NF1-related diagnostic criteria except for axillary or inguinal freckling.

A heterozygous pathogenic variant in SPRED1 with a variant allele fraction of 50% in apparently normal tissue or a parent with Legius disease.

What are the criteria for neurofibromatosis type 2?
- Bilateral eighth nerve palsy confirmed by computed tomography or magnetic resonance imaging (MRI)
- A parent, sibling, or child with NF type 2 and either unilateral eighth nerve mass or any two of the following: neurofibroma, meningioma, glioma, schwannoma, or juvenile posterior subcapsular lenticular opacity.

Blockade of vascular endothelial growth factor with bevacizumab improves hearing in some patients (not all) with NF type 2 and has been associated with a reduction in the volume of most growing vestibular schwannomas.

What is the significance of the Lisch nodules?
Lisch nodules are melanocytic hamartomas that appear as well-defined, dome-shaped elevations projecting from the surface of the iris and are clear to yellow and brown. The incidence increases with age: at the age of 5 years, only 22% have Lisch nodules, whereas at the age of 20 years, 100% have them. Therefore, older patients who do not have Lisch nodules are also unlikely to have NF type 1. They are an important tool in establishing the diagnosis of NF type 1 and in providing accurate genetic screening.

What is the histology of the skin tumours?
The peripheral nerve tumours are of two types:
- Schwannomas: arise in cranial and spinal nerve roots and also in peripheral nerve trunks
- Neurofibromas: composed of a proliferation of all elements of the peripheral nerve including neuritis, Schwann cells, and fibroblasts. In sensory nerve twigs, they appear as subcutaneous nodules, while in peripheral nerve trunks, they may appear as a fusiform enlargement or a plexiform neurofibroma.

Is a biopsy of the neurofibromas required to make a diagnosis?
No, as the diagnosis is usually evident on clinical grounds.

What are the associated abnormalities of neurofibroma?
- Lung cysts
- Retinal hamartomas
- Skeletal lesions: rib notching and other erosive bony defects, intraosseous cystic lesions, subperiosteal bony cysts, dysplasia of the skull, bowed legs, and pseudarthrosis of the tibia
- Intellectual disability
- Aqueductal stenosis
- Epilepsy
- Sarcomatous change.

Is phaeochromocytoma common in this condition?
In NF type 1, phaeochromocytoma is relatively rare (<5%). Because of this, routine screening for the tumour is not generally recommended. Genetic testing in members of an affected family is possible. Phaeochromocytomas in affected individuals usually produce both adrenaline and noradrenaline.

What do you know about the inheritance of the two types?
Both are autosomal dominant syndromes, type 1 being carried on chromosome 17q11.2 and type 2 on chromosome 22. The gene for NF type 1 encodes a protein called neurofibromin (GTPase-activating protein), which downregulates the function of the p21 Ras oncoprotein. Learning disabilities have been ascribed to abnormal brain development, resulting from deficiency in neurofibromin signalling. The gene for type 2 NF (locus is 22q11) also encodes a tumour suppressor protein (merlin or schwannomin), which links integral membrane proteins of the cytoskeleton. How this protein is involved in tumorigenesis is not clear. Family members at risk for type 2 NF should be screened regularly with hearing tests and brainstem auditory evoked responses.

What screening would you do annually for these patients?
Asymptomatic adults with NF1 would usually require annual screening depending on the individual. MRI of plexiform neurofibromas, screening for phaeochromocytoma in suspected cases of hypertension, mammograms for women, dual-energy X-ray absorptiometry (DEXA) scan for osteoporosis, and depression assessment.

What is the risk of a further child being affected in a family?
If one parent is affected, then there is a 50% chance that another child will be affected, whereas when neither parent is affected, then the risk of another child being affected is no more than the standard risk in the normal population.

Further Information
The first case reports of probable neurofibromatosis appeared in the 16th century.

The first review of this condition was published in 1849 by Robert W. Smith, Professor of Surgery in Dublin, who suggested that the tumours originated from connective tissue surrounding small nerves.

Friedreich Daniel von Recklinghausen (1833–1910) was Professor of Pathology successively at Könisberg, Wüurzburg, and Strasbourg. He also described another disease, arthritis deformans neoplastica, to which his name is attached. Von Recklinghausen in 1882 was the first to recognize that the characteristic tumours arise from nervous tissue. He described in the report of his second case: 'His [a 47-year-old male] most striking abnormality consisted of innumerable tumours, running close to a thousand altogether, in the outer skin layer. …The patient could only report that he had had them as long as he could remember…and that they had increased markedly after his fifteenth year…my interest turned understandably to the externally palpable peripheral nerve trunks. …I was soon able clearly to recognise thickenings of these in their gross distribution'.

The elephant man, John Merrick, is commonly believed to have suffered from neurofibromatosis, but according to Wallace (1994) a rare condition, Proteus syndrome, is the more likely diagnosis.

Professor Lisch first described the association of the Lisch nodule with neurofibromatosis in 1937 (Lisch, 1937). These nodules were first described by Waardenburg in 1918, but he did not appreciate the association with neurofibromatosis.

CHAPTER 137

Onycholysis

Instruction
Examine this patient's hands.

Salient Features
HISTORY
- History of excessive exposure to detergents, alkalis and keratolytic agents, and demeclocycline-induced photolysis
- History of psoriasis
- History of thyrotoxicosis
- History of diabetes (fungal infection).

EXAMINATION
- Distal separation of the nail plate from the nail bed (Fig. 137.1)

Proceed as follows:
- Look for nail pitting and silvery white plaques (psoriasis).
- Glance at the neck for goitre and tell the examiner that you would like to exclude thyrotoxicosis, hypothyroidism, and diabetes mellitus.
- Tell the examiner that you would like to exclude a fungal infection.

Diagnosis
This patient has onycholysis (lesion), probably caused by thyrotoxicosis, as evidenced by tachycardia, exophthalmos, and goitre (aetiology).

Questions

What nail changes are associated with psoriasis?
Yellow, friable nails with pitting and onycholysis (lifting of nail from the bed), distal subungual hyperkeratosis.

How would you manage these nail lesions?
- Manicure and careful debridement
- Reduction of exposure to irritants (detergents, bleaches, alkalis)
- Intradermal steroids in the area of nail matrix (these are very painful injections).
- Nonsurgical removal of dystrophic nails using urea ointments.

501

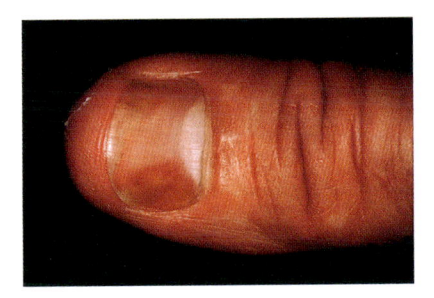

Fig. 137.1 Onycholysis.

What are Plummer nails?

This term refers to the onycholysis that occurs in hyperthyroidism and typically occurs in the fourth finger.

Further Information

S. Plummer (1874–1936), physician at the Mayo Clinic, Rochester, Minnesota, also described Plummer–Vinson syndrome (iron-deficiency anaemia and dysphagia).

CHAPTER 138

Palmar Xanthomata

Instruction
Examine this patient's hands.

Salient Features
HISTORY
- Family history of hyperlipidaemia and coronary artery disease.

EXAMINATION
- Yellowish-orange discolorations over the palmar and digital creases (Fig. 138.1)
- Look for the following signs:
  - Xanthelasmata around the eyes (see Fig. 155.1)
  - Tuboeruptive xanthomata around the elbows and knees (see Fig. 156.1F)
  - Signs of primary biliary cirrhosis.
- Tell the examiner that this patient probably has a type III hyperlipidaemia.

Note: A more generalized form may be associated with monoclonal gammopathy of myeloma or lymphoma.

Remember: Xanthomas are usually not present in mild to moderate hypertriglyceridaemia; when present, they do not help to distinguish the various hypertriglyceridaemic disorders.

Questions

How would you classify hyperlipidaemia?
Fredrickson classification, depending on laboratory findings:
- Type I: raised levels of chylomicrons and triglycerides, normal cholesterol concentration (pancreatitis, eruptive xanthomata, and lipaemia retinalis)
- Type IIa: raised low-density lipoprotein (LDL) and cholesterol levels, normal concentration of triglycerides (premature coronary artery disease, tendon xanthomata, and arcus corneae)
- Type IIb: raised levels of LDL, very-low-density lipoprotein (VLDL), cholesterol, and triglycerides (premature coronary artery disease)
- Type III: raised β-VLDL (cholesterol-rich) remnants, cholesterol, and triglycerides (premature coronary artery disease, peripheral vascular disease, palmar, and tuberous xanthomata)
- Type IV: raised VLDL and triglycerides, normal cholesterol (premature coronary artery disease: in some forms, risk of developing chylomicronaemia syndrome)
- Type V: raised chylomicrons, VLDL, cholesterol, and triglycerides (pancreatitis, eruptive xanthoma, lipaemia retinalis).

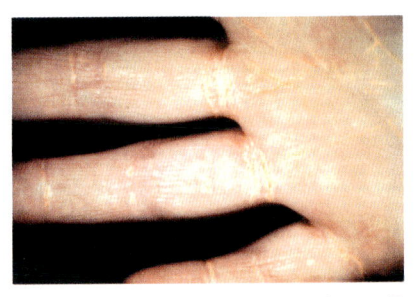

Fig. 138.1 Striate palmar xanthomata. (With permission from Durrington, P., 2003. Dyslipidaemia. Lancet 362, 717–731.)

What are the causes of hypercholesterolaemia?
- Primary hypercholesterolaemia: familial hypercholesterolaemia, familial combined hyperlipidaemia, polygenic hypercholesterolaemia
- Secondary hypercholesterolaemia: biliary cirrhosis, hypothyroidism, nephrotic syndrome, diet, drugs (thiazides, beta-blockers, oestrogens).

What is the histology of xanthomas?
Xanthomas are collections of foamy histiocytes within the dermis. These cells have abundant and finely vacuolated cytoplasm, giving it a foamy appearance. Cholesterol (both free and esterified), triglycerides, and phospholipids are present within the cell. Often, the cells are surrounded by inflammatory cells and fibrosis around the central zone of lipid-laden cells.

CHAPTER 139

Peutz–Jeghers Syndrome

Instruction
Look at this patient's face.

Salient Features
HISTORY
- Pain in the abdomen as a result of intestinal intussusception
- Haemorrhage in the upper gastrointestinal (GI) tract or rectal bleeding
- Family involvement (autosomal dominant).

EXAMINATION
- Pigmented freckles around the lips (Fig. 139.1A).

Proceed as follows:
- Look in the mouth for similar pigmentation (Fig. 139.1B) and anaemia.

Diagnosis
This patient has pigmented freckles around the lips (lesions) caused by Peutz–Jeghers syndrome (aetiology).

Questions

What are the types of colonic polyp?
There are numerous types of colonic polyps or polyp formations with different clinical behaviours, prognosis, and risk of dysplasia and malignancy. Some types of colonic polyps are:
- adenomas (with different endoscopic classifications and histological characteristics)
- hamartomas
- serrated and hyperplastic polyps
- other polypoid lesions: haemangiomas, lipomas, fibromas, endocrine tumours, perineuromas.

What is the histology of polyps in Peutz–Jeghers syndrome?
The polyps, which are large and pedunculated (can be >5 cm in diameter), histologically are hamartomas. They show an arborizing network of connective tissue and well-developed smooth muscle that extends into the polyp and surrounds; normal abundant glands are lined by normal intestinal epithelium rich in goblet cells. At endoscopy, their number varies from 1 to 20 per bowel segment and are more common in the small bowel but can also appear in the stomach and colon.

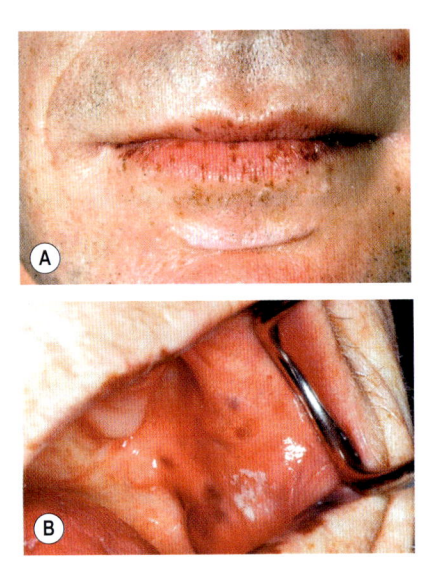

Fig. 139.1 Peutz–Jeghers syndrome. **(A)** Cutaneous pigmentation on the lips. **(B)** Pigment changes in the buccal mucosa. (With permission from Winship, I.M., Dudding, T.E., 2008. Lessons from the skin: cutaneous features of familial cancer. Lancet Oncol. 9, 462–472.)

What do you know about the genetics of Peutz-Jeghers syndrome?
The gene has been identified and encodes the serine threonine kinase LKB1 (STK11). Studies of the original kindred described by Peutz found an inactivating germline mutation in *LKB1*. The clinical features included GI polyposis, mucocutaneous pigmentation, nasal polyps, and rectal polyps. Family longevity was reduced by intestinal obstruction and malignant transformation.

What polyposis syndromes do you know?
- *Familial adenomatous polyposis* (FAP) is an autosomal dominant condition with the defect localized to *APC* on chromosome 5q21. There are several thousand polyps in the colon, which start to appear between the ages of 10 and 35 years. The potential malignant change is 100% by the age of 40 years. Hence, all relatives should be screened annually from the age of 12 years and all patients should have prophylactic colectomy by the age of 30.
- *Gardner syndrome*. This is a variant of FAP in which affected members develop extraintestinal soft tissue tumours (osteomas, lipomas, dermoid tumours) and pigmentation of fundi.
- *Turcot syndrome*. In this variant, central nervous system gliomas may also develop. Disruption of any of three genes—*APC, hMLH1*, or *hPMS2*—can lead to Turcot syndrome.
- *Familial juvenile polyposis* is an autosomal dominant condition occurring in children and teenagers. It causes GI bleeds, abdominal pain, diarrhoea, and intussusception. There is an increased incidence of malignant change in the interspersed adenomatous polyps. The affected genes are *Smad4 (DPC4), BMPR1A*, and *PTEN*.
- *Peutz-Jeghers syndrome* is an autosomal dominant condition characterized by mucocutaneous melanosis with GI hamartomas. The intestinal polyps may give rise to haematemesis, melaena or rectal bleeding, anaemia, or intussusception depending on their location. These polyps are usually found in the ileum and jejunum and they rarely undergo malignant change. However, affected people tend to have an increased incidence of other malignancies, both of GI tract (stomach and duodenum) and other viscera (lung, breasts, pancreas, and gonads).

- *Cronkhite–Canada syndrome* comprises sporadic, colonic, small bowel or gastric polyps associated with ectodermal changes such as hyperpigmentation, nail atrophy, and alopecia.
- *Cowden's disease* is an autosomal dominant condition characterized by multiple GI hamartomas with warty papules on the mucosa and by skin malformations. The affected genes are *PTEN (MMAC1, DEP1)*.
- *Bannayan–Riley–Ruvalcaba syndrome* comprises microcephaly, hamartomatous polyps, fibromatosis, speckled penis, and haemangiomas. The affected gene is *PTEN*.

Further Information

Morrison (1993) showed a classic picture of a patient with Peutz–Jeghers syndrome.

This condition was originally described by J.L. Peutz of Holland in 1921 and rediscovered by H.J. Jeghers et al. of the United States in 1949 (Jeghers, McKusick, Katz, 1949).

E.J. Gardner (1909–1989), US geneticist and Professor of Zoology at Utah University.

J. Turcot, Canadian surgeon, J.-P. Després, and F. St. Pierre first described Turcot syndrome in 1959. In 1949, H.W. Crail had described a similar syndrome (Crail, 1949).

L.W. Cronkhite, physician, Massachusetts General Hospital.

CHAPTER 140

Phlebitis Migrans

Instruction

Look at this patient's leg: he has had similar such lesions at different sites previously.

Salient Features

HISTORY

- Time course, pain, and tenderness of skin lesions
- Ask the patient about:
  - local trauma (including intravenous infusions)
  - gastrointestinal malignancies (pancreatic or gastric cancer)
  - history of oral contraceptives.

EXAMINATION

- Inflamed superficial leg veins.

Proceed as follows:
- Tell the examiner that you would like to investigate for the underlying malignancy, usually carcinoma of the pancreas or stomach.

Diagnosis

This patient has migratory phlebitis (lesion) and I would like to investigate for an underlying pancreatic or gastric malignancy (aetiology).

Questions

In which other condition is superficial phlebitis a prominent sign?
Thromboangiitis obliterans.

Is superficial thrombophlebitis associated with deep vein thrombosis?
It may be associated with occult deep vein thrombosis in about 20% of cases, although pulmonary emboli are rare.

Is phlebitis more frequently associated with plastic venous catheters or with steel intravenous needles?
It is more likely to be associated with plastic catheters, but this may be caused by the catheter remaining in the vein for longer periods (Fig. 140.1).

140 — PHLEBITIS MIGRANS

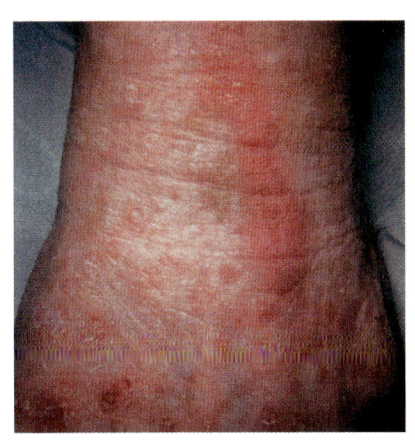

Fig. 140.1 Venous flare reaction overlying access vein of the forearm. (With permission from Abeloff, M.D., Armitage, J.O., Niederhuber, J.E., et al., 2008. Abeloff's Clinical Oncology, fourth edn. Churchill Livingstone, Edinburgh.)

How is superficial phlebitis treated?
- Local heat, elevation of the leg, and nonsteroidal antiinflammatory drugs
- When very extensive or in proximity to the saphenofemoral junction, ligation and division of the saphenous vein at the saphenofemoral junction (as pulmonary embolism may result if the phlebitis of the saphenous vein extends into the deep vein)
- Septic thrombophlebitis, which is usually caused by *Staphylococcus aureus*, requires excision of the involved vein up to its junction with an uninvolved vein in order to control infection.

What other dermatoses complicate pancreatic disease?
- Panniculitis
- 'Bronze' pigmentation of haemochromatosis
- 'Necrolytic migratory erythema' of glucagonoma syndrome
- Cutaneous haemorrhage of acute pancreatitis: 'bruising' of the left flank (Grey Turner's sign) or umbilicus (Cullen's sign).

Further Information

Armand Trousseau (1801–1867), physician at the Hôtel-Dieu in Paris, noted the sign as his death warrant, confirming his suspicion of an underlying malignancy in 1865. (Trousseau, 1872).

G. Grey Turner (1877–1951), Professor of Surgery, Hammersmith Hospital, London.

T.S. Cullen (1868–1953), Canadian born, Professor of Gynaecology, Johns Hopkins Hospital, Baltimore, USA.

CHAPTER 141

Pretibial Myxoedema

Instruction
Look at this patient's legs.

Salient Features
HISTORY
- Easy irritability, nervousness, insomnia
- Fatigue
- Weight loss with increased appetite
- Frequent defecation
- Oligomenorrhoea
- Dislike for hot weather, heat intolerance, excessive sweating
- Palpitations, dyspnoea
- Family history of thyroid disease
- Proximal muscle weakness, muscle atrophy, periodic paralysis (particularly in patients of East Asian ethnicity).

EXAMINATION
- Red thickened swellings above the lateral malleoli (peau d'orange appearance), which progresses to thickened nonpitting oedema of the feet
- Examine the following:
  - The hands for acropachy, palmar erythema, and warm, sweaty palms
  - The neck for goitre and thyroidectomy scar
  - The eyes for exophthalmos (see Fig. 79.1)
  - The pulse for tachycardia and atrial fibrillation.
- Tell the examiner that you would like to know whether or not the patient has had any treatment, in particular radioactive iodine.

> **Remember:**
> - Almost all cases of thyroid dermopathy are associated with relatively severe ophthalmopathy.
> - Usually, ophthalmopathy appears first and dermopathy much later.

Diagnosis
This patient has pretibial myxoedema (lesion) caused by Graves disease (aetiology) with ophthalmopathy and signs of thyrotoxicosis (functional status).

Questions

What investigations would you do?
Serum thyroxine (T_4), triiodothyronine (T_3), and thyroid-stimulating hormone (TSH).

How are these lesions treated?
- Mild and high-potency steroids applied topically
- Smoking cessation
- Compression stockings for lymphoedema
- Cytotoxic therapy, immunosuppression, systemic steroids, plasmapheresis, and immunoglobulin are some treatments that have been reported.
- Octreotide.

Note: Surgical excision should be avoided because surgical scars may aggravate the dermopathy and precipitate recurrence.

What are the types of pretibial myxoedema?
Three major classes of thyroid dermopathy have been identified (pretibial myxoedema; Fig. 141.1):
- Nonpitting oedema accompanied by hyperkeratosis, pigmentation and pinkish, brownish red or yellowish discoloration of the skin, plaque formation, and nodularity characteristically absent in this group
- Plaque form, consisting of raised, discrete, or confluent plaques
- Nodular form, characterized by nodule formation.

Less common types:
- Elephantiasic form
- Polypoid form.

Note: Almost all patients tend to have ophthalmopathy, which is usually severe.

What is the histology of pretibial myxoedema?
- Characteristic features include fraying and oedematous appearance on routine staining with haematoxylin and eosin and an increase in mucinous material staining with Alcian blue–periodic acid–Schiff, with resultant connective tissue fibre separation.
- Review of pathology reports does not show any distinguishing microscopic characteristics for various clinical forms of this dermopathy.

What is the pathogenesis of pretibial myxoedema?
- All patients with localized myxoedema have high serum concentrations of TSH receptor antibodies, indicating the severity of the autoimmune condition.
- Occurrence of thyroid dermopathy in areas other than pretibial skin indicates a systemic process.
- Similar to Graves eye disease, TSH receptors in the connective tissue may be the antigen responsible for the immune process.
- Both humoral and cellular immune mechanisms are involved in the stimulation of fibroblasts and the production of large amounts of glycosaminoglycans.
- Localization in the pretibial area relates to mechanical factors and dependent position.

What are the recommendations for screening thyroid dysfunction?
It is not proven yet if a screening programme for the general population is beneficial in the absence of clinical suspicion of thyroid disease. Routine screening is not currently offered. The indication

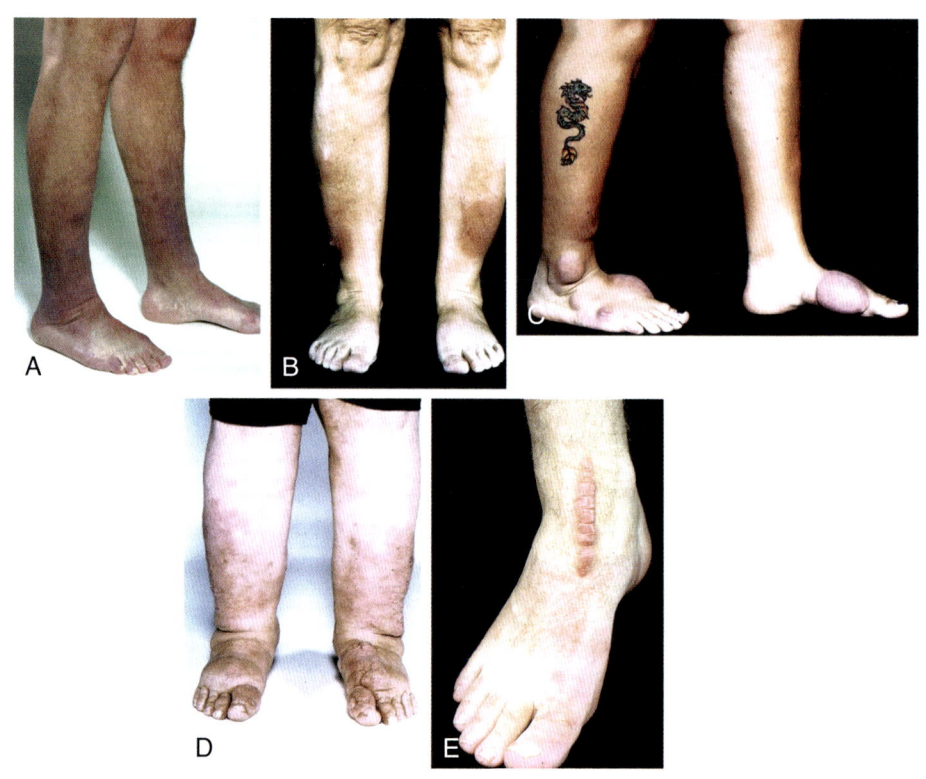

Fig. 141.1 Thyroid dermopathy (localized myxedema) in five patients. **(A)** Nonpitting oedema form in pretibial area. **(B)** Plaque form in pretibial area. **(C)** Nodular form in ankle and foot. **(D)** Elephantiasic form. **(E)** Occurrence of thyroid dermopathy in scar tissue. (With permission from Schwartz, K.M., Fatourechi, V., Ahmed, D.D., Pond, G.R., 2002. Dermopathy of Graves' disease (pretibial myxedema): long-term outcome. J. Clin. Endocrinol. Metab. 87, 438–446.)

for screening is particularly compelling in women, but it may also be justified in men as a relatively cost-effective measure in the context of periodic health examination.

How can hyperthyroidism present in the elderly?

Thyrotoxicosis can present in the elderly with atrial fibrillation and such patients may lack other common signs of thyrotoxicosis; this is known as apathetic hyperthyroidism. Also, low serum TSH is a risk factor for atrial fibrillation in the elderly. Osteoporosis may be the result of subclinical thyrotoxicosis.

CHAPTER 142

Pseudoxanthoma Elasticum

PATIENT 1

Instruction
Look at this patient's fundus.

Salient Features
HISTORY
- Family history (either autosomal recessive, the most common, or autosomal dominant; the gene for both forms has been mapped to chromosome 16)
- Upper gastrointestinal (GI) haemorrhage, myocardial infarction, stroke and intermittent claudication, visual loss
- Hypertension (from involvement of renal vasculature)
- Intracranial haemorrhage.

EXAMINATION
- Fundus shows angioid streaks: linear grey or dark red streaks with irregular edges lying beneath the retinal vessels (Fig. 142.1) (roughly 50% of patients with angioid streaks have pseudoxanthoma elasticum, whereas 85% of those with pseudoxanthoma have angioid streaks).

Proceed as follows:
- Look at the neck (Fig. 142.2), antecubital fossae, axillae (Fig. 142.3), groin, and periumbilical region for loose 'chicken skin' appearance of skin.
- Examine the peripheral pulses: absent pulses from peripheral arterial involvement but acral ischaemia is uncommon because of development of collaterals.

Diagnosis
This patient has angioid streaks on fundoscopy and 'chicken-skin' appearance in the neck and axillae (lesions) caused by pseudoxanthoma elasticum (aetiology).

PATIENT 2

Instruction
Look at this patient.

513

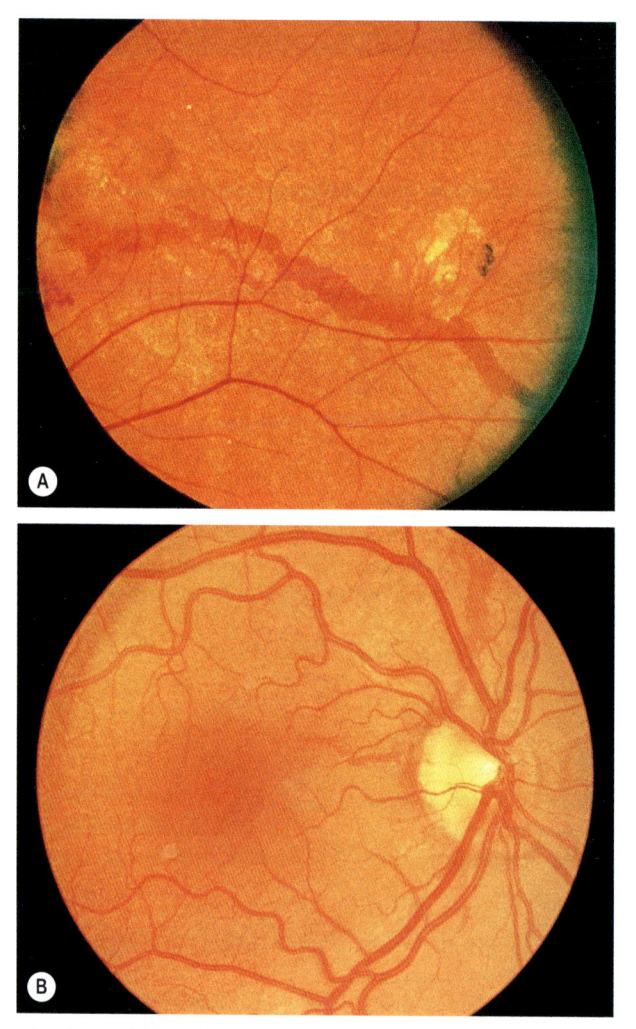

Fig. 142.1 Fundus showing angioid streaks.

Salient Features

EXAMINATION

- Small yellow papules arranged in a linear or reticular pattern in plaques on the neck, axillae, cubital fossae, periumbilical region, and groin.

Proceed as follows:
- Tell the examiner that you would like to examine the fundus.

Diagnosis

This patient has 'chicken-skin' appearance in the neck and axillae (lesions) caused by pseudoxanthoma elasticum (aetiology).

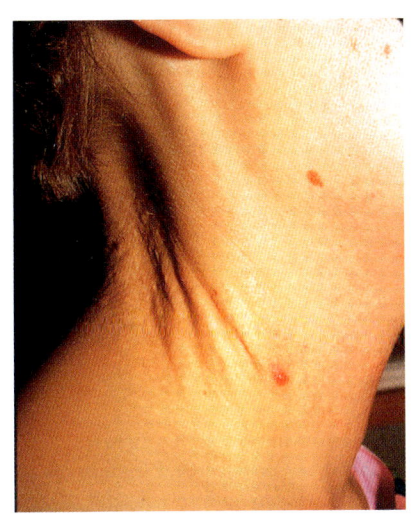

Fig. 142.2 'Chicken skin' appearance of neck.

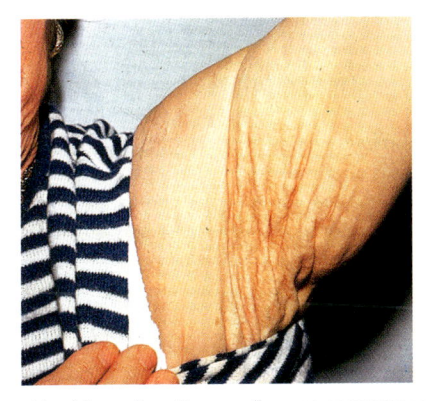

Fig. 142.3 Thickened sagging skin of the axilla with peau d'orange appearance.

Questions

In which other conditions are angioid streaks seen?
- Paget disease
- Haematological conditions like sickle cell disease, spherocytosis, and thalassaemias
- Ehlers–Danlos syndrome
- Other conditions: alpha-beta lipoproteinaemia, hyperphosphataemia, lead poisoning, trauma, pituitary disorders, and intracranial disorders.

What causes angioid streaks?
They are caused by abnormal elastic tissue in Bruch's membrane of the retina.

Which fundal finding is virtually pathognomonic of pseudoxanthoma elasticum?
'Leopard skin spotting' changes, which consist of yellowish mottling of the posterior pole temporal to the macula. These may antedate angioid streaks.

What is the triad of pseudoxanthoma elasticum, angioid streaks, and vascular abnormalities known as?
Groenblad–Strandberg syndrome.

What are the cardiovascular manifestations of this condition?
- Mitral valve prolapse
- Restrictive cardiomyopathy
- Renovascular hypertension
- Premature coronary artery disease resembling accelerated atherosclerosis from calcification of the internal elastic laminae of arteries. Arterial grafts should not be used for coronary artery bypass surgery in these patients because of possible calcification of the internal elastic laminae of the internal mammary artery.
- Peripheral vascular disease.

What are the gastrointestinal manifestations of this disease?
GI haemorrhage, particularly during the first decade. Bleeding complications can be prevented by avoiding aspirin in patients with pseudoxanthoma elasticum.

What are the causes of visual loss in pseudoxanthoma elasticum?
Macular involvement by a streak, disciform scarring secondary to choroidal haemorrhage or traumatic macular haemorrhage.

What are cutaneous histological features of pseudoxanthoma elasticum?
The histological diagnosis is made by doing a 4-mm punch biopsy of scars or flexural skin of the neck or axillae in patients who have angioid streaks on fundoscopy but no visible skin lesions. The Verhoeff–van Gieson stain (for elastic tissue) reveals characteristic fragmentation and clumping of elastic tissue in the middle and deep dermis. The von Kossa stain (for calcium) shows staining of calcified elastic tissue in the middle and deep dermis. Calcified elastic tissue is the hallmark of pseudoxanthoma elasticum. An arteriolar sclerosis develops in the media of muscular arteries and arterioles and as a result the lumen may become progressively and concentrically narrowed.

What do you know about the genetics of this disorder?
A mutation affecting *ABCC6* encoding the multidrug resistance-associated protein MRP6 is the cause in 80%. This protein is a homologue of the cellular export pumps of the adenosine triphosphatase-binding cassette transporter superfamily. *ABCC6* is primarily expressed in the liver and kidneys, suggesting that pseudoxanthoma elasticum may be a metabolic disorder.

Which heritable connective-tissue disorders are associated with the presence of intracranial aneurysm and subarachnoid haemorrhage?
Polycystic kidney disease, Ehlers–Danlos syndrome (type IV), pseudoxanthoma elasticum, and fibromuscular dysplasia.

Further Information

K.W.L. Bruch (1819–1884), Professor of Anatomy at Giessen, Germany.
E.E. Groenblad, Swedish ophthalmologist and J. Strandberg, Swedish dermatologist.
T.L. Terry (1899–1946), Head of Ophthalmology at Harvard University, described angioid streaks in Paget disease.

CHAPTER 143

Psoriasis

Instruction
Look at this patient.
Do a general examination.

Salient Features
HISTORY
- Symptoms (itching, pain, flexural intertrigo, limitation of manual dexterity), cosmetic problems, or both
- Joint pains (psoriatic arthropathy; psoriatic arthritis may be found in 10%–15% of patients)
- Family history (30% of patients have family history)
- Aggravating factors (emotional stress, overuse of alcohol, streptococcal infections, drugs such as beta-blockers, lithium, or tumour necrosis factor-α therapies).

EXAMINATION
- Well-demarcated salmon pink plaques with silvery white scales (Fig. 143.1) over extensor surfaces, scalp, naval, and natal cleft. They often tend to have a pink or red line in the intergluteal fold.
- A white blanching ring, known as *Woronoff's ring*, may be observed in the skin surrounding a psoriatic plaque.

Proceed as follows:
- Look at the nails for pitting (Fig. 143.2) and onycholysis (separation of the nail plate from the bed).

Diagnosis
This patient has silvery white scales and nail pitting (lesion) caused by psoriasis (aetiology), with considerable itching (functional status).

Questions

What are the characteristics of psoriasis?
Psoriasis is a papulosquamous disease with variable morphology, distribution, severity, and course. Papulosquamous diseases are characterized by scaling papules (raised lesions <1 cm in diameter) and plaques (raised lesions >1 cm in diameter). Other papulosquamous diseases include tinea infections, pityriasis rosea, and lichen planus.

The lesions of psoriasis are distinct and are classically very well circumscribed, circular, red papules, or plaques with a grey or silvery-white dry scale. In addition, the lesions are typically distributed symmetrically on the scalp, elbows, knees, lumbosacral area, and in the body folds.

517

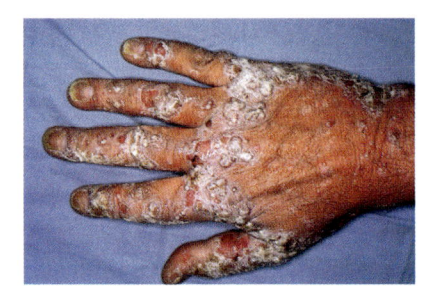

Fig. 143.1 Psoriasis.

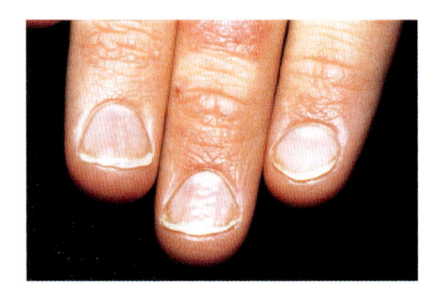

Fig. 143.2 Nail pitting.

How common is this condition?
It affects 1% to 2% of the population of the United Kingdom.

What are the typical features of psoriatic plaques?
Distinguishing features include:
- silvery colour of the scaling
- moist red surface on removal of the scales (*Bulkeley's membrane*)
- capillary bleeding when the individual silvery scales are plucked from the plaque (*Auspitz's sign*)
- new skin lesions at the site of trauma (*Koebner's phenomenon*).

How is the severity of involvement usually estimated?
- The patient's own perception of the disability
- Objective assessment of disability.

It is usually estimated by using the *Psoriasis Area and Severity Index*, which takes into consideration the area of involvement, thickness, redness, and scaling. The maximal score on this index is 72, with mild, moderate, and severe having scores of <10, 10 to 50, and >50, respectively.

What are the types of psoriasis?
Depending on the natural history:
- Type 1: young patients with a strong family history have a more aggressive disorder
- Type 2: older patients with no family history have a more indolent course.

Depending on the nature of skin lesion:
- *Chronic plaque psoriasis*. With gradual peripheral extension, plaques may develop different configurations, including:
    - psoriasis gyrata, in which curved linear patterns predominate
    - annular psoriasis, in which ring-like lesions develop secondary to central clearing

- psoriasis follicularis, in which minute scaly papules are present at the openings of pilosebaceous follicles.
- *Rupioid* and *ostraceous*, which relate to distinct morphological subtypes of plaque psoriasis:
    - Rupioid plaques are small (2–5 cm in diameter) and highly hyperkeratotic, resembling limpet shells.
    - Ostraceous plaques are hyperkeratotic with relatively concave centres, similar in shape to oyster shells.
- *Inverse psoriasis*: plaques evolve in the intertriginous areas and therefore lack the typical silver scale appearance because of moisture and maceration.
- *Guttate psoriasis*: numerous small papular lesions with silvery scaling evolve suddenly over the body surface, often the trunk, upper arms, and thighs. Often precipitated by streptococcal infection. Commonly spontaneously clears completely.
- *Pustular psoriasis*: can be localized or generalized; superficial pustules may stud the plaques.
- *Erythrodermic psoriasis*: generalized erythema and scaling; can be life threatening.

What do you know about the genetics of psoriasis?
- Clear identification of the causative gene has been difficult because of the extensive linkage disequilibrium (i.e. genes on one chromosome are inherited together and are not easily separable by recombination events) observed within the major histocompatibility complex (MHC).
- The major genetic determinant of psoriasis is *PSORS1*, which probably accounts for 35% to 50% of the heritability of the disease in multiple genome-wide studies. *PSORS1* is located within the MHC on chromosome 6p. Guttate psoriasis (an acute-onset form usually occurring in adolescents) is strongly associated with *PSORS1*, whereas late-onset cases of psoriasis vulgaris (usually in persons >50 years of age) and palmoplantar pustulosis are not associated with *PSORS1*.
- In a genome-wide association study, polymorphisms in the genes for interleukin-12 (*IL12B*) and interleukin-23 (*IL23R*) were associated with psoriasis. These interleukins are cytokines that induce naive CD4 T cells to differentiate into type 1 helper T cells (Th1 cells) and type 17 helper T cells (Th17 cells), respectively; they have been identified as key mediators of psoriasis.

What do you know about the pathology of plaque psoriasis?
- Hyperproliferation of the epidermis
- Inflammation of the epidermis and dermis.

What do you understand by the term Koebner phenomenon?
Injury or irritation of psoriatic skin tends to provoke lesions of psoriasis in the site of trauma in some patients: this is known as the Koebner phenomenon.

Mention a few exacerbating factors.
- Drugs: beta-blockers, angiotensin-converting enzyme inhibitors, lithium, indomethacin, antimalarials, alcohol
- Psychological factors
- Infection: β-haemolytic streptococci, HIV (Preexisting psoriasis may become more refractory to therapy and plaque psoriasis may change to the guttate form in HIV-positive patients.)
- Injury to the skin: mechanical injury, sunburn.

How would you manage a patient with psoriasis?
- Educate the patient that there is no cure and that only suppression of the disease is possible.
- Weight loss and smoking cessation may lower the risk or severity of psoriasis. Avoiding alcohol excess may also reduce severity.

- Indications for treatment include symptoms (itching, pain, flexural intertrigo, limitation of manual dexterity), cosmetic problems, or both.
- Initial treatment is topical when <20% of the body is involved.
- Topical therapy in some form is usually the mainstay of treatment and includes:
    - emollients (soft yellow paraffin or aqueous cream)
    - keratolytic agents (salicylic acid)
    - coal tar, which is usually used in combination with ultraviolet B phototherapy: *Goeckerman treatment*
    - dithranol used on plaques for 10 to 30 min a day before removal and washed off can be effective in short courses. It is staining and irritable to normal skin so should be used with care.
    - topical steroids, such as betamethasone ointment
    - calcipotriol (vitamin D), which is known to act locally to increase extracellular calcium concentrations, which leads to increased keratinocyte differentiation and decreased proliferation and scaling; it is an excellent alternative to steroids.
- Systemic therapy:
    - Phototherapy (ultraviolet B radiation): narrowband ultraviolet B has replaced broadband ultraviolet B as it induces longer remissions and fewer burns.
    - Photochemotherapy (methotrexate with ultraviolet A therapy)
    - Methotrexate
    - Etretinate and acitretin (vitamin A derivatives), retinoids
    - Systemic steroids
    - Ciclosporin, tacrolimus, or mycophenolate mofetil.
- Biological therapies:
    - Anti-CD4 monoclonal antibody, e.g. ibalizumab
    - Biologic agents that block both interleukin-12 and interleukin-23, e.g. ustekinumab; interleukin-17 inhibitors such as secukinumab
    - Agents that selectively block tumour necrosis factor-α, e.g. etanercept, adalimumab, infliximab
    - There are few head-to-head trials between these biological therapies, but meta-analyses suggest that whilst all are very effective compared with placebo and methotrexate, adalimumab, secukinumab, and ustekinumab had the best tolerability.

What are the indications for systemic treatment?
- Failure of topical therapy
- Repeated hospital admissions for topical treatment
- Extensive plaque psoriasis in the elderly
- Generalized pustular or erythrodermic psoriasis
- Severe psoriatic arthropathy.

What underlying condition would you suspect when psoriasiform lesions are seen on the nose, ears, fingers, and toes?
Such lesions are paraneoplastic eruptions associated with squamous cell carcinoma of the oropharynx, tracheobronchial tree, and oesophagus: this is known as *Bazex syndrome*.

Further Information

B. Russell, in 1950, proposed that psoriasis be known by the eponym Willan–Plumbe syndrome. The first clear descriptions were by Willan (1808) and Plumbe (1824) and ended hundreds of years of confusion and laid the foundation for establishing psoriasis as a disease entity that is separate from leprosy.

CHAPTER 144

Purpura

Instruction
Examine this patient's skin.

Salient Features
HISTORY
- Drug history: steroids, anticoagulants, carbimazole, phenylbutazone, chloramphenicol, gold salts
- Age (senile purpura)
- History of chronic liver disease (thrombocytopenia)
- History of mouth ulcers (severe neutropenia).

EXAMINATION
- Small circumscribed bleeding into the skin from small blood vessels, purpura, or larger lesions, bruises, or ecchymoses (Fig. 144.1). Lesions begin as 1- to 3-mm papules, which increase in size and become palpable. They may coalesce to form plaques; in some instances, they may ulcerate.

Proceed as follows:
- Look for an underlying cause.
- Comment on the patient's age: consider senile purpura.
- Comment on the distribution: Henoch–Schönlein purpura is seen over the buttocks and lower limbs.
- Look for the following signs:
  - Rheumatoid arthritis where purpura is drug induced (steroids, gold)
  - Anaemia (leukaemia, marrow aplasia, or infiltration)
  - Chronic liver disease
  - Ulcers in the mouth (severe neutropenia)
  - Bleeding gums, corkscrew hair, and perifollicular haemorrhages of scurvy (particularly in the elderly)
  - Stigmata of Ehlers–Danlos syndrome
  - Bleeding from multiple venepuncture sites (disseminated intravascular coagulation).

Tell the examiner that you would like to examine the spleen, liver, and lymph nodes.

Diagnosis
This patient has purpura (lesion) that is caused by ingestion of steroids (aetiology) and is cosmetically unacceptable to the patient (functional status).

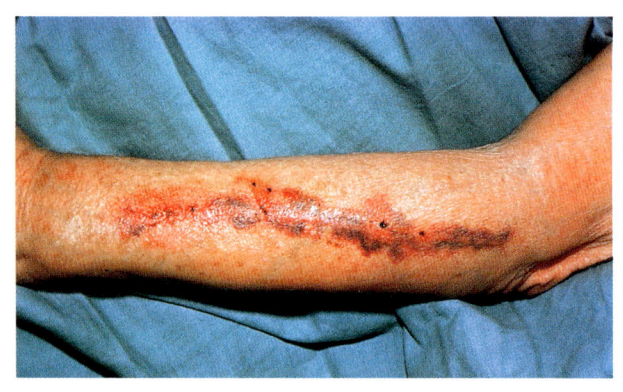

Fig. 144.1 Purpura.

Questions

What are the common causes of purpura?
- Senile purpura, as a result of age-related or sun damage changes in the vessel walls in skin
- Purpura induced by steroids or anticoagulants
- Thrombocytopenia caused by:
  - Primary autoimmune thrombocytopenia
  - Leukaemia and marrow aplasia
  - Chronic liver disease and splenomegaly
  - Heparin-induced thrombocytopenia: antiplatelet antibodies induce platelet plugs which block capillaries.

What are causes of bruising?
- Thrombocytopenia: idiopathic thrombocytopenic purpura, marrow replacement by leukaemia, or secondary infiltration
- Vascular defects: senile purpura, steroid-induced purpura, Henoch–Schönlein purpura, scurvy (vitamin C deficiency), von Willebrand disease, uraemia
- Coagulation defects: haemophilia, anticoagulants, Christmas disease
- Drugs: thiazides, sulphonamides, phenylbutazone, sulphonylureas, sulindac, barbiturates.

What do you know about Moschcowitz syndrome?
Moschcowitz syndrome or thrombotic thrombocytopenic purpura is an acute disorder characterized by thrombocytopenic purpura, microangiopathic haemolytic anaemia, transient and fluctuating neurological features, fever, and renal impairment.

Further Information

E. Moschcowitz (1879–1964), New York physician.

In 1951, William Harrington, then a trainee in haematology at the Barnes Hospital in St. Louis, Missouri, had severe thrombocytopenia immediately after voluntarily receiving plasma from a patient with the disease, establishing beyond doubt that a plasma factor causes the destruction of platelets in chronic idiopathic thrombocytopenic purpura.

CHAPTER 145

Pyoderma Gangrenosum

Instruction
Look at this patient's skin.

Salient Features
HISTORY
- Diarrhoea (inflammatory bowel disease)
- Joint pains (rheumatoid arthritis)
- Leukaemia, multiple myeloma.

EXAMINATION
- Necrotic ulcer with purplish overhanging edges, usually seen on the lower limbs or trunk (Fig. 145.1).

Diagnosis
These are necrotic ulcers (lesions), which are a feature of pyoderma gangrenosum (aetiology). I would like to investigate for underlying inflammatory bowel disease.

Questions

How is the diagnosis of pyoderma gangrenosum established?
Pyoderma gangrenosum is a clinical diagnosis, based on history and the appearance of the ulcer, and biopsy is performed only to exclude other conditions if there is clinical doubt. Clinical criteria have been proposed and they are as follows:
- Major criteria that must be present to achieve a diagnosis:
  - Rapid progression of a painful, necrotic, cutaneous ulcer with irregular, violaceous, and undermined border, and all other causes of cutaneous ulceration excluded.
- Minor criteria (two out of four must be present):
  - History suggestive of pathergy or clinical finding of cribriform scarring, systemic disease associated with the lesion, histopathologic findings, treatment response (rapid response to systemic glucocorticoid treatment).

Except for the lower limbs, can pyoderma gangrenosum appear in other body sites?
Variants have been described based on the location of the lesion or the associated process, the skin lesion being similar to the classic pyoderma gangrenosum:
- Peristomal pyoderma gangrenosum at the site of ileostomy (Fig. 145.2) or colostomy in ulcerative colitis or Crohn's disease
- Vulvar pyoderma gangrenosum

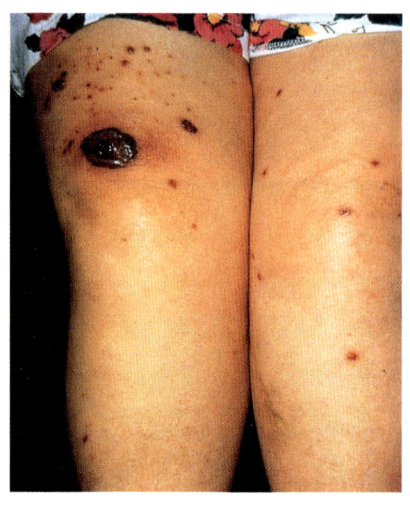

Fig. 145.1 Pyoderma gangrenosum.

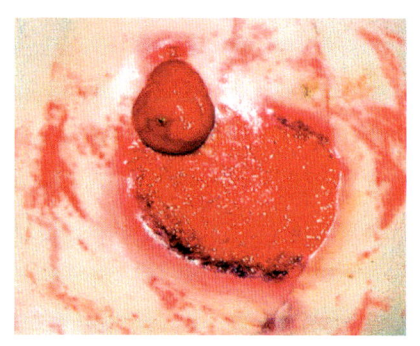

Fig. 145.2 Pyoderma gangrenosum at ileostomy site. (With permission from Ennis, O., Feroz, A., Stephenson, B.M., Allison, M.C., 2001. Para-ileostomy pyoderma gangrenosum. Lancet. 358, 533.)

- Penile or scrotal in adolescent adults
- Pyostomatitis vegetans is an oral variant with chronic pustular and, eventually, vegetative lesions in the mucous membrane of the mouth.

What is the histology in this condition?
Nonspecific features including massive neutrophilic infiltration, haemorrhage, and necrosis of the epidermis.

How would you evaluate these patients?
- Detailed history and physical examination
- Skin biopsy (with cultures for bacteria, fungus, and virus)
- Gastrointestinal (GI) studies
- Serology for antineutrophil cytoplasmic antibodies (ANCAs), antinuclear antibodies, antiphospholipid antibody, and serum protein electrophoresis
- Complete blood count, peripheral smear, and bone marrow examination.

In which conditions can pyoderma gangrenosum be seen?
- Ulcerative colitis
- Crohn's disease
- Chronic active hepatitis
- Rheumatoid arthritis, seronegative arthritis associated with GI symptoms
- Acute and chronic myeloid leukaemia, myelocytic leukaemia, hairy cell leukaemia
- Polycythaemia rubra vera
- Multiple myeloma
- Immunoglobulin A monoclonal gammopathy
- PAPA syndrome (pyogenic arthritis, pyoderma gangrenosum, and acne).

How would you manage these lesions?
- Topical steroids
- Intralesional steroids
- Topical calcineurin inhibitors
- Topical therapy, including dressings, limb elevation, rest
- Surgery is avoided
- Systemic therapy with corticosteroids or steroid sparing agents used in more extensive or refractory disease
- Treatment of the underlying cause.

What conditions can be mistaken for pyoderma gangrenosum?
Six broad disease categories may simulate pyoderma gangrenosum:
- Vascular occlusive or venous disease: anti-phospholipid antibody syndrome, livedoid vasculopathy, venous stasis ulceration, small-vessel occlusive arterial disease, type I cryoglobulinaemia, Klippel–Trénaunay–Weber syndrome
- Vasculitis: Wegener granulomatosis, polyarteritis nodosa, cryoglobulinaemic (mixed) vasculitis, Takayasu arteritis
- Infection: herpes simplex virus, cutaneous tuberculosis, *Entamoeba histolytica* (amoeba cutis), deep fungal infections such as *Penicillium marneffei*, sporotrichosis, aspergillosis, cryptococcosis, and zygomycosis
- Malignancy: lymphoma, Langerhans cell histiocytosis, leukaemia cutis
- Exogenous tissue injury: drug induced or direct injury
- Other inflammatory disorders.

How would you exclude these lesions?
- History. Markedly painful ulcer, rapid progression of ulceration, type of skin lesion preceding the ulcer (papule, pustule, or vesicle), minor trauma (pathergy) preceding development of the ulcer, symptoms of an associated disease (e.g. inflammatory bowel disease or arthritis)
- Medication history (e.g. bromides, iodide, hydroxyurea, or granulocyte–macrophage colony-stimulating factor)
- Examination. Characteristic features of ulcer: tenderness, necrosis, irregular violaceous border, undermined, rolled edges
- Skin biopsy. Elliptical incisional biopsy preferable to punch biopsy (include inflamed border and ulcer edge at a depth that includes subcutaneous fat). The inflamed border is examined for routine histology (haematoxylin and eosin) and microorganisms (Gram, methenamine silver, and Fite stains). The edge of ulcer is cultured in appropriate media to detect bacteria, fungi, and atypical mycobacteria.

- Laboratory investigations. Complete blood count, erythrocyte sedimentation rate, blood chemistry (liver and kidney function tests), protein electrophoresis, coagulation panel (including anti-phospholipid antibody screening), ANCA, cryoglobulins
- Venous and arterial function studies
- Chest radiography
- Colonoscopy.

Further Information

Pyoderma gangrenosum was first described in 1930 by Brunsting, Goeckerman, and O'Leary, with five cases (Brunsting, Goeckerman and O'Leary, 1930).

CHAPTER 146

Raynaud's Phenomenon

Instruction
Examine this patient's hands.

Salient Features
HISTORY
Ask the patient about the following:
- Whether precipitated by cold, emotion, and relieved by heat
- The different phases change: in idiopathic Raynaud disease, the cold dead-white hands (ischaemia) become blue (stasis) and finally red (reactive hyperaemia) and painful
- Sensory changes secondary to vasospasm (numbness, stiffness, aching pain)
- Occupation (polishing tools, vibrating tools)
- Dysphagia (CREST syndrome)
- Butterfly rash, arthralgia, xerostomia (systemic lupus erythematosus (SLE), collagen vascular disorder)
- Use of electrically heated gloves.

EXAMINATION
- Hands may be painful: ask the patient.
- The hands and fingers are cyanosed and cold, or may be warm and red or blue (Fig. 146.1). The thumbs are rarely affected.

Proceed as follows:
- Examine the hands carefully for signs of scleroderma (tightening of skin, telangiectasia).
- Examine the face for tightening of skin around the mouth (scleroderma), butterfly rash (SLE).
- Tell the examiner that you would like to examine upper limb pulses and blood pressure in both upper limbs (useful in the detection of cervical rib).

Diagnosis
This patient has cold, blue hands (lesion) caused by Raynaud's phenomenon (aetiology) and is unable to continue in her occupation, which requires using a vibratory hand drill (functional status).

Questions
How is primary differentiated from secondary Raynaud's phenomenon?
- Primary:
  - Attacks symmetric
  - No tissue necrosis, ulceration, or gangrene

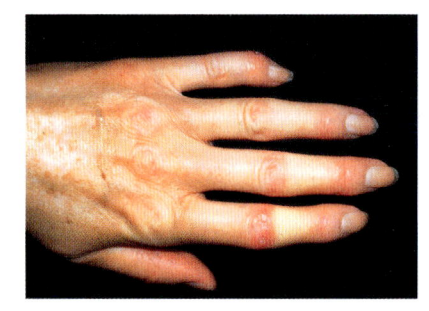

Fig. 146.1 Scleroderma showing Raynaud's phenomenon: pallor, cyanosis, and often rubor of the skin, in response to cold or emotional stimuli.

- No secondary cause on the basis of a patient's history and general physical examination
- Normal nailfold capillaries
- Negative result when tested for antinuclear antibody
- Normal erythrocyte sedimentation rate (ESR).
- Secondary:
  - Age at onset of >30 years
  - Episodes intense, painful, asymmetric, or associated with ischaemic skin lesions
  - Clinical features suggestive of a connective-tissue disease (e.g. arthritis and abnormal lung function)
  - Specific autoantibodies
  - Evidence of microvascular disease on microscopy of nailfold capillaries.

What are the causes of Raynaud's phenomenon?
- Immunological and connective tissue disorders:
  - Scleroderma
  - SLE
  - Dermatomyositis
  - Rheumatoid arthritis
  - Mixed connective tissue disorders.
- Obliterative arterial disease:
  - Atherosclerosis
  - Thoracic outlet syndrome, cervical rib.
- Occupational:
  - Vibration, causing white fingers
  - Cold injury, e.g. from handling frozen commodities
  - Vinyl chloride.
- Drugs:
  - Beta-blockers
  - Bromocriptine
  - Sulphasalazine
  - Ergot alkaloids
  - Combination of bleomycin and vincristine (as for testicular cancer).

- Miscellaneous:
  - Cold agglutinins
  - Cryoglobulins
  - Idiopathic.

Note: Raynaud disease is diagnosed if the phenomenon persists for greater than 3 years without evidence of associated disease.

What investigations would you do to look for autoimmune rheumatic disease in a patient with Raynaud's phenomenon?
- Full blood count, ESR
- Total immunoglobulin and electrophoresis strip
- Urine analysis
- Chest radiography
- Renal and liver function tests
- Test for antinuclear antibody
- Hand radiography.

What drugs have been used to treat Raynaud syndrome?
Nifedipine, nitrates, stanazolol, inositol nicotinate, naftidrofuryl oxalate, prostaglandin 12, thymoxamine, guanethidine, prazosin.

What is the role of surgery in treating Raynaud disease?
In patients resistant to medical therapy with severe, frequent attacks and if trophic changes have occurred interfering with work, dorsal sympathectomy may be indicated.

Do you know of any other vasospastic conditions?
- White finger syndrome
- Livedo reticularis
- Erythromelalgia
- Chilblains.

Further Information

Auguste-Maurice Raynaud (1834–1881) described the sign in 1862. He was a physician at Hôpital Lariboisière, Paris. He died of an attack of angina pectoris.

CHAPTER 147

Rosacea

Instruction
Look at this patient's face.

Salient Features
HISTORY
- Age (typically occurs between the ages of 30 and 50 years)
- Intermittent facial flushing
- Blushing of the face with caffeine, alcohol, or spicy foods
- History of unilateral headaches (an increased incidence of migrainous headaches accompanying rosacea has been reported).

EXAMINATION
- Red patch with telangiectasia, acneiform papules, and pustules overlying the flush areas of the face: cheeks, chin, and nose (Fig. 147.1). The papules and pustules distinguish it from the rash of systemic lupus erythematosus.
- Comment on the following:
  - Rhinophyma or 'whiskey nose' or 'rum blossom' (Fig. 147.2) (irregular thickening of the skin of the nose with enlarged follicular orifices caused by hyperplasia of the sebaceous glands and hyperplasia of connective tissue); although rhinophyma is often referred to as 'end-stage rosacea', it may occur in patients with few or no other features of rosacea.
  - Blepharitis, conjunctivitis.
- Tell the examiner that you would like to obtain an ophthalmological evaluation for chalazion and progressive keratitis, which can lead to scarring and blindness.

Diagnosis
This patient has a red patch on the face with papules and pustules (lesion) caused by rosacea (aetiology), which is cosmetically disfiguring (functional status).

Questions

How do you diagnose rosacea?
The diagnosis of rosacea is a clinical one. There is no confirmatory laboratory test. Biopsy is warranted only to rule out alternative diagnoses because histopathological findings are not diagnostic. Diagnostic phenotypes are rosacea with phymatous changes or fixed centrofacial erythema. Major phenotypes are papulopustular rosacea, flushing, telangiectasia, and ocular rosacea. Minor symptoms include burning, oedema, and itching. One diagnostic or two major phenotypes are required to establish the diagnosis.

147—ROSACEA

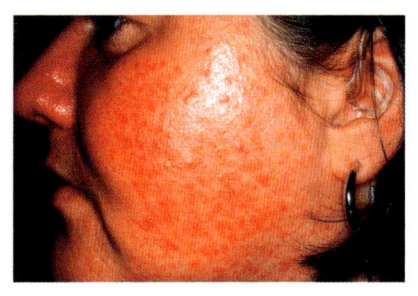

Fig. 147.1 Papulopustular rosacea.

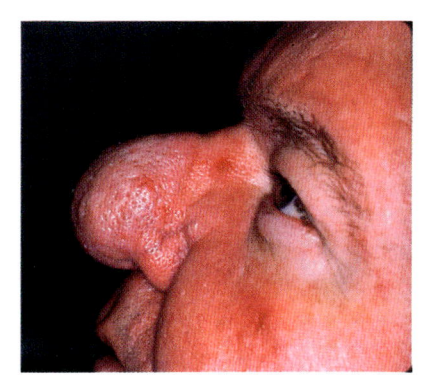

Fig. 147.2 Rhinophyma.

How would you distinguish rosacea from acne?
Rosacea is distinguished from acne by age (middle-aged and older people), the presence of a vascular component (i.e. rosy hue, erythema, and telangiectasia), and the absence of comedones.

How would you manage such a patient?
- Avoid factors that provoke facial flushing.
- Avoid the sun; use sunscreens to limit photodamage.
- Avoid oil-based creams.
- Topical therapy includes metronidazole, sodium sulfacetamide, azelaic acid; these are usually effective in eliminating erythematous papules and pustules.
- Use oral tetracycline in those who fail to respond to topical therapy; also useful in ameliorating nodular lesions and eye symptoms.
- Use retinoids in resistant disease.
- Use yellow light laser for telangiectasia.
- Perform surgical removal for rhinophyma.

What are the causes of red face in an adult?
- Malar rash of systemic lupus erythematosus (SLE)
- Heliotrope rash of dermatomyositis
- Seborrheic dermatitis
- Perioral dermatitis.

Further Information
It has been suggested that the painter Rembrandt had rosacea, which he depicted in his self-portrait (Espinel, 1997).

CHAPTER 148

Seborrhoeic Dermatitis

Instruction
Comment on this patient's skin.

Salient Features
HISTORY
- History of itching
- Oily skin
- History of psoriasis
- History of immunosuppression
- Parkinson disease or other neurological diagnosis (stroke, epilepsy).

EXAMINATION
- Greasy scales overlying erythematous plaques or patches affecting the face (eyebrows, eyelids, glabella, nasolabial folds, or ears) (Fig. 148.1), submammary folds, gluteal clefts
- Occasionally generalized
- Severe dandruff on the scalp.

Proceed as follows:
- Tell the examiner that you would like to look for the underlying disorder (Parkinson disease, HIV, and stroke).

> **Remember:**
> - The name is misleading and the condition is unrelated to seborrhoea (excess sebum production).
> - Distinguishing severe seborrhoeic dermatitis from early facial psoriasis can be particularly difficult.

Diagnosis
This patient has seborrhoeic dermatitis (lesion) with Parkinson disease and finds the lesion cosmetically unacceptable (functional status).

Questions
Name some conditions that are associated with development of seborrhoeic dermatitis in adults.
- Parkinson disease, epilepsy, facial nerve palsy
- Immunosuppression (HIV, transplant, lymphoma)
- Psoriasis treatment.

148 — SEBORRHOEIC DERMATITIS

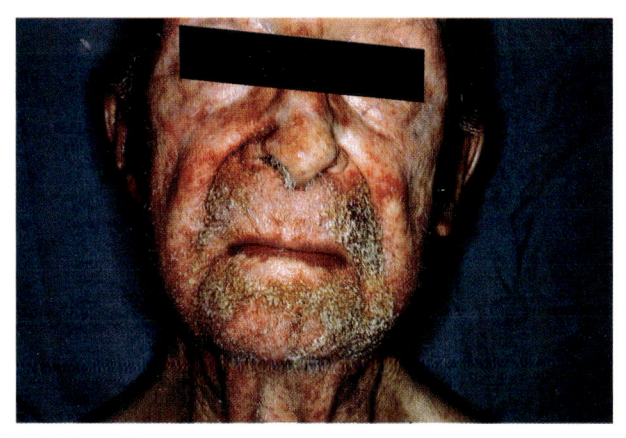

Fig. 148.1 Seborrhoeic dermatitis.

What is the aetiology of this disorder?
It is based on a genetic predisposition mediated by several factors including nutritional status, infection, and hormones. Its response to antifungal agents has suggested that it represents an inflammatory reaction to *Pityrosporum ovale* yeasts present in the scalp of humans.

Mention some clinical variants.
- Adult variants:
  - Pityriasis capitis (dandruff)
  - Blepharitis
  - Pityriasiform seborrhoeic dermatitis: rare form involving the trunk and limbs
  - Flexural seborrhoeic dermatitis: involves any body folds, especially the retroauricular areas, the inner thighs, the genitalia, and the breast folds, with intertriginous, sometimes oozing lesions
  - *Pityrosporum (Malassezia)* folliculitis: itchy, erythematous follicular papules, sometimes pustules, typically in sites rich in sebaceous glands; often occurs in immunocompromised hosts
  - Erythroderma (exfoliative dermatitis): generalized redness and scaling of the skin with systemic manifestations.
- Infantile variants:
  - Scalp seborrhoeic dermatitis (cradle cap): red-yellow plaques covered by scales on the scalp of infants; develops after a few weeks of age
  - Leiner disease: poorly defined entity that includes a primary immunodeficiency syndrome not related to seborrhoeic dermatitis
  - Pityriasis amiantacea: thick, asbestos-like scales adhering to tufts of scalp hairs; may be associated with psoriasis, atopic dermatitis, or tinea capitis.
- HIV-related seborrhoeic dermatitis:
  - Occurs particularly in those with CD4 cell counts $<400 \times 10^6$ cells/L
  - Is usually more severe, diffuse, and inflammatory than in otherwise healthy persons.
- Drug-related seborrhoeic-like dermatitis:
  - Common in patients treated with erlotinib or sorafenib
  - Also reported in patients treated with recombinant interleukin-2, psoralen plus ultraviolet A.

How would you treat these skin lesions?
- Topical antifungals, including ketoconazole, bifonazole, and ciclopirox olamine, which are available in different formulations such as creams, gels, foams, and shampoos
- Topical glucocorticoids (avoid fluorinated preparations on the face)
- Shampoos containing coal tar and salicylic acid
- Selenium sulfide shampoos for the scalp
- Eyelid margins respond to gentle cleaning with undiluted Johnson and Johnson baby shampoo using a cotton swab.
- Oral ketoconazole is invaluable in the persistent seborrhoeic dermatitis of AIDS but should rarely be used otherwise.
- Topical lithium succinate and lithium gluconate are effective alternatives for the treatment of seborrhoeic dermatitis in areas other than the scalp.
- Topical 1% pimecrolimus or similar calcineurin inhibitors.

What is the prognosis of this condition?
There is a tendency to lifelong recurrences.

CHAPTER 149

Sturge–Weber Syndrome (Encephalotrigeminal Angiomatosis)

Instruction

Look at this patient's face.

Salient Features

HISTORY

- History of seizures (focal or generalized)
- Hemiparesis, hemisensory disturbance
- Ipsilateral glaucoma
- Learning disability.

EXAMINATION

- A port-wine stain is present on the face in the distribution of the first and second division of the trigeminal nerve (Fig. 149.1).
- Hypertrophy of the involved area of the face.

Proceed as follows:
- Look for haemangiomas of the episclera and iris.

Tell the examiner that you would like to:
- examine the fundus for unilateral choroidal haemangiomata: the so-called haemangioma is in almost all cases on the side of the facial naevus flammeus and is so diffuse that the colour change it causes is commonly called a 'tomato ketchup' fundus (Fig. 149.2)
- consider brain computed tomography (CT) (Fig. 149.3) for intracranial 'tramline' calcification, particularly in the parieto-occipital lobe (caused by mineral deposition in the cortex beneath the intracranial angioma)
- check blood pressure: may be associated with phaeochromocytoma.

Diagnosis

This patient has a port-wine stain on the face in the distribution of the first two divisions of the trigeminal nerve (lesion), which is probably caused by Sturge–Weber syndrome (aetiology).

Questions

What is the inheritance in such patients?

This is the only syndrome of the phacomatoses that does not have a hereditary tendency. It occurs sporadically and has no sexual predilection. It is due to a sporadic somatic mutation of the gene GNAQ.

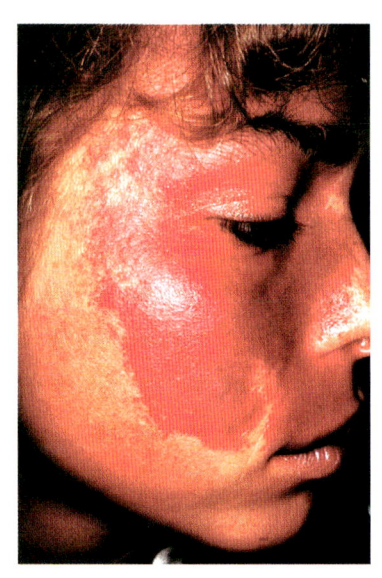

Fig. 149.1 Sturge–Weber syndrome.

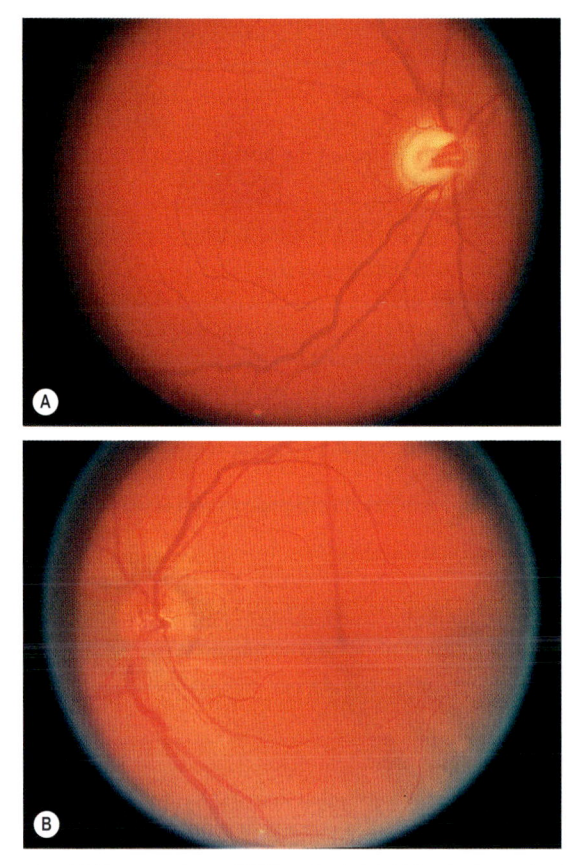

Fig. 149.2 Diffuse choroidal haemangioma. **(A)** The affected right fundus has saturated red colour and a large deep cup of optic disc. **(B)** The uninvolved left fundus, with more orange coloured choroid and a normal optic disc. (With permission from Yanoff, M., Duker, J.S., 2008. Ophthalmology, third edn. Mosby, Philadelphia, PA.)

149—STURGE–WEBER SYNDROME (ENCEPHALOTRIGEMINAL ANGIOMATOSIS)

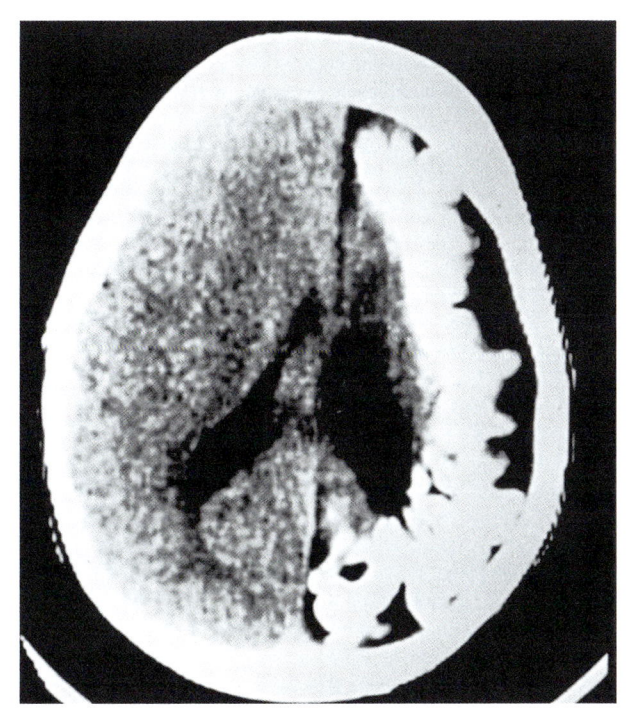

Fig. 149.3 Computed tomography scan showing unilateral calcification and underlying atrophy of a cerebral hemisphere. (With permission from Kliegman, R.M., Behrman, R.E., Jenson, H.B., Stanton, B.F., 2007. Nelson Textbook of Pediatrics, eighteenth edn. Saunders, Philadelphia, PA.)

What are the neurological manifestations in such patients?
Jacksonian epilepsy, contralateral hemianopia, hemisensory disturbance, hemiparesis and hemianopia, learning and behavioural difficulties.

What other ocular manifestations do you know?
Choroidal angioma, glaucoma (in 30%), buphthalmos (large eye), optic atrophy.

What is the histology of port-wine stains?
They are composed of networks of ectatic vessels in the outer dermis, under a normal dermis.

Does the location of the port-wine stain predict Sturge–Weber syndrome?
Patients who do not have port-wine stain in the distribution of the first two branches of the trigeminal nerve are unlikely to have neuro-ophthalmological manifestations of the syndrome.

How would you treat such a patient?
- Treatment is aimed at the pharmacological control of seizures.
- The patient should be referred to the ophthalmologist for management of increased intraocular pressure or choroidal angioma.
- Photothermolysis to treat the port-wine stains.

Name some other vascular malformation syndromes.
- Proteus (rare syndrome with a wide range of clinical expressions, with vascular malformations and tissue overgrowth)

- Klippel–Trenaunay (heterogenous group of diseases characterized by capillary, venous, lymphatic malformations, and tissue overgrowth)
- Parkes (capillary malformation and bone hypertrophy in one limb).

Further Information

William A. Sturge (1850–1919), a London physician, described this condition in 1879. He was attached to the Royal Free Hospital, London, and founded the Society of Prehistoric Archaeology in East Anglia.

Otto Kalischer, a German pathologist, described postmortem findings in a case as early as 1901.

Frederick Parkes Weber (1863–1962), a London physician, was the first to describe the radiological appearances in this condition. Two other syndromes to which Weber's name is attached are Weber–Christian disease (relapsing, febrile, nodular, nonsuppurative panniculitis) and Osler–Weber–Rendu syndrome (hereditary haemorrhagic telangiectasia).

CHAPTER 150

Tuberous Sclerosis (Bourneville or Pringle Disease)

Instruction

Look at this patient who has a history of seizures and learning difficulties.

Salient Features

HISTORY

- Family history (autosomal dominant inheritance with variable penetrance)
- Seizures
- Cognitive deficits
- Reddened nodules (adenoma sebaceum) on the face from childhood
- History of cardiac disease.

EXAMINATION

- Angiofibromas (adenoma sebaceum) distributed in a butterfly pattern over the cheeks (Fig. 150.1), chin, and forehead
- Shagreen patches: leathery thickenings in localized patches over the lumbosacral region
- Ash-leaf patches: hypopigmented areas (Fig. 150.2)
- Subungual fibromas (Fig. 150.3)
- Examine the fundus (retinal glial hamartomas).

Diagnosis

This patient has adenoma sebaceum (lesions) caused by tuberous sclerosis (aetiology). I would like to perform a full clinical examination and determine his functional status.

Questions

What other lesions may be present?
- Hamartomas within the central nervous system occurring as cortical tubers and subependymal hamartomas
- Renal angiomyolipomas
- Cardiac rhabdomyomas and pulmonary myomas
- Cysts in the liver, kidney, and pancreas.

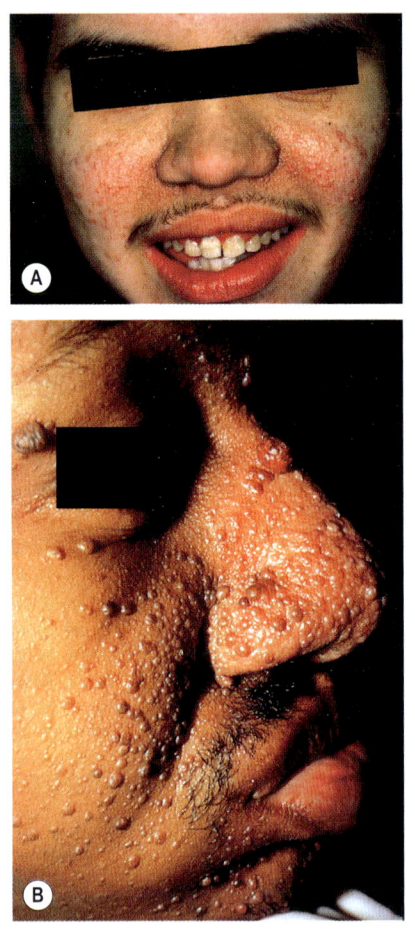

Fig. 150.1 Tuberous sclerosis: angiofibromas in a butterfly pattern over the cheeks, chin, and forehead.

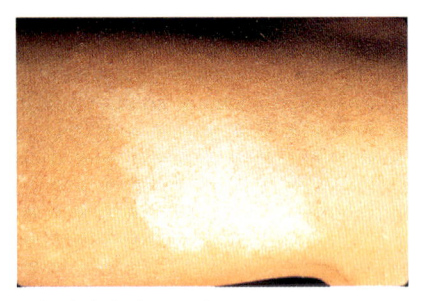

Fig. 150.2 Hypopigmented macules (ash-leaf pattern).

Give some examples of the appearance of clinical manifestations at distinct developmental points.
- Hypopigmented macules (formerly known as ash-leaf spots) are usually detected in infancy or early childhood.
- Shagreen patch is identified with increasing frequency after the age of 5 years.

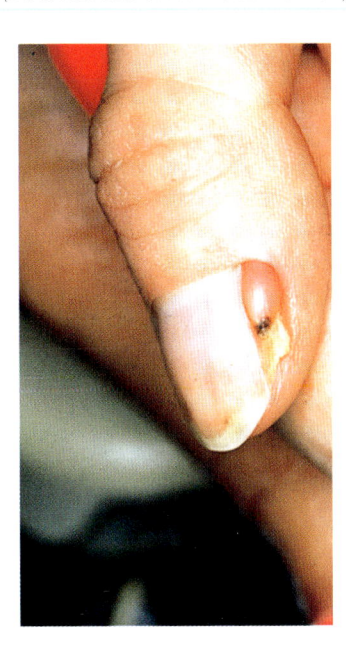

Fig. 150.3 Subungual fibromas.

- Ungual fibromas characteristically appear after puberty and may develop in adulthood.
- Facial angiofibromas (formerly called adenoma sebaceum) may be detected at any age but are generally more common in late childhood or adolescence.
- Cortical tubers and cardiac rhabdomyomas are typical findings in infancy because they form during embryogenesis.
- A subependymal giant cell tumour of the brain may develop in childhood or adolescence.
- Renal cysts can be detected in infancy or early childhood.
- Angiomyolipomas develop in childhood, adolescence, or adulthood.
- Pulmonary lymphangiomyomatosis is found in adolescent girls or women.

What is the prevalence of tuberous sclerosis?
Population-based studies in the United Kingdom estimate a frequency of 1 in 12,000 to 1 in 14,000 in children <10 years of age. Improved methods of determination have detected individuals who are not severely affected by tuberous sclerosis, increasing the estimates of its frequency: the disorder has a birth rate of 1 in 5000 to 1 in 10,000 births.

What are the diagnostic criteria for tuberous sclerosis?
A combination of genetic and clinical criteria exists to diagnose tuberous sclerosis.
Genetic criteria: Identification of a responsible mutation (TSC1 or TSC2) from nonlesional tissue suffices to establish the diagnosis of tuberous sclerosis, without the aid of any clinical combinations described later.
Clinical criteria are divided into major and minor:
- *Major features*:
    - Facial angiofibromas or forehead plaque, pits in dental enamel
    - Nontraumatic ungual or periungual fibroma (two or more)
    - Hypomelanotic macules (three or more, at least 5 mm diameter)
    - Shagreen patch (connective tissue nevus) migration lines

- Multiple retinal hamartomas
- Cortical dysplasias
- Subependymal nodule
- Subependymal giant cell astrocytoma
- Cardiac rhabdomyoma, single or multiple
- Lymphangiomyomatosis
- Angiomyolipomas (two or more).
- *Minor features*:
  - Confetti skin lesions
  - Nonrenal hamartomas
  - Multiple renal cysts
  - Retinal achromic patch
  - Intraoral fibromas (two or more)
  - Dental enamel pits (three or more).

Establishing the existence of one major and two minor clinical features makes the diagnosis of tuberous sclerosis possible, whereas the presence of two major and two minor clinical features give a definite clinical diagnosis of tuberous sclerosis.

How would you manage such patients?

- Symptomatically, with anticonvulsant therapy for seizures, and genetic counselling. When severe epilepsy and intellectual disability are present, the prognosis for life beyond the third decade is poor. Death is usually from seizures, associated neoplasms, or intercurrent illness.
- Regular, at least annual, assessment for the development of associated neuropsychiatric disorders, three-monthly screening for dental complications, annual screening for intraabdominal lesions, in the form of intraabdominal imaging, regular echocardiogram every 1 to 2 years, regular ophthalmology and dermatology examination, regular pulmonary function tests and imaging if required, regular dermatologic evaluation with or without laser therapy, or surgical removal for identified lesions.
- Regular follow-up with imaging for brain lesions: The growth of angiomyolipomas or subependymal giant cell tumours requires regular follow-up. Periodic imaging of the brain and abdomen to monitor the growth of lesions in the brain and kidney should occur at least every 3 years and more often in patients with lesions that have progressive growth. Annual magnetic resonance imaging (MRI) of the brain is suggested until patients are at least 21 years of age, and then MRI should be done every 2 to 3 years both to diagnose and to monitor subependymal giant cell tumours. Treatment of identified brain tumours can be achieved with surgical resection or alternatively medical therapy with everolimus in patients who are not surgical candidates.

Do you know on which chromosome the gene is localized?

Tuberous sclerosis is an autosomal dominant disorder, although two-thirds of patients have sporadic mutations. The genes in which abnormalities are found are called *TSC1* and *TSC2*. Both have been studied by multigenerational linkage analysis and have been localized to chromosome 9 (*TSC1*) and chromosome 16 (*TSC2*).

What do you know about the benign metastasis hypothesis?

The 'benign metastasis' hypothesis for the pathogenesis of lymphangiomyomatosis proposes that histologically benign cells with mutations in *TSC1* or *TSC2* may have the ability to travel to the lungs from angiomyolipomas in the kidney.

What do you know about the pathogenesis of tuberous sclerosis?
Several downstream protein cascades from tuberin and hamartin might be affected, for example the mammalian target of rapamycin (mTOR) pathway, which detects signals of nutrient availability, hypoxia, or growth factor stimulation. The mTOR pathway is stimulated by a small G-protein of the Ras superfamily RHEB (Ras homologue enriched in brain). Rheb is active when bound to guanine triphosphate (GTP). Tuberin and hamartin form intracellular complexes that activate GTPase, thus reducing the stimulation of mTOR. Whether Rheb is the sole downstream effector or mTOR is the only clinically relevant target of Rheb remains to be characterized.

Further Information

D.M. Bourneville (1840–1909), a French neurologist, described tuberous sclerosis in 1880 (Bournville, 1880). J.J. Pringle (1855–1922), an English dermatologist who was also the editor of the *British Journal of Dermatology*. The Eker rat is an animal model of tuberous sclerosis.

CHAPTER 151

Urticaria

Instruction
Look at the skin of this patient, who has recurrent lesions.

Salient Features
HISTORY
- Determine the physical causes that could have precipitated this response: cold urticaria, dermatographism (Fig. 151.1), pressure, sunlight, exercise, hot shower
- Drug history: aspirin, nonsteroidal antiinflammatory drugs (NSAIDs), morphine, codeine, penicillin, sulphonamides
- Duration of lesions
- Food allergy: strawberries, seafood, nuts, chocolate
- Blood products causing these lesions
- Wasp or bee stings
- Viral infections and febrile illnesses
- Ask if the patient has recurrent angioedema.
- Obtain a history of atopy.

EXAMINATION
- Wheals that are smooth, oedematous, pink, or red and surrounded by a bright-red flare. Clearing of the central area may leave an annular pattern.
- Associated scratch marks, indicating the wheals are itchy.

Proceed as follows:
Tell the examiner that you would like to exclude infections (hepatitis, chronic sinusitis) and connective tissue disorders.

Diagnosis
This patient has wheals (lesion) caused by chronic urticaria and dermatographism (aetiology), complicated by severe itching (functional status). Tell the examiner that you would like to exclude urticarial vasculitis before making a firm diagnosis.

> **Notes:**
> - Systemic lupus erythematosus and Sjögren syndrome may present with urticarial lesions, which are usually urticarial vasculitis.
> - Chronic urticaria is the occurrence of daily or almost daily widespread itchy wheals for at least 6 weeks. This includes urticarial vasculitis and physical urticaria.

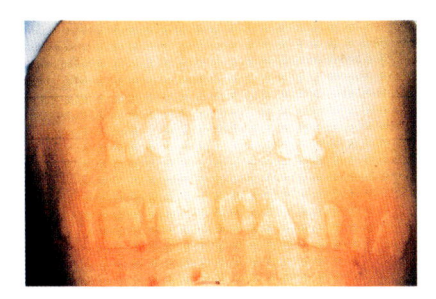

Fig. 151.1 Urticaria.

Questions

How do you diagnose urticaria?
The diagnosis of urticaria is a clinical one. There are no diagnostic tests that would help with confirming a diagnosis, and a biopsy is not helpful or needed. However, once the clinical diagnosis is established, a series of other investigations may be helpful to elicit possible causative agents or exclude an underlying generalized disorder associated with urticaria if other symptomatology is present.

What do you understand by the term dermatographism?
It is the presence of itchy, linear wheals with a surrounding bright-red flare at sites of scratching or rubbing.

Which systemic disorder is associated with urticaria?
- Hashimoto disease is the only systemic disorder with a clear and common association with chronic urticaria and angioedema.
- Less common is an association with Graves disease.

How would you investigate a patient with chronic urticaria?
- Full blood count and white count, if eosinophilia is present
- Examination of the stool for ova and parasites
- Physical urticaria must be assessed by appropriate challenge testing.
- Peanut-specific Ig-E when peanut allergy is suspected
- Serum complement C4 when there is a history of repeated cutaneous or mucosal angioedema
- Thyroid function tests because of diagnostic overlap between chronic urticaria and thyroid disease. The percentage of patients with chronic urticaria who have antithyroglobulin antibody, antimicrosomal antibody, or both is 27%; 19% have abnormal thyroid function.

How would you manage patients with chronic urticaria?
- Identify avoidable cause such as food additives. Challenge testing for food additives should be avoided in patients with a history of severe angioedema, asthma, or episodes of anaphylaxis.
- Antihistamines: about 85% of cutaneous histamine receptors are of the H_1 subtype, and the remaining 15% are H_2 receptors. The addition of an H_2-receptor antagonist to an H_1-receptor antagonist augments the inhibition of a histamine-induced wheal-and-flare reaction once H_1-receptor blockade has been maximized.

- Corticosteroids merit consideration in patients who have had little response to even a combination of H_1- and H_2-receptor blockers. Ciclosporin is the best studied immunosuppressive therapy for chronic urticaria.
- Other treatments for refractory cases include leukotriene antagonists and immunotherapy.
- All patients should be advised to avoid aspirin and other NSAIDs, angiotensin-converting enzyme inhibitors, macrolide antibiotics, and imidazole antifungal agents.

CHAPTER 152

Urticaria Pigmentosa

Instruction
- Look at this patient's skin.

Salient Features
HISTORY
- Urticaria with pruritus on trauma, rubbing, or heat: *Darier's sign*
- Headache
- Diarrhoea
- Itching.

EXAMINATION
- Itchy reddish-brown macules and papules (Fig. 152.1)
- Telangiectasia.

Proceed as follows:
- Look for hepatosplenomegaly.

Diagnosis
- This patient has itchy reddish-brown macules with telangiectasia and Darier's sign (lesions) indicating urticaria pigmentosa (aetiology).

Questions

What do you know about urticaria pigmentosa?
- It is the cutaneous manifestation of systemic mastocytosis, also called maculopapular cutaneous mastocytosis.

What is the histology of urticaria pigmentosa?
It varies from an increase in the number of spindle-shaped and stellate mast cells about the superficial dermal vessels to large numbers of tightly packed round to oval mast cells in the upper and mid dermis. Variable fibrosis, oedema, and a small number of eosinophils may also be present.

What do you know about systemic mastocytosis?
It is a condition characterized by mast cell hyperplasia that, in most cases, is neither clonal nor neoplastic. It can occur at any age and is slightly more common in men. Four forms have been recognized:
- Indolent form: this does not alter life expectancy and constitutes the majority of cases.
- Associated with frank leukaemia or dysmyelopoiesis: the prognosis is determined by the underlying haematological disorder.

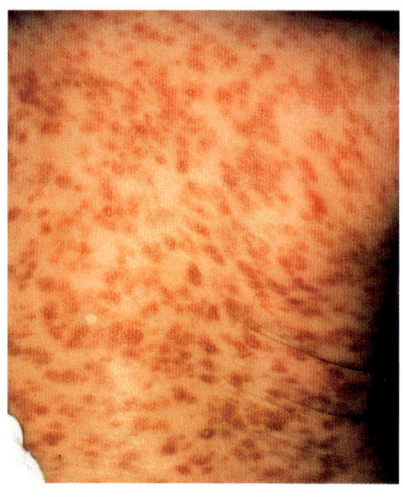

Fig. 152.1 Urticaria pigmentosa: reddish-brown macules and papules.

- Aggressive form: the prognosis is determined by the extent of organ involvement.
- Mast cell leukaemia: rare, invariably fatal.

What diagnostic tests would you order?
- Urinary histamine is elevated in most cases (an elevated urinary histamine level is not a required finding for a diagnosis of mastocytosis; there is poor correlation between the urinary histamine content and the severity of symptoms in mastocytosis).
- Serum tryptase is elevated in most cases (the tryptase level is elevated in >83% of patients and is highly specific for this disease).
- Coagulation defects may occur as a result of the release of mast-cell heparin.
- Bone marrow biopsy is often diagnostic (revealing the focal infiltration of mast cells).
- Immunohistochemical analysis with monoclonal antibodies against the mast-cell markers tryptase and CD117 is used to confirm the diagnosis.

How would you manage such patients?
Treatment is based on blocking mast cell products, including histamine, prostaglandin D_2, and leukotrienes:
- Antihistamines
- Steroid creams
- Phototherapy.

Further Information
F.J. Darier (1856–1938), a French dermatologist.

CHAPTER 153

Venous Ulcer

Instruction
Look at this patient's leg.

Salient Features
HISTORY
- Varicose veins; duration
- History of venous thromboembolism
- Duration of ulceration and whether this is the first episode or recurrent
- Pain (lack of pain suggests neuropathic aetiology)
- Rheumatoid arthritis (remember, up to half the patients with rheumatoid arthritis have venous leg ulcers rather than as a result of rheumatoid arthritis)
- Ankle swelling
- Skin discolouration.

EXAMINATION
- Ulcer located on the medial aspect of leg (around the ankles) with pigmentation
- Surrounding dermatitis and excoriation from pruritus (stasis dermatitis)
- White atrophy with scars in the overlying skin
- The ulcer may be secondarily infected (cellulitis or thrombophlebitis)
- Look for varicose veins (Fig. 153.1)
- The range of hip, knee, and ankle movement should be determined
- Sensation should be tested with a monofilament to exclude peripheral neuropathy (neuropathic arthritis or Charcot joints).

Diagnosis
This patient has a venous ulcer (lesion) caused by disturbed venous flow and stasis (aetiology), which has caused severe pigmentation and dermatitis around the ankles (functional status).

Questions
What causes the surrounding pigmentation?
It results from extravasation of red blood cells and haemosiderin deposition.

What causes the white atrophy (atrophie blanche)?
It results from hyalinization of skin vessels, leading to scars in the overlying skin.

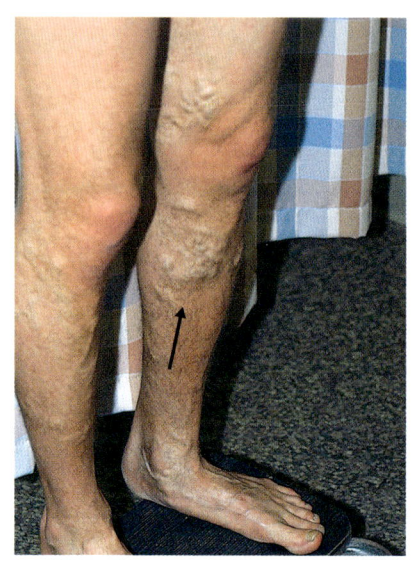

Fig. 153.1 Varicose veins of the leg *(arrow)*. (With permission from Kumar, V., Abbas, A.K., Fausto, N., Aster, J., 2009. Robbins and Cotran Pathologic Basis of Disease, eighth (professional) edn. Saunders, Philadelphia, PA.)

What is the pathogenesis of venous ulcer?

Disturbed venous flow patterns and chronic inflammation probably underlie all the clinical manifestations of the disease.

How is the diagnosis confirmed?

The diagnosis of a venous ulcer is a clinical one, based on the history, clinical examination findings, and characteristic appearance of a venous ulcer in combination with identifying the risk factors for venous insufficiency. Further testing is sometimes warranted to confirm the diagnosis, exclude coexisting diagnoses, and determine causative factors and appropriate treatment options. These tests may be in the form of duplex ultrasonography, venography, and plethysmography.

How would you manage such an ulcer?

- Reduction of venous hypertension and oedema. Elevation of the limbs, wearing support bandages, weight reduction in the obese. The mainstay of community management of venous ulcers is graduated compression bandaging (in these patients the ankle brachial pressure index must be at least 0.8). The healing rate depends on the initial size of the ulcer, but 65% to 70% of venous ulcers heal within 6 months.
- Control the surrounding inflammation. Use wet compresses and topical steroids.
- For infection, use antibiotics for cellulitis.
- For dermatitis, use zinc and salicylic acid paste.
- Skin on the lower leg must be kept moist: emollient such as simple aqueous cream or 50:50 liquid paraffin.
- For ulcers, cleaning with potassium permanganate and wound debridement and skin grafting are performed as needed.
- Treatment of varicose veins. Long saphenous or short saphenous incompetence in the presence of normal deep veins may benefit from surgery to correct venous abnormality in the leg and allow ulcer healing. Patients with refluxing deep veins would benefit from compression bandaging.
- In resistant cases, therapies such as hyperbaric oxygen and radiofrequency ablation may be considered.

Is recurrence common?
The 5-year recurrence rate of healed venous ulcers is about 40%; it is about 69% in noncompliant patients compared with 19% in patients wearing class 2 compression hosiery.

Are varicose veins in the absence of skin changes indicative of chronic venous insufficiency?
Varicose veins in the absence of skin changes are not indicative of chronic venous insufficiency. Chronic venous disease encompasses the full spectrum of signs and symptoms associated with all the CEAP (clinical, etiologic, anatomical, and pathophysiological classification; used to grade chronic venous disease) classes, whereas the term 'chronic venous insufficiency' is generally restricted to disease of greater severity (i.e. classes C4–C6). The CEAP uses clinical signs in the affected legs to place the venous disease into seven classes, C0 to C6. Leg symptoms associated with chronic venous disease include aching, heaviness, a sensation of swelling, and skin irritation; limbs categorized in any clinical class may be symptomatic (S) or asymptomatic (A).

What are the factors that influence venous pressure in the legs?
Pressure in the veins of the leg is determined by three components.
- Hydrostatic component is related to the weight of the column of blood from the right atrium to the foot (during standing without skeletal muscle activity, venous pressures in the legs are determined by the hydrostatic component and capillary flow, and they may reach 80–90 mm Hg).
- Hydrodynamic component is related to pressures generated by contractions of the skeletal muscles of the leg and the pressure in the capillary network (skeletal muscle contractions, as during ambulation, transiently increase pressure within the deep leg veins).
- Venous valve component, if effective, ensures that venous blood flows towards the heart, thereby emptying the deep and superficial venous systems and reducing venous pressure, usually to <30 mm Hg. Both hydrostatic and hydrodynamic effects are profoundly influenced by the action of the venous valves. Even very small leg movements can provide important pumping action. In the absence of competent valves, the decrease in venous pressure with leg movements is attenuated. If valves in the perforator veins are incompetent, the high pressures generated in the deep veins by calf muscle contraction can be transmitted to the superficial system and to the microcirculation in skin.

What are the causes of lower extremity ulcers?
- Cardiovascular disease
- Diabetic nephropathy
- Arterial insufficiency
- Trauma
- Vasculitis
- Sickle cell anaemia
- Malignancy infection
- Pyoderma gangrenosum.

Name some conditions that are associated with venous ulcers.
- Hypertension
- Venous thromboembolism
- Multiple pregnancies
- Varicose veins
- Lower limb surgery
- Obesity.

What factors are associated with poorly healing ulcers?
- Large initial size (>20 cm^2)
- Duration of time before compression treatment (>1 year)
- Combined arterial insufficiency
- Poor improvement in first 4 weeks of compression treatment
- Age.

CHAPTER 154

Vitiligo

Instruction
Look at this patient.

Salient Features
HISTORY
- Age of onset (about half the patients present before the age of 20 years)
- Whether or not it runs in the family (familial in 36% of cases)
- About other autoimmune disorders (hypothyroidism, hyperthyroidism, thyroiditis, Addison disease, diabetes mellitus, pernicious anaemia).

EXAMINATION
- Hypopigmented patches (Fig. 154.1) that are distributed symmetrically; sometimes, the border may be hyperpigmented. The distribution often includes wrists, axillae, perioral, periorbital, and anogenital skin.
- White hairs in the vitiliginous area
- Some spontaneous re-pigmentation in the sun exposed regions (in a third of cases).

Proceed as follows:
- Look at the scalp for alopecia and white hair.

Note: Scratching when the disease is active may induce lesions along the scratch marks; this is termed isomorphic response or Koebner's phenomenon. It is also seen in response to the friction or pressure resulting from common activities such as brushing hair, drying skin with a towel, and wearing a belt or watch.

Diagnosis
This patient has vitiligo (lesion), which is of autoimmune origin (aetiology).

Questions
Mention some associated conditions.
Organ-specific autoimmune conditions:
- Thyroid disease: Graves disease, myxoedema, Hashimoto disease
- Pernicious anaemia
- Diabetes mellitus
- Alopecia areata
- Addison disease.

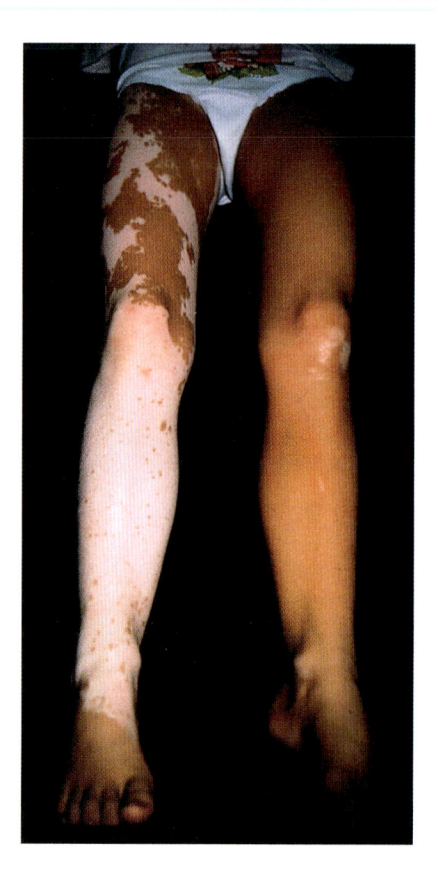

Fig. 154.1 Vitiligo.

What are the types of vitiligo?
Nonsegmental vitiligo—white patches that are often symmetric and that usually increase in size over time, corresponding to a substantial loss of functioning epidermal melanocytes, and sometimes hair-follicle melanocytes. The key precipitating factors include immunologic factors, oxidative stress, or a sympathetic neurogenic disturbance. Accounts for 85% to 90% of all cases of vitiligo.

Segmental vitiligo—unilateral distribution that may completely or partially match a dermatome. In most patients, there is one unique segment of depigmentation. Rarely, two or more segments with ipsilateral or contralateral distribution may occur. A neurogenic sympathetic disturbance is considered a key precipitating factor. This is seen in autoimmune diseases.

Which fungal condition can be mistaken for vitiligo?
Pityriasis versicolor (caused by the fungus *Malassezia furfur*).

How would you confirm the diagnosis?
Vitiligo is a clinical diagnosis and no further tests are needed. Examination is with a Wood's lamp in a completely dark room after the examiner's eyes have adapted to the darkness (it is less useful in patients with darker skin types). It is a hand-held ultraviolet A irradiation device that emits at approximately 365 nm. Wood's lamp provides bright reflection of white patches and

enhanced details on intermediate pigment tones. Lamps that incorporate a magnifying lens are useful in evaluating terminal and vellus pigmentation of hair. A complete examination should include inspection of the genitalia and areas of skin folds as these areas can be easily overlooked.

Are there any systems to assess severity?
Two scoring systems are available for assessing severity but do not have a role in clinical practice: Vitiligo Area Scoring Index and the Vitiligo European Task Force system. Both of them are mainly used to monitor disease for the purpose of clinical research.

How would you manage such patients?
- Cosmetics are useful for concealing disfiguring patches
- Sun protection with high sun protection factor (SPF) sunscreen
- Topical steroids
- Topical tacrolimus
- Phototherapy
- Segmental vitiligo or stable nonsegmental vitiligo in a limited area (<200 cm^2): epidermal autografts and cultured epidermis combined with psoralen plus ultraviolet A (split-thickness skin grafting, punch grafting, suction blister epidermal grafting, noncultured epidermal cell suspension grafting)
- Depigmentation therapy.

Note: On the whole, treatment of vitiligo remains unsatisfactory.

Mention a few conditions in which hypopigmentation is common.
- Hypopituitarism
- Albinism
- Phenylketonuria
- Leprosy
- Burns
- Radiodermatitis
- Piebaldism (an autosomal dominant condition manifested by a white forelock)
- Ash leaf spots (tuberous sclerosis)
- Leukoderma (occurs as a complication of lichen planus, lichen simplex chronicus, atopic dermatitis, and discoid lupus erythematosus).

What is the histology of vitiligo?
Characteristically, there is partial or complete loss of pigment-producing melanocytes in the epidermis. In contrast, some forms of albinism have melanocytes, but no melanin pigment is produced because of lack of, or a defect in, the tyrosinase enzyme.

CHAPTER 155

Xanthelasma

Instruction
Examine this patient's eyes.

Salient Features
HISTORY
- Jaundice, generalized pigmentation, itching (primary biliary cirrhosis)
- Family history of hyperlipidaemia
- History of diabetes, hypertension
- Symptoms of hypothyroidism
- History of oral contraceptives.

EXAMINATION
- Xanthelasmata (flat yellow nodules or plaques) seen on eyelids and around both eyes, particularly on the inner canthus (Fig. 155.1)
- Look for the following signs:
  - Corneal arcus
  - Jaundice, generalized pigmentation, scratch marks (primary biliary cirrhosis)
  - Tendon xanthomata
  - Palmar xanthomata.

Tell the examiner that you would like to check the following:
- Urine sugar
- Blood pressure
- Pulse and ankle jerks (hypothyroidism).

Diagnosis
This patient has xanthelasmata on the eyelids (lesions) and I would like to test serum lipids to exclude an underlying lipid disorder (aetiology).

Questions

Mention a few secondary causes of hyperlipidaemia.
Diabetes mellitus, hypothyroidism, nephrotic syndrome, cholestatic jaundice, excess alcohol intake, oral contraceptives.

How would you manage a patient with hyperlipidaemia?
- Lifestyle advice
- Control of reversible cardiovascular risk factors
- Lipid-lowering drugs.

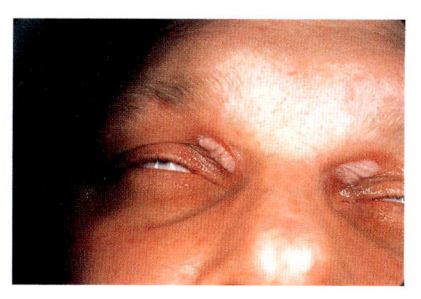

Fig. 155.1 Xanthelasma. Multiple, soft, yellow plaques involving the eyelid.

Mention a few lipid-lowering drugs.
- Ion-exchange resin: cholestyramine
- Fibrates: bezafibrate, gemfibrozil
- Sitostanol-ester margarine (a plant sterol that reduces serum cholesterol concentration by inhibiting cholesterol absorption)
- Hydroxymethylglutaryl coenzyme A reductase inhibitors: simvastatin, pravastatin, atorvastatin. These drugs block the endogenous synthesis of cholesterol and reduce levels of low-density lipoprotein cholesterol.
- Ezetimibe: inhibits absorption of cholesterol at the small intestine brush border via Niemann-Pick C1-Like1 (NPC1L1) transporter
- Nicotinic acid derivatives: nicotinic acid, probucol.

Why are all statins best given in the evening?
Because the rate of endogenous cholesterol synthesis is higher at night.

CHAPTER 156

Xanthomata

Instruction

Look at this patient's hands.

Salient Features

HISTORY

- Family history of hyperlipidaemia
- History of premature coronary artery disease.

EXAMINATION

- Tendon xanthomata seen on the extensor tendons and becoming more prominent when the patient clenches his fist (Fig. 156.1B).

Proceed as follows:
- Look at other tendons, particularly the patellar and Achilles tendon (Fig. 156.1A).
- Look at the eyes for xanthelasmata (see Fig. 155.1) and corneal arcus.

Tell the examiner that you would like to:
- check fasting lipids, in particular for an increase in cholesterol level
- screen family members for hypercholesterolaemia
- examine the heart for aortic valve stenosis caused by lipid deposition.

Diagnosis

This patient has tendon xanthomata (lesion) caused by hypercholesterolaemia (aetiology).

Questions

What are the different types of xanthomas and what is their association with lipid profile?
- Xanthelasma: soft, yellow velvety lesions in the inner surface of the eyelids, usually symmetrical, that may or not be associated with hyperlipidaemia (Fig. 155.1)
- Tendon xanthoma: subcutaneous nodules on tendons, associated with hypercholesterolaemia and increased low-density lipoprotein (LDL) levels (Fig. 156.1B).
- Eruptive xanthoma: small red plaques in the extensor surfaces, associated with hypertriglyceridaemia (Figs 156.1H and 116.1)
- Palmar xanthoma: flat papules on the hands, associated with type III hyperlipidaemia (dysbetalipoproteinaemia) (Fig. 156.1E).

What is familial hypercholesterolaemia?
It is a genetic disease, characterized by high blood levels of LDL cholesterol (LDL-C) and increased risk of early onset coronary artery disease.

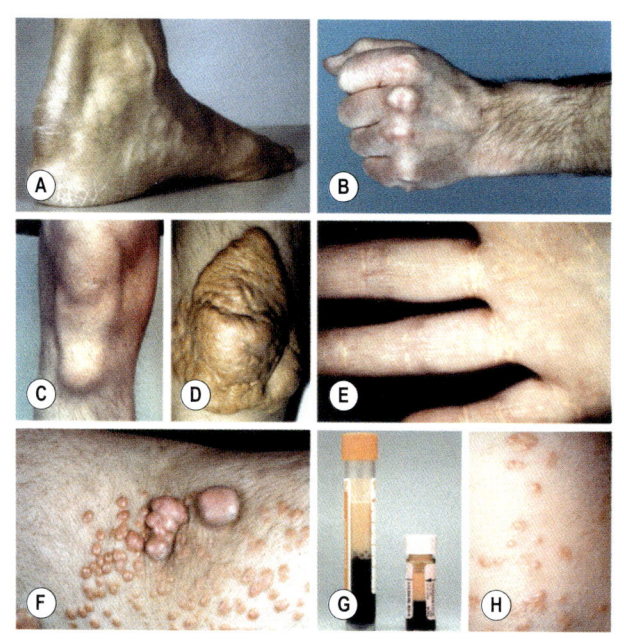

Fig. 156.1 Clinical manifestations of hyperlipidaemia. **(A)** Achilles tendon xanthoma (heterozygous familial hypercholesterolaemia). **(B)** Tendon xanthomata on dorsum of hand (heterozygous familial hypercholesterolaemia). **(C)** Subperiosteal xanthomata (heterozygous familial hypercholesterolaemia). **(D)** Planar xanthoma in antecubital fossa (homozygous familial hypercholesterolaemia). **(E)** Striate palmar xanthomata (type III hyperlipoproteinaemia). **(F)** Tuberoeruptive xanthomata on elbow and extensor surface of arm (type III hyperlipoproteinaemia). **(G)** Milky plasma from patient with acute abdominal pain (severe hypertriglyceridaemia). **(H)** Eruptive xanthomata on extensor surface of forearm (severe hypertriglyceridaemia). (With permission from Durrington, P., 2003. Dyslipidaemia. Lancet 362, 717731.)

Defects in genes encoding for lipoprotein receptors result in reduced clearance of lipoproteins; defects in the gene that encodes for the proprotein convertase subtilisin/kexin type 9 protease (PCSK9) result in receptor destruction. Both mutations result in elevated plasma levels of LDL-C and total cholesterol.

Diagnosis can be made with a combination of clinical history and cholesterol levels, using diagnostic criteria/tools; however, genetic testing can be used, which has the additional advantage of identifying the exact mutation.

How is familial hypercholesterolaemia treated?
All patients should receive lipid-lowering therapy with statins being the first-line treatment. If second-line treatment is needed to pursue acceptable cholesterol levels, then a different lipid-lowering agent may be used.

SECTION X

Neurology and Elderly Care Medical Cases

SECTION OUTLINE

157 Neurology Case
158 Headache
159 Memory Loss
160 Lower Urinary Tract Symptoms
161 Abnormal Gait
162 Argyll Robertson Pupil
163 Muscular Dystrophy
164 Spastic Paraplegia
165 Bitemporal Hemianopia
166 Brown-Séquard Syndrome
167 Carpal Tunnel Syndrome
168 Central Scotoma
169 Cerebellar Syndrome
170 Cerebellar Dysarthria
171 Cerebellopontine Angle Tumour
172 Charcot–Marie–Tooth Disease (Peroneal Muscular Atrophy)
173 Chorea
174 Lateral Popliteal Nerve Palsy, L4, L5 (Common Peroneal Nerve Palsy)
175 Expressive Dysphasia
176 Facioscapulohumeral Dystrophy (Landouzy–Déjérine Syndrome)
177 Friedreich's Ataxia
178 Hemiballismus
179 Hemiplegia
180 Homonymous Hemianopia

181 Internuclear Ophthalmoplegia
182 Jerky Nystagmus
183 Limb-Girdle Dystrophy
184 Motor Neurone Disease
185 Multiple Sclerosis
186 Multiple System Atrophy
187 Myasthenia Gravis
188 Myotonia Congenita
189 Myotonic Dystrophy
190 Parkinson Disease
191 Peripheral Neuropathy
192 Proximal Myopathy
193 Pseudobulbar Palsy
194 Ptosis and Horner Syndrome
195 Radial Nerve Palsy
196 Seventh Cranial Nerve Palsy
197 Sixth Cranial Nerve Palsy
198 Syringomyelia
199 Tetraplegia
200 Third Cranial Nerve Palsy
201 Tremor
202 Deformity of a Lower Limb
203 Ulnar Nerve Palsy
204 Wallenberg Syndrome (Lateral Medullary Syndrome)
205 Wasting of the Small Muscles of the Hand
206 Long Thoracic Neuropathy
207 Anxiety
208 Back Pain
209 Pruritus
210 Speech Disturbance
211 Unsteadiness

CHAPTER 157

Neurology Case

Instruction

Please examine this patient's neurological system.

HISTORY

- Note the mnemonic SHOVE:
  Syncope, speech defect, swallowing difficulty
  Headache
  Ocular disturbances: diplopia, field defects
  Vertigo
  Epilepsy: seizures.
- History pertaining to motor and sensory components of the cranial nerves and limbs (e.g. pain, paraesthesia, weakness, incoordination).

Examination of the Cranial Nerves

FIRST CRANIAL NERVE

- Ask the patient, 'Have you noticed any change in your sense of smell recently?' 'Can you differentiate between the odour of tea, coffee and bananas?'
- If the examiner requires you to test the sense of smell, use an odour that can be readily identified, such as soap or clove oil. If the patient has frequent nasal troubles, the value of this examination is limited.

SECOND CRANIAL NERVE

- First check visual acuity with a pocket Snellen's chart and finger counting.
- Make sure that the patient is wearing their spectacles should they use them, as one is not concerned with refractive errors.
- Check visual fields with a white hat pin (10 mm in diameter); your instructions to the patient should be clear and precise. Smaller hat pins (5 mm in diameter) are used for detecting small scotomata. Red hat pins, for reasons that are not clear, are useful in the detection of pregeniculate lesions and are therefore useful in compression of the optic nerve, optic chiasm, or optic tract.
- Comment on the pupils (size, shape, or inequality) and test their reaction to light (direct and indirect reaction) and to accommodation. The popular acronym PERRLA (pupils equal, round and reactive to light, and accommodation) is a convenient description of normal pupillomotor function.

- Examine the fundus in a definite sequence: retina, retinal vessels, optic nerve, and macula.

THIRD, FOURTH, AND SIXTH CRANIAL NERVES

Test eye movements:
- The Parks–Bielschowsky three-step test is used to determine which muscle is weak in a patient who has a vertical deviation because of a weakness in a single muscle:
    - Step 1: determine which eye is hypertropic; paralysis of the superior oblique is one cause of hypertropia.
    - Step 2: determine whether the hypertropia is greater in left or right gaze; hypertropia caused by superior oblique paralysis is greater on gaze to the contralateral side.
    - Step 3: determine whether the hypertropia is greater in left or right head tilt; hypertropia caused by superior oblique paralysis is greater in a head tilt to the ipsilateral side.
    - A further step 4 can confirm that the correct muscle has been identified and helps to rule out other causes of vertical deviation: determine whether the hypertropia is worse in upgaze or downgaze.
- Remember to ask the patient if they see a double image: this is the most sensitive sign of defective eye movement and may be present even when there is no apparent weakness of extraocular muscle or an abnormality of gaze.
- Saccadic movements are tested by asking the patient to look voluntarily to the right and left and up and down. Note whether these movements are carried out rapidly to the extremes of gaze.
- Pursuit movements are examined by asking the patient to follow an object moved to the right and left and up and down.

Note whether these movements are carried out smoothly without interruption.
- Remember to comment on nystagmus: nystagmus is a repetitive drift of the eyeball away from the point of fixation, followed by a fast corrective movement towards it.
- Comment on ptosis if present (seen in third nerve palsy).

FIFTH CRANIAL NERVE

- Test the masseters: 'Clench your teeth'; take care to palpate the muscles.
- Test the pterygoids: 'Open your mouth'; note the jaw deviates to the side of the lesion.
- Test corneal (not conjunctival) sensation by touching a wisp of cotton wool to the cornea while the patient looks upwards and away from the examiner.
- Test facial sensation: keep in mind that this nerve supplies not only the face but also the anterior half of the scalp. Impairment of sensation limited to the face only is usually psychogenic in origin.
- Test jaw jerk: ask the patient to have his or her mouth half open; place your thumb over the patient's chin and lightly tap on the thumb. A mild jaw jerk or absent jerk is seen in normal individuals. In upper motor neuron lesions above the cervical cord, the jaw will manifest a marked jerk with this procedure.

SEVENTH CRANIAL NERVE

Remember that the facial nerve is a motor nerve:
- Test the lower half of the face: 'Show me your teeth'. Note the nasolabial fold, which often disappears in mild facial palsy.
- Test the upper half of the face: 'Screw your eyes tightly shut and don't let me open them'.

- Ask the patient to wrinkle his or her forehead and note the movement of the muscles of the forehead.

Note: Taste may be lost on the anterior two-thirds of the tongue, but this is not usually tested.

EIGHTH CRANIAL NERVE

- Test by bringing a watch from beyond auditory acuity into the zone of hearing.
- Occlude each external auditory meatus with your finger and whisper short phrases, asking the patient to repeat them.
- Perform Rinne's and Weber's tests (use a tuning fork with a frequency of 256 or 512 cycles/s). Normally, air conduction is better than bone conduction:
    - Rinne's test: in obstructive deafness bone conduction is better; in nerve deafness the normal relations are kept (i.e. air conduction is greater than bone conduction in the deaf ear).
    - Weber's test: if the base of the tuning fork is placed on the middle of the forehead of a person with an obstructive deafness, he or she will hear it better in the deaf ear; with a nerve deafness, the fork will be heard better in the normal ear.

NINTH AND TENTH CRANIAL NERVES

- Ask the patient 'Open your mouth and say "aah"'; observe the soft palate with a torch (the soft palate is pulled to the normal side on saying 'aah').
- Tell the examiner that you would like to check the gag reflex. An absence of gag reflex is significant only if it is unilateral.

ELEVENTH CRANIAL NERVES

- Ask the patient 'Shrug your shoulders'; try to push him or her down simultaneously (this tests the trapezii muscles).
- Test the sternomastoids by the patient's ability to resist lateral movement of the neck. Keep in mind that one rotates the head to the right by use of the left sternomastoid muscle.

TWELFTH CRANIAL NERVE

- Ask the patient, 'Open your mouth'; comment on fasciculations of the tongue while in the mouth. Comment on wasting.
- Ask the patient, 'Stick out your tongue'; the tongue will deviate to the side of the lesion but a slight deviation of the tongue can be disregarded.

Neurological Examination of the Upper Limbs

1. Introduce yourself to the patient and ask him to take his top off so that both his arms are well exposed. If the patient is female, cover her breasts with suitable clothing so that she is decent.
2. Comment on wasting, tremor, fasciculations.
3. Assess tone: 'Let your arms go loose and let me move them from you':
    - Flex and extend wrists passively: cogwheel rigidity is elicited by this method.
    - Flex and extend at the elbows, pronate, and supinate at the forearm: lead-pipe rigidity and clasp-knife spasticity are elicited by these methods.

4. Test power: 'I am going to test the strength of the muscles of your arms'. Ask the patient the following, evaluating strength on a scale of 0 to 5:
   - 'Hold your arms stretched out in front of you and then close your eyes': observe for drift, action tremor.
   - 'Hold your arms outwards at your sides (like this) and keep them up; don't let me stop you': shoulder abduction, the chief movers are the deltoids, C5. (**Note:** Supraspinatus is responsible for the initiation of abduction and for the first 60 degrees of this movement, but this method of testing only assesses the power of the deltoids.)
   - 'Push your arms in towards you and don't let me stop you': shoulder adduction, chief movers are the pectoral muscles, C6 to C8.
   - 'Bend your elbows and pull me towards you; don't let me stop you': elbow flexion, chief mover is the biceps, C5.
   - 'Straighten your elbows and push me away; don't let me stop you': elbow extension, chief mover is the triceps, C7.

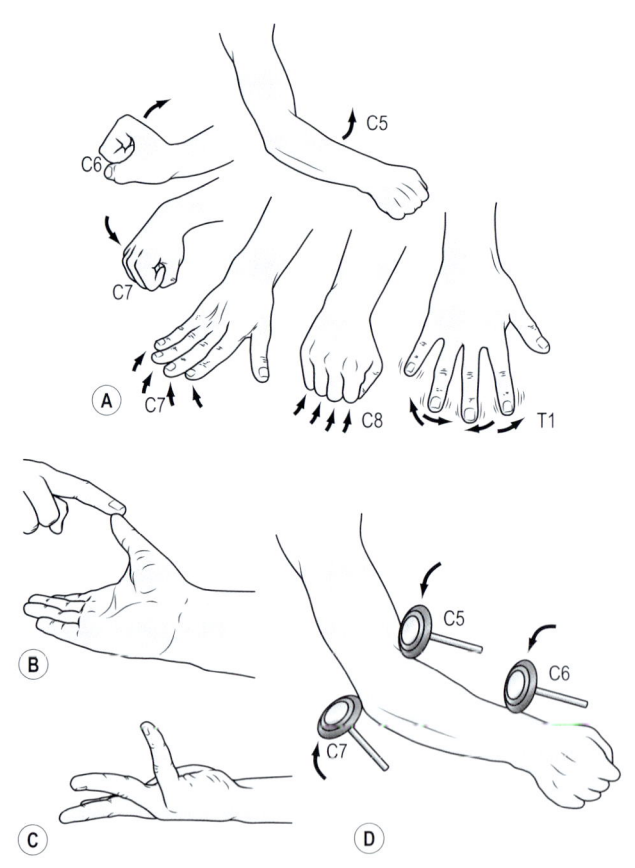

Fig. 157.1 Examination of the upper extremities. **(A)** Muscle groups, designated by their respective nerve root innervation. These are C5, elbow flexion; C6, wrist extension; C7, finger extension; C8, finger flexion; and T1, finger abduction. **(B, C)** Motor innervation of muscles of the hand. **(B)** Thumb abduction tests median motor nerve function. **(C)** Little finger flexion at the metacarpophalangeal joint with simultaneous interphalangeal joint extension tests ulnar motor nerve function. **(D)** Stretch reflexes and nerve roots of origin.

- 'Clench your fist and cock your wrists up; don't let me stop you': wrist extension, chief mover is C7.
- 'Now push the other way': wrist flexion, chief mover is C7 (Fig. 157.1).
- 'Spread your fingers wide apart and don't let me push them together': finger abduction, chief movers are the dorsal interossei, T1 (ulnar nerve). (**Note: D**orsal interossei **ab**duct mnemonic, DAB).
- 'Hold this piece of paper between your fingers and don't let me snatch it away': finger adduction, chief movers are the palmar interossei, T1 (ulnar nerve). (**Note: P**almar interossei **ad**duct mnemonic, PAD).
- 'Hold your palms facing the ceiling and now point your thumb towards the ceiling; don't let me stop you': thumb abduction, chief mover is the abductor pollicis brevis, C8, T1 (median nerve).
- 'Grip these two fingers of mine tightly and don't let them go': flexion of fingers, chief movers are the long and short flexors of the fingers, C8.

Notes:
- The median nerve supplies the lateral two **l**umbricals, **o**pponens pollicis, **a**bductor pollicis brevis, **f**lexor pollicis brevis (mnemonic, LOAF).
- The ulnar nerve supplies all other small muscles of the hand.
- The lumbricals are responsible for flexion at the metacarpophalangeal joint when the interphalangeal joints are in extension.
- Power is graded from 0 to 5:
  0, absence of movement
  1, flicker of movement on voluntary contraction
  2, movement present when gravity is eliminated
  3, movement against gravity but not against resistance
  4, movement against resistance but not full strength
  5, normal power.

5. Test deep tendon reflexes (Fig. 157.1D):
   - Biceps jerk, C5, C6
   - Triceps, C7
   - Supinator, C5, C6.

Notes:
- If the reflexes are absent, test after reinforcement: ask the patient to clench his or her teeth
- Inversion of the supinator reflex. When the supinator jerk is elicited, the normal response is a slight flexion of the fingers, contraction of the brachioradialis and flexion at the elbow joint. The jerk is said to be 'inverted' when finger flexion is the sole response, with contraction of the brachioradialis and elbow flexion being absent. There is associated absence of the biceps jerk and exaggeration of the triceps jerk.
- The inverted jerk indicates a lower motor neuron lesion at the fifth cervical level and an upper motor neuron lesion below this level. It could be caused by cervical spondylosis, trauma to the cervical cord, spinal cord tumours at this level, and syringomyelia.

6. Finger reflexes:
   - Hoffman sign: the examiner holds the patient's wrist in the horizontal pronated position with the fingers and wrists relaxed. Then the distal phalanx of the patient's middle finger is forcibly flexed. Normally, no reflex occurs unless the patient is under emotional tension. In upper motor neuron lesions, the patient's thumb undergoes a quick flexion–adduction–opposition movement while the other fingers move in flexion–adduction. This response is labelled as a 'positive' Hoffman sign.

- Wartenberg sign: the patient places his or her hand in partial supination resting on a table with the fingers slightly flexed. Then the examiner places his or her middle and index fingers on the volar surface of the patient's four fingers and taps his or her own fingers briskly with the tendon hammer. The response is one of flexion of the patient's four fingers and the distal phalanx of the thumb.
- Mayer sign: with the patient's thumb abducted and the hand relaxed, the proximal phalanx of the middle finger is forcibly flexed towards the palm. Normally, the thumb adducts. In upper motor neuron lesions, the thumb usually remains in the position of abduction.

7. Test coordination:
   - Finger–nose–finger test: 'Touch your nose with your index finger and now touch my finger'.
   - Rapid alternating movement of one hand over the other.
8. Test sensation:
   - Light touch: use cotton wool and check each dermatome.
   - Pinprick: demonstrate first the sharp end and then the blunt end on the sternum; then check each dermatome for sharp or blunt sensation with the eyes closed.
   - Joint position sense: check in the distal interphalangeal joint of the thumb.
   - Vibration sense: use a tuning fork of 128 cycles/s (although some authorities believe that a fork of 64 cycles/s is more accurate). First test on the sternum so that the patient can recognize the vibration and then check over the fingers, moving proximally if the vibration sense is absent distally. Pallaesthesia is the ability to perceive the presence of vibration when an oscillating tuning fork is placed over certain bony prominences. Loss of vibratory perception is referred to as pallanaesthesia.

Remember:
- Joint sense and vibration sense are carried in the dorsal columns.
- Pain and temperature are carried in the lateral spinothalamic tracts.
- Light touch is carried in both the aforementioned tracts.

Neurological Examination of the Lower Limbs

1. Introduce yourself and then ensure that the lower limbs are well exposed. It is important to ensure that the patient is decent—cover the genital area with a towel or any suitable clothing.
2. Inspect for wasting, fasciculations (tap the muscles of the leg and thigh to elicit fasciculations if not seen).
3. Assess tone:
   - Ask the patient, 'Let your leg go loose and lax, and let me move it for you'; then passively flex and extend the leg at the knee and hip:
     - Roll the extended leg, feeling for resistance.
     - Put your hand behind the knee and pull it upwards, observing the foot to check whether or not it flops.
     - If there is spasticity or increased tone, then test for ankle clonus and patellar clonus.
   - Patellar clonus—with the patient in the supine position, grasp the upper edge of the patella between the thumb and index finger and apply a quick constant pressure in a downward direction. Avoid prolonging this manoeuvre as it is often painful to the patient. In upper motor neuron lesions, the patella may manifest a few jerks (unsustained clonus) or a constant jerking as long as the pressure is applied (sustained clonus).

157 — NEUROLOGY CASE

- Ankle clonus—ensure that the patient's knee is semiflexed and the foot relaxed. The foot is suddenly pushed dorsally with moderate force and held there. In upper motor neuron lesions, the posterior muscles of the leg will enter into a persistent contraction.

4. Test power (begin at the hips): 'I am going to test the strength of the muscles of your legs'; then ask the patient to:
   - 'lift your leg straight up and keep it there; don't let me stop you': hip flexion, chief mover is iliopsoas, L1, L2.
   - 'push your leg downwards into your bed and don't let me stop you': hip extension, chief movers are glutei, L4, L5.
   - 'push your thigh inwards against my hand': chief movers are adductors of the thigh, L2–L4 (Fig. 157.2A).
   - 'bend your knee and pull your heel towards you; don't let me stop you': knee flexion, chief movers are the hamstrings, L5, S1.
   - 'straighten your knee and don't let me stop you': knee extension, chief movers are quadriceps, L3, L4.
   - 'push your foot downwards against my hand': plantar flexion of the ankle, chief mover is the gastrocnemius, S1.
   - 'move your foot up and don't let me stop you': dorsiflexion of the ankle, chief movers are the tibialis anterior and long extensors, L4, L5.
   - 'push your foot inwards against my hand': inversion of the foot, chief movers are tibialis anterior and posterior, L4.

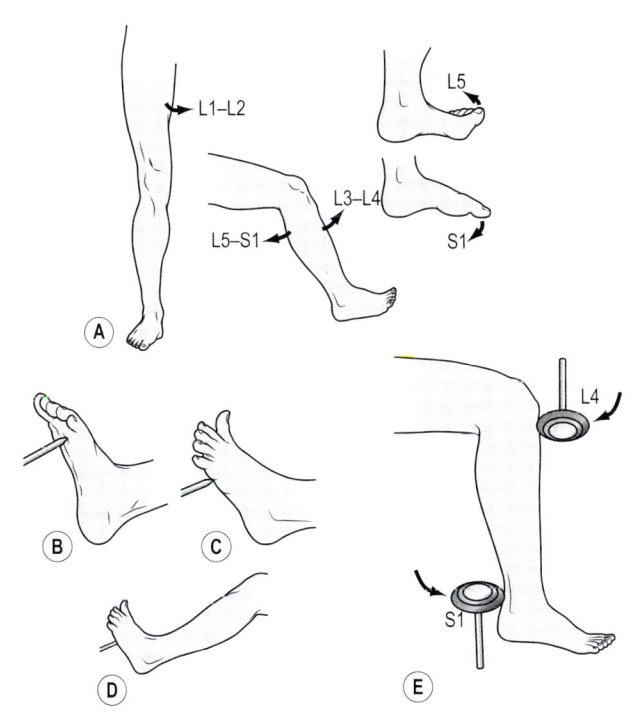

Fig. 157.2 Examination of the lower extremities. **(A)** Muscle groups, designated by their respective nerve root innervation: *L1–L2*, hip abductors; *L3–L4*, knee extension; *L5–S1*, knee flexion; *L5*, great toe extension; *S1*, great toe flexion. **(B)** Plantar reflex. **(C)** Babinski sign. **(D)** Triple flexion response. **(E)** Stretch reflexes and nerve roots of origin.

- 'push your foot outwards against my hand': eversion of the foot, chief movers are the peronei, S1.
- 'pull your toe upwards and don't let me stop you': extension of the great toe, chief mover is the extensor hallucis longus, L5.

5. Test the plantar response (Fig. 157.2B): 'I am going to tickle the bottom of your foot'; use an orange stick to stimulate the outer portion of the sole and then across the ball to the base of the big toe. Always describe the response as either downgoing or upgoing. Normally, the response is downgoing (i.e. all the toes flex towards the plantar surface). Upgoing plantars or the Babinski response (Fig. 157.2C) is a feature of upper motor neuron lesions where the four small toes fan and turn towards the sole while the big toe extends dorsally. There is associated slight flexion of the hip and knee. The contraction of the tensor fasciae lata is referred to as the Brissaud reflex and is a part of the spinal defence reflex mechanism. Other responses to plantar stimulation include the quick avoidance response, the grasp reflex, and the support reaction. Remember that if the feet are cold (when outside the bedclothes for long), the response may be equivocal.

6. Test deep tendon reflexes (Fig. 157.2E):
   - Knee jerk, L4
   - Ankle jerk, S1. In the elderly, the plantar-strike technique is said to be more reliable than the tendon-striking method for eliciting ankle jerks. The plantar-strike technique of eliciting ankle jerks is as follows: the patient's legs are side by side and the foot is passively dorsiflexed; the reflex hammer strikes the examiner's own fingers, which are placed over the plantar surface.
   - When the reflexes are absent, reinforce by asking the patient to pull outwards his or her clasped hands (Jendrassik manoeuvre). Do not tie your hands into a knot while testing the left ankle jerk from the patient's right-hand side. Avoid jabbing the patient while eliciting reflexes.

Notes:
- By convention, deep tendon reflexes are graded as follows:
  0, no response, abnormal
  1+, slight but definitely present response which may be normal or abnormal
  2+, brisk response, normal
  3+, very brisk response, which may be normal or abnormal
  4+, a tap elicits clonus, abnormal
- Asymmetry of reflexes suggests abnormality.

7. Test coordination:
   - Heel–shin test. Have the patient place the heel of one foot upon the knee of the opposite leg and then move the heel downwards along the tibia. In a positive test, the patient has difficulty placing or holding the heel on the opposite knee or cannot keep the heel firmly on the tibia as the heel is moved downwards.
8. Test sensation. Avoid testing in a given rhythm where the patient can expect to be stimulated at a given time. Always compare sensory responses in different areas of the same side of the body, as well as the two sides of the body:
   - Light touch
   - Pinprick: test irregularly with the pin-point and pin-head, asking the patient whether the perceived sensation is sharp or blunt.
   - Joint position sense: hold the lateral aspect of the patient's big toe (not the dorsum of the toe) while eliciting this and move the toe gently up and down; the examiner's fingers

157 — NEUROLOGY CASE

should not rub against the skin of the adjoining toe during this test and the joint should not be put in the extreme position of flexion during the test.
- Vibration sense.

Note: When there is weakness of the limbs, tell the examiner that you would like to check sensation in the sacral area.

9. Romberg's test: 'Please stand up with your legs together and now close your eyes'. Take care to protect the patient if he or she sways or tends to fall. A positive test result is shown by pronounced swaying of the trunk. Sometimes, functional cases will sway without having a true Romberg. This may be proved by diverting the attention of the patient by instituting the finger–nose test at the same time as Romberg is being tested. In functional cases, the 'rombergism' will usually disappear.
10. Check gait, and if the heel–shin test is affected, then test tandem walking (asking the patient to walk along a straight line with one heel in front of the other foot). *Candidates frequently forget to check the gait when asked to examine the legs.*
11. Special manoeuvres in suspected upper motor neuron lesions:
    - Rossolimo's sign: the undersurface of the patient's toes are tapped with the examiner's fingers to produce abrupt extension (dorsiflexion) of the toes. In normal individuals, there is no response, whereas in patients with upper motor neuron lesions, all the toes respond with a quick plantar flexion.
    - In upper motor neuron lesions, the big toe will often dorsiflex (i.e. upgoing toe) when any of the following manoeuvres is conducted:
        - Gordon reflex: on applying pressure to the muscle of the calf
        - Oppenheim sign: on applying heavy pressure with the thumb and index finger to the shin, stroking downwards from below the knee down to the ankle
        - Bing reflex: when the dorsum of the toe is pricked with a pin
        - Schaefer reflex: pinching the Achilles tendon enough to cause pain
        - Chaddock reflex: on stroking the lateral side of the foot, beginning below the malleolus and extending anteriorly along the dorsum of the foot to the base of the big toe
        - Gonda reflex: grasping the small toes between the fingers, slowly and forcibly flex the toe and then suddenly release the toe.

Approach to a Myopathic Patient

There are six key questions:
1. Does the patient have negative or positive signs and symptoms?
   - Negative: weakness, fatigue, atrophy
   - Positive: pain, cramps, contractures, stiffness, hypertrophy.
2. What is the timing of the weakness, pain, or stiffness?
   - Constant or episodic
   - Monophasic or relapsing
   - Age at onset
   - Lifelong
   - Progressive or nonprogressive.
3. What is the distribution of weakness?
   - Proximal arms/legs
   - Distal arms/legs
   - Proximal and distal

- Neck
- Cranial: ocular, pharyngeal, facial, atrophy/hypertrophy.
4. Are there triggering events?
    - During or immediately after exercise
    - After brief or prolonged exercise
    - After exercise followed by rest
    - After carbohydrate meal
    - Relieved by exercise drugs/toxins
    - Temperature (internal/external).
5. Family history of myopathy?
6. Any associated medical conditions?
    - Rash
    - Baldness
    - Fever
    - By organ system.

Further Information

H.A. Rinne (1819–1868), German ear, nose, and throat physician.

F.E. Weber-Liel (1832–1891), a German otologist.

J.J. Babinski (1857–1932), of Polish origin, graduated from the University of Paris with a thesis on multiple sclerosis. The Babinski response refers to upgoing plantars in upper motor neuron lesions. He described adiposogenitalis a year before Frolich.

CHAPTER 158

Headache

Instruction

This patient presents with recurrent episodes of headaches for the last few months. Please take a history and advise on further management.

Salient Features

HISTORY

- Age
- Onset of headache
    - Sudden
    - Gradual
    - Thunderclap.
- Duration of each episode of headache
    - Minutes
    - Hours
    - Days.
- Severity
    - Severity compared to previous headaches, severity in scale 1 to 20, and progression of headache throughout its total duration
    - Waking up from sleep because of headache.
- Site
    - Occipital, frontal, temporal, cervical, retroorbital
    - Unilateral, bilateral.
- Radiation
    - Neck, shoulders.
- Character
    - Throbbing/pulsatile
    - Shooting
    - Tightness
    - Pressure-like
    - Different to headaches that patient usually has.
- Frequency
    - Constant
    - Daily
    - In clusters
    - Weekly
    - Every morning
    - Headache diary.

573

- Aggravating factors
  - Posture
  - Exercise
  - Cough
  - Sleep deprivation
  - Stress
  - Food triggers
  - Menstruation
  - Fasting
  - Alcohol.
- Relieving factors
  - Dark room
  - Pain relief
  - Posture.
- Associated symptoms
  - Fever
  - Neurological deficit (weakness or sensory loss)
  - Cognitive dysfunction
  - Change in personality
  - Seizures
  - Eye lacrimation, rhinorrhea, autonomic features, conjunctival injection
  - Ptosis, miosis
  - Aura
  - Visual disturbances
  - Scalp tenderness, jaw claudication
  - Nausea, vomiting
  - Weight loss, systemic symptoms
  - Neck pain
  - Phonophobia, photophobia
  - Facial pain
  - Rash.
- Medical history
  - Recent trauma
  - History of headaches prior to this presentation
  - Chronic sinusitis
  - Immunosuppression or other systemic illness
  - Pregnancy.
- Drug history
  - Medications used for any cause
  - Analgesics used for any cause
  - Analgesics used for headache
  - Illicit drug use.

EXAMINATION

- Fundoscopy
- Cranial nerves, cerebellar, and peripheral nerve examination
- Palpation of temples, neck, shoulder, spine.

Diagnosis

This patient gives a history consistent with cluster headache. Because of the recent onset in combination with the age of the patient, I would like to request imaging to exclude secondary causes of a cluster headache.

Questions

Name some red-flag symptoms of headache and their associations.
- Fever (systemic illness: giant cell arteritis; infection: meningitis)
- Thunderclap headache (subarachnoid haemorrhage, cerebral sinus thrombosis)
- Recent head trauma (intracranial bleeding, artery dissection)
- Headache exacerbated by lying, bending, cough, or sneeze (raised intracranial hypertension)
- Orthostatic (spontaneous intracranial hypotension)
- Acutely painful red eye and halo with nonmiotic pupil (acute closure glaucoma).

Describe the main clinical characteristics of the common primary headaches: migraine, tension headache, and cluster headache.
Migraine can be unilateral or bilateral headache of gradual onset over hours, described as throbbing or pulsatile in character with moderate intensity. It can get worse with physical activity and patients usually want to rest in a darkroom without noises. It can last up to 3 days and patients can sometimes describe associated features before the headache and during the headache, as well as identify specific triggers (e.g. specific food).

Tension is a mild- to moderate-intensity bilateral headache, described like pressure or tightness around the head, lasting from 30 min to a week, constant or with episodes where it is relieved and episodes where it exacerbates. It is unusual for this type of headache to have accompanying symptoms and there is no neurology described with it.

Cluster is a unilateral, excruciating headache, usually around the eye, behind the eye, and in the ipsilateral temporal region. It comes in clusters of 15 min to 3 hours, and characteristically, it does not last longer than that. The patient, contrasting to migrainous headache, is usually restless during the episode. It can be associated with red and teary eyes, runny or stuffy nose, miosis, and ptosis, but neurological deficits other than ipsilateral Horner syndrome are rare.

Depending on duration and frequency characteristics, all aforementioned types of headache can be classified as chronic or episodic.

For these main types of primary headaches, can you mention acute treatment and prophylactic treatment choices?
Migraine is treated acutely with an oral triptan with or without the addition of simple analgesia and antiemetic.

Tension is treated acutely with simple analgesia (paracetamol, aspirin, or nonsteroidal antiinflammatory drugs (NSAIDs)).

Cluster is not treated with simple analgesia. Instead, a combination of triptan and high-flow oxygen should be given.

Verapamil is used for the prevention of cluster.

Both amitriptyline and propranolol can be used for the prevention of migraine.

Riboflavin may be effective in reducing frequency and intensity of migraine.

No medication has proven to be effective in preventing tension headache but acupuncture may be helpful.

What do you know of trigeminal neuralgia?
Trigeminal neuralgia does not cause headache, but facial pain (with or without headache). However, the clinical symptom may only reveal itself during history taking, as many patients will call their facial pain 'headache'. Trigeminal neuralgia is typically a neuropathic type pain characterized by repetitive sharp pains with or without dysesthesia across the distribution of the trigeminal nerve often described as 'electric shocks'. Trigeminal neuralgia is an important differential of a primary headache, as patients with primary headaches may also experience facial pains, but they are not expected to have characteristics of neuralgia. Trigeminal neuralgia usually responds well to carbamazepine.

What is the clustertic syndrome?
It is a term used to describe the combination of cluster headache with trigeminal neuralgia. It is relevant in a patient presenting with cluster headache because it requires treatment of both conditions in order for the patient to find symptomatic relief, but controlling the episodes is very difficult as patients may not respond to either treatment.

What do you know of medication-overuse headache?
Medication-overuse headache is caused by analgesia taken regularly for other types of headaches. Medications that have been mainly associated with overuse headache are opioids but other analgesics can lead to overuse headache, such as triptans, aspirin, and NSAIDs. The diagnosis is made clinically when there is a positive history of regular use of symptomatic analgesics for three months or more. Usually a diagnosis of a primary headache has preceded this presentation as this is the reason patients have been prescribed the causative analgesics. The headache description may mimic cluster headache, occurs daily or almost daily but lasts more than a typical cluster episode. The treatment is to abruptly stop the offending medications warning the patient that the headaches initially will worsen upon stopping the medication, but eventually withdrawing of the causative agent will result in improvement of symptoms.

CHAPTER 159

Memory Loss

Instruction
This patient is increasingly forgetful. Take a history and perform a focused examination.

Salient Features

HISTORY

- Older person: prevalence increases dramatically with age
- Alzheimer disease presents with a progressive decline in cognition over years, including in the following areas:
    - Loss of retention of new information: patient may repeat questions multiple times over a short time.
    - Unable to complete complex tasks, including cooking, paying bills, and driving
    - Orientation: getting lost in familiar places including in own house
    - Language: word finding difficulties
    - Behaviour: walking with purpose, agitation, aggression, poor motivation
    - Recognition: unable to recognize new acquaintances, then friends/distant family, then children and spouse
    - Reasoning: poor judgement, unable to weigh risk
    - Self-care: leads to neglect in personal appearance, grooming, continence.
- Vascular dementia: history of vascular risk factors
    - Classically associated with stepwise deterioration
    - Often patchy cognitive impairments, may have frontal lobe features
    - Emotional lability common.
- Lewy body dementia:
    - Visual hallucinations
- Frontotemporal dementia (previously referred to as Pick disease):
    - Earlier age of onset, marked behavioural change
- History of head injury, stroke, diabetes, depression, alcohol abuse, delirium, Parkinson disease
- Family history of early dementia
- Drug history including anticholinergics.

EXAMINATION

- Look for evidence of reversible causes of delirium.
- Examine for evidence of vascular disease: stroke, peripheral vascular disease.
- Examine for signs of parkinsonism.
- Examine gait, looking for 'marche a petit pas' (small stepping gait) in vascular dementia, Parkinsonian gait, or broad-based 'foot stuck to the floor' gait of normal pressure hydrocephalus.

- Check for signs of depression: low affect, poor eye contact, low voice.
- Offer to measure cognitive function (Mini Mental State Examination, Montreal Cognitive Assessment); ask the patient to draw a clock.

Diagnosis

This elderly man has a progressive history of short-term memory loss with a change in behaviour, suggesting Alzheimer disease (lesion and aetiology). This is now affecting his ability to self-care (functional status).

Questions

What investigations would you do in this patient?
The main purpose of investigations is to look for reversible causes; therefore, the following should be completed:
- Full blood count: looking for anaemia, infection
- Renal function
- Thyroid-stimulating hormone: hypothyroidism
- Calcium: hypercalcaemia
- B_{12}: low level is associated with short-term memory loss.
- Syphilis serology: only if specific risk factors
- Cerebrospinal fluid (CSF) serology: only if rapidly progressive symptoms suggestive of Creutzfeldt–Jakob disease (CJD).

What is the role of neuroimaging?
Should be considered in any patient with sudden onset or rapid progression, those with focal neurology, and if there is a high risk of malignancy or subdural haematoma. Those with moderate to severe dementia with a clear clinical diagnosis may not need structural imaging, but in reality, most patients will undergo computed tomography (CT) or magnetic resonance imaging (MRI) of the brain as part of the standard workup for suspected dementia.
- CT is the usual modality: signs of infarcts, small vessel ischaemia, and atrophy may be seen.
- MRI: look for subcortical vascular changes.
- Single-photon emission computed tomography (SPECT): this can be useful if the diagnosis is in doubt and can help distinguish between Alzheimer disease and vascular and frontotemporal dementia.

What are the most common causes of dementia?
- Alzheimer disease: 50% to 60%, rising to 80% in older patients
- Vascular: 10% to 20%
- Mixed Alzheimer and vascular: 10% to 20%
- Lewy body dementia, Parkinson disease with dementia: 5% to 10%.

What are the treatment options for Alzheimer disease?
- Acetylcholinesterase (ACh) inhibitors (donepezil, rivastigmine, galantamine) are recommended for mild to moderate Alzheimer disease.
- N-Methyl-D-aspartate (NMDA) receptor antagonist (memantine) is licensed for moderate to severe Alzheimer disease, often given together with ACh inhibitor.
- Aducanumab, a monoclonal antibody directed against beta amyloid, has been given approval in the United States for mild Alzheimer disease, but is not available in the United Kingdom or Europe.

- Social, physical, and emotional support for both the person with the diagnosis of dementia, their families, and carers to promote and maintain independence and dignity for as long as possible. May benefit from 'memory cafes' providing reminiscence therapies and structured group cognitive stimulation, other support groups. Advice may be needed regarding legal issues including driving, finances, advocacy.
- As the disease progresses, continence care, assistance with mobility, and advance care planning and end-of-life care become increasingly important.
- Nonpharmacological interventions should be used in the first instance for those with behaviour that challenges, including reassurance, distraction, and therapeutic use of music. Pharmacological options including antipsychotics should be used only in the cases of severe distress or an immediate risk of harm to themselves or others.

Modifiable vascular risk factors should be treated for those with mixed and vascular dementia.

How would you differentiate between Lewy body dementia and Parkinson disease dementia?
If the symptoms of Parkinson disease precede those of dementia by a year or more, the diagnosis is Parkinson disease with dementia. Around 75% of people with Parkinson disease will develop a degree of dementia, with those who develop early hallucinations at high risk. In Lewy body dementia, motor and cognitive symptoms develop within 1 year of each other. They have similar clinical and pathological features, including visual hallucinations, fluctuating cognitive impairment, rapid eye movement sleep disorder, episodes of reduced consciousness, and problems with executive functions and attention. Lewy bodies (spherical, eosinophilic inclusion bodies) are found throughout the brain, including in the basal ganglia and limbic system.

What is the association between depression, delirium, and dementia?
- A previous history of depression and delirium are risk factors for dementia.
- Delirium can unmask previous unrecognized dementia, but also occasionally, some people do not fully recover from delirium and their cognition progressively declines. Dementia can be diagnosed 6 months after onset of delirium if cognition does not improve.
- Depression can mimic dementia, so this should be screened for in those presenting with progressive decline in memory. If diagnosis is uncertain, depression should be treated in the first instance to look for any reversibility.
- Depression coexists in up to a quarter of patients with dementia or mild cognitive impairment.

Name some rare causes of dementia.
Frontotemporal dementia:
- Due to abnormal processing of tau protein
- Predominantly affects the frontal and anterior temporal lobes
- Insidious onset. Memory usually relatively spared initially. Early features: personality change, emotional blunting, loss of insight, disinhibition, impulsivity, incontinence.

Normal pressure hydrocephalus:
- Rare but potentially reversible cause of cognitive impairment
- Characteristic triad of gait disturbance, subcortical cognitive impairment, and urinary incontinence
- Raised intracranial fluid pressure (idiopathic or secondary to meningitis, subarachnoid haemorrhage, tumour) leads to enlarged ventricles and sulcal effacement seen on CT scan.
- Removal of 40 to 50 mL of CSF and reassessing gait speed and cognition is used to assess those who may benefit from ventriculoperitoneal shunting.

Prion disease:
- Most well known is CJD.
- Others include Gerstmann–Sträussler–Scheinker disease, Kuru, fatal familial insomnia.
- Caused by a build-up of an infectious pathogen which contains protein but lacks nucleic acid
- Some forms of prion disease seem to be genetic.
- There is currently no treatment.

Is there a genetic predisposition to Alzheimer disease?
A number of genes are implicated in familial autosomal dominant Alzheimer disease, which is the cause of less than 1% of Alzheimer disease. These include apolipoprotein E4 allele on chromosome 19, presenilin 1 on chromosome 14, presenilin 2 on chromosome 1, and amyloid precursor protein on chromosome 21. These genes all enhance the accumulation of amyloid proteins leading to beta-amyloid plaques and neurofibrillary tangles, resulting in neuronal cell death.

Cerebral autosomal dominant arteriopathy with subcortical infarcts and leukoencephalopathy (CADASIL) is caused by mutations in the *NOTCH3* gene on chromosome 19 and encodes the NOTCH3 receptor protein, expressed in adults by vascular smooth muscle cells and pericytes. This causes small vessel disease, including subcortical infarcts and progressive cognitive decline.

Should we screen for dementia?
There is little evidence for general population screening for dementia. Those with evidence of mild cognitive impairment should be followed up and reassessed as 50% will develop dementia. Those with a family history of familial autosomal dominant Alzheimer disease or frontotemporal dementia, CADASIL, or Huntington disease should be offered genetic counselling.

Further Information

Alois Alzheimer, a German psychiatrist, first published a case report of a young (51-year-old) woman with memory, behaviour, and language deficits in 1907 following her postmortem, showing neurofibrillary tangles and amyloid plaques.

Arnold Pick (1851–1924), a Czech neurologist, described a series of patients in 1892 displaying cognitive disturbance, personality change, aphasia, and apraxia.

CHAPTER 160

Lower Urinary Tract Symptoms

Instruction
This man has difficulty passing urine; take a history and proceed to abdominal examination.

Salient Features

HISTORY
- Obstructive symptoms: hesitancy, straining, weak stream, dribbling, nocturia, sensation of incomplete bladder emptying, acute retention, chronic retention with overflow incontinence
- Overactive symptoms: frequency, urgency, nocturia
- Haematuria
- Signs of infection: dysuria, frequency, nocturia, urgency or urge incontinence
- History of diabetes, stroke, multiple sclerosis, or urological or gynaecological surgery
- Number of pregnancies.

EXAMINATION
- Abdominal examination to look for palpable bladder
- Offer to perform:
  - Genital examination: in men looking for phimosis, in women for vaginal atrophy or prolapse
  - Rectal examination: for faecal loading, which can precipitate urinary retention, for anal tone, and for examination of prostate size and texture in men.
- Neurological examination: for evidence of stroke, multiple sclerosis, which could cause neurogenic bladder.

Differential Diagnosis

With obstructive symptoms:
- Neurogenic causes
- Enlarged prostate either benign or malignant
- Constipation
- Medications.

With irritable symptoms:
- Infection
- Detrusor overactivity: spontaneous contractions of detrusor muscle
- Bladder calculus or tumour
- Atrophic vaginitis
- *Candida* infection
- Caffeine, citrus drinks.

581

With polyuria:
- Poorly controlled diabetes
- Nocturnal oedema resorption
- Hypercalcaemia.

With stress symptoms: rise in abdominal pressure (e.g. after coughing, laughing) causes small leaks:
- Pelvic muscle and ligament laxity: usually after childbirth.

Questions

What investigations would you perform?
- Urinalysis: haematuria, infection
- Urea and electrolytes
- Glucose: hyperglycaemia causes urinary frequency
- Prostate-specific antigen (PSA); it is important to discuss with patient as to the risks and benefits of further investigations and treatment prior to checking PSA. For every 100,000 men at age 50 years offered screening, 748 would end up being treated. Those who accept screening would have their lives extended on average by a day. However, as a result of the treatment, 274 men would be made impotent, 25 incontinent, and 17 would have rectal problems.
- Post-void bladder scan: for residual volume
- Ultrasound scan renal tract: for evidence of hydronephrosis, residual volume, bladder mass, or debris, prostate volume
- Cystoscopy: if haematuria for bladder stone or tumour
- Computed tomography of the kidneys, ureters, and bladder: to investigate for renal stones.

How would you treat benign prostatic hypertrophy?
- Watchful waiting: if symptoms are mild. Risk of acute urinary retention is 1% to 2% per year.
- Alpha-blockers (e.g. tamsulosin): act by relaxing smooth muscle of prostate to increase flow rate. Side effects include postural hypotension.
- 5-Alpha reductase inhibitors (e.g. finasteride): prostate size is reduced by inhibiting prostatic testosterone metabolism. Side effects include gynaecomastia, erectile dysfunction, and loss of libido.
- Minimally invasive surgical treatments carried out in clinic such as prostatic urethral lift, water vapour thermal therapy, and transurethral microwave therapy.
- Surgery: if severe symptoms not responding to medical management. Transurethral resection of the prostate has over 90% success rates. Complications include incontinence and erectile dysfunction; 10% need further surgery.

When would you catheterize a patient with problems micturating?
- Acute urinary retention
- Chronic retention: contributory causes should be treated including infection and constipation. If trials without a catheter fail long-term, urethral catheter may be required, or intermittent catheterization.

Which drugs worsen obstructive symptoms?
Those with high anticholinergic effects, including tricyclic antidepressants and antimuscarinics for overactive bladder.

CHAPTER 161

Abnormal Gait

Instruction

Look at this patient walking.
Test this patient's gait.

Salient Features

EXAMINATION

There are several types of abnormal gait.

Cerebellar Gait

The patient has a broad-based gait, reeling and lurching to one side:
- Proceed by telling the examiner that you would like to examine the patient for other cerebellar signs.

Parkinsonian Gait

Steps are small and shuffling, and the patient walks in haste (festinating gait). The entire body stoops forwards, knees bent, head hunched forward, and the feet must hurry to keep up, as if trying to catch up with the centre of gravity. There is associated loss of arm swing and mask-like facies.

Hemiplegic Gait

Gait is slow, spastic, and shuffling. With each step, the pelvis is tilted upward on the involved side to aid in lifting the foot off the ground, and the entire affected limb is circumducted; rotated in a semicircle at the pelvis. The upper limb is flexed and adducted and does not swing, and the lower limb is extended.

Sensory Ataxia

The feet stamp, the movement of the legs bearing no relation to the position of the legs in space since proprioception is impaired or absent. The patient has to look down at the ground to compensate for the loss of proprioception. The patient walks on a wide base; the feet are lifted too high off the ground and are brought down too vigorously. The clinician should perform a full neurological examination including Romberg's sign, vibration, and joint position sense. As sensory ataxia may be caused by tabes dorsalis and subacute degeneration of the cord, relevant signs should be sought for, e.g. Argyll-Robertson pupil and signs of anaemia.

High Stepping Gait

Usually unilateral and results from foot drop. The patient has to lift the foot high in order to avoid dragging the forefoot. It is seen in
- peroneal nerve palsy
- poliomyelitis

- Charcot–Marie–Tooth disease
- lead or arsenic poisoning.

Scissor Gait

Seen in spastic paraplegia. The adductor spasm may be so severe as to lead to the legs crossing in front of one another. Short steps with the front of the feet clinging to the ground result in a wearing out of the toes of shoes. Common aetiologies are cord compression, multiple sclerosis, and cerebral palsy.

Waddling Gait

The legs are held wide apart and the patient shifts weight from one side to the other when walking:
- Comment on the lumbar lordosis.
- Waddling gait is seen in advanced pregnancy and proximal weakness (Cushing syndrome, osteomalacia, thyrotoxicosis, polymyositis, diabetes, hereditary muscular dystrophies).

Questions

What do you understand by the term astasia abasia?

This is seen in psychogenic disturbances in which the patient is unable to walk or cannot stand. The patient falls far to the side on walking but usually regains balance before hitting the ground. The legs may be thrown out wildly or the patient may kneel with each step.

What do you understand by the term marche à petit pas?

This is to describe a gait in which the movement is slow and the patient walks with very short, shuffling and irregular steps with loss of associated movements. It is seen in normal-pressure hydrocephalus. This gait bears some resemblance to that seen in Parkinson disease.

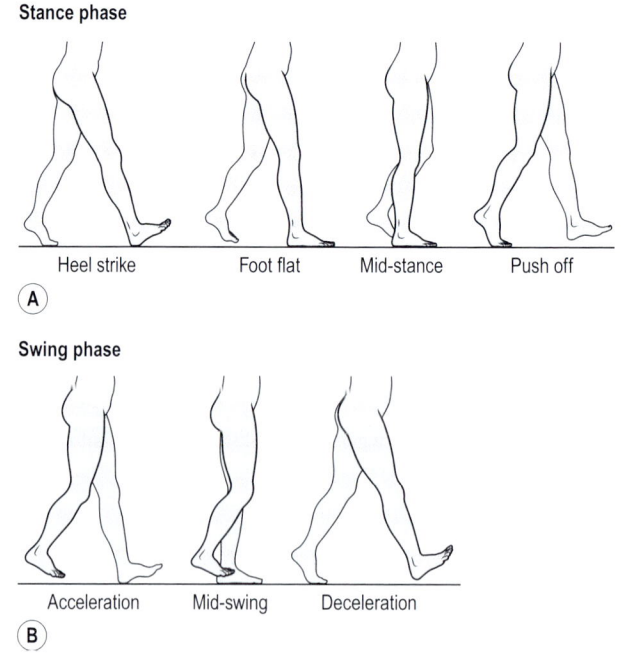

Fig. 161.1 The phases of the normal gait cycle.

What are the phases of normal gait?
The phases of gait are (Fig. 161.1):
1. *Heel strike*: the lateral calcaneus makes contact with the ground and the muscles, tendons, and ligaments relax, providing for optimal energy absorption.
2. *Midstance*: the foot is flat and is able to adapt to uneven terrain, maintain equilibrium, and absorb the shock of touchdown; the calcaneus is just below the ankle, keeping the front and back of the foot aligned for optimal weight bearing.
3. *Heel rise*: the calcaneus lifts off the ground; the foot pronates; the muscles, tendons, and ligaments tighten; and the foot regains its arch.
4. *Toe push-off*: the foot leaves the surface.

CHAPTER 162

Argyll Robertson Pupil

Instruction

Examine this patient's eyes.

Salient Features

HISTORY

- History of lancinating pains
- History of multiple sclerosis, sarcoidosis, or syphilis
- Difficulty in walking (remember the gait in tabes dorsalis).

EXAMINATION

- The pupils are small and irregular.
- Light reflex is absent.
- Accommodation reflex is intact.
- There may be depigmentation of the iris.
- Bilateral ptosis and marked overcompensation by frontalis muscle (in tabes dorsalis)
- Examination for vibration and position sense, Romberg's sign, and decreased deep tendon reflexes
- Argyll Robertson pupils show little response to atropine, physostigmine, or methacholine.

Diagnosis

This patient has Argyll Robertson pupil (lesion) and I would like to investigate for underlying neurosyphilis or luetic infection (aetiology).

Questions

What are the causes of Argyll Robertson pupil?
- Neurosyphilis: tabes dorsalis
- Diabetes mellitus and other conditions with autonomic neuropathy
- Pinealoma
- Brainstem encephalitis
- Multiple sclerosis
- Lyme disease
- Sarcoidosis
- Syringobulbia
- Tumours of the posterior portion of the third ventricle.

162—ARGYLL ROBERTSON PUPIL

What do you know about the nerve pathways of the light reflex?
- The afferent is through the optic nerve and the efferent limb is through the third cranial nerve. Among the relevant optic nerve fibres responsible for the light reaction, those responsible for the perception of light terminate in the pretectal region of the midbrain, from whence a further relay passes to the Edinger–Westphal nucleus.
- Disturbances of the pupillary light reflex occur when there is involvement of the following:
    - Superior colliculus
    - Decussation of Meynert
    - Edinger–Westphal nucleus (supplies the constrictor muscles of the iris).

Where is the lesion in Argyll Robertson pupil?
Damage to the pretectal region of the midbrain is believed to be responsible for the Argyll Robertson pupil of neurosyphilis. This, however, does not explain the small irregular pupils and it has been suggested that local involvement of the iris is a separate lesion.

Which muscle in the eye is responsible for the accommodation reflex?
Paralysis of accommodation occurs when the ciliary muscle is involved. Remember that accommodation is a much more potent stimulus for constriction of the pupils than light, as there are more nerve fibres mediating the accommodation reflex than the light reflex.

Mention a few causes of a small pupil.
- Senile miosis
- Pilocarpine drops in the treatment of glaucoma.

What is 'reversed' Argyll Robertson pupil?
The pupils react to light but not to accommodation; this is seen in parkinsonism caused by encephalitis lethargica.

What do you understand by the term anisocoria?
Anisocoria is gross inequality of the pupils. Causes include:
- third nerve palsy
- iritis
- blind or amblyopia in one eye (pupil larger in the affected eye)
- cerebrovascular accidents
- severe head trauma
- hemianopia caused by optic tract involvement.

Anisocoria occurs also in about 20% of normal individuals.

Eccentric pupil occurs when the pupil is not in the centre of the iris. It may result from trauma or iritis, and need not be pathognomonic of neurological disease.

Further Information

Douglas M.C.L. Argyll Robertson (1837–1909) of Edinburgh described these pupils in 1869 with neurosyphilis (Argyll Robertson, 1869). His studies on the effects of the extracts of the Calabar bean (*Physostigma venenosum*) on the pupil were widely acclaimed. He was the President of the Royal College of Surgeons, Edinburgh.

CHAPTER 163

Muscular Dystrophy

Instruction

This patient is having difficulty walking. Please examine his muscles.

Salient Features

HISTORY

- Know whether there is a family history of the condition
- Age of onset (Duchenne muscular dystrophy presents earlier in life than Becker muscular dystrophy)
- Shortness of breath (heart failure as a result of cardiomyopathy)
- History of learning difficulties.

EXAMINATION

- Male patient
- Proximal weakness of the lower extremities (in later stages more generalized muscle involvement)
- Pseudohypertrophy of calves
- Facial muscle weakness characteristically absent or insignificant
- Kyphoscoliosis in late stages.

Diagnosis

This young patient has proximal muscle weakness and pseudohypertrophy (lesion) caused by Becker dystrophy (aetiology). The patient has mild disability and the condition is usually progressive (functional status).

Questions

What is the difference between Duchenne and Becker muscular dystrophy?
By definition, patients with Becker muscular dystrophy can ambulate beyond the age of 15 years. The onset in Becker muscular dystrophy is usually between the ages of 5 and 15 years, but onset can occur in the third or fourth decades or even later. The majority survive into the fourth or fifth decades. Early symptoms of Becker muscular dystrophy include falls, walking on toes, and difficulties rising from the floor. Becker muscular dystrophy is less common (3 per 100,000 live male births) and has a more variable presentation of skeletal muscle weakness (Fig. 163.1). Behavioural and cognitive difficulties are also less common with Becker muscular dystrophy.

163—MUSCULAR DYSTROPHY

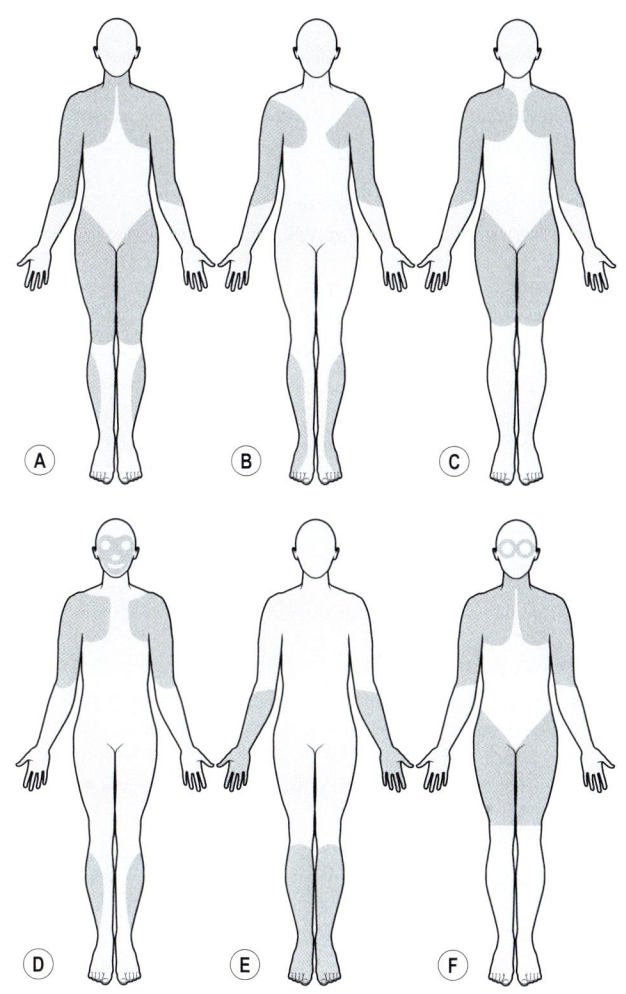

Fig. 163.1 Distribution of predominant muscle weakness *(shaded)* in different types of dystrophy. **(A)** Duchenne and Becker types; **(B)** Emery–Dreifuss; **(C)** limb girdle; **(D)** facioscapulohumeral; **(E)** distal; **(F)** oculopharyngeal.

Is there any difference between the genetics of Duchenne and Becker muscular dystrophy?

No, both Duchenne and Becker muscular dystrophy are caused by mutations in the same gene, located at Xp21. Dystrophin, its protein product, is usually absent in patients with Duchenne muscular dystrophy but is reduced in amount or abnormal in size in people with Becker's muscular dystrophy. Another protein, utrophin, closely related to dystrophin, is encoded by a second gene on chromosome 6. In normal muscle, utrophin is located predominantly in the neuromuscular junction, whereas dystrophin is found in the sarcolemmal surface.

How would you confirm the clinical diagnosis of Becker dystrophy?
- Raised creatine kinase and myoglobin levels
- Western blot analysis of muscle biopsy samples, demonstrating abnormal or reduced dystrophin
- Molecular genetic karyotyping.

Mention other X-linked myopathies.
- X-linked tubular myopathy linked to Xq28
- McLeod syndrome, where the responsible gene has been localized to Xp21 and the phenotype is characterized by mild, even subclinical, myopathy, acanthocytosis, and haemolytic anaemia. The definitive diagnosis rests on determination of the Kell red cell antigen phenotype
- Emery–Dreifuss muscular dystrophy, first described in a large family in Virginia by Emery and Dreifuss in 1966. Known association with deutan colour blindness led to localization of the gene on Xq28. The weakness presents in early childhood and is slowly progressive. The distribution of weakness is unique: an early humeral–peroneal pattern eventually evolves into a scapulo–humero–pelvi–peroneal distribution. Marked focal atrophy of the humeral and peroneal muscles is a consistent feature. Pseudohypertrophy is absent, except in extensor digitorum brevis.

How would you clinically differentiate Becker from limb-girdle muscular dystrophy?
Limb-girdle muscular dystrophy (LGMD) is also a group of genetically inherited disorders that affect skeletal muscles but they are autosomal. They present with progressive proximal muscle weakness. One of the clinical differences is that calf muscle hypertrophy is not a prominent feature of LGMD.

What is the role of antisense-mediated exon skipping in Duchenne muscular dystrophy?
Antisense-mediated exon skipping induces dystrophin synthesis in selected patients with Duchenne muscular dystrophy. The skipping of the additional exon restores the reading frame of the mRNA, allowing new production of dystrophin. The dystrophin that is produced is not normal but probably retains considerable function and therefore improves quality of life (as seen in patients with clinically milder Becker muscular dystrophy, who have similar or identically modified dystrophins). They form current treatment options for patients with Duchenne or Becker muscular dystrophy.

What is the role of myogenic stem cell transplant in muscle degenerative disorders?
Prospectively isolatable muscle-forming stem cells are present in adult skeletal muscle, and experimental studies have demonstrated the efficacy of myogenic stem cell transplant in therapy of muscle degenerative disease. In particular, satellite cells reside beneath the basal lamina of skeletal muscle fibres and include cells that act as precursors for muscle growth and repair. Although they share a common anatomical localization and typically are considered a homogeneous population, satellite cells actually exhibit substantial heterogeneity. Cell-surface marker expression was utilized to purify from the satellite cell pool a distinct population of skeletal muscle precursors that function as muscle stem cells. When purified, these precursor cells were engrafted into muscle of dystrophin-deficient *Mdx* mice and were found to contribute up to 94% of myofibres, restoring dystrophin expression and significantly improving muscle histology and contractile function. Transplanted skeletal muscle precursors also entered the satellite cell compartment, renewed the endogenous stem cell pool, and participated in subsequent rounds of injury repair. Further research is ongoing in animal models.

Further Information

Edward Meryon described Duchenne muscular dystrophy in 1852, 10 years before the French neurologist Guillaume Benjamin Amand Duchenne, with remarkably prescient pathological observations: '…the sarcolemma or tunic of the elementary fibre was broken and destroyed…' (Emery and Emery, 1995).

P.E. Becker, Professor of Human Genetics at the University of Göttingen, Germany.

Duchenne is reported to have designed a version of the modern muscle biopsy needle, which he kept in alcohol to prevent rusting. He could not have known that this also prevented sepsis.

Newton Morton, a geneticist, was the first to introduce discriminant and segregation analysis into modern human genetics as a part of a large population study of Duchenne muscular dystrophy. Tony Murphy used the disease to develop Bayesian risk-analysis procedures.

CHAPTER 164

Spastic Paraplegia

Instruction

This patient presents with difficulty walking. Please carry out a neurological examination of this patient's lower limbs.

Salient Features

HISTORY

- Onset, duration, and course of symptoms
- Back pain: whether localized
- Radicular pain
- Numbness and paraesthesia, particularly below the level of lesion
- Weakness: whether gradual or sudden
- Sphincter control and bladder sensation (differentiates cauda equina from cord compression)
- Functional status: wheelchair transfers, walking aids, orthotic shoes, and whether the house has been modified for the patient's disability
- Family history (hereditary spastic paraplegia)
- History of birth anoxia (cerebral palsy)
- History of urinary infections, pressure sores, and deep venous thrombosis (as complications of the condition).

EXAMINATION

- Increased tone in both lower limbs (in reality, patients who have had spastic paraplegia for years, the tone diminishes with time, so they may have normal or decreased tone on examination)
- Hyperreflexia bilaterally
- Ankle clonus
- Weakness in both lower limbs
- Wasting.

Additional examination findings:
- Sensory level
- Spinal tenderness or deformity
- Sacral sensation
- Upper limb involvement
- Cerebellar signs (multiple sclerosis, Friedreich's ataxia).

The following clinical signs reveal the level of the lesion:
- Spasticity of the lower limb alone: lesion of thoracic cord (T2–L1)
- Irregular spasticity of lower limbs with flaccid weakness of scattered muscles of lower limbs: lesion of lumbosacral enlargement (L2–S2)

164 — SPASTIC PARAPLEGIA

- Radicular pain: useful early in the disease, with time becomes diffuse and ceases to have localizing value
- Superficial sensation: not good for localizing as the level of sensory loss may vary greatly in different individuals and in different types of lesions.

Diagnosis

This patient has bilateral spastic paraparesis (lesion) at L1 spinal level. This is evident by the bilateral weakness of upper motor neuron type in the lower limbs, with bilateral hypertonia, hyperreflexia, clonus, and bilateral extensor plantar response. It is probably caused by spinal trauma (aetiology) as there is evidence of previous spinal surgery on the lower back; it is complicated by bladder involvement (functional status).

Questions

What are the causes of spastic paraparesis?
- Trauma (motor vehicle or diving accident)
- Spinal cord tumour (meningioma, neuroma, metastasis)
- Vascular causes (infarction, bleeding, spinal arteriovenous malformation)
- Infective causes (HIV, Lyme disease, tabes dorsalis)
- Motor neurone disease
- Syringomyelia
- Subacute combined degeneration of the cord (associated peripheral neuropathy)
- Transverse myelitis (viral, autoimmune, multiple sclerosis)
- Hereditary (familial spastic paraplegia, Friedreich's ataxia, apolipoproteinaemias).

What intracranial cause for spastic paraparesis do you know?
Parasagittal falx meningioma.

What do you know about transverse myelitic syndrome?
- Causes include trauma, compression by bony changes or tumour, vascular disease.
- All the tracts of the spinal cord are involved.
- It can present with radicular pain at onset.
- The chief clinical manifestation is spastic or flaccid paralysis.
- The lesion can be incomplete cord compression or total cord transection.

	Total Cord Transection	*Incomplete Cord Compression*
Paraplegia-in-flexion	+	+
Paralysis	Symmetrical	Asymmetrical
Flexor–withdrawal reflex	+ Without return (withdrawal phase only)	Associated with return to original position
Other	Vasomotor and sphincter changes	Variable area of anaesthesia that is not consistent with motor loss

What do you know about paraplegia-in-flexion?
Paraplegia-in-flexion is seen in partial transection of the cord where the limbs are involuntarily flexed at the hips and knees because the extensors are more paralyzed than the flexors. In complete transection of the spinal cord the extrapyramidal tracts are also affected hence no voluntary movement of the limb is possible, resulting in paraplegia-in-extension.

What investigations would you do?
- Full blood count for anaemia, corrected calcium, inflammatory markers, autoimmune screen, B_{12} and folate levels, prostate-specific antigen, serology for syphilis and HIV, serum protein electrophoresis
- Magnetic resonance imaging (MRI) of the spine
- Computed tomography (CT) myelography or plain CT
- CT of the head to exclude parasagittal meningiomas
- Cerebrospinal fluid (CSF) for oligoclonal bands.

Where is the lesion in patients with spastic weakness of one leg?
The lesion may be localized to the spinal cord or the brain. Progression to involve the arm does not help to differentiate between the spinal cord and the brain. Similarly, spread to the opposite leg does not necessarily indicate that the lesion is in the spinal cord. Investigation would include CT, MRI, and magnetic resonance angiogram (MRA) to exclude spinal dural arteriovenous fistula.

What do you know about hereditary spastic paraplegia?
Hereditary spastic paraplegia is not a single condition. It is a group of hereditary neurological disorders that share the features of spastic paraplegia of the lower limbs. The first entity was described by Seeligmuller and Strumpell in 1883, in which spasticity is more striking than muscular weakness. Since then, multiple cases have been described, with heterogeneity in clinical presentation and differences in inheritance and genetics. The age of onset is variable and the condition has a relatively benign course, with life expectancy usually not affected. When the onset is in childhood, there may be shortening of the Achilles tendon, often requiring surgical lengthening. There is usually no sensory disturbance. The mode of inheritance and genetics vary widely. An autosomal dominant form of hereditary spastic paraplegia is associated with mutations in the mitochondrial import chaperonin HSP60. An autosomal recessive form of hereditary spastic paraplegia is the result of mutations in the gene *SPG7*, which encodes paraplegin, a mitochondrial protein similar to yeast metalloproteases.

What do you know about tropical spastic paraplegia?
This is seen in Japan, the Caribbean, and parts of western Africa and South America where women, more often than men, in their third and fourth decade have spastic paraparesis with neurogenic bladder. Viral infection with human T-lymphotropic virus 1 has been implicated as a cause of this disorder.

How do you localize the lesion to the second and third lumbar root level?
- Muscular weakness: hip flexors and quadriceps
- Deep tendon reflexes affected: knee jerk
- Radicular pain/paraesthesia: anterior aspect of thigh, groin, and testicle
- Superficial sensory deficit: anterior thigh.

How do you localize the lesion to the fourth lumbar root level?
- Muscular weakness: quadriceps, tibialis anterior, and posterior
- Deep tendon reflexes affected: knee jerk
- Radicular pain/paraesthesia: anteromedial aspect of the leg
- Superficial sensory deficit: anteromedial aspect of the leg.

How do you localize the lesion to the fifth lumbar root level?
- Muscular weakness: hamstrings, peroneus longus, extensors of all the toes
- Deep tendon reflexes affected: none

- Radicular pain/paraesthesia: buttock, posterolateral thigh, anterolateral leg, dorsum of the foot
- Superficial sensory deficit: dorsum of the foot and anterolateral aspect of the leg.

How do you localize the lesion to the first sacral root level?
- Muscular weakness: plantar flexors, extensor digitorum brevis, peroneus longus, and hamstrings
- Deep tendon reflexes affected: ankle jerk
- Radicular pain/paraesthesia: buttock, back of thigh, calf, and lateral border of the foot
- Superficial sensory deficit: lateral border of the foot.

How do you localize the lesion to the lower sacral root level?
- Muscular weakness: none
- Deep tendon reflexes affected: none (but anal reflex impaired)
- Radicular pain/paraesthesia: buttock and back of thigh
- Superficial sensory deficit: saddle and perianal areas.

What are the clinical features of spinal cord compression from epidural metastasis?
The initial symptom is progressive axial pain, referred or radicular, which may last for days to months. Recumbency frequently aggravates the pain, unlike the pain of degenerative joint disease, where it is relieved. Weakness, sensory loss, and incontinence typically develop after the pain. Once a neurological deficit appears, it can evolve rapidly to paraplegia over a period of hours to days. In suspected cases, MRI of the whole spine must be performed urgently. About 50% of cases in adults arise from breast, lung, or prostate cancer. Compression usually occurs in the setting of disseminated disease. It is at the thoracic level in 70% of cases, lumbar in 20%, and cervical in 10%, and it occurs at multiple, noncontiguous levels in less than half of the cases. The tumour usually occupies the anterior or anterolateral spinal canal. CSF findings are nonspecific in metastatic epidural compression. The cell count is usually normal, but protein levels may be raised because the flow of CSF is impeded. Lumbar puncture has been known to worsen the neurological deficit, presumably caused by impaction of the cord.

CHAPTER 165

Bitemporal Hemianopia

Instruction

Examine this patient's eyes.
Examine this patient's visual fields.

Salient Features

HISTORY

- Insidious onset of defects in visual field. Involvement of the macula is late and is associated with abrupt visual failure as the presenting feature.,
- Hypogonadism (may precede the visual failure many years): males have impotence and females have amenorrhoea.

EXAMINATION

- Bitemporal hemianopia, which is caused by a median lesion of the optic chiasma (see Fig. 180.1).
- Proceed by examining the hands and face for acromegaly.
- Signs of hypopituitarism. The probable causes are:
  - pituitary tumour (endocrine symptoms precede the visual symptoms; the upper temporal fields affected first and then defect spreads down)
  - craniopharyngioma (bitemporal hemianopia initially worse in the lower quadrants)
  - suprasellar meningioma
  - aneurysms
  - metastases
  - glioma.

Diagnosis

This patient has bitemporal hemianopia (lesion) and I would like to investigate for a median mass lesion compressing the optic chiasma.

Questions

How would you investigate this patient?
- Formal field testing: perimetry
- Serum prolactin
- Skull radiography (calcification of craniopharyngioma and size of the pituitary fossa, which is best seen in the lateral skull radiograph)
- Computed tomography or magnetic resonance imaging of the head.

CHAPTER 166

Brown-Séquard Syndrome

Instruction
Examine this patient's neurological system.

Salient Features

HISTORY
- Weak leg that feels normal, whereas the other leg is moving perfectly but the patient cannot feel pain and temperature sensation (Fig. 166.1)
- Trauma to the spine, e.g. stab injury
- History of degenerative spine disease or multiple sclerosis
- Bladder and bowel symptoms.

EXAMINATION
Deficits below the level of the lesion include:
- Ipsilateral monoplegia or hemiplegia
- Ipsilateral loss of joint position and vibration sense
- Contralateral loss of spinothalamic (pain and temperature) sensation; the latter is sometimes localized to one or two segments below the anatomical level of the lesion.

Deficits in the segment of the lesion:
- Ipsilateral lower motor neuron paralysis
- Ipsilateral zone of cutaneous anaesthesia and a zone of hyperaesthesia just below the anaesthetic zone
- Segmental signs such as muscular atrophy, radicular pain, or decreased tendon reflexes are usually unilateral.

External examination of the spine should take place, as well as a full neurological examination looking for signs consistent with multiple sclerosis.

Diagnosis
This patient has Brown-Séquard syndrome (or hemisection of the spinal cord) at the level of T8 (lesion) which is probably the result of a compressive or destructive lesion of the spinal cord (aetiology). The patient is limited by the weakness in one limb (functional status).

Question
What are the causes of hemisection of the spinal cord?
- Syringomyelia
- Cord tumour
- Haematomyelia

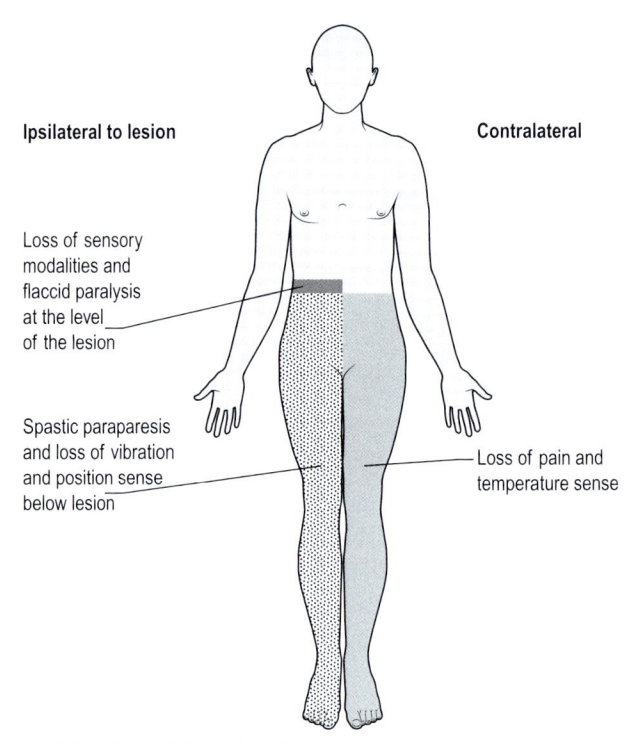

Fig. 166.1 Sensory deficit in Brown-Séquard syndrome.

- Bullet or stab wounds
- Degenerative disease of spine
- Multiple myeloma.

Further Information

Charles-Edouard Brown-Séquard (1817–1894) was Professor of Physiology in Virginia, United States, at the National Hospital, Queen Square, London, at Harvard, and finally in Paris. He was the first physician-in-chief of the National Hospital in Queen Square, which was founded in 1860. Several nations lay claim to Brown-Séquard: he was born in Mauritius, then a British colony, the son of a French woman and an American sea captain. He is said to have crossed the Atlantic more than 60 times and set up residence in the United States four times, France six, and England once.

CHAPTER 167

Carpal Tunnel Syndrome

Instruction
Examine this patient's hands.

Salient Features
HISTORY

- Nocturnal pain (commonest cause of hand pain at night). Often, the pain wakes up the patient and the patient shakes the hand to ameliorate symptoms: 'wake and shake'.
- Pain, tingling, burning, numbness, or some combination of these symptoms on the palmar aspect of the thumb, index finger, middle finger, and radial half of the ring finger (no such symptoms affect the fifth finger even on detailed questioning).
- History of oral contraceptives, rheumatoid arthritis, myxoedema, acromegaly, chronic renal failure, or sarcoidosis.
- Family history (abnormally small size of carpal tunnel runs in families).

EXAMINATION

- Wasting of the thenar eminence (Fig. 167.1A)
- Weakness of flexion, abduction, and opposition of thumb
- Diminished sensation over lateral three and half fingers.

A targeted question to ask the patient is 'What do you actually do with your hand(s) when symptoms are at their worst?' If the patient makes flicking movement of the wrist and hand, similar to that employed in shaking down a clinical thermometer (the 'flick sign'), this had both a sensitivity and a specificity >90% in one study.

- Scar of previous surgery (hidden by the crease of the wrist)
- On percussion over the course of the median nerve in the forearm the patient may experience tingling — Tinel sign (Fig. 167.1A). The sensitivity of Tinel sign ranges from 25% to 60%, although its specificity is higher (67%–87%).
- Hyperextension of the wrist for 1 min may bring on symptoms (dysaesthesia over the thumb and lateral two and half fingers): Phalen test (Fig. 167.1B).
- Associated and relevant clinical findings:
  - Signs of underlying causes such as myxoedema, acromegaly, and rheumatoid arthritis
  - Cervical spondylosis, frozen shoulder, and tennis elbow (these may be associated)
  - Cimino–Brescia fistula for haemodialysis.

Diagnosis

This patient has median nerve involvement of the hand with Tinel sign (lesion) caused by carpal tunnel syndrome as a complication of chronic haemodialysis (aetiology). The patient has disabling tingling and pain at night (functional status).

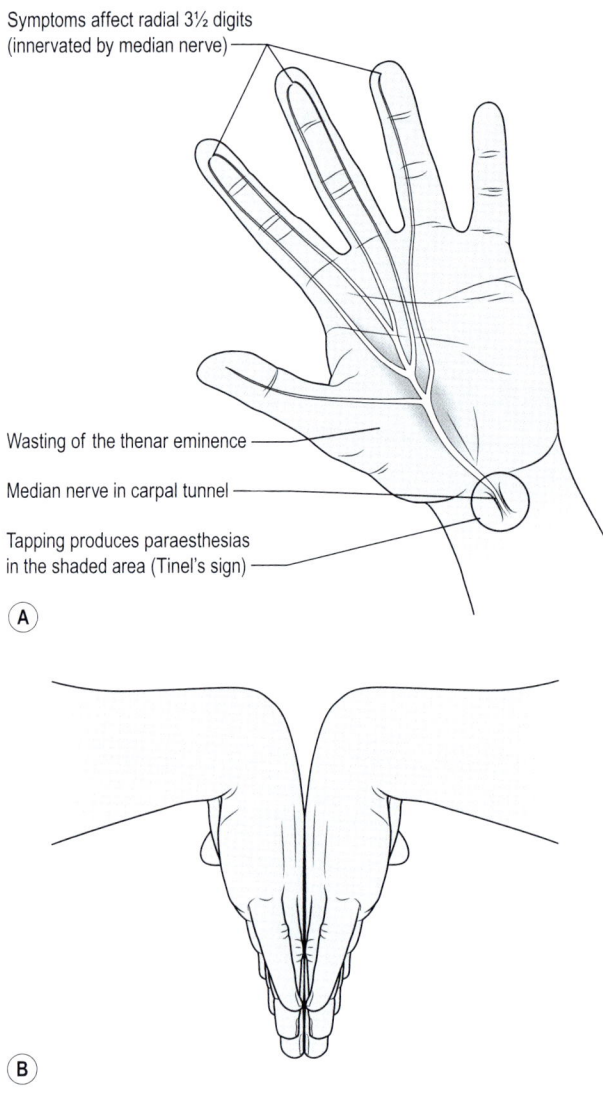

Fig. 167.1 Carpal tunnel syndrome. **(A)** Distribution of pain and/or paraesthesia *(shaded area)* when the median nerve is compressed by swelling in the wrist (carpal tunnel). **(B)** Phalen's test.

Questions

Mention a few causes of carpal tunnel syndrome.
- Pregnancy
- Oral contraceptives
- Rheumatoid arthritis
- Myxoedema
- Acromegaly
- In patients with chronic renal failure on long-term dialysis, it is caused by β_2-microglobulin as amyloid deposition

- Sarcoidosis
- Hyperparathyroidism
- Amyloidosis (e.g. caused by multiple myeloma).

How would you treat this condition?
- For mild disease with symptoms limited to numbness and tingling, with no sensory loss or pain, no sleep disturbance, and no loss of hand function, nonsurgical measures can be tried first, such as glucocorticoid injections and nocturnal wrist splinting in the neutral position, oral steroids, and occupational therapy techniques.
- For clinically moderate to severe disease with disturbing nocturnal symptoms, pain, or even developed weakness and loss of function in the hand, then surgical decompression is the treatment of choice. Surgical decompression is also the treatment of choice for severe disease, demonstrated by nerve conduction studies or electromyography.

List some clinical predictors of failure of conservative treatment
- Positive Phalen's sign
- Long duration of symptoms
- Age >50 years old
- Constant paraesthesia
- Impaired two point discrimination.

How would you confirm the diagnosis?
Nerve conduction studies: increased latency at the wrist on stimulation of the median nerve; the muscle action potential from abductor pollicis brevis is a valuable diagnostic sign. Rarely, the proximal latency may be normal with a prolonged distal latency caused by an anastomosis between the ulnar and median nerves in the forearm. Therefore, a negative test does not rule the syndrome out absolutely but calls it into question.

Mention a few clinical diagnostic tests.
- Wrist extension test: the patient is asked to extend the wrists for 1 min; this should produce numbness or tingling in the distribution of the median nerve.
- Phalen's test: the patient is asked to keep both hands with the wrist in complete palmar flexion for 1 min; this produces numbness or tingling in the distribution of the median nerve (Fig. 167.1B). Sensitivity and specificity range widely from 40% to 80%.
- Tourniquet test: the symptoms are produced when the blood pressure cuff is inflated above the systolic pressure.
- Pressure test: pressure placed where the median nerve leaves the carpal tunnel causes pain.
- Luthy's sign: this is regarded as positive if the skinfold between the thumb and index finger does not close tightly around a bottle or cup because of thumb abduction paresis.
- Durkan's test: direct pressure over the carpal tunnel (the carpal compression test); this is more sensitive and specific than Tinel's and Phalen's signs.

Mention other entrapment neuropathies.
- Meralgia paraesthetica: lateral cutaneous nerve of the thigh trapped under the inguinal ligament
- Elbow tunnel syndrome: ulnar nerve trapped in the cubital tunnel
- Common peroneal nerve trapped at the head of the fibula
- Morton's metatarsalgia: trapped medial and lateral plantar nerves causing pain between third and fourth toes
- Tarsal tunnel syndrome: trapped posterior tibial nerve

- Suprascapular nerve trapped in the spinoglenoid notch
- Radial nerve trapped in the humeral groove
- Anterior interosseous nerve trapped between the heads of the pronator muscle.

Further Information

Jules Tinel (1879–1952), a French neurologist, described it as the 'sign of formication' in his book on nerve wounds. He took an active part in the French resistance.

T.G. Morton (1835–1903), a US surgeon, described this syndrome in 1859.

CHAPTER 168

Central Scotoma

Instruction
Examine this patient's visual fields.

Salient Features

HISTORY
- Sudden onset
- Patient notices a 'hole' in the vision while reading a poster or looking at a clock
- Difficulty in performing reading, driving, walking, and recognizing faces.

EXAMINATION
- Central scotoma (allow the patient to find the defect by moving the white hat pin in his or her own visual field). Then determine:
  - the size and shape of the defect by moving the pin in and out of the blind area
  - whether the defect crosses the horizontal midline (vascular defects of retina do not do so)
  - whether the defect crosses the vertical midline (defects caused by pathway damage have a sharp vertical edge at the midline)
  - whether the defect extends to the blind spot: so-called caecocentral scotoma (seen in glaucoma, vitamin B_{12} deficiency) (Fig. 168.1)
  - whether there is a similar defect in the other eye (to exclude homonymous hemianopic scotomas).

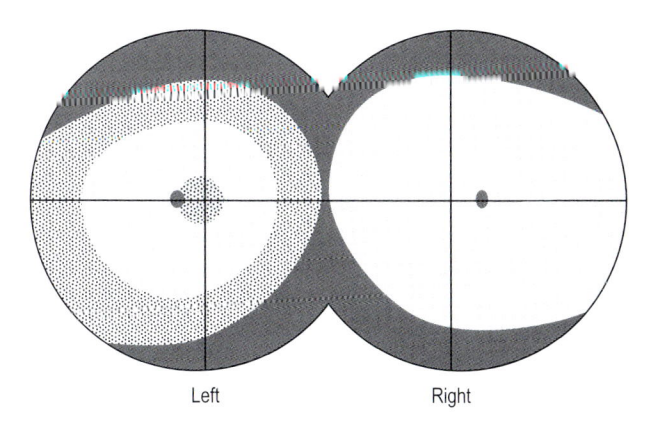

Fig. 168.1 Compressive optic neuropathy causing contraction of left visual field and caecocentral scotoma. Right visual field is normal.

- Fundoscopy; the optic discs may be:
  - pale (optic atrophy)
  - normal (retrobulbar neuritis)
  - swollen and pink (papillitis).

Diagnosis

This patient has a central scotoma (lesion) caused by optic atrophy (aetiology).

Questions

What do you understand by the term scotoma?
It is a small patch of visual loss within the visual field.

Mention a few underlying causes for central scotoma.
- Demyelinating disorders (multiple sclerosis)
- Optic nerve compression by tumour, aneurysm
- Glaucoma
- Toxins: methanol, tobacco, lead, arsenical poisoning
- Ischaemia, including central retinal artery occlusion caused by thromboembolism, temporal arteritis, syphilis, idiopathic acute ischaemic neuropathy
- Hereditary disorders: Friedreich ataxia, Leber optic atrophy
- Paget disease
- Vitamin B deficiency
- Secondary to retinitis pigmentosa
- Late age-related macular degeneration: the patient usually has enough vision to be ambulatory because the peripheral visual field around a central scotoma is intact
- Valsalva retinopathy, which is characterized by a painless, sudden loss of vision in an otherwise healthy patient with no ocular history after activities such as vomiting, coughing, and weight lifting. (The sudden rise in intrathoracic pressure increases the intraocular venous pressure, causing the rupture of perifoveal capillaries.) Visual loss can be marked but spontaneous recovery usually occurs
- Bungee jumping.

CHAPTER 169

Cerebellar Syndrome

Instruction

Examine this patient, who presented with a history of falling to one side. Demonstrate the cerebellar signs.

Salient Features

HISTORY

- Onset of symptoms (acute versus chronic) will point towards possible differentials (stroke would present with acute symptomatology, whereas a congenital cause would be more a progressive or chronic process. Multiple causes can present subacutely—over a period of weeks—such as demyelinating disease).
- Symptoms caused by cerebellar syndrome: falls, tremor, difficulty in walking, difficulty in coordination, difficulty standing up with feet together
- Symptoms that could point towards the anatomical lesion causing the cerebellar syndrome: vertigo (midline structures), irregular speech (hemispheres), unilateral symptomatology (ipsilateral lesion)
- Symptoms that could accompany a systemic illness that can cause cerebellar ataxia, symptoms or history of malignancy, previously diagnosed retinopathies that may point towards mitochondrial disorders, symptoms of autoimmune disease or sarcoidosis, detailed alcohol, and occupational and drug history
- If suspected or diagnosed stroke, risk factors should be explored (smoking, hypertension, stroke history, history of atrial fibrillation, diabetes, hypercholesterolaemia).
- If aforementioned causes have not revealed any helpful differentials, then other causes should be excluded: drug toxicity like phenytoin, alcohol abuse, lead poisoning and solvent abuse, history of intracranial tumours (posterior fossa including cerebellopontine angle tumour), history of hypothyroidism (a reversible cause), history of lung cancer (paraneoplastic manifestation).
- Family history (Friedreich's ataxia and other hereditary ataxias) and birth defects (congenital malformations at the level of the foramen magnum).

EXAMINATION

- Speech assessment (staccato, irregular type of speech)
- Rebound phenomenon on outstretched hands
- Examination for rapid alternating movements with the hand
- Finger–nose test to look for past-pointing and intention tremor
- Heel–shin test to look for dysmetria and incoordination
- Gait, in particular tandem walking. If ataxia is not marked, the patient's gait may be tested with the eyes closed; patients will often veer to the side of the lesion.
- Eye examination for eye movements, nystagmus, and saccadic movements

- Fundoscopy for optic atrophy as demyelination is the commonest cause of cerebellar signs.
- Dysarthria—the speech may be scanning or staccato. Articulation may be uneven; words may be slurred and variations in pitch and loudness can occur.

Diagnosis

This patient has a cerebellar syndrome with optic atrophy (lesion) caused by multiple sclerosis (aetiology) and he is markedly ataxic (functional status).

Questions

How may cerebellar signs manifest?
- Disorders of movement:
  - Nystagmus: coarse horizontal nystagmus with lateral cerebellar lesions and its direction is towards the side of the lesion
  - Scanning dysarthria: a halting, jerking dysarthria, which is usually a feature of bilateral lesions
  - Lack of finger–nose coordination (past-pointing): movement imprecise, in force, direction, and distance (dysmetria)
  - Rebound phenomenon: inability to arrest strong contraction on sudden removal of resistance (known as Holmes rebound phenomenon)
  - Intention tremor
  - Dysdiadochokinesia: impairment of rapid alternating movements (clumsy)
  - Dyssynergia: movements involving more than one joint are broken into parts
  - Dysarthria.
- Hypotonia
- Absent reflexes or pendular reflexes
- Lack of coordination of gait: patient tends to fall towards the side of the lesion
- The classic clinical triad of cerebellar disease is ataxia, atonia, and asthenia
- The cerebellum is not primarily responsible for motor function. It is developed phylogenetically from a primary vestibular area and is involved in modulation of motor activity. It receives afferents from the vestibular nuclei, spinal cord, and cerebral cortex via the pontine nuclei.

What are the causes of cerebellar syndrome?
- Demyelination (multiple sclerosis)
- Brainstem vascular lesion
- Phenytoin toxicity
- Alcoholic cerebellar degeneration (there is atrophy of the anterior vermis of the cerebellum)
- Space-occupying lesion in the posterior fossa including cerebellopontine angle tumour
- Hypothyroidism (a reversible cause)
- Paraneoplastic manifestation of bronchogenic carcinoma
- Friedreich's ataxia and other hereditary ataxias
- Congenital malformations at the level of the foramen magnum.

A useful way of remembering the different causes of cerebellar syndrome is to categorize them into groups of diseases.
- Neoplasia related (metastatic cancer to the cerebellum, paraneoplastic syndrome caused by extracerebellar malignancy, primary lesion in the cerebellum)

- Toxic and metabolic (alcohol, phenytoin and other antiepileptics, electrolyte disturbances such as low calcium, low magnesium, and vitamin deficiencies, such as B_{12} deficiency and vitamin E deficiency)
- Vascular causes (stroke, thrombotic episode or haemorrhagic stroke, vertebrobasilar insufficiency syndrome)
- Congenital and genetic (Arnold Chiari malformation, mitochondrial disorders, Refsum disease. There is a long list of congenital causes for cerebellar ataxia).

How are cerebellar signs localized?
- Gait ataxia (inability to do tandem walking): anterior lobe (palaeocerebellum)
- Truncal ataxia (drunken gait, titubation): flocculonodular or posterior lobe (archicerebellum)
- Limb ataxia, especially upper limbs and hypotonia: lateral lobes (neocerebellum).

What is the difference between sensory ataxia and cerebellar ataxia?

	Cerebellar Ataxia	*Sensory Ataxia*
Site of lesion	Cerebellum	Posterior column or peripheral nerves
Deep tendon	Unchanged or pendular	Lost or diminished reflexes
Deep sensation	Normal	Decreased or lost
Sphincter disturbances	None	Decreased when posterior column involved, causing overflow incontinence

If you were allowed to do one investigation, which one would you choose in a patient with a suspected cerebellar lesion?
Magnetic resonance imaging.

Further Information

Sir Gordon M. Holmes (1876–1965) was a consultant neurologist at the National Hospital for Nervous Diseases, London; his observations on wartime gunshot wounds allowed him to study cerebellar disease (Holmes, 1939). He was the editor of the journal *Brain*.

Luigi Luciani (1840–1919), an Italian physiologist, described the cerebellar triad in his landmark publication in 1891.

CHAPTER 170

Cerebellar Dysarthria

Instruction
Ask this patient a few questions.

Salient Features
EXAMINATION
- The speech may be scanning (enunciation is difficult, words are produced slowly and in a measured fashion) or staccato (in bursts). Scanning speech is more common in multiple sclerosis, whereas staccato speech is more common in Friedreich ataxia.
- Articulation is uneven, words are slurred, and variations in pitch and loudness occur.
- A full neurological examination should be carried out for further cerebellar signs.

Diagnosis
This patient has scanning speech (lesion) caused by cerebellar involvement secondary to chronic alcohol abuse (aetiology).

Questions

What do you understand by the term dysarthria?
Dysarthria is impaired articulation of speech. It may result from lesions of muscles, myoneural junctions, or motor neurons of lips, tongue, palate, and pharynx. Common causes include mechanical defects such as ill-fitting dentures or cleft palate. Dysarthria may also result from impaired hearing, which begins in early childhood.

How would you test the different structures responsible for articulation?
- Lips: ask the patient to say, 'me, me, me'.
- Tongue: ask the patient to say, 'la, la, la'.
- Pharynx: ask the patient to say, 'kuh, gut'.
- Palate, larynx, and expiratory muscles: ask the patient to say, 'ah'. In palatal paralysis, the patient's speech is worse when the head is bent forwards.

Articulation can also be tested by asking the patient to repeat the following:
- British constitution
- Hippopotamus
- Methodist episcopal
- Constantinople is the capital of Turkey.

What do you understand by 'top of the basilar' syndrome?
Emboli to the rostral portion of the basilar artery usually produce this syndrome, with a myriad of possible symptoms characterized by visual, oculomotor, and behavioural abnormalities, often

without significant motor dysfunction. A 'top of the basilar syndrome' is characterized by somnolence and, sometimes, stupor; inability to make new memories; small, poorly reactive pupils; and defective vertical gaze. Patients with cerebellar infarcts often have dizziness, sometimes in conjunction with frank vertigo, blurred vision, difficulty walking, and vomiting. These patients often veer to one side and cannot sit upright or maintain an erect posture without support. They may have hypotonia of the arm on the side of the infarct, a sign best elicited by having them hold their arms straight ahead and then rapidly lower them, quickly braking the movement. The hypotonic arm overshoots on both descent and rapid ascent. Nystagmus is common. Patients with pure cerebellar infarcts *do not* have hemiparesis or hemisensory loss.

What parts of the brain does the vertebrobasilar artery supply?
The vertebrobasilar arterial system supplies the brainstem (medulla, pons, and midbrain), cerebellum, occipital lobes, posterior temporal lobes, and thalamus. The vertebrobasilar arterial system consists of the extracranial and intracranial vertebral arteries; these unite to form the basilar artery, which runs midline along the ventral surface of the brainstem, feeding it with small, deep perforators until it merges with the circle of Willis to give off the posterior cerebral arteries.

What is the significance of anti-Yo antibodies in a patient with cerebellar syndrome?
The presence of anti-Yo antibodies in the serum of a woman with cerebellar symptoms is virtually conclusive evidence that she has paraneoplastic cerebellar degeneration and gynaecologic, usually ovarian, cancer.

What is the role of chaperones in cerebellar tumours?
A chaperone complex (which typically maintains cellular protein assembly and function) mediates the assembly of the von Hippel–Lindau tumour suppressor protein; when this protein is not assembled correctly, its tumour-suppressing activity is lost, permitting the development and growth of tumours. A mutation in or deletion of part of this tumour-suppressor protein is associated with von Hippel–Lindau disease (characterized by phaeochromocytoma, renal carcinoma, and densely vascularized retinal and cerebellar tumours).

What is the role of the Sonic hedgehog *Shh* pathway in the pathogenesis of medulloblastoma?
Medulloblastoma arises through abnormalities of developmental pathways in a population of progenitor cells. These tumours aberrantly express multiple regulatory genes known to mediate the proliferation of neural stem cells. Activity in the *Shh* pathway is important for the self-renewal of progenitor cells and the proliferation of their progeny and in the initiation of brain tumours. Medulloblastoma cells die rapidly when cultured with cyclopamine, an antagonist of the hedgehog family of signalling pathways.

CHAPTER 171

Cerebellopontine Angle Tumour

Instruction
Examine this patient's cranial nerves.

Salient Features
EXAMINATION
- Damage to the seventh and eighth cranial nerves is the hallmark of this lesion in this region.
- History of hearing loss and tinnitus
- Rarer symptoms include vertigo, headache, facial hypaesthesia, and diplopia.
- Cerebellopontine angle tumours rarely cause facial weakness.
- Examination of the corneal reflex and the trigeminal nerve.

Tell the examiner you would like to examine for the following:
- Cerebellar signs
- Signs of neurofibromatosis type 2
- Papilloedema (seen uncommonly as a result of raised intracranial pressure).

Diagnosis
This patient has features of cerebellopontine angle tumour (lesion), usually caused by an acoustic neuroma (aetiology), and has severe hearing loss and disabling tinnitus (functional status).

Questions

Mention a few causes of cerebellopontine angle lesions.
- Acoustic neuroma (now known as vestibular schwannoma) accounts for 85% of cerebellopontine angle tumours.
- Meningioma, cholesteatoma, haemangioblastoma, aneurysm of the basilar artery
- Pontine glioma
- Sarcomas of the clivus and lateral skull base
- Medulloblastoma and astrocytoma of the cerebellum
- Carcinoma of the nasopharynx
- Local meningeal involvement by syphilis and tuberculosis.

What do you understand by the term cerebellopontine angle?
It is the shallow triangular fossa lying between the cerebellum, lateral pons, and the inner third of the petrous temporal bone. It extends from the trigeminal nerve (earlier) to the glossopharyngeal nerve (see later). The abducens nerve runs along the medial edge, whereas the facial and auditory cranial nerves traverse the angle to enter the internal auditory meatus. There is a wide range of pathologic processes within the cerebellopontine angle. These processes may present because of

mass effect on local structures, such as the fifth to twelfth cranial nerves, or because of mass effect on the pons or cerebellum, which may result in fourth ventricular obstruction.

What is the histology of acoustic neurofibroma?
It consists of elongated cells similar to spindle fibroblasts with much collagen and reticulum. They are believed to arise from Schwann cells and are also known as schwannomas. These lesions most often arise from the inferior vestibular nerve within the internal auditory canal and present with hearing loss or tinnitus. Schwannomas can be entirely intracanalicular or have intracanalicular and cisternal components, resulting in the description of an 'ice-cream cone' tumour (Fig. 171.1).

How would you investigate such patients?
- Magnetic resonance imaging (MRI) (Fig. 171.1) with gadolinium contrast with fluid-attenuated inversion recovery and diffusion-weighted imaging
- Computed tomography
- Serology for syphilis

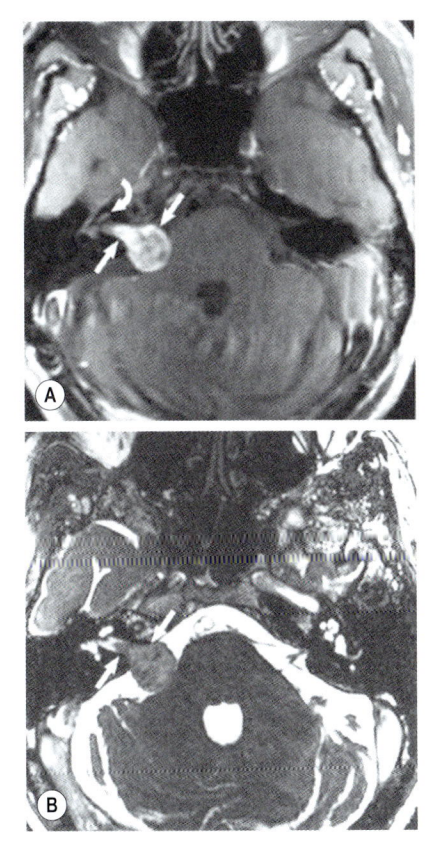

Fig. 171.1 **(A)** Axial T_1-weighted, postcontrast, fat-saturated imaging demonstrates a heterogeneously enhancing classic 'ice-cream cone' vestibular schwannoma of the right cerebellopontine angle and internal auditory canal *(arrows)*. **(B)** Axial fast imaging using steady-state acquisition, thin-slice, T_2-weighted imaging of the same lesion *(arrows)* shows the contours of the schwannoma, clearly delineated from hyperintense CSF and with a 'cap' of CSF between the schwannoma and the cochlea. (With permission from Lakshmi, M., Glastonbury, C.M., 2009. Imaging of the cerebellopontine angle. Neuroimaging Clin. North Am. 19, 393–406.)

- Audiological testing
- Caloric test (which will reveal that the labyrinth is destroyed)
- Vertebral angiography
- Cerebrospinal fluid (CSF) may be abnormal or have raised protein concentration.

What is the treatment in this condition?
- Stereotactic radiosurgery. Techniques include gamma knife, linear accelerator (LINAC), and fractionated radiotherapy
- Microsurgical resection
- Conservative approach is increasingly popular with a recognition that tumours are largely slow growing. Yearly MRI scanning is recommended, with approximately 20% of patients going to further treatment.

Mention some tumours that occur in families with familial adenomatous polyposis.
Papillary thyroid carcinoma, sarcomas, hepatoblastomas, pancreatic carcinomas, and medulloblastomas of the cerebellar–pontine angle of the brain.

Further Information

F.T. Schwann (1810–1864), a German anatomist, was Professor of Anatomy in Louvain. He was one of the first to demonstrate that fermentation was associated with living organisms. Independently from Schleiden, he concluded that plants are formed of cells; this is known as the Schleiden–Schwann cellular theory. Schwann also discovered that the upper oesophagus contains striated muscle. He discovered pepsin and showed that bile was essential for digestion.

The first surgical removal of an acoustic neuroma was performed in 1894.

L. Leksell was the first to use radiosurgery in 1969, what he called the 'gamma knife' (Leksell, 1971).

CHAPTER 172

Charcot–Marie–Tooth Disease (Peroneal Muscular Atrophy)

Instruction

Examine this patient's legs.

Salient Features

EXAMINATION

- Wasting of the muscles of calves and thighs that stops abruptly, usually in the lower third of the thigh, and is described as 'stork' or 'spindle' legs, 'fat bottle' calves, and 'inverted champagne bottles' (Fig. 172.1)
- Pes cavus (high-arched foot) or pes planus (flat foot), clawing of toes, contractures of the Achilles tendon
- Weakness of dorsiflexion, foot drop
- Absent ankle jerks, plantars downgoing or equivocal
- Mild sensory impairment or no sensory loss. Some patients have decreased responses to pain in the stocking distribution.
- Lateral popliteal nerve thickening felt on palpation (seen in some cases only)
- Small muscle wasting and clawing of the hands
- Gait impairment.

There are two distinctive clinical features of this disease:
1. The muscular atrophy begins in the distal portions of the affected muscles in the lower and upper limbs, unlike the global atrophy of motor neurone disease or muscular dystrophy. The atrophy then creeps upwards, involving all muscles.
2. The degree of disability is minimal in spite of marked deformity.

Diagnosis

This patient has 'inverted champagne bottle' legs with sensory neuropathy (lesion), which is caused by hereditary Charcot–Marie–Tooth disease (CMT) (aetiology). She has severe foot drop and requires calipers (functional status).

Questions

What are the phenotypic types of Charcot–Marie–Tooth disease?

CMT is divided into two major phenotypic types according to electrophysiological, clinical, and nerve biopsy evaluations:
- Glial myelinopathy (type 1): a demyelinating neuropathy (marked slowing of conduction in motor nerves; absent deep tendon reflexes)
- Neuronal axonopathy (type 2): an axonal neuropathy (little or no slowing of nerve conduction; normal deep tendon reflexes).

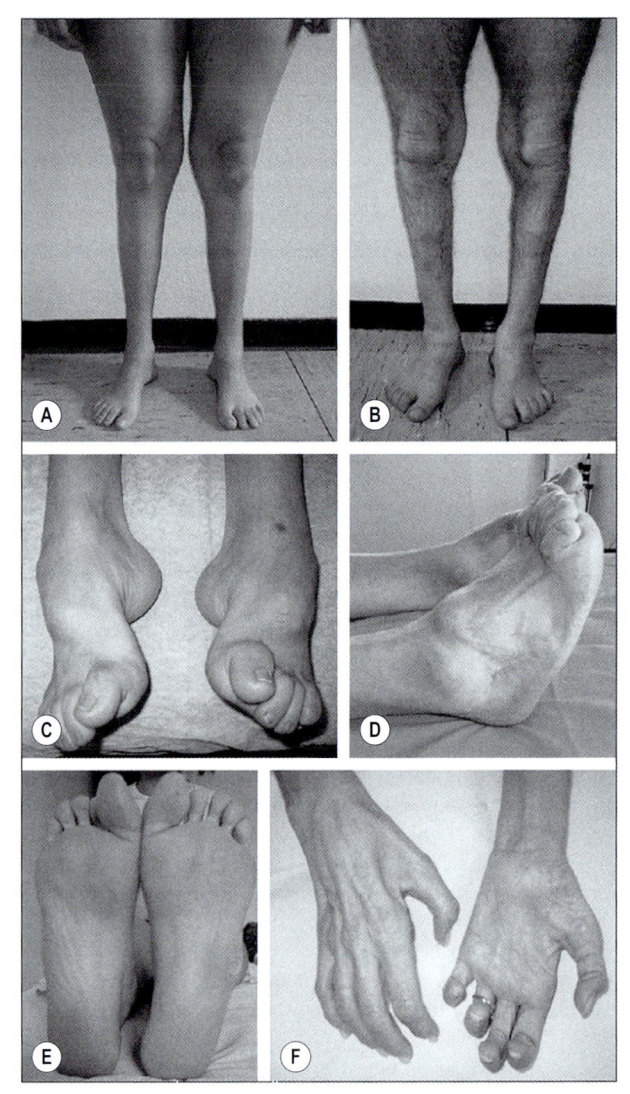

Fig. 172.1 CMT disease. **(A** and **B)** Muscle wasting of the legs and the lower third of the thigh. **(C–E)** Foot deformities of different severities, with high arches, hammer toes, and callosities. **(F)** Severe atrophy of intrinsic hand muscles (main en griffe, claw hand). (With permission from Pareyson, D., Marchesi, C., 2009. Diagnosis, natural history, and management of Charcot–Marie–Tooth disease. Lancet Neurol. 8, 654–667.)

What is the mode of inheritance?
Each type can be inherited in a dominant, recessive, or X-linked fashion. There are also autosomal dominant intermediate forms of CMT that can have features of both axonal and demyelinating neuropathies. Mutations in 31 known genes and additional unidentified loci can produce CMT:
- Some common genes include *PMP22, MPZ, PRX, GDAP1,* and *EGR2.*

- *MPZ* (encoding myelin protein zero is a member of the immunoglobulin superfamily; it may be important not only in forming myelin but also in cell signalling), *GDAP1* and *GJB1* are known to be associated with CMT type 1, but select mutations in these genes can also cause CMT type 2.
- *NEFL* is known to be associated with CMT type 2, but select mutations convey a CMT type 1 phenotype.
- Dominant intermediate forms of CMT have been reported to be associated with *MPZ* mutations.
- Specific recessive alleles related to CMT have also been reported for *EGR2* and *PMP22*.
- Two mutations in *SH3TC2* (encoding the SH3 domain and tetratricopeptide repeats 2) cause autosomal recessive CMT.
- Of the 31 genes in 39 known CMT loci, only 15 are currently available for clinical testing.
- Current evidence-based clinical guidelines for distal symmetric polyneuropathy recommend genetic testing consisting of screening for common mutations, including the *CMT1A* duplication copy-number variant and point mutations of the X-linked *GJB1*.
- Whole-genome sequencing is emerging to be the diagnostic tool in this condition.

What other uncommon features may these patients have?
Optic atrophy, retinitis pigmentosa, spastic paraparesis.

In which other progressive conditions is pes cavus seen?
Pes cavus, which is the Latin translation for 'hollow foot' can be idiopathic in 10% of the general population, but as it accompanies hereditary neuropathies like CMT, it is a 'spy sign' that should alert the physician to suspect a possible underlying neurological pathophysiology. Another progressive neurological condition that pes cavus is seen is Friedreich's ataxia.

How does the forme fruste of the disease manifest?
The forme fruste may be seen in family members of patients with CMT and manifests as pes cavus and absent ankle jerks.

Mention other hereditary neuropathies.
- Roussy–Lévy syndrome (where features of progressive muscular atrophy may be combined with tremor and ataxia)
- Hereditary amyloidosis
- Refsum disease (phytanic acid accumulates in the central and peripheral nervous systems)
- Fabry disease (where there is a deficiency of α-galactosidase)
- Tangier disease
- Bassen–Kornzweig disease (abetalipoproteinaemia, absence of low-density lipoprotein, and vitamin E deficiency)
- Metachromatic leukodystrophy (where galactosyl sulfatide accumulates in the central and peripheral nervous systems).

Mention a few conditions that Charcot is credited to have described for the first time.
- Ankle clonus
- Tabes dorsalis and Charcot joints
- Multiple sclerosis
- Peroneal muscular atrophy
- Multiple cerebral aneurysms, called Charcot–Bouchard aneurysms
- Hysteria.

Further Information

The syndrome was originally described by J.M. Charcot (1825–1923) and P. Marie (1853–1940) in 1886 at the Salpêtrière in Paris and independently by H. H. Tooth at St Bartholomew's Hospital and the National Hospital for Nervous Diseases, Queen Square, London.

P. Marie was a world-famed neurologist. He published extensively on aphasia. He succeeded Charcot lineage of Raymond, Brissaud, and Dejerine at the Salpêtrière in 1918.

CHAPTER 173

Chorea

PATIENT 1: SYDENHAM'S CHOREA

Instruction
Look at this patient.

Salient Features

HISTORY
- History of sore throat if the patient is an adolescent, particularly if female; rheumatic fever should raise suspicion of Sydenham's chorea (St. Vitus' dance)
- Family history (especially in the middle-aged adult) for Huntington disease
- Oral contraceptive use in a young woman or recent pregnancy (chorea gravidarum).

EXAMINATION
- Irregular, jerking, ill-sustained, unpredictable, quasipurposeful movements of the upper limbs
- The patient is clumsy and keeps dropping objects. Patients with mild disease may show increased fidgeting or restlessness
- Abnormal grip of the hands: when the patient squeezes the doctor's hands, a squeezing and relaxing motion occurs, which has been described as a 'milkmaid's grip'.
- Examination of the tongue for any involuntary movements: known as 'jack-in-the box' tongue or 'bag of worms'
- Deep tendon reflexes may be normal or 'pendular' or 'hung-up' reflexes.

Diagnosis
This young patient has Sydenham's chorea (lesion) secondary to streptococcal sore throat (aetiology); this condition is usually self-limiting (functional status).

Questions

Mention a few more causes of acquired chorea.
- Systemic lupus erythematosus
- Polycythaemia vera
- Chorea gravidarum, seen in pregnancy
- Idiopathic hypoparathyroidism; hyperthyroidism
- Focal vascular lesion in basal ganglia
- Drug-induced, e.g. levodopa
- Kernicterus.

What is the cause of Sydenham's chorea?
Sydenham's chorea, also known as rheumatic chorea, is a complication of rheumatic fever.

What is the prognosis of patients with Sydenham's chorea?
Most patients recover within 1 to 3 months; a few may have relapses. A small proportion may develop valvular heart disease and hence should receive penicillin prophylaxis to prevent recurrence of rheumatic fever. Severe cases of Sydenham's chorea have been reported (chorea paralytica) and these cases may need immunosuppression or more invasive treatments.

Is there any haematological disorder associated with chorea?
- Polycythaemia vera
- Neuroacanthocytosis or 'chorea–acanthocytosis', where >15% of the red blood cells are acanthocytes.

PATIENT 2: HUNTINGTON DISEASE
Instruction
Look at this patient and ask him a few questions.

Salient Features
HISTORY
- Family history of dementia and chorea.

EXAMINATION
- Young adult (aged 30–50 years)
- Chorea
- Cognitive impairment.

Diagnosis
This patient has chorea (lesion) caused by Huntington disease and is severely limited by the disease and chorea.

Questions
What do you know about Huntington disease?
Huntington disease is the most common cause of hereditary chorea. It is an autosomal dominant disorder with a full penetrance characterized by progressive chorea and dementia in middle life. These characteristic findings are the result of severe neuronal loss, initially in the neostriatum and later in the cerebral cortex. The defect is on the small arm of chromosome 4. There is associated random repetition of a sequence of trinucleotides (CAG; normal chromosomes contain about 11–34 copies of this repeat). In Huntington disease, the greater the number of CAG repeats, the earlier the onset of disease. The protein product for the gene has been termed huntingtin. It has been proposed that the huntingtin protein is cleaved to fragments that are conjugated with ubiquitin and carried to the proteasome complex. This huntingtin and proteasome component then

translocates to the nucleus, where it forms intranuclear inclusions; over time, this process leads to cell death. There is a marked reduction in acetylcholine, substance P, and γ-aminobutyric acid activity in the corpus striatum, whereas dopamine activity is normal and somatostatin is increased.

Using neuropeptide immunochemistry, the chorea has been shown to be associated with damage to the lateral globus pallidus, whereas the parkinsonian signs are caused by additional damage in projections of the medial globus pallidus.

What is the advantage of assessing CAG expansion in persons at risk for Huntington disease?
It is a direct test allowing more accurate assessment of genetic risk, without the need to obtain DNA from family members. This also allows privacy and confidentiality to be maintained because of the reduced need for blood samples from relatives. However, since the misdiagnosis of other illnesses as Huntington disease may occur, the testing of DNA from at least one affected relative is recommended to confirm that CAG expansion is present in other affected persons in the family. This finding will allow the correct interpretation of a normal number of CAG repeats in a person at risk.

What do you know of transcriptional dysregulation and mitochondrial impairment in Huntington disease?
- Transcriptional dysregulation and mitochondrial impairment are two important mechanisms in Huntington disease.
    - *Transcriptional dysregulation.* Mutant huntingtin may alter the complement of proteins that are synthesized in a cell, a change that may lead to the pattern of neurodegeneration that characterizes Huntington disease (it binds and sequesters the binding protein for cyclic AMP response-element-binding protein (CREB)), which alters the expression of genes regulated by the transcription factor CREB. In a similar way, mutant huntingtin interferes with Sp1-mediated gene transcription.
    - *Mitochondrial impairment.* Activities of mitochondrial electron transport complexes II, III, and IV are reduced in Huntington disease. Peroxisome proliferator-activated receptor-γ coactivator 1α (PGC-1α) is a transcriptional coactivator that controls many metabolic processes, including mitochondrial biogenesis, oxidative phosphorylation, and adaptive thermogenesis (the body's response to cold temperatures). PGC-1α regulated gene transcription is defective. As a result, there is reduced expression of mitochondrial and antioxidant genes regulated by PGC-1α.

Are any other diseases known to be associated with increased numbers of triplet repeats?
Yes, these include myotonic muscular dystrophy, spinocerebellar ataxia type 1, FRAXE syndrome, and hereditary dentatorubral pallidoluysian atrophy.

How would you manage this patient?
Management progresses from clinical suspicion and genetic testing. Once a diagnosis is confirmed, the treatment is symptomatic plus support for depression. A combination of valproate and olanzapine may help in relieving the psychosis and movement disorders associated with Huntington disease. Tetrabenazine, amantadine, or riluzole can also be considered. Research is ongoing into the role of deep brain stimulation as a treatment for Huntington's chorea.

Further Information

Thomas Sydenham (1624–1689) was a Puritan from Dorset and in 1666 published his first work on fevers, which he dedicated to Robert Boyle. *Chorea* in Greek means dance.

Gustav Mahler was diagnosed with a cardiac valve anomaly in 1907 and died of subacute bacterial endocarditis in 1911. It is possible that the composer suffered from rheumatic disease in childhood with carditis and

- Sydenham's chorea, which may have left him with cardiac valve disorder, obsessive–compulsive personality, and persistent chorea.
- George Summer Huntington (1851–1916) first documented (in 1909) the clinical and hereditary features of this condition in a family from Suffolk settled in Long Island in New York.
- Sydenham's chorea is also known as St. Vitus' dance. The term stems from the middle ages when patients affected with the disease would go to the chapels of St. Vitus' to be cured.

CHAPTER 174

Lateral Popliteal Nerve Palsy, L4, L5 (Common Peroneal Nerve Palsy)

Instruction

Examine this patient's legs.
Test this patient's gait.

Salient Features

HISTORY

- History of trauma to the nerve particularly when it winds around the neck of the fibula where it is protected by only skin and fascia
- Symptoms may occur after sitting crossed leg for prolonged periods
- Recent weight loss, particularly in those who have been confined to bed rest (nerve more vulnerable because the protective fat and muscle is lost)
- Plasters around the knee
- History of diabetes, polyarteritis nodosa, collagen vascular diseases (all causes of mononeuritis multiplex).

EXAMINATION

- Wasting of the muscles on the lateral aspect of the leg, namely the peronei and tibialis anterior muscle
- Weakness of dorsiflexion and eversion of the foot
- Foot drop
- High-stepping gait
- Loss of sensation on the lateral aspect of the leg and dorsum of the foot. If the deep peroneal branch is affected, the sensory loss may be limited to the dorsum of the web between the first and second toes.
- Ankle jerk
    - Absent ankle jerk: S1 lesion
    - Normal jerk: common peroneal nerve palsy
    - Brisk jerk: upper motor neuron lesion.
- Calliper shoes or splints may be by the bedside.

Diagnosis

This patient has wasting of the lateral aspect of the leg and sensory loss (lesion) caused by common nerve palsy after trauma to the head of the fibula (aetiology) and has to wear callipers (functional status).

Questions

Mention a few causes of lateral popliteal nerve palsy.
- Compression resulting from application of a tourniquet or plaster of Paris casts. The nerve is vulnerable at the head of the fibula, where it lies on the surface of the hard bone with a covering of only skin. Compression from knee-high boots can also result in this injury.
- Direct trauma to the nerve, including knee dislocation
- Leprosy (commonest cause worldwide)
- Ganglion arising from the superior tibiofibular joint may compress the nerve.
- Compression of the nerve by the tendinous edge of the peroneus longus
- Causes of mononeuropathy including diabetes, alcohol.

How would you manage such a patient?
- Nerve conduction studies: there may be a local conduction block or slowing in the region of the head of the fibula. There may be denervation in the tibialis anterior and extensor digitorum profundus.
- If the intact nerve is severed surgery is performed.
- If the nerve is intact and not functioning, the patient may benefit from nonsurgical measures including physiotherapy, 90-degree splint at night, calliper shoes with a 90-degree stop, and galvanic or faradic stimulation to maintain the bulk of the muscle until the nerve recovers.
- For refractory cases and those with compressive masses, surgical decompression may be required. If this fails, tendon and nerve transfer may help.

What other types of nerve injury do you know?
- Neurapraxia: concussion of the nerve, after which a complete recovery occurs
- Axonotmesis: the axon is severed but the myelin sheath is intact; recovery may occur.
- Neurotmesis: the nerve is completely severed and the prognosis for recovery is poor.

What are other causes of foot drop?
- Peripheral neuropathy
- L4, L5 root lesion
- Motor neurone disease
- Sciatic nerve palsy
- Lumbosacral plexus lesion.

CHAPTER 175

Expressive Dysphasia

Instruction
Ask this patient a few questions.

Salient Features
HISTORY
- Patient has difficulty in finding the appropriate words.

EXAMINATION
- Patient's ability to find appropriate words is impaired, whereas comprehension is intact (e.g. asking the patient to name geometric shapes, parts of the body, or components of common objects such as a pen).
- Repetition may or may not be intact.
- A full neurological examination of the patient should be carried out looking for signs of a right-sided stroke.

The neurologic basis of language is controlled by a network of neocortical areas centred in the perisylvian regions of the left hemisphere of the brain. This language network is almost always located in the left hemisphere of the brain and includes the perisylvian portions of the inferior frontal and temporoparietal regions, known as Broca's and Wernicke's areas, respectively, as well as surrounding regions of the frontal, parietal, and temporal cortex. The term dysphasia denotes a disorder in language processing caused by damage to this network.

Diagnosis
This patient has expressive dysphasia (lesion) caused by a right-sided stroke (aetiology).

Questions

Where is the lesion?
In Broca's area, which is located in the posterior portion of the third left frontal gyrus. It is the motor association cortex for face, tongue, lips, and palate. It contains the motor patterns necessary to produce speech.

How would you manage this patient?
- Computed tomography or magnetic resonance imaging (MRI) head scan to localize the affected area
- Antiplatelets and secondary prevention medication
- Referral to the speech therapist
- Multidisciplinary rehabilitation and modification of risk factors.

623

What do you understand by stuttering?
- Stuttering is a disorder of fluency of speech characterized by the involuntary repetition or prolongation of sounds, syllables, words, or phrases, as well as frequent pauses, impeding the rhythmic flow of speech.
- Onset is typically between 3 and 6 years of age, and ~5% of preschool children may stutter. The majority of young children who stutter go on to make a full recovery. The disorder may continue unabated in some, resulting in a prevalence of about 1% among adults.

What is the commonest sign of primary progressive aphasia?
The commonest clinical feature of primary progressive aphasia is anomia (the inability to retrieve the right word in conversation or to name objects as requested by an examiner). The early stages of anomia can be detected by asking the patient to name geometric shapes, parts of the body, or components of common objects (the cap of a pen or the wristband of a watch). Many patients remain in an anomic stage through most of the course of the disease, with a gradual intensification of word-finding deficits, almost to the point of mutism. Occasionally, distinct forms of agrammatism or deficits in word comprehension develop.

What do you understand by the term agrammatism?
Agrammatism refers to inappropriate word order and the misuse of word endings, prepositions, pronouns, conjunctions, and verb tenses.

What do you know about the genetics of speech?
- Linkage studies of prevalent types of speech and language disorders have implicated several regions of the genome, most notably on chromosomes 3, 13, 16, and 19. The putative risk genes underlying these linkages have yet to be identified.
- Mutation in *FOXP2*, which is located in chromosomal band 7q31 and encodes a transcription factor, has been described in a British family with autosomal dominant transmission of oral motor and speech dyspraxia. These patients have problems sequencing the precise movements of tongue, lips, jaw, and palate that contribute to intelligible speech (known as verbal dyspraxia or childhood apraxia of speech). They also have difficulties with learning and production of nonspeech sequences involving the orofacial musculature (orofacial dyspraxia) and have a broad profile of linguistic deficits in expressive and receptive domains—problems that affect both oral and written language. The protein product, FOXP2, downregulates the expression of *CNTNAP2*, a gene that encodes a neurexin protein. The general relevance of *CNTNAP2* to speech dyspraxia remains to be determined. *CNTNAP2* is probably associated with disorders associated with nonsense-word repetition (e.g. autism).
- Genes at 7q11.23 are exquisitely sensitive to dosage alterations, which can influence human language and visuospatial capabilities.

Genetic factors have been implicated in stuttering, with linkage to markers on chromosome 12 and variations in genes governing lysosomal metabolism.

What do you understand by the term dysphasia?
Dysphasia is a disorder of the content of speech, which usually follows a lesion of the dominant cortex. The type of dysphasia indicates the site of the lesion in the cortex:
- Expressive, nominal, or motor dysphasia: site is the posterior inferior part of the dominant frontal lobe of the cortex (i.e. Broca's area).
- Sensory or receptive dysphasia: site is the superior temporal lobe or Wernicke's area.

Sites associated with speech function are variably located along the cortex and can go well beyond the classic anatomical boundaries of Broca's area. These sites typically involve an area contiguous with the face–motor cortex; however, they can be located several centimetres from the Sylvian fissure.

What do you understand by the term dysarthria?
Dysarthria is an inability to articulate properly caused by local lesions in the mouth or disorders of speech muscles or their connections. There is no disorder of the content of speech. The causes of dysarthria are:
- stutter
- paralysis of cranial nerves: Bell's palsy, ninth, tenth, and eleventh nerves
- cerebellar disease: staccato, scanning speech
- Parkinson's disease: slow, quiet, slurred, monotonous
- pseudobulbar palsy: monotonous, high-pitched 'hot potato' speech
- progressive bulbar palsy: nasal.

What are the components of speech?
- Phonation: abnormality is called dysphonia.
- Articulation: abnormality is called dysarthria.
- Language: abnormality is called dysphasia.

What are the other dominant hemisphere functions?
- Right–left orientation
- Finger identification
- Calculation.

What are the nondominant hemisphere functions?
- Drawing ability
- Topographic ability
- Construction
- Dressing
- Facial recognition
- Awareness of body and space
- Motor persistence.

What are the parietal lobe signs?
- Loss of accurate localization of touch, position, joint sense, and temperature appreciation
- Loss of two-point discrimination
- Astereognosis
- Dysgraphaesthesia
- Sensory inattention
- Attention hemianopia, homonymous hemianopia, or lower quadrantic hemianopia.

What do you understand by the term agnosia?
Agnosia is a failure to recognize objects despite the fact that the sensory pathways for sight, sound, or touch are intact. This is tested by asking the patient to feel, name, and describe the use of certain objects.

What are the different types of agnosia?
- Tactile agnosia and astereognosis: the patient is unable to recognize objects placed in his or her hands despite the fact that the sensory system of the hands and fingers is intact and

there is adequate motor function to allow examination of the object. The lesion is in the parietal lobe.
- Prosopagnosia: the inability to recognize a familiar face. The lesion is in the parietooccipital lobe.
- Visual agnosia: the inability to recognize objects despite the fact that the main visual pathways to the occipital cortex are preserved. The lesion is in the parietooccipital lobe.
- Anosognosia: the lack of awareness or realization that the limbs are paralyzed or weak or have impaired sensation. The lesion is usually in the nondominant parietal lobe.

What do you understand by the term apraxia?
Apraxia is the inability to perform purposeful volitional movements in the absence of motor weakness, sensory deficits, or severe incoordination. Usually, the defect is in the dominant parietal lobe, with disruption of connections to the motor cortex and to the opposite hemisphere.

What are the different types of apraxia?
- Dressing apraxias: patient is unable to put on his or her clothes correctly.
- Gait apraxia: there is difficulty in walking, although patients may show intact leg movements when examined in bed.
- Ideomotor apraxia: patients are unable to perform movements on command, although they may do this automatically, e.g. lick their lips.
- Ideational apraxias: patients have difficulty in carrying out a complex series of movements, e.g. to take a match from a box to light a cigarette.
- Constructional apraxia: patient has difficulty in arranging patterns on blocks or copying designs.

What do you know about dyslexia?
Reading difficulties, including dyslexia, occur as a part of a continuum that also includes normal reading ability. It is not an all-or-none phenomenon but, like hypertension, occurs in degrees. It has been defined as a disorder that is manifested by difficulty in learning to read despite conventional instruction, adequate intelligence, and sociocultural opportunity.

Further Information

Sir Charles Sherrington (1857–1952), Oxford University, and Lord Edgar Douglas Adrian (1889–1977), Cambridge University, were awarded the Nobel Prize in 1932 for their discoveries regarding the functions of neurons.

Pierre Paul Broca (1824–1880) was Professor of Surgery in Paris. His notable achievements were in anthropology, and his suggestion of cerebral localization of speech was first made at a French Anthropological Society meeting in 1861. He is reported to have described muscular dystrophy (before Duchenne), venous spread of cancer (before Rokitansky), and rickets as a nutritional disorder (before Virchow).

CHAPTER 176

Facioscapulohumeral Dystrophy (Landouzy–Déjérine Syndrome)

Instruction
Perform a neurological examination of this patient's cranial nerves and upper limbs.

Salient Features

HISTORY
- Age of onset (usually between 10 and 40 years of age)
- Family history (parents or siblings may only have facial weakness)
- Weakness begins in the face and affects the shoulder girdle subsequently (particularly the lower trapezii, pectoralis, triceps, and biceps).

EXAMINATION
- In the face:
  - Prominent ptosis
  - Difficulty in closing the eyes
  - Marked facial weakness, resulting in a dull expressionless face with lips open and slack, and inability to whistle or puff the cheeks
  - Speech is impaired owing to difficulty in articulation of labial consonants.
- In the neck:
  - Wasted sternomastoids and marked weakness of neck muscles.
- In the shoulder girdle (Figs 176.1 and 176.2):
  - Winging of the scapula
  - Lower pectorals and lower trapezii severely affected
  - Weakness of triceps and biceps
  - True hypertrophy of deltoids to compensate for other muscles
  - Absent biceps and triceps jerk.
- In the trunk:
  - Weakness (lower abdominal muscles are weaker than upper abdominal muscles), resulting in the *Beevor sign*; a physical finding very specific for this condition, which is a marked upward movement of the umbilicus following neck flexion of the patient in a lying position.
- Uncommon features: congenital absence of pectoralis, biceps, or brachioradialis; tibialis anterior may be the only muscle involved outside the shoulder girdle.

On identification of these signs, patients will need evaluation for:
- high-frequency hearing loss (in ~75%)
- retinal telangiectasias (in ~60%)
- sleep apnoea.

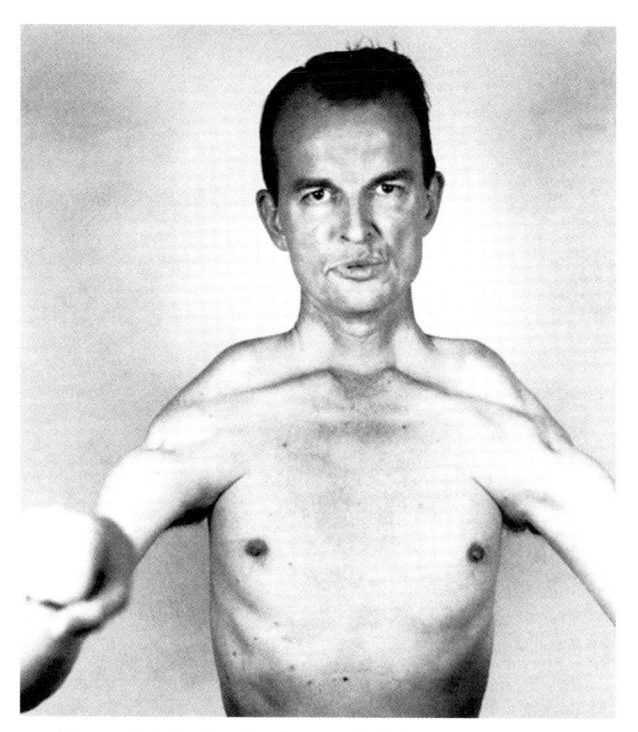

Fig. 176.1 Facioscapulohumeral dystrophy: the downward-sloping clavicles and bulge in the region of the trapezius muscle are caused by the scapula being displaced upwards on attempted elevation of the arms. The patient is also attempting to purse his lips. (With permission from Bradley, W.G., Daroff, R.B., Fenichel, G., Jankovic, J., 2008. Neurology in Clinical Practice, fifth edn. Butterworth-Heinemann, Oxford.)

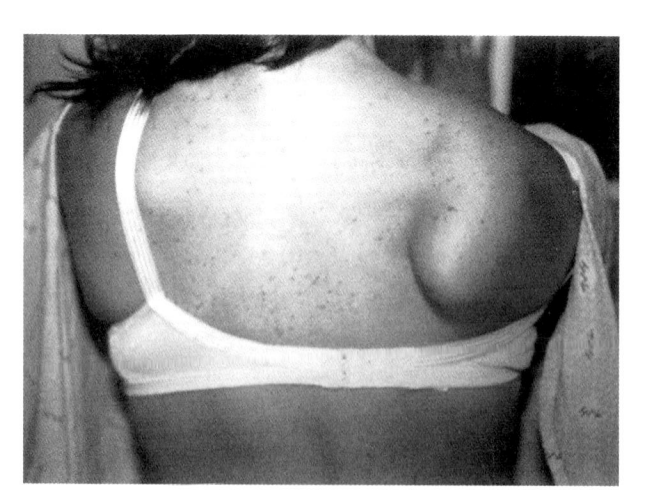

Fig. 176.2 Asymmetrical scapular winging in facioscapulohumeral muscular dystrophy. (With permission from Bradley, W.G., Daroff, R.B., Fenichel, G., Jankovic, J., 2008. Neurology in Clinical Practice, fifth edn. Butterworth-Heinemann, Oxford.)

Diagnosis

This patient has weakness of the muscles of the face, neck, and shoulder girdle (lesion) caused by inherited facioscapulohumeral dystrophy (aetiology).

Questions

What is the mode of inheritance?
Autosomal dominant; both sexes are equally affected. The gene responsible (DUX4) has been localized to the long arm of chromosome 4.

Are higher mental functions affected in this condition?
The IQ is normal in such patients.

What is the lifespan in such a patient?
Normal.

What is the age of onset of this disorder?
Between 10 and 40 years of age.

Are levels of muscle enzymes raised in this condition?
The enzyme levels remain normal usually. About half of those affected show a slight to moderate increase.

Can you name some atypical phenotypes of this condition?
- Limb-girdle muscular dystrophy
- Scapulohumeral dystrophy
- Focal monomelic upper limb atrophy
- Early onset (infantile).

What do you know about the genetics of this condition?
In most cases (more than 95%), it results from a partial deletion of an integral number of 3.3 kb polymorphic D4Z4 repeats, within the subtelomeric region of chromosome 4q. Whereas healthy individuals normally have *Eco*RI digestion fragments of D4Z4 consisting of 11 to 150 U, patients with facioscapulohumeral dystrophy have fragments of 1 to 10 U. However, it has been noted that, although molecular diagnosis of the disease is often cited to be 98% accurate, the search for the gene during testing is sometimes hampered by sequence homologies between the suspected 4q35 region and other chromosomal regions. Although the genetic lesion is well described, the causal gene and the protein products are not known.

Further Information

Louis Théophile Joseph Landouzy (1845–1917), Professor of Therapeutics in Paris; although remembered for the description of the syndrome which bears his name, his major research interest was tuberculosis.

Joseph Jules Déjérine (1849–1917), a French neurologist, was a pioneer in the localization of function in the brain. This syndrome was described in 1885.

Charles Edward Beevor (1854–1908) first documented the finding of an upwards deflection of the umbilicus on flexion of the neck in spinal cord injury at or below the level of Th10. Apart from positive Beevor's sign as a result of spinal cord lesions, positive Beevor's sign has also been described in patients with facioscapulohumeral muscular dystrophy.

CHAPTER 177

Friedreich's Ataxia

Instruction
Perform a neurological examination of this patient's legs.

Salient Features
HISTORY
- Age of onset (usually the same in each family and ranges from 8 to 16 years of age)
- High-arched foot in childhood in the family (Friedreich's foot) (Fig. 177.1)
- Scoliosis developing in childhood
- Cerebellar dysarthria and ataxia.

EXAMINATION
- Pes cavus
- Pyramidal weakness in legs
- Cerebellar signs, ataxia being a constant sign
- Impaired vibration and joint sense
- Romberg's sign positive
- Absence of deep tendon reflexes (caused by degeneration of peripheral nerves)
- Distal muscle wasting (in 50% of cases), especially in the hands
- Nystagmus (present in 25% of the cases), scanning speech, intention tremor
- Signs of hypertrophic cardiomyopathy
- Optic atrophy (present in 30% of cases)
- Kyphoscoliosis of the spine
- Signs of diabetes.

Friedreich's ataxia is the most common genetic cause of ataxia, affecting approximately 1 in 30,000 people. Symptoms that affect mobility include ataxia, spasticity, and peripheral neuropathy.

Diagnosis
This patient has kyphoscoliosis, pes cavus, and a combination of pyramidal, cerebellar, and sensory deficits (lesions) in the lower limbs caused by Friedreich's ataxia (aetiology); he is severely disabled by his deformity (functional status).

Questions
What is the mode of inheritance?
Autosomal recessive or rarely sex linked.

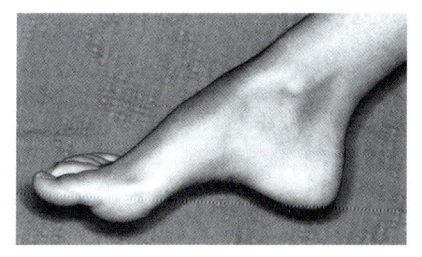

Fig. 177.1 Foot deformity in Friedreich ataxia. (With permission from Bradley, W.G., Daroff, R.B., Fenichel, G., Jankovic, J., 2008. Neurology in Clinical Practice, fifth edn. Butterworth-Heinemann, Oxford.)

Why are the deep tendon reflexes absent even though plantars are upgoing?
This is caused by a combination of pyramidal weakness with peripheral neuropathy.

In which other condition is there a mixture of cerebellar, pyramidal, and dorsal column signs?
Multiple sclerosis.

Mention a few conditions with absent knee jerks and upgoing plantars.
- Peripheral neuropathy in a stroke patient
- Motor neurone disease
- Conus medullaris: cauda equina lesion
- Tabes dorsalis
- Subacute combined degeneration of the spinal cord.

On which chromosome is the gene for this disorder localized?
The disease is caused by triplet repeat expansions on chromosome 9. The causative mutation is a GAA trinucleotide repeat expansion in the first intron of the gene *FRDA* (or *X25*), which encodes frataxin. The mitochondrial localization of frataxin and decreased oxidation activity suggest that this is a mitochondrial disease. Frataxin is involved in iron metabolism and may protect mitochondria from oxidative damage. Excessive free iron may damage proteins containing iron–sulphur groups, including complexes I, II, and III and aconitase, a Krebs cycle enzyme.

What are the clinical criteria for diagnosis of Friedreich's ataxia?
Harding's criteria are:
- Essential criteria are onset before the age of 25 years, ataxia of limbs and gait, absent knee and ankle jerks, extensor plantars, autosomal recessive inheritance, motor conduction velocity greater than 40 m/s, small or absent sensory nerve action potentials, and dysarthria within 5 years of onset.
- Additional criteria (present in two-thirds) are scoliosis, pyramidal weakness of lower limbs, absent upper limb reflexes, loss of vibration and joint position sense in the legs, abnormal electrocardiogram (ECG), and pes cavus.
- Other features (present in <50%) are nystagmus, optic atrophy, deafness, distal muscle wasting, and diabetes.

What is the prognosis of Friedreich's ataxia?
Friedreich's ataxia usually progresses slowly, and few patients live longer than 20 years after the onset of symptoms. Occasionally, it may appear to be arrested, and abortive cases may be encountered in apparently healthy relatives of affected patients. Most patients will lose their ability to

walk, stand, or sit without support within 10 to 15 years of disease onset. The mean life expectancy is around the age of 40 and the cause of death is usually a cardiovascular complication.

What are the pathological changes in Friedreich's ataxia?
- Marked loss of cells in the posterior root ganglia
- Degeneration of peripheral sensory fibres
- Involvement of the posterior and lateral columns of the cord.

What is the role of idebenone in Friedreich's ataxia?
Therapy with idebenone, an antioxidant, is associated with improvement in neurological function and activities of daily living in patients with Friedreich's ataxia. Idebenone also functions as an electron transport carrier (like coenzyme Q) and has various other effects, including stimulation of nerve growth factor production and blockade of voltage-sensitive calcium channels. In the murine conditional-knockout model of Friedreich's ataxia, oxidative stress is not observed, but idebenone exerts effects on cardiac measures and increases lifespan. Idebenone also enhances the viability of Friedreich's ataxia fibroblasts in vitro.

Name a few syndromes with spinocerebellar degeneration.
- Roussy–Lévy disease: hereditary spinocerebellar degeneration with atrophy of lower limb muscles and loss of deep tendon reflexes
- Refsum disease
- Bassen–Kornzweig syndrome: caused by cellular deficiency of vitamin E (α-tocopherol) resulting from a defect in the α-tocopherol-transfer protein, and abetalipoproteinaemia associated with a defect of very-low-density lipoprotein
- Olivopontocerebellar degeneration: first described in 1882. This has an autosomal dominant inheritance and has been mapped to the human leukocyte antigen loci on the short arm of chromosome 6 where a highly polymorphic CAG repeat sequence occurs. The CAG repeat sequence is longer than normal and unstable in affected patients.
- Machado–Joseph disease: dominant inheritance, first described in families of Portuguese origin. Clinical features include progressive ataxia, ophthalmoparesis, spasticity, dystonia, amyotrophy, and parkinsonism. This disorder has been linked to chromosome 14 and is caused by the expansion of unstable CAG repeat sequences.
- Dentatorubral pallidoluysian atrophy is similar to Machado–Joseph disease but maps on the short arm of chromosome 12. The abnormally expanded CAG repeat sequences identified in the gene for olivopontocerebellar degeneration, Machado–Joseph disease, and dentatorubral pallidoluysian atrophy each result in the expression of a specific ataxin.

Further Information

Nikolaus Friedreich (1825–1882), Professor of Pathology and neurologist in Heidelberg, described this condition, in a series of papers from 1861 to 1876.

G. Roussy (1874–1948), a French neuropathologist.

G. Lévy (b. 1881), a French neurologist.

Sigvald Refsum (1907–1991), a Norwegian neurologist, was successively Professor of Neurology at Bergen University and at the National Hospital in Oslo.

Anita Harding (1953–1995), Professor of Neurology at the National Hospital, Queen Square, London, died at the age of 42 years from colonic cancer.

CHAPTER 178

Hemiballismus

Instruction
Look at this patient.

Salient Features
HISTORY
- Sudden onset
- Cardiovascular disease for source of emboli: atrial fibrillation, valvular heart disease, or severe left ventricular dysfunction.

EXAMINATION
- Unilateral, involuntary, flinging movements of the proximal upper limbs.

Diagnosis
This patient has hemiballismus (lesion) caused by a stroke (aetiology) and has severe exhaustion (functional status).

Questions

Where is the lesion?
It is often thought that hemiballismus is caused most commonly by a lesion in the contralateral subthalamic nucleus, but the localization is usually elsewhere. It may result from lesions affecting the afferent or efferent pathways of the subthalamic nucleus, corpus striatum, thalamus, parieto-temporal, or frontal cerebral cortex.

What is the underlying cause?
- Vascular event, usually an infarct
- Rarely tumour, abscess, multiple sclerosis, arteriovenous malformation, cerebral trauma.

What investigations would you do?
- Electrocardiogram for atrial fibrillation
- Echocardiogram to rule out source of emboli
- Computed tomography scan, but this is usually unhelpful because the lesion is small
- Magnetic resonance imaging of the brain may be useful.

What is the prognosis?
The prognosis for recovery is usually good and most patients recover within 6 weeks. Hemiballismus may occasionally prevent the patient from eating and can be exhausting or even life-threatening. It can result in injuries to limbs.

Which drugs are usually used in ameliorating this condition?
Tetrabenazine, haloperidol, or levetiracetam are useful. Prolonged and medically intractable hemiballism can be treated with contralateral thalamotomy or pallidectomy.

CHAPTER 179

Hemiplegia

Instruction

This patient presents with difficulty walking. Please carry out a neurological examination of his peripheral nervous system.

Salient Features

HISTORY

- History of headache, seizures, and loss of consciousness (more common in subarachnoid haemorrhage or intracerebral bleeds than in cerebral infarction)
- Onset, duration, and progression of symptoms (sudden onset may signify a vascular event, progressive symptoms may signify demyelination or space-occupying lesion)
- History of speech defects, sensory loss, weakness of face and limbs, and other associated cortical symptomatology (aphasia, agnosia, neglect)
- History of trauma (associated with intracranial haemorrhage)
- Risk factors for intracerebral vascular events: hypertension, smoking, diabetes mellitus
- Family history (conditions associated with ruptured aneurysm, such as adult polycystic kidney disease)
- History of functional status: swallowing, mobility, pressure sores, independence in activities of daily living, visual difficulties (for visual field defects).

EXAMINATION

- Unilateral upper motor neuron seventh nerve palsy
- The arm is held to the side, the elbow is flexed, and the fingers and wrist are flexed on to the chest.
- The leg is extended at both the hip and knee, while the foot is plantar flexed and inverted.
- Weakness of the upper and lower limbs on the same side with upper motor neuron signs: increased tone, hyperreflexia, and upgoing plantar response
- Hemiplegic weakness of the upper limbs affects the shoulder abductor, elbow extensors, wrist and finger extensors, and small muscles of the hand.
- Hemiplegic weakness of the lower limbs affects hip flexors, knee flexors, and dorsiflexors and evertors of the foot
- Sensory signs and in particular joint sensation are important in rehabilitation.
- Hypertension and signs of diabetes.

Other possible signs:
- Homonymous hemianopia and sensory inattention
- Horner syndrome: contralateral to hemiplegia suggests carotid dissection
- Carotid bruits
- Speech defects

635

- Atrial fibrillation
- Heart murmurs
- Previous craniotomy scar.

Diagnosis

This patient has had a stroke, causing a right or left hemiplegia (lesion), which can be the result of either a vascular event, such as thrombosis, embolism, or haemorrhage, or a neoplasm of the brain (aetiology). This patient is limited by hemiplegia and hemianopia (functional status).

Questions

What are the causes of stroke?

About 80% of all strokes are caused by cerebral infarction resulting from thrombotic or embolic occlusion of a cerebral artery. The remaining 20% are caused by either intracerebral or subarachnoid haemorrhage.

Aside from vascular events, other conditions that can cause hemiplegia or mimic a stroke include space-occupying lesions, trauma and subdural haematoma, infections, demyelination, and connective tissue disorders with vasculitis.

How would you manage a patient with stroke during the hyperacute phase?

Early hospital admission to a dedicated stroke unit leads to long-term reductions in death, dependency, and need for institutional care. Urgent radiological confirmation and immediate treatment with intravenous thrombolysis and/or mechanical thrombectomy depending on the scenario are the immediate treatment options in tertiary centres. Other therapies and investigations in the acute phase are:
- Aspirin given within 48 hours of ischaemic stroke reduces the risk of death and recurrent stroke.
- Blood tests should be obtained for full blood count including platelet count, serum glucose, serum electrolytes, renal function, and coagulation screen.
- Electrocardiogram should be performed on presentation and any arrhythmia should be treated appropriately.
- Carotid Doppler prior to endarterectomy, presurgical evaluation of saccular aneurysm
- Control of immediate risk factors: hypertension, hyperlipidaemia, hypoxia, and diabetes
- Involvement of the multidisciplinary team (physiotherapy, occupational therapy, dietetics, and speech and language therapy) and secondary prevention are part of the on-going management after a stroke.

What is the role of imaging in acute stroke?

Stroke is a clinical diagnosis. Immediate neuroimaging in the form of computed tomography (CT) is crucial to differentiate between ischaemia and haemorrhage. Magnetic resonance imaging (MRI) with diffusion-weighted sequences allows early detection. MRI has a much higher sensitivity than CT for acute ischaemic changes, especially in the posterior fossa and in the first hours after an ischaemic stroke. However, as CT is easily available and immediately accessible in most centres, it is the imaging of choice in the acute evaluation of a patient presenting with stroke, in order to exclude haemorrhage and proceed to thrombolysis if appropriate.

Discuss the importance of blood pressure reduction in a patient with acute ischaemic stroke.

Randomized clinical trials have suggested that patients with acute ischaemic stroke treated with antihypertensive agents may have an adverse clinical outcome and increased mortality.

In acute ischaemic stroke, maintaining adequate systemic blood pressure is essential to maintain blood flow in the brain. The blood pressure during the acute phase of an ischaemic stroke should be maintained between 120 mm Hg and 200 mm Hg, as studies have demonstrated a U-shaped relationship between blood pressure and adverse outcomes (both high and low blood pressure associated with adverse outcomes). Therefore, current guidelines suggest that the blood pressure should be monitored, but not actively treated, unless it rises above 200 mm Hg or falls below 120 mm Hg. Antihypertensives can be safely started or restarted if the patient has persistent hypertension 48 hours after the acute phase and remains neurologically stable. An exception to this approach is when the patient is a candidate to receive intravenous thrombolysis. In this case, the blood pressure should be maintained lower than 185/110 mm Hg.

Name some tools used to determine the outcome after an acute stroke.
Some of the standard measures include the following:
- Barthel index: measure of the ability to perform activities of daily living such as eating, bathing, walking, and using the toilet.
- Modified Rankin Scale: simplified overall assessment of function in which a score of 0 indicates the absence of symptoms and a score of 5 shows severe disability
- Glasgow Outcome Scale: global assessment of function in which a score of 1 indicates good recovery; a score of 2, moderate disability; a score of 3, severe disability; a score of 4, survival but in a vegetative state; and a score of 5, death
- National Institute of Health Stroke Scale: a serial measure of neurological deficit using a 42-point scale that quantifies neurological deficits in 11 categories. For example, a mild facial paralysis is given a score of 1 and complete right hemiplegia with aphasia, gaze deviation, visual field deficit, dysarthria, and sensory loss is given a score of 25. Normal function without neurological deficit is scored as 0.

What is the role of thrombolysis in acute stroke?
Treatment with intravenous tissue plasminogen activator (tPA) when administered within 4.5 hours after onset of the ischaemic event (and in the absence of any sign of brain injury on CT) improves clinical outcome at 3 to 6 months. Even within the 4.5 hour window, any delay in administering thrombolysis can lead to an increase in adverse stroke outcomes so alteplase (tPA) should be administered as soon as possible once contraindications have been excluded. A number of anatomical and clinical factors can affect the response to thrombolysis, but as a generality, recanalization is associated with reduced mortality and improved function in acute ischaemic stroke.

A patient presents patient presents to you 60 min after the onset of a left hemispheric stroke, how long do you have to initiate thrombolytic therapy?
The correct answer is 1 min, not 2 hours! Time is neurons saved!

What is the role of anticoagulants in the immediate treatment of acute ischaemic stroke?
Anticoagulants (including unfractionated heparin, low-molecular-weight heparin, or specific thrombin inhibitors) offer no short- or long-term benefits in the immediate treatment of acute ischaemic stroke. Although the risks of deep venous thrombosis or pulmonary embolus are significantly reduced, these benefits are offset by a dose-dependent increased risk of intracranial or extracranial bleeding. If anticoagulation is needed to prevent venous thromboembolism (VTE) in the acute stroke phase (and after 24 hours of thrombolysis), then low-dose low-molecular-weight heparin is preferred. Compression stockings are not to be used for prevention of VTE in acute stroke as they have not been shown to prevent VTE.

What are the important principles of rehabilitation after a stroke?
- Long-term use of aerobic training
- Exercises to enhance flexibility, balance, and coordination
- Resistance exercises within daily activities.

What are the clinical features that would interest you for the rehabilitation of a stroke?
- Independence in activities of daily living: bathing, dressing, toileting, transferring, continence, and feeding
- Independence in more complex activities such as meal preparation, shopping, financial management, housekeeping, transportation, medication-taking, and laundering.

What are key goals before and after discharge of a stroke patient?
- Before discharge the patient should be able to:
  - Provide reliable yes and no responses to questions
  - Express himself or herself in short phrases
  - Use the unaffected hand effectively for self-care
  - Walk 50 m slowly with hands-on supervision (with the aid of a cane and/or ankle–foot orthosis).
The patient would be expected to require some physical help for self-care.
- After discharge:
  - Physical, occupational, and speech therapy with a focus on training in skills needed to increase independence for activities of daily living both at home and in the community; successful learning of such personal skills may require 20 or more hours of practice.
  - Conduct formal training of caregivers.
  - Depression should be identified and treated.
  - Improvement in movement and language skills is possible with further practice at any time after stroke (because of the plasticity of neural pathways that remain intact).

What is the prognosis in a patient with acute ischaemic stroke?
About 20% of stroke patients are dead within a month; about 30%, by 6 months; and 50%, by 1 year. The overall 10-year survival of a patient after a stroke is around 70%. Prognosis is worse when it is caused by intracerebral and subarachnoid haemorrhage, where the 1-month mortality is close to 50%. Of those who survive the acute event, about half will experience some disability after 6 months.

What is the significance of carotid artery stenosis?
Carotid artery stenosis is an important predisposing factor for cerebrovascular ischaemic events, with the risk increasing with the severity of the stenosis and the presence of symptoms.

For *severe symptomatic stenosis* (>70% narrowing), carotid endarterectomy is recommended.

For *severe symptom-free stenosis*, optimal management has yet to be defined: one meta-analysis of trials showed only a small absolute benefit from surgery in reducing the odds of ipsilateral stroke. Also, 45% of strokes in patients with asymptomatic stenosis with 60% to 99% narrowing are attributable to lacunae or cardioembolism. Hence, carotid endarterectomy cannot be routinely recommended.

For *mild to moderate symptomatic stenosis* (<70% narrowing), an antiplatelet agent such as aspirin is recommended. Persistent symptoms may necessitate use of other agents such as ticlopidine or clopidogrel, which reduce the relative risk for further ischaemic events slightly more than aspirin or anticoagulation with aspirin.

How would you manage a patient with a transient ischaemic attack (TIA)?
- Advise to stop smoking.
- Aspirin

- Duplex ultrasonography of the carotid vessels
- Carotid artery digital subtraction angiography
- MRI scan of the head with diffusion-weighted imaging. It has been argued that all patients with TIA should be scanned since permanent damage may be seen in the brain on MRI in about 25% of patients with TIAs.

What do you know of the ABCD2 score?
The ABCD2 scoring system used to be calculated in order to inform the clinician of the urgency of the investigations and prevention therapies, as it was used to calculate the risk of subsequent stroke within a week after the initial TIA. It is not currently used to risk stratify these patients as it is suboptimal and high risk patients could be missed. It is still used though sometimes to inform the clinician of patients that may need dual antiplatelet therapy.
- **A**ge ≥60 years: 1 point
- **B**P elevation at first assessment (≥140/90 mm Hg): 1 point
- **C**linical feature of TIA: unilateral weakness: 2 points; speech impairment without weakness: 1 point
- **D**uration of TIA: 10 to 59 min: 1 point; ≥60 min: 2 points
- **D**iabetes: 1 point.

What do you understand by the term TIA?
An acute loss of focal cerebral or ocular function with symptoms lasting <24 hours.

Why is it important to differentiate a carotid TIA from a vertebrobasilar attack?
Carotid TIAs may be amenable to surgery. Furthermore, a TIA in the anterior circulation is generally of more serious prognostic significance than a TIA in the posterior circulation.

What are the features of a carotid TIA?
Hemiparesis, aphasia, or transient loss of vision in one eye only (amaurosis fugax).

What are the features of a vertebrobasilar TIA?
- Vertigo, dysphagia, ataxia, and drop attacks (at least two of these should occur together)
- Bilateral or alternating weakness or sensory symptoms
- Sudden bilateral blindness in patients aged over 40 years.

What are the risk factors for stroke?
Hypertension, ischaemic heart disease, atrial fibrillation, peripheral vascular disease, diabetes, smoking, previous TIA, cervical bruit, hyperlipidaemia, raised haematocrit, oral contraceptive pill, and cardiomyopathy.

Why is it important to treat TIAs?
Prospective studies have shown that within 5 years of a TIA:
- 1 in 6 patients will have suffered a stroke.
- 1 in 4 patients will have died (from either stroke or heart disease).

What is the role of carotid endarterectomy in patients with a carotid TIA?
- For patients with severe stenosis (70%–99% of cases), the risks of surgery are significantly outweighed by the later benefits.
- For patients with mild stenosis (0%–50% of cases), there is little 3-year risk of ipsilateral ischaemic stroke, even in the absence of surgery; consequently, any 3-year benefits of surgery are small and outweighed by its early risks.

- For patients with moderate stenosis (50%–69% of cases), the balance of surgical risk and eventual benefit is still being evaluated.

What is the role of carotid angioplasties in patients with recent carotid artery TIAs who have severe stenosis of the ipsilateral carotid artery?

Carotid angioplasty has not been adequately assessed in patients with recent carotid artery TIAs or nondisabling ischaemic stroke and severe stenosis of the ipsilateral carotid artery, and hence, it is not recommended. However, registry data suggest that carotid artery stenting may be useful in carefully selected patients. The results of the CREST (Carotid Revascularization Endarterectomy versus Stenting Trial) (randomized trial funded by the National Institutes of Health examining the role of carotid stenting) showed similar net outcomes with carotid artery stenting and carotid endarterectomy for the treatment of carotid stenosis. On the other hand, the International Carotid Stenting Study interim safety results at 120 days appeared to favour carotid artery stenting over carotid endarterectomy for patients with symptomatic carotid stenosis only.

What to you understand by 'RIND'?

Reversible ischaemic neurological disease, in which symptoms and signs reverse within 1 week but not within 24 hours.

What are lacunar infarcts?

Lacunar infarcts are seen in hypertensive patients and consist of small infarcts in the region of the internal capsule (causing partial hemiparesis or hemisensory impairment), pons (ataxia of cerebellar type, partial hemiparesis), basal ganglia, or thalamus. They are often multiple. Lacunae are thought to be caused by occlusion of small branch arteries or by rupture of Charcot–Bouchard microaneurysms, producing a small haematoma that resolves, leaving an area of infarction.

What are the deficits supplied by the anterior carotid artery?

The anterior carotid artery supplies the frontal lobes and the medial cerebral hemispheres with the exception of the visual cortex of the occipital lobes. Cortical areas supplied by this artery include the motor and sensory areas of the lower limbs, a 'micturition centre', and the supplementary motor cortex. Ischaemia in the territory of one anterior carotid artery produces weakness and mild sensory deficits in the opposite lower limb. Some patients with left anterior carotid artery ischaemia have a mild transient aphasia.

What do you understand by the term stroke?

Stroke is characterized by rapidly progressive clinical symptoms and signs of focal, and at times global, loss of cerebral function lasting >24 hours or leading to death, with no apparent cause other than that of vascular origin.

How do you classify stroke?

The Bamford clinical classification of stroke has the following.
  Total anterior circulation syndrome:
  - Unilateral motor deficit of face, arm, and leg
  - Homonymous hemianopia
  - Higher cerebral dysfunction (e.g. aphasia, neglect).

  Partial anterior circulation syndrome has any two of the following features:
  - Unilateral motor and/or sensory deficit
  - Ipsilateral hemianopia or higher cerebral dysfunction
  - Higher cerebral dysfunction alone or isolated motor and/or sensory deficit restricted to one limb or the face.

Posterior circulation syndrome has one or more of the following features:
- Bilateral motor or sensory signs not secondary to brainstem compression by a large supratentorial lesion
- Cerebellar signs, unless accompanied by ipsilateral motor deficit (ataxic hemiparesis)
- Unequivocal diplopia with or without external ocular muscle palsy
- Crossed signs, e.g. left facial and right limb weakness
- Hemianopia alone or with any of previous the four items.

Lacunar syndromes can be pure motor, pure sensory, ataxic hemiparesis, or sensorimotor:
- Pure motor stroke:
  - Unilateral, pure motor deficit
  - Clearly involving two of three areas (face, arm, and leg)
  - With the whole of any limb being involved.
- Pure sensory stroke:
  - Unilateral pure sensory symptoms (with or without signs)
  - Involving at least two of three areas (face, arm, and leg)
  - With the whole of any limb being involved.
- Ataxic hemiparesis:
  - Ipsilateral cerebellar and corticospinal tract signs
  - With or without dysarthria
  - In the absence of higher cerebral dysfunction or a visual field defect.
- Sensorimotor stroke:
  - Pure motor and pure sensory stroke combined (i.e. unilateral motor or sensory signs and symptoms)
  - In the absence of higher cerebral dysfunction or a visual field defect.

Further Information

Hippocrates first described stroke symptoms but called the symptoms 'apoplexy'—literally 'struck down with violence'.

CHAPTER 180

Homonymous Hemianopia

Instruction

Examine this patient's eyes.
Examine this patient's visual fields.

Salient Features

HISTORY

- Patient bumps into things on one side and may have a history of traffic accidents where one side of the car is damaged without the patient realizing.
- Patient may insist that they have one 'bad' eye (however, blindness in one eye causes impairment of perceiving distances, but the normal eye will provide a full field of vision on both sides and hence patient will not bump into objects).
- Reading difficulty (suggests that the visual defect splits the midline: if the defect is on the right side, patient is unable to scan along the line to the next word and hence reading is almost impossible, whereas when the defect is on the left side, the patient cannot find the beginning of the next line).
- Clinician should determine whether the patient is aware of his/her defect (if the patient is aware of the visual defect, it is likely the defect 'splits' the macula and bisects the central field; if the patient is unaware and bumps into things, then the defect is either macular sparing or an attention hemianopia).

EXAMINATION

- Homonymous hemianopia examination includes:
  - Testing for an attention field defect using both hands of the examiner and asking the patient to determine which finger is moving
  - Testing the whole field in each eye using a white hat pin
  - Reevaluation of the field in each eye to determine whether there is macular sparing or macular splitting using a hat pin. If you are unable to determine, then tell the patient that you would like to do formal field testing with a tangent screen or using a perimeter.
- Visual acuity and examination of the fundus
- Full neurological examination should be performed to look for an underlying cause: stroke, intracranial tumour.

Homonymous hemianopic visual field defects with normal visual acuity are the hallmark of a unilateral retrochiasmal lesion.

Diagnosis

This patient has a homonymous hemianopia (lesion) for which I would like to determine the aetiology, such as a stroke or tumour.

642

180 — HOMONYMOUS HEMIANOPIA

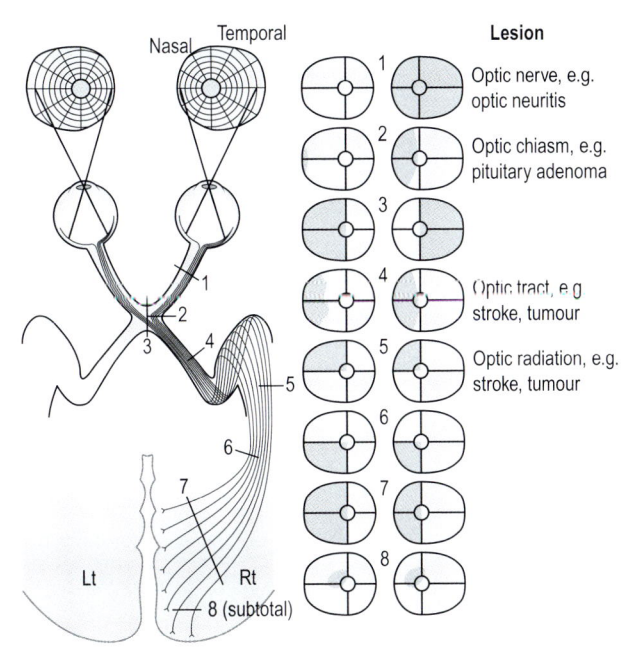

Fig. 180.1 Visual fields that accompany damage to the visual pathways. See the list given in the text for details.

Questions

Where is the lesion?
The lesion is in the optic tract and beyond (visual acuity is intact when the macula is spared). Fig. 180.1 shows the sites of the lesions and the visual field effects.

	Site	Type of Homonymous Hemianopia
1	Optic nerve	Unilateral amaurosis
2	Lateral optic chiasm	Grossly incongruous, contralateral
3	Central optic chiasm	Bitemporal hemianopia
4	Optic tract	Incongruous, incomplete
5	Temporal lobe	Superior quadrantic defect, congruous partial or complete (contralateral)
6	Posterior parietal lobe	Inferior quadrantic defect, congruous partial or complete
7	Complete parietooccipital interruption of the optic radiation	Complete congruous homonymous hemianopia with shift of foveal point, often sparing central vision
8	Incomplete damage to the visual cortex	Congruous homonymous scotomas, usually encroaching at least acutely on central vision

What further investigations would you do?
- Formal field testing: perimetry is particularly important if the patient holds a driving licence.
- Magnetic resonance imaging or computed tomography.

CHAPTER 181

Internuclear Ophthalmoplegia

Instruction
This lady has developed blurred vision. Please examine her eyes.

Salient Features

HISTORY
- Diplopia
- History of multiple sclerosis, stroke, nutritional deficiencies
- Neurofibroma (causing pontine gliomas)
- Drugs (phenytoin, carbamazepine, tricyclic antidepressants, opiates).

EXAMINATION
- Nystagmus is more prominent in the abducting eye (Harris' sign).
- Diverging squint
- Abduction in either eye is normal, whereas adduction is impaired (Fig. 181.1): there is dissociation of eye movements. On covering the abducting eye, the adduction in the other eye is normal.
- Other signs of demyelination should be sought for: optic atrophy, pale discs, pyramidal signs.

Multiple sclerosis and microvascular brainstem ischaemia are the most common causes of internuclear ophthalmoplegia. The two causes may be distinguished by age at presentation, with younger patients likely to have demyelination, and older patients, ischaemia.

Diagnosis
This patient has internuclear ophthalmoplegia (lesion), which is probably caused by multiple sclerosis (aetiology).

Questions

Where is the lesion?
In the medial longitudinal bundle or fasciculus, which connects the sixth nerve nucleus on one side to the third nerve nucleus on the opposite side of the brainstem. The eye will not adduct because the third nerve and, therefore, the medial rectus have been disconnected from the lateral gaze centre and sixth nucleus of the opposite side.

181 — INTERNUCLEAR OPHTHALMOPLEGIA

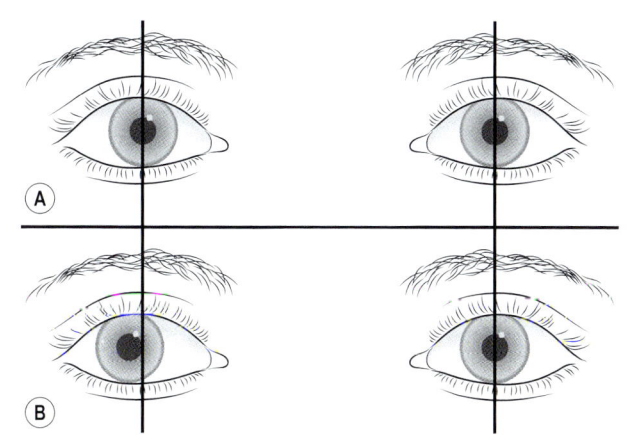

Fig. 181.1 Internuclear ophthalmoplegia. **(A)** Gaze straight ahead. **(B)** Attempted right gaze, the right abducting eye achieves the target earlier than the left adducting eye. *The vertical line* indicates the midpupillary point; the left pupil does not move off this when the gaze changes.

What are the causes?
- Multiple sclerosis
- Vascular disease
- Tumour (pontine glioma)
- Inflammatory lesions of the brainstem
- Drugs (phenytoin, carbamazepine, opiates, tricyclic antidepressants).

How would you manage this patient?
- Magnetic resonance imaging (MRI) scan
- Edrophonium (Tensilon) test to exclude myasthenia
- Treatment of the underlying cause.

What are the mechanisms to elicit conjugate gaze?
There are four mechanisms for eliciting conjugate gaze in any direction.
- *The saccadic system* involves voluntary gaze (even when the eyes are shut). Pathways mediating saccadic gaze arise in the frontal lobe and pass to the pontine gaze centre.
- *The pursuit system* allows the subject to follow a moving object. Pathways mediating pursuit movements arise in the parietooccipital lobe and pass to the pontine gaze centre.
- *The optokinetic system* involves the restoration of gaze despite movements from the outside world (e.g. while a subject is sitting in a railway train and looking out of the window, the eyes move slowly as the train moves, to be followed by rapid corrective movement back to the initial position of gaze). This is tested with a hand-held drum bearing vertical black and white stripes. Optokinetic nystagmus is often disturbed even before damage to the pursuit system is apparent.
- *The vestibuloocular system* involves correction of gaze for movements of the head. This is achieved by inputs from the labyrinths and neck proprioceptors to the brainstem. The patient is asked to fixate to the examiner's face and the head is briskly rotated by the examiner from side to side or up and down (doll's head manoeuvre). In supranuclear gaze palsy,

these vestibuloocular reflex eye movements are preserved, despite the absence of both saccadic and pursuit movements. Caloric tests are used to demonstrate the vestibuloocular reflex.

Notes:
1. Diplopia is not a feature of defects in conjugate gaze.
2. The centres for saccadic and pursuit movements in the cerebral hemispheres control deviation of the eyes towards the opposite side of the body. These pathways descend towards the brainstem and cross before they reach the pons.
3. The centres for conjugate vertical gaze lie in the midbrain.
4. The centres for conjugate downward vertical gaze are not well localized, and lesions both in the midbrain and at the level of the foramen magnum can cause defects of voluntary downgaze.

What do you know about 'Fisher's one and a half syndrome'?
It is a syndrome in which horizontal eye movement is absent and the other eye is capable only of abduction—one and a half movements are paralyzed. The vertical eye movements and the pupils are normal. The cause is a lesion in the pontine region involving the medial longitudinal fasciculus and the parapontine reticular formation on the same side. This results in failure of conjugate gaze to the same side, impairment of adduction of the eye, and nystagmus on abduction of the other eye. One and a half syndrome is most often caused by multiple sclerosis, brainstem stroke, brainstem tumours, and arteriovenous malformations.

Further Information

Internuclear ophthalmoplegia was first reported by Bielschowsky (1902) and then subsequently by Lhermitte in 1922.

Spiller, in 1924, described the necropsy findings, implicated the median longitudinal fasciculus, and suggested the name 'ophthalmoplegia internuclearis anterior'.

CHAPTER 182

Jerky Nystagmus

Instruction
Examine this patient's eyes.
Test the patient's eye movements.

Salient Features
HISTORY
- Symptoms suggesting cerebellar syndrome: multiple sclerosis, alcohol, etc.
- Ear infections (vestibular involvement).

EXAMINATION
- Horizontal nystagmus with fast components to right or left side (When eliciting nystagmus, take care to keep your finger at least 2 ft (60 cm) away from the patient and avoid going laterally beyond the extent of binocular vision.)
- Cerebellar signs
- Fundoscopy for optic atrophy (multiple sclerosis).

If the patient has vertical nystagmus in addition to horizontal nystagmus, it is more likely to be vestibular nystagmus or brainstem disease.

Diagnosis
This patient has a jerky nystagmus with optic atrophy (lesion) caused by multiple sclerosis (aetiology). I would like to examine her neurological system to evaluate the disability (functional status).

Questions
What do you understand by the term nystagmus?
Nystagmus is a series of involuntary, rhythmic oscillations of one or both eyes. It may be horizontal, vertical, or rotator.

What are the types of nystagmus?
- Congenital
- Dissociated
- Gaze evoked
- Vestibular.

What is pendular nystagmus?
In pendular nystagmus, the oscillations are equal in speed and amplitude in both directions of movement. It may be seen on central gaze when the vision is poor, as in severe refractive error or macular disease.

What do you understand by the term jerky nystagmus?
Jerky or phasic nystagmus is a condition in which eye movement in one direction is faster than that in the other. This is usually seen in the horizontal plane and is brought out by lateral gaze to one or both sides. It is seen with lesions of the cerebellum, vestibular apparatus, or their connections in the brainstem.

What is dissociated nystagmus?
Dissociated or ataxic nystagmus is irregular nystagmus in the abducting eye. It is bilateral in multiple sclerosis, brainstem tumour, or Wernicke's encephalopathy. It is unilateral in vascular disease of the brainstem. It is caused by a lesion in the medial longitudinal fasciculus (which links the sixth nerve nucleus on one side to the medial rectus portion of the third nerve on the other).

Where is the lesion in vestibular nystagmus?
It may be in one of two locations:
- Peripheral (labyrinth or vestibular nerve), as in labyrinthitis, Ménière syndrome, acoustic neuroma, otitis media, head injury
- Central (affecting vestibular nuclei), as in stroke, multiple sclerosis, tumours, alcoholism.

What do you know about 'downbeat' and 'upbeat' nystagmus?
Downbeat nystagmus is associated with brainstem lesions, meningoencephalitis, and hypomagnesaemia. Upbeat nystagmus is caused by lesions of the anterior vermis of the cerebellum.

Further Information

K. Wernicke (1848–1904) graduated from the University of Breslau; although aware that a toxic factor was important in the aetiology, he did not realize that this syndrome was caused by a nutritional deficiency.

P. Ménière (1799–1862), French ear, nose, and throat specialist.

CHAPTER 183

Limb-Girdle Dystrophy

Instruction

Perform a neurological examination of this patient's upper and lower limbs.

Salient Features

HISTORY

- Age of onset (between 10 and 30 years of age)
- Onset may be in either the pelvic or shoulder girdle
- It may remain confined to the pelvic or shoulder girdle and may be static for years before peripheral weakness and wasting occur.

EXAMINATION

Upper limbs (Fig. 183.1):
- Biceps and brachioradialis are involved late; wrist extensors are first involved when it extends to the wrist.
- Deltoids may show pseudohypertrophy and are spared until late.

Lower limbs (Fig. 183.1):
- In the early stages of the disease, hip flexors and glutei are weak.
- There is early wasting of medial quadriceps and tibialis anterior.
- Lateral quadriceps and calves may show hypertrophy.

The face is never affected.

Diagnosis

This patient has weakness of the proximal muscles of the arms and legs (lesion) caused by limb-girdle dystrophy (aetiology).

Questions

What is the mode of inheritance?
The limb-girdle muscular dystrophies (LGMDs) have been identified to be inherited in either an autosomal dominant (type 1) or autosomal recessive (type 2) pattern. Six subtypes of the dominant LGMDs (1A–1F) and 11 subtypes of the recessive LGMDs (2A–2K) have been reported. In four of the limb-girdle dystrophies (2C–2F), mutations affecting the *sarcoglycan complex of proteins* have been identified. These membrane proteins interact with dystrophin through another transmembrane protein, β-dystroglycan. Dysferlin is a sarcolemmal protein, and its deficiency causes proximal and distal forms of recessively inherited muscular dystrophies, designated as LGMD type 2B.

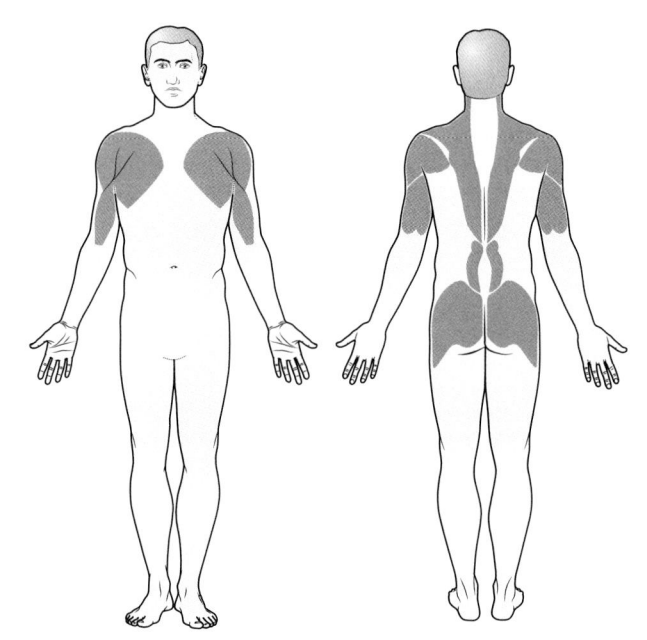

Fig. 183.1 Pattern of weakness in limb-girdle dystrophy.

LGMD2A, the most prevalent form, accounts for at least 30% of all cases and is caused by mutations in *CAPN3* (also called *p94*), which encodes CAPN3, the largely skeletal muscle-specific member of the calpain superfamily. These patients have symmetrical and selective involvement of proximal limb-girdle muscles. They have normal intelligence and no cardiac or facial disturbances. The disease shows wide intrafamilial and interfamilial clinical variability. A dystrophic or myopathic process is seen on muscle biopsy. During the active phase, the serum level of creatine kinase is moderately or markedly increased; however, patients with a normal serum level of creatine kinase or a neurogenic pattern on electromyography have also been reported, suggesting that there is a spectrum of variability in this calpainopathy. Intramuscular administration of the synthetic calpain inhibitor leupeptin to dystrophic *Mdx* mice can prevent decreases in muscle fibre diameter. Calpain inhibitors, therefore, have the potential of being beneficial in this condition.

What is the age of onset?
Between 10 and 30 years of age, causing disability 10 to 20 years after onset.

How is the intelligence affected?
It is unaffected and IQ is normal.

Is the lifespan affected?
No.

What happens to the serum enzymes?
Levels of serum enzymes are slightly affected or normal.

Further Information

John Walton, Professor of Neurology at Oxford and Newcastle, was made a peer following his retirement and carried the title of Lord Walton of Detchant. His chief interest was muscular diseases.

Sir Roger Bannister, Master of Pembroke College at Oxford, worked at the National Hospital for Nervous Diseases, Queen Square, and St Mary's Hospital, London, and his main interest was chronic autonomic failure. He was the first person to run the 4-min mile.

CHAPTER 184

Motor Neurone Disease

Instruction

Examine this patient's cranial nerves.
Examine this patient's upper limbs.
Examine this patient's lower limbs.

Salient Features

HISTORY

- Fasciculations and cramps: these may precede other symptoms by months.
- Painless, asymmetrical weakness of muscles of the upper limb or lower limb
- Dysarthria and dysphagia
- Emotional lability if there is bulbar involvement.

EXAMINATION

- Fasciculations, absent reflexes, and weakness in the upper limbs
- Spasticity, exaggerated reflexes, and upgoing plantars in lower limbs
- Sluggish palatal movements, absent gag reflex, and brisk jaw jerk
- Tongue fasciculations
- Neck muscle weakness; head droop is seen when there is weakness of the thoracic and cervical paraspinal muscles.
- A combination of the aforementioned signs may be seen.

Diagnosis

This patient has a combination of upper and lower motor neurone signs (lesions) caused by motor neurone disease (aetiology), although I would like to exclude cervical cord compression. The patient is wheelchair bound as a result of the disease (functional status).

Questions

What important cause should be ruled out before making a firm diagnosis of motor neurone disease?
Cord compression may produce a similar clinical picture, and hence, it is important to do a magnetic resonance imaging scan of the spine to exclude it.

What are the symptoms attributable to motor neurone disease?
- Direct (owing to motor neuronal degeneration):
  - Weakness and atrophy
  - Fasciculations and muscle cramps

- Spasticity
- Dysarthria
- Dysphagia
- Dyspnoea
- Emotional lability.
- Indirect (as a result of primary symptoms):
  - Psychological disturbances
  - Sleep disturbances
  - Constipation
  - Drooling
  - Thick mucous secretions
  - Symptoms of chronic hypoventilation
  - Pain.

What are the characteristic features of this disease?
- It rarely begins before the age of 40 years.
- There is presence of upper and lower motor neuron involvement of a single spinal segment and motor dysfunction involving at least two limbs or one limb and bulbar muscles.
- Sensory symptoms or signs are not seen.
- Ocular movements are not affected.
- There are never cerebellar or extrapyramidal signs.
- Sphincters are involved late, if at all.
- Remission is unknown and the disease is fatal within 5 to 7 years (caused by bronchopneumonia).

What are the clinical patterns of motor neurone disease?
- Bulbar: bulbar or pseudobulbar palsy (in 25%)
- Amyotrophic lateral sclerosis (ALS; in 50%), also known as Lou Gehrig disease: flaccid arms and spastic legs
- Progressive muscular atrophy (in 25%): a lesion in the anterior horn cells affecting distal muscles. Characteristically, there is retention of deep tendon reflexes in the presence of severe muscular atrophy.
- Primary lateral sclerosis (rare): signs progress from an upper motor neurone to a lower motor neurone type.

Which other conditions affect the lower motor neurons?
- Werdnig–Hoffman disease: presents in the neonatal period as a 'floppy infant' and known as infantile progressive spinal muscular atrophy
- X-linked spinal muscular atrophy: the patient has associated testicular atrophy resulting in oligospermia and gynaecomastia; it is associated with the amplification of a trinucleotide repeat in the coding sequence of the androgen receptor gene and disease severity is directly related to the number of repeats present.
- Spinal muscular atrophy: linked to locus on the large arm of chromosome 5.

What are the other types of motor neurone disease?
- Madras motor neurone disease, common in southern India, where the onset is early (before the age of 30 years), with asymmetrical limb weakness and wasting; bulbar and facial involvement occurs along with sensorineural deafness. The course is more benign than the disorder observed in Europe and America.

- ALS associated with a parkinsonism–dementia complex in Guam. It also tends to have an earlier onset and a more protracted course than the sporadic cases seen in Europe and America.

What are the criteria for diagnosis of ALS?
Summary of revised El Escorial criteria ('Gold Coast criteria'):
Progressive lower and upper motor neuron signs and symptoms in one limb or body segment, or progressive lower motor neuron signs in two body segments.
Absence of evidence of other disease processes that could explain the symptoms in neuroimaging, electrophysiological studies, and laboratory findings.

What is the pathology of motor neurone disease?
The clinical manifestations result from degeneration of Betz cells, pyramidal tracts, cranial nerve nuclei, and anterior horn cells. Both upper and lower motor neurons may be involved, but sensory involvement is not seen.

What is the explanation for fasciculation?
It is the result of spontaneous firing of large motor units formed by branching fibres of surviving axons that are striving to innervate muscle fibres that have lost their nerve supply.

What are the cerebrospinal fluid changes in the disease?
Usually normal; protein may be slightly raised.

What do you know about the heredity of ALS?
Most cases are sporadic, but 5% to 10% are familial. Familial ALS is linked to a gene on the long arm of chromosome 21, with various missense mutations identified in different families. This genetic locus appears to encode a copper–zinc-binding superoxide dismutase (SOD). Therapies that ameliorate symptoms in the *Sod1* mutant mouse have consistently failed in humans suggesting other mechanisms. It has been shown that a muscle-specific microRNA (miR-206) in the *Sod1* mouse delays disease progression and promotes regeneration of neuromuscular synapses by boosting the secretion of a growth factor-binding protein into the extracellular matrix indirectly; this, in turn, potentiates growth factors that promote presynaptic innervation at the neuromuscular junction. MicroRNAs are endogenous, small RNAs (~22 nucleotides in length) that target and downregulate, in a sequence-specific manner, messenger RNA.
Mutations in additional genes (encoding alsin, angiogenin, dynactin 1, senataxin, and vesicle-associated protein B) have also been associated with a motor neurone disease (although often not a typical ALS phenotype) in a few families.

How are DNA chips (microarrays) used in genetic analysis?
The DNA chip or the microarray is able to genotype hundreds of thousands of single-nucleotide polymorphisms (SNPs) simultaneously in a single experiment. (SNPs are single-nucleotide variations in the DNA sequence that can be used as markers for neighbouring genetic variation.) Comparing the prevalence of a specific SNP in patients and controls, the chromosomal region represented by the SNP associated with a disease can be determined. This approach is known as a high-density genome-wide association study. Using one such study, a recent group of investigators reported that variants of *FLJ10986* may confer susceptibility to sporadic ALS. *FLJ10986* and 50 other candidate loci warrant further investigation for their potential role in conferring susceptibility to the disease.

Is there any treatment for motor neurone disease?
Riluzole has proved to improve survival in specific types of motor neurone disease. Patients often require treatment for painful muscle cramps, constant drooling, severe fatiguability, sleep problems, incipient contractures, subluxation of the shoulder joint, dysphagia, and neuralgia—all of which can be ameliorated. Patients often have extreme lability of emotion, particularly in the early stages of ALS. In order to alleviate distress before or during respiratory failure, which is usually the terminal event, narcotic drugs should not be withheld.

What is the rationale for using riluzole?
The suggestion is that accumulation of toxic levels of glutamate at synapses may cause neuronal death through a calcium-dependent pathway. It is thought that riluzole reduces glutamate toxicity in three ways: inhibition of glutamic acid release, blockade of *N*-methyl-D-aspartate receptor responses, and action on the voltage-dependent sodium channel. Riluzole has been shown to be useful in patients with disease of bulbar onset but not in those with disease of spinal onset. The risk of death or tracheostomy is lower with 100 mg riluzole than placebo in limb or bulbar onset disease, but it is debatable whether this translates into an improved quality of life.

What is the course of palliative care in motor neurone disease?
1. Counselling on diagnosis
2. Treatment of symptoms:
   - *Fasciculations*:
     - Mild: magnesium, vitamin E
     - Severe: quinine, carbamazepine, phenytoin.
   - *Spasticity*:
     - Support: ankle–foot orthoses, wheelchair, home modification
     - Drug treatment: baclofen, tizanidine, memantine, tetrazepam.
   - *Drooling*:
     - Amitriptyline, transdermal hyoscine patches, glycopyrrolate, atropine, benztropine.
   - *Pathological laughing or crying*:
     - Amitriptyline, fluvoxamine, lithium, levodopa.
   - Riluzole for disease of bulbar onset.
3. Support for vital functions:
   - Assisted ventilation
   - Nutritional support: percutaneous endoscopic or radiologically inserted gastrostomy.
4. End-of-life palliative care (advanced directive?).

What is the role of magnetic cortical stimulation in ALS?
Magnetic cortical stimulation uses time-varying magnetic fields to induce electrical currents within the brain painlessly. It is said to activate cortical motor neurons transsynaptically through thalamocortical and corticocortical afferents and allows detection of degeneration of cortical Betz cells. In patients with ALS, the sensitivity of this technique to detect upper motor neuron involvement in those with clinical signs is high, but the sensitivity of the technique in those without clinical signs is unknown.

Is there any animal model for ALS?
Transgenic mouse model possessing mutations in the gene encoding the cytosolic form of the enzyme copper–zinc SOD.

A patient presents on the acute medical take with weakness and slurred speech. On general inspection he has gynaecomastia with facial muscle wasting and on examination he has symmetrical distal and proximal muscle weakness. The only past medical history of note is that he is under investigations for infertility. Can you think of a motor neuron disease form that this male patient may be suffering from?

Kennedy disease (spinal bulbar muscular atrophy).

Further Information

Charcot gave a detailed clinical and pathological description of ALS in 1865.

Lou Gehrig, the American baseball player, died of ALS 50 years ago.

Professor Stephen Hawking (1942–2018), the Cambridge theoretical physicist, was the most famous sufferer of motor neurone disease in recent times. It also claimed the lives of the actor David Niven, the football manager Don Revie, and the wartime pilot Sir Leonard Cheshire, VC.

CHAPTER 185

Multiple Sclerosis

PATIENT 1
Instruction

Examine this patient's eyes.

Salient Features
HISTORY

- Remissions and relapses
- Diplopia, visual disturbances
- Sensory and motor problems
- Paraesthesia and pain
- Speech disturbances
- Balance problems, cerebellar ataxia, and gait disturbances
- Bowel and bladder dysfunction
- Fatigue
- History of other autoimmune conditions
- Depressive symptoms and detailed social history
- Medication history, side effects, and compliance.

EXAMINATION

- Optic atrophy
- Nystagmus
- Internuclear ophthalmoplegia (see Fig. 181.1)
  - Features of cerebellar syndrome.

Diagnosis

This patient has optic atrophy (lesion) caused by demyelinating disorder, likely multiple sclerosis (MS) (aetiology). She is registered blind (functional status).

PATIENT 2
Instruction

Examine this patient's legs.

657

Salient Features

HISTORY

- Remissions and relapses: weakness, incoordination, pain, paraesthesias, urinary urgency, impotence. Steinberg's triad is history of incontinence of bladder, impotence, or constipation.

EXAMINATION

- Spastic paraparesis (increased tone, upgoing plantars, weakness, brisk reflexes, and ankle or patellar clonus). Spasticity is quantified using the Ashworth scale, which scores muscle tone on a scale of 0 to 4, with 0 representing normal tone and 4 severe spasticity.
- Impaired coordination on heel–shin test (if there is marked weakness, this test may be unreliable)
- Diminished abdominal reflexes
- In such patients, spinal cord compression should be excluded before making a diagnosis of MS.
- Patients with demyelinating disease may present with a mixture of combination of the aforementioned signs on examination. Be prepared to demonstrate as many as possible in the examination room and reach a unifying diagnosis.

Diagnosis

This patient has spastic paraparesis (lesion) caused by a demyelinating disorder (MS) and is wheelchair bound (functional status).

Questions

What investigations would you consider?
MS is a clinical diagnosis and is based on clinical presentation, based on agreed diagnostic criteria demonstrating lesions disseminated in space and time. Even for a typical clinical presentation, a series of blood tests needs to be performed to exclude alternative diagnoses.

- Obtain full blood count, inflammatory markers, basic biochemistry (liver, renal function tests, and electrolytes, including calcium and magnesium), thyroid function tests, glucose, vitamin B_{12}, and HIV serology.
- On suspicion of a diagnosis of MS, a spinal and brain magnetic resonance imaging (MRI) is requested to demonstrate lesions spread in time and space (Fig. 185.1).
- Clinical presentation and MRI should be enough to diagnose MS, especially for typical presentations. Other tests that can be utilized if needed in equivocal cases are cerebrospinal fluid (CSF) sample for oligoclonal bands, and visual evoked potentials.
- Visual evoked potentials: despite normal visual function, there may be prolonged latency in cortical response to a pattern stimulus. This indicates a delay in conduction in the visual pathways.
- Lumbar puncture: total protein may be raised, and oligoclonal bands will be positive in 90% to 95% of patients with MS.

Mention a few causes of bilateral pyramidal lesions affecting the lower limbs.
- Cord compression
- MS
- Cervical spondylosis

185 — MULTIPLE SCLEROSIS

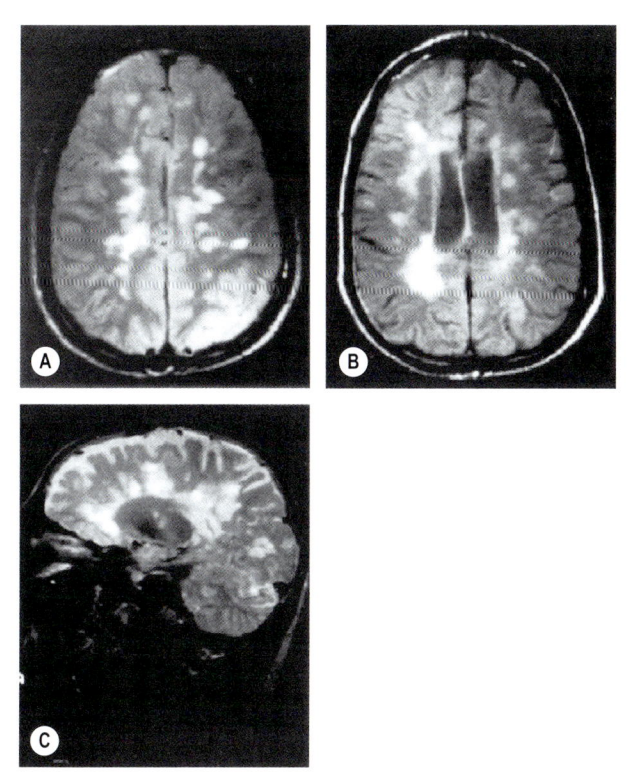

Fig. 185.1 MRI in MS. **(A)** Multifocal lesions in the centrum semiovale (proton density image). **(B)** Multiple, at times confluent, white matter lesions abutting the lateral ventricles (proton density image). **(C)** Lesions distributed in a radiating fashion from the corpus callosum (Dawson fingers) plus significant cerebral atrophy with ventriculomegaly and cortical atrophy (T_2-weighted image). (With permission from Bradley, W.G., Daroff, R.B., Fenichel, G., Jankovic, J., 2008. Neurology in Clinical Practice, fifth edn. Butterworth-Heinemann, Oxford.)

- Transverse myelitis
- Motor neurone disease
- Vitamin B_{12} deficiency
- Cerebrovascular disease.

How common is MS?
The prevalence in the United Kingdom is about 1 in 800 people, with an annual incidence of 2 to 10 per 100,000. The age of onset varies but peaks between 20 and 40 years of age. It affects approximately 100,000 people in the United Kingdom. Prevalence varies geographically.

What are the main ways in which MS can present?
- Optic neuritis (in 40%), resulting in partial loss of vision
- Weakness of one or more limbs
- Tingling in the extremities caused by posterior column involvement
- Diplopia
- Nystagmus, cerebellar ataxia
- Vertigo.

What is the natural history of MS?
The course of the disease is extremely variable and patients with MS face enormous prognostic uncertainty. The onset may be acute, subacute, or insidious. The course may be rapidly downhill, or may spontaneously remit for periods lasting from days to years before a second exacerbation.

What are the clinical categories of MS?
Clinically isolated syndrome: the first episode that has characteristics of demyelination and could prove to be MS in the future

Relapsing–remitting: episodes of acute worsening with recovery and a stable course between relapses

Secondary progressive: gradual neurologic deterioration with or without superimposed acute relapses in a patient who previously had relapsing–remitting MS

Primary progressive: gradual, nearly continuous neurologic deterioration from the onset of symptoms.

What is Lhermitte's sign?
A tingling or electric shock-like sensation that radiates to the arms, down the back, or into the legs on flexion of the patient's neck. It has also been called the 'barber's chair' sign. It indicates disease near the dorsal column nuclei of the higher cervical cord. Causes include MS, cervical stenosis, and subacute combined degeneration of the cord.

What is Uhthoff's symptom?
The exacerbation of symptoms of MS during a hot bath.

What do you know of the diagnostic criteria for MS?
The revised McDonald's criteria are based on the clinical attacks and lesions initially, attempting to establish dissemination in time and place for lesions identified clinically and on MRI. Primary importance is placed on clinical attacks but if the clinical features do not fit the criteria exactly, MRI can substitute for one of these clinical episodes. The criteria should only be used if MS is suspected and should not be used to aid in differentiating MS from other pathologies.

What is the role of steroids in acute attacks of MS?
In acute disabling attacks, treatment is initiated with a short course of steroids. Different regimens are used, intravenously or orally. The treatment of the acute attack aims at reducing the episode of the acute exacerbation but does not have a prognostic benefit on the overall progression of the disease.

Does pregnancy affect the clinical features of MS?
Pregnancy itself may have a mildly protective effect, but there is an increased risk of relapse during the puerperium; overall, the effect on the course of the disease is probably negligible.

What is the role of exercise in the treatment of such patients?
Patients should be encouraged to keep active during remission and to avoid excessive physical exercise during relapses.

What is the role of MRI in MS?
MRI cannot replace clinical suspicion but can support the diagnosis, as it can help establishing a diagnosis in up to 80% of patients with MS. T_2-weighted images show hyperintense focal periventricular lesions. Although periventricular white matter lesions are typical of MS, they are not

pathognomonic. Small infarcts, disseminated metastases, moyamoya disease, and inflammatory diseases can produce a similar picture. MRI may provide useful prognostic information in patients who present with an acute clinically isolated syndrome suggestive of MS.

Mention some other demyelinating disorders.
- Leukodystrophies
- Devic disease: optic neuritis with acute myelitis with MRI changes that extend over at least three segments of the spinal cord. It is associated with a specific antibody marker (neuromyelitis optica (NMO)–immunoglobulin G) targeting the water channel aquaphorin-4.
- Tuberous sclerosis (patchy demyelination)
- Schilder disease (diffuse cerebral sclerosis; may present with cortical blindness when the occipital cortex is involved).

What does the National Institute for Health and Clinical Excellence recommend about modifiable risk factors for MS?
- Encourage regular exercise.
- Live vaccinations may be contraindicated with the concurrent use of disease-modifying drugs (DMTs).
- Advise against smoking.

Name some medications that help with symptom control in MS.
- Amantadine for fatigue
- Baclofen for spasticity
- Fampridine for mobility
- Gabapentin for oscillopsia
- Amitriptyline for emotional lability.

What are the prognostic markers that predict more severe MS?
- Progressive disease from the onset of symptoms
- Frequent relapses in the first 2 years
- Motor and cerebellar signs at presentation to neurologist
- Short interval between the first two relapses
- Male sex
- Poor recovery from relapse
- Multiple cranial lesions on T_2-weighted MRI at presentation.

Women and patients with predominantly sensory symptoms and optic neuritis have a more favourable prognosis.

What is the differential diagnosis of MS?
- Disorders affecting one anatomical site and with either a relapsing–remitting or progressive course (especially, tumours and other structural lesions)
- Systemic diseases complicated by CNS involvement that follow a relapsing–remitting course (e.g. vasculitis)
- Monophasic disorders affecting several neuroanatomical locations (e.g. acute disseminated encephalomyelitis)
- Diseases of the spinal cord and brain confined to selected physiological systems and usually following a progressive course (e.g. the hereditary cerebellar ataxias)
- Nonorganic symptoms that, intentionally or otherwise, mimic the clinical features of MS (so-called functional or somatization disorders).

Is there any treatment for MS?
Therapies that alter prognosis: There is no curative treatment for MS, however, there are DMTs that have been shown to reduce both the relapse rate and the brain lesions. The DMTs that are currently used for MS are monoclonal antibodies (e.g. natalizumab, rituximab, alemtuzumab), interferons (interferon-β1b, interferon-β1a), other injectables (e.g. glatiramer acetate), and oral medications (e.g. teriflunomide, fingolimod, and dimethylfumarate). All of these therapies have been proven to reduce rate of relapse and the rate of the brain lesions, and the choice of DMT will depend on individual needs.

Acute relapses: Intravenous methylprednisolone may hasten recovery from acute relapses but has no effect in the long term. Intravenous methylprednisolone is no better than equivalent oral doses of methylprednisolone for acute relapses and steroid regimens are multiple.

Miscellaneous:
- Fatigue is modestly reduced by amantadine.
- Bladder dysfunction usually consists of combined detrusor hyperreflexia and incomplete emptying volumes, with <100 mL urine remaining in the bladder after micturition, and is managed with oxybutynin or tolterodine; retention of volumes >100 mL require clean, intermittent self-catheterization.
- Sexual dysfunction may be helped with the phosphodiesterase inhibitor sildenafil citrate or alpha-adrenergic blockers.
- Limb spasticity requires a multidisciplinary approach ensuring correct posture, prevention of skin ulceration from pressure, management of bladder and bowel dysfunction, as well medications such as tizanidine, an $α_2$-adrenoreceptor antagonist antispastic agent. Tizanidine reduces spasticity but there is no beneficial effect on mobility.

There is no evidence to suggest that any treatment alters the long-term outcome in MS.

A patient has been diagnosed with MS during the coronavirus pandemic (SARS-CoV-2). What is recommendation for starting DMTs?
Given the potentially life-threatening effect of COVID-19 infection in patients with MS, the recommendation is that vaccination is likely more important than medication. The major vaccine manufacturers have advised that the vaccine can be given concurrently with the majority of DMTs. Exceptions to this are for sphingosine-1-phosphate receptor modulators, alemtuzumab, cladribine, anti-CD20 monoclonal infusions, and ofatumumab, where vaccination is recommended 4 weeks before initiation.

What do you know about the two-hit model in the pathogenesis of MS?
Grey matter atrophy proceeds three times faster in MS than in unaffected persons, and with progressive neurologic disability, this rate of atrophy increases to 14 times faster in affected patients than in unaffected persons. Grey matter atrophy correlates with physical disability and cognitive disability more strongly than white matter atrophy. The two-hit model for cortical demyelination posits that two separate pathogenic 'hits'—an activation hit and a demyelination hit—trigger the pathologic process in the cortex. An immune-mediated inflammation targets contactin 2 (expressed in specialized regions of myelinated fibres by oligodendrocytes, Schwann cells, and the axons of a subpopulation of neurons, including those in the hippocampus and spinal cord) on or near grey matter endothelial cells to open the blood–brain barrier or alter endothelial cells in the grey matter, permitting effectors of demyelination (such as antibodies to myelin proteins) to gain access to grey matter.

Three patterns of demyelinating lesion have been described in the brain cortex in patients with MS:
    I: lesions involve both white and grey matter.
    II: lesions are small perivascular areas of cortical demyelination.
    III: lesions are bands of cortical demyelination below the pial surface that often cover several gyri and stop at cortical layer three or four.

What do you understand by the Pulfrich effect?

The Pulfrich effect is a stereo-illusion resulting from latency disparities in the visual pathways. It is a feature of optic neuritis but is also to be found with other conditions. The symptoms are often difficult for the patient to explain and for the physician to understand. Symptoms may be sufficiently disturbing to significantly interfere with activities of daily living (e.g. prevention of driving, crossing the road or playing ball games). Treatment with the use of monocular tints is simple and effective.

Further Information

J.L. Lhermitte (1877–1959), a French neurologist and neuropsychiatrist, wrote exclusively on spinal injuries, myoclonus, internuclear ophthalmoplegia, and chorea.

William Ian McDonald (1933–2006), native of New Zealand, was Head of the Department of Neurology at Queen Square, London. He delineated the pathophysiology of demyelination of peripheral nerves in 1963 (McDonald, 1963).

CHAPTER 186

Multiple System Atrophy

Instruction
Perform a neurological examination on this patient.

Salient Features

HISTORY
- Dizziness when standing up (caused by postural hypotension)
- Dysphagia
- Ataxia
- Symptoms of Parkinson disease
- Impotence, bladder disturbances
- Anhidrosis.

EXAMINATION
- Mask-like facies and other features of bradykinesia
- Increased tone (rigidity)
- Hyperreflexia
- Camptocormia (severe anterior flexion of the spine)
- Cerebellar signs.

Proceed as follows:
- Look for postural hypotension (a fall in systolic blood pressure (BP) of at least 20 mm Hg or in diastolic BP of at least 10 mm Hg within the 3 min after standing), the hallmark of this condition (caused by autonomic failure).
- Look for signs of autonomic dysfunction (pupillary asymmetry, Horner syndrome).

Diagnosis
This patient has cerebellar signs and parkinsonism (lesion) caused by multiple system atrophy, a degenerative disorder (aetiology), and has marked disability including incontinence (functional status).

Questions

What are the types of multisystem atrophy (MSA)?
Striatonigral degeneration. Clinical picture resembles Parkinson disease but without tremor. These patients do not respond to antiparkinsonian medications and often develop adverse reactions to these agents.
Shy–Drager syndrome. Clinical picture consists of Parkinson disease combined with severe autonomic neuropathy (particularly postural hypotension). Other important clinical features are impotence and bladder disturbances.

Olivopontocerebellar atrophy. Combination of extrapyramidal manifestations and cerebellar ataxia. Patients may also have autonomic neuropathy and anterior horn cell degeneration.
Parkinsonism and motor neurone disease. Rare.

What is the pathology in Shy–Drager syndrome?
In 1960, Shy and Drager described changes in the brainstem and ganglia; subsequently, loss of neurons has been shown in the autonomic nervous system and in the cells of the intermediolateral column of the spinal cord. Positron emission tomography (PET) shows decreased uptake of dopamine in the putamen and caudate lobe.

What factors can lower BP in these patients?
Standing up: orthostatic hypotension, a hallmark of this condition.
Food and exercise can produce hypotension even in the supine position.

What is the morbidity of this condition?
It tends to disable most patients severely after 5 to 7 years. An older age of onset is associated with more rapid deterioration.

How would you treat these patients?
Treatment is symptomatic and supportive for hypotension and neurological deficits. Symptoms of postural hypotension may be ameliorated by antigravity stockings and fludrocortisone.

How does pure autonomic failure differ from MSA?
Pure autonomic failure differs in its lack of any sensory, cerebellar, pyramidal, or extrapyramidal dysfunction. Afferent pathways and somatic neurons are not affected. It is less progressive than MSA, and patients usually have a prolonged and sometimes stable course. Pure autonomic failure affects postganglionic neurons and autonomic impairment is the principal clinical feature (orthostatic hypotension, bladder incontinence, and impotence in men are the major signs).

What are the radiological signs of MSA?
- The more common typical radiological findings in MSA include atrophy of the cerebellum, most prominently in the vermis, middle cerebellar peduncles, pons, and lower brainstem.
- In addition to putaminal atrophy, a characteristic hypointense signal in T_2 with hyperintense rim, corresponding to reactive gliosis and astrogliosis, can be observed in the external putamen and is termed the 'slit-like void sign' (Fig. 186.1B). This combination of hypointense and hyperintense putaminal signal change is specific for MSA and its finding can be used to differentiate MSA from progressive supranuclear palsy and Parkinson disease.
- The 'hot-cross bun' sign is characterized by cruciform signal hyperintensity on T_2-weighted images in mid pons (Fig. 186.1A). This finding is said to correspond to the loss of pontine neurons and myelinated transverse cerebellar fibres with preservation of the corticospinal tracts. However, this sign is not specific to MSA and has been reported in other conditions such as spinocerebellar ataxia.
- Hypointensity alone without hyperintense rim is a sensitive radiological feature but non-specific for MSA.

What are the diagnostic criteria for *probable* MSA?
A sporadic, progressive, adult-onset (aged >30 years) disease characterized by:
- Autonomic failure involving urinary incontinence (with erectile dysfunction in males) *or*
- Orthostatic decrease of BP within 3 min of standing by at least 30 mm Hg systolic or 15 mm Hg diastolic *and either*

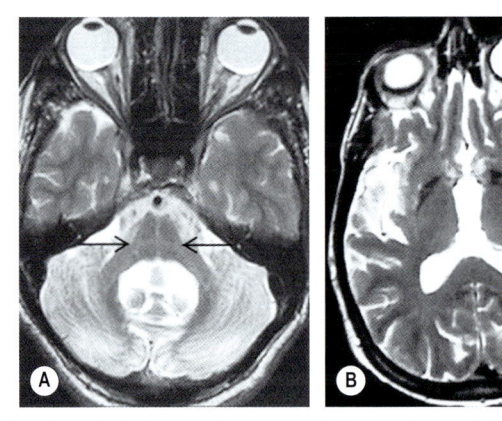

Fig. 186.1 Axial T$_2$-weighted MR images showing the 'hot-cross bun sign' **(A)** and the 'slit-like void sign' **(B)**. (With permission from Ling, H., Lees, A.J., 2010. How can neuroimaging help in the diagnosis of movement disorders? Neuroimaging Clin. North Am. 20, 111–123.)

- Poorly levodopa-responsive parkinsonism (bradykinesia with rigidity, tremor, or postural instability) *or*
- A cerebellar syndrome (gait ataxia with cerebellar dysarthria, limb ataxia, or cerebellar oculomotor dysfunction).

What are the diagnostic criteria for *possible* MSA?
A sporadic, progressive, adult-onset (aged >30 years) disease characterized by:
- Parkinsonism (bradykinesia with rigidity, tremor, or postural instability) *or*
- A cerebellar syndrome (gait ataxia with cerebellar dysarthria, limb ataxia, or cerebellar oculomotor dysfunction) *and*
- At least one feature suggesting autonomic dysfunction (otherwise unexplained urinary urgency, frequency or incomplete bladder emptying, erectile dysfunction in males, or significant orthostatic BP decline that does not meet the level required in probable MSA) *and*
- At least one of the additional features:
  - Possible MSA-P or MSA-C (parkinsonian subtype or cerebellar dysfunction subtype, respectively, see later)
  - Babinski's sign with hyperreflexia
  - Stridor.

Possible MSA-P is indicated by:
- Rapidly progressive parkinsonism
- Poor response to levodopa
- Postural instability within 3 years of motor onset
- Gait ataxia, cerebellar dysarthria, limb ataxia, or cerebellar oculomotor dysfunction
- Dysphagia within 5 years of motor onset
- Atrophy on magnetic resonance imaging (MRI) of putamen, middle cerebellar peduncle, pons, or cerebellum
- Hypometabolism on fluorodeoxyglucose PET (FDG-PET) in the putamen, brainstem, or cerebellum.

Possible MSA-C is indicated by:
- Parkinsonism (bradykinesia and rigidity)
- Atrophy on MRI of putamen, middle cerebellar peduncle, or pons
- Hypometabolism on FDG-PET in putamen

- Presynaptic nigrostriatal dopaminergic denervation on single-photon emission computed tomography (SPECT) or PET.

What are features supporting a diagnosis of MSA?
- Orofacial dystonia
- Disproportionate antecollis
- Camptocormia (severe anterior flexion of the spine) with or without Pisa syndrome (severe lateral flexion of the spine)
- Contractures of the hands or feet
- Inspiratory sighs
- Severe dysphonia
- Severe dysarthria
- New or increased snoring
- Cold hands and feet
- Pathological laughter or crying
- Jerky, myoclonic postural, or action tremor.

What are features that do not support a diagnosis of MSA?
- Classic pill-rolling rest tremor
- Clinically significant neuropathy
- Onset after age 75 years
- Family history of ataxia or parkinsonism
- Dementia
- White matter lesions that suggest multiple sclerosis
- Hallucinations not induced by drugs.

What do you know about the pathogenesis of MSA?
In transgenic mouse models of oligodendroglial α-synucleinopathy, sickle-shaped glial cytoplasmic inclusions composed of misfolded α-synuclein can be seen. The dying neuron contains condensed chromatin; the nuclear membrane is disrupted and there is cell shrinkage. These findings indicate three possible pathogenic pathways in multiple system atrophy:
- Inclusions could trigger microglial activation, which causes chronic oxidative stress and ultimately leads to neuronal cell death.
- Inclusions could exacerbate susceptibility to exogenous oxidative stress and lead to neuronal cell death in striatonigral and olivopontocerebellar systems.
- Inclusions could lead to secondary axonal α-synuclein aggregation or oligodendroglial mitochondrial dysfunction, which eventually leads to neuronal cell death.

Further Information

Bradbury and Eggleston in 1925 first described the combination of postural hypotension, incontinence, impotence, and abnormality of sweating (anhidrosis). Neurological manifestations were identified later.

G.A. Drager (1917–1967), a US neurologist.

G.M. Shy (1919–1967), a US neurologist who obtained his MRCP in London in 1947.

In 1969, Graham and Oppenheimer introduced the term multiple system atrophy to combine the entities of striatonigral degeneration, olivopontocerebellar ataxia, and Shy–Drager syndrome.

CHAPTER 187

Myasthenia Gravis

Instruction
This patient complains of drooping of the eyelids in the evenings; examine this patient.

Salient Features

HISTORY
- Weakness in muscles is more marked in the evening.
- Muscle weakness increases with exercise (remember that *fatigability* is the hallmark of myasthenia gravis) and is painless.
- Muscle weakness affects smiling (Fig. 187.1), chewing, speaking, muscles of the neck, walking, breathing, movements at the elbow, and hand movements.
- Obtain history of thyrotoxicosis, diabetes mellitus, rheumatoid arthritis, systemic lupus erythematosus (SLE), and thymoma.
- Ask about D-penicillamine treatment for rheumatoid arthritis (myasthenia gravis is sometimes caused by D-penicillamine).

EXAMINATION
- The patient may have obvious ptosis.
- Check for worsening of ptosis after sustained upward gaze for at least 45 s.
- Check extraocular movements for diplopia and variable squint.
- Comment on snarling face when the patient attempts to smile.
- Weakness without loss of reflexes or alteration of sensation or coordination. The weakness may be generalized; it may affect the limb muscles, often proximal in distribution, as well as the diaphragm and neck extensors.
- Speech is nasal.
- Muscle wasting is rare and when present indicates late disease.
- Ask the patient to count to 50 (voice may deteriorate).

Proceed as follows:
- Tell the examiner that myasthenia is associated with thyrotoxicosis, diabetes mellitus, rheumatoid arthritis, SLE, and thymoma.
- Perform ice pack test by the bedside.

Diagnosis
This patient has diplopia at the end of each day with ptosis; the weakness is marked on repeated exertion of the muscle (lesion) and is caused by myasthenia gravis (aetiology).

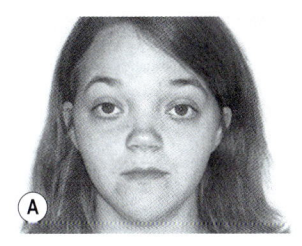

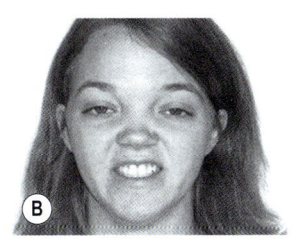

Fig. 187.1 Typical myasthenic facies. **(A)** At rest, there is slight bilateral lid ptosis, which is partially compensated for by raising the right eyebrow. **(B)** During attempted smile, there is contraction of the medial portion of the upper lip and horizontal contraction of the corners of the mouth without the natural upward curling, producing a 'sneer'. (With permission from Bradley, W.G., Daroff, R.B., Fenichel, G., Jankovic, J., 2008. Neurology in Clinical Practice, fifth edn. Butterworth-Heinemann, Oxford.)

Questions

At what age is myasthenia common?
The incidence has two age peaks, with one peak in the second and third decades affecting mostly women and another peak in the sixth and seventh decades affecting mostly men.

What groups of muscles are commonly involved?
Muscles affected are as follows, in order of likelihood: extraocular, bulbar, neck, limb girdle, distal limbs, and trunk.

What investigations would you like to do in this patient?
- Ice pack test should form part of the examination by the bedside.
- Vital capacity (forced vital capacity should be closely monitored in suspected myasthenic crisis)
- Imaging of the mediastinum: chest radiography, computed tomography, or magnetic resonance imaging of the chest
- Serum acetylcholine receptor antibodies (AchR-Ab) would be present in >80% of cases. 50% of patients have antibodies directed against muscle-specific kinase receptors (MuSK-Ab). Occasionally patients may have low-density lipoprotein receptor-related protein 4 (LRP4) antibodies. Around 10% of patients with myasthenia have seronegative disease, which means antibodies will not be detectable with the current available assays.
- Thyroid function tests (to rule out an associated thyroid disorder)
- Anti-striated muscle antibody (seen in association with thymoma)
- Antinuclear antibody, rheumatoid factor, and antithyroid antibodies may be positive.
- Tuberculin test if immunosuppressive therapy is contemplated
- Electromyography (EMG): abnormalities include a decremental response to tetanic train stimulation at 5 to 10 Hz, and evidence of neuromuscular blockade in the form of jitter and blocking of motor action potentials in single-fibre EMG. Single-fibre EMG is the most sensitive of these studies, with a sensitivity around 95%.

What is the differential diagnosis?
- Botulism
- Eaton–Lambert syndrome
- Myotonic dystrophy
- Thyroid ophthalmoplegia
- Cranial nerve mononeuritis
- Motor neurone disease.

Any neurological disease that can mimic the signs of generalized or ocular myasthenia can pose a differential of myasthenia gravis.

What are the treatment modalities available?
- Symptomatic treatment entails administration of an anticholinesterase drug (e.g. pyridostigmine) given up to five times per day.
- Definitive treatment entails immunosuppression, e.g. steroids, azathioprine, cyclosporin, mycophenolate mofetil, rituximab, plasmapheresis, intravenous immunoglobulin, and thymectomy.

Mention a drug that can cause myasthenia.
D-Penicillamine therapy given for rheumatoid arthritis.

Why may a gin and tonic exacerbate myasthenia?
The quinine in tonic water causes muscle weakness.

If this patient develops an infection, which group of antibiotics would you avoid?
Aminoglycosides.

Mention a few exacerbating features.
Fatigue, exercise, infection, emotion, change of climate, pregnancy, magnesium enemas, and drugs (aminoglycosides, propranolol, morphine, barbiturates, procainamide, quinidine).

How is the myasthenia graded?
The Osserman grading has five stages:
   I: Involves focal disease (e.g. restricted to ocular muscles, ocular myasthenia)
   II: Mild generalized myasthenia with slow progression, no crises, and drug responsive
   III: Moderate generalized myasthenia with severe skeletal and bulbar involvement but no crises; drug response less satisfactory
   IV: Acute fulminating myasthenia with rapid progression of severe symptoms of respiratory crises and poor drug response; high incidence of thymoma and high mortality rate
   V: Late severe myasthenia; same as grade III but takes 2 years to progress from class I to II; crises; high mortality rate with life-threatening respiratory impairment.

The Newsom–Davies clinical grading has three subgroups:
1. Patients with thymoma, equal sex incidence, peak age of onset 30 to 50 years, no human leukocyte antigen (HLA) association, and poor response to thymectomy
2. Young onset (aged <40 years), typically female, thymic medullary germinal centres present, strong association with *HLA-B8* and *HLA-DR3*, and usually a good response to thymectomy
3. Older onset (aged >40 years), more common in males, thymic involution, an association with *HLA-B7* and *HLA-DR9*, and doubtful response to thymectomy.

What do you know about Eaton–Lambert syndrome?
Eaton–Lambert syndrome is a myasthenic disorder associated with malignancy. It is associated with small-cell carcinoma of the bronchus. Weakness of the truncal and proximal limb muscles is common. The pelvic girdle and thighs are almost invariably involved. Deep tendon reflexes are absent. Transient improvement in muscle strength and deep tendon reflexes may follow brief exercise. Unlike myasthenia, bulbar symptoms are rare. Antibodies to calcium channels may be detected. EMG is diagnostic. In rested muscle, there is marked depression of neuromuscular transmission after a single submaximal stimulus and marked facilitation of response during

repetitive stimulation at rates greater than 10 per second. Assays for P/Q-type calcium channel antibodies are positive.

What is myasthenic crisis?
Exacerbation of myasthenia. The need for artificial ventilation occurs in about 10% of patients with myasthenia. Those with bulbar and respiratory involvement are prone to respiratory infection. The crisis can be precipitated by respiratory infection and surgery. Such patients should be closely monitored for pulmonary function. Those with artificial ventilation are not given cholinergics as this avoids stimulation of pulmonary secretions and uncertainties about overdosage.

How does a cholinergic crisis manifest?
Excessive salivation, confusion, lacrimation, miosis, pallor, and collapse. It is important to avoid edrophonium in such patients.

Mention a few associated disorders.
Thyroid disorders (thyrotoxicosis, hypothyroidism), rheumatoid arthritis, diabetes mellitus, dermatomyositis, pernicious anaemia, SLE, Sjögren disease, sarcoidosis, pemphigus.

What is the role of thymectomy in such patients?
In the case of thymoma, thymectomy is necessary to prevent tumour spread, although most thymomas are benign. In the absence of a tumour, thymectomy has been found to be beneficial in 85% of patients and 35% go into drug-free remission. The improvement is noticed for 1 to 10 years after surgery. The role of thymectomy in ocular myasthenia, in adults over 55 years of age and in children, is still under debate.

What is the role of immunomodulation in myasthenia gravis?
Intravenous immunoglobulin seems as efficacious as plasma exchange.

Further Information

Myasthenia gravis was first described by Oxford physiologist Thomas Willis in 1672 and by Erb in 1878. It was also known as Hoppe–Goldflam disease after H.H. Hoppe (1867–1919), a US neurologist (Hoppe, 1892), and S.V. Goldflam (1852–1932), a Polish neurologist. In 1895, F. Jolly named the disease myasthenia gravis pseudoparalytica (Jolly, 1895).

L.M. Eaton (1905–1958), Professor of Neurology at the Mayo Clinic, Rochester, Minnesota.

E.H. Lambert (b. 1915), Professor of Physiology, University of Minnesota.

Sir Samuel Wilks (1824–1911), physician, Guy's Hospital, London. Myasthenia gravis was known as Wilks syndrome.

CHAPTER 188

Myotonia Congenita

Instruction
Look at this patient.

Salient Features
HISTORY
- Ask the patient whether or not there is any seasonal variation in symptoms: myotonia is worse in winter from the cold.
- Take a family history (inheritance is usually autosomal dominant; gene on long arm of chromosome 7).

EXAMINATION
- Diffuse muscle hypertrophy
- Myotonia, which may be apparent while shaking hands with the person. (The myotonia displays a *warm-up phenomenon*, in which the myotonia decreases or vanishes completely when repeating the same movement several times.)

Know the phenotypic patterns of muscle disorders.

Diagnosis
This patient has diffuse muscular hypertrophy with myotonia (lesion) caused by Thomsen disease (aetiology).

Questions

How is the disease recognized in infancy?
Myotonia is present from birth and may be recognized by the child's peculiar cry. Also noticed in early infancy are difficulty in feeding and inability to reopen the eyes while having the face washed.

When does muscle hypertrophy manifest?
It is usually apparent in the second decade.

What is the cause of muscle hypertrophy?
It is caused by almost continual involuntary isometric exercise.

What is the life expectancy in such patients?
These patients have a normal life expectancy.

What drugs would you use to ameliorate the myotonia?
Procainamide, quinidine.

What do you know about the genetics of this disease?
It can be inherited as either an autosomal dominant (Thomsen disease) or recessive (Becker myotonia) trait, with close to 130 currently known mutations. Myotonia congenita is a specific inherited disorder of muscle membrane hyperexcitability caused by reduced sarcolemmal chloride conductance as a result of mutations in *CLCN1*, the gene coding for the main skeletal muscle chloride channel ClC-1.

In which other conditions is myotonia seen?
Myotonia can be a presenting sign of:
- Myotonic dystrophy
- Nondystrophic myotonias, in which myotonia is caused by dysfunction of:
    - channels for chloride (in myotonia congenita)
    - sodium channels (in paramyotonia congenita, potassium-aggravated myotonia, and hyperkalaemic periodic paralysis with myotonia).
- Myopathies (acid maltase deficiency, polymyositis, myotubular myopathy)
- Administration of drugs such as clofibrate, colchicine
- Rarely, denervation of any cause.

Further Information

A.J.T. Thomsen (1815–1896) was a Danish physician who described this condition in his family and himself in 1876.

CHAPTER **189**

Myotonic Dystrophy

Instruction

Look at this patient's face.
Examine this patient's cranial nerves.

Salient Features

HISTORY

- Onset usually in the third and fourth decades. However, if the mother is the carrier, then the disease may manifest in infancy and undergo rapid deterioration at the usual age of onset.
- Onset dominated by weakness or myotonia or both
- Difficulty in releasing grip
- Leg weakness (difficulty in kicking a ball)
- 'Pseudo-drop attacks' (caused by weakness of quadriceps muscle)
- Ask the patient if they have dysphagia (oesophageal involvement).
- Impotence (caused by gonadal atrophy)
- Recurrent respiratory infections (caused by weakness of muscles of bronchioles)
- Excessive urge to sleep (daytime somnolence is common).

EXAMINATION

- While shaking hands with the patient, note the myotonia.
- Frontal baldness (the patient may be wearing a wig and it is important to mention if this is so)
- Ptosis (bilateral or unilateral) with a *smooth* forehead
- Cataracts (posterior capsular cataracts) or evidence of surgery for cataracts
- Difficulty in opening the eyes after firm closure
- Expressionless face ('hatchet face'; Fig. 189.1) with wasting of temporalis, masseters, and sternomastoids and 'swan neck' caused by thinning of the neck.

Proceed as follows:
Test:
- Sternomastoids
- Distal muscles of the upper limbs, wasting, percussion myotonia over thenar muscles, and weakness
- Deep tendon jerks (depressed)
- Examine precordium for evidence of permanent pacemaker.
- Examine for evidence of diabetes/insulin use.

Tell the examiner that you would like to do the following:
- Check the urine for sugar (diabetes mellitus).
- Test higher intellectual function (low IQ).
- Examine for gynaecomastia and testicular atrophy.

Respiratory failure is the commonest cause of death.

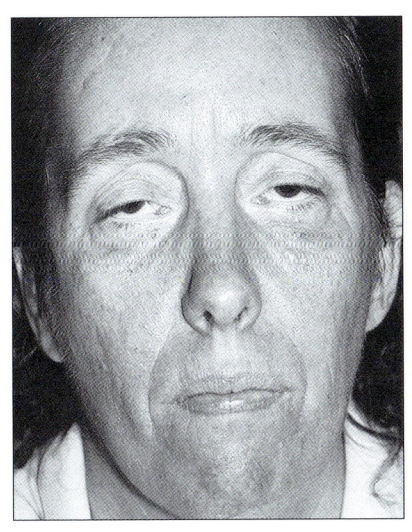

Fig. 189.1 Muscle wasting in myotonic dystrophy gives the characteristic drawn appearance of 'hatchet facies'. (With permission from Yanoff, M., Duker, J.S., 2008. Ophthalmology, third edn. Mosby, Philadelphia, PA.)

Diagnosis

This patient has frontal balding, myotonia, cataracts, and wasting of the sternomastoids (lesion) caused by dystrophia myotonica (aetiology). He has dysphagia and severe muscular weakness (functional status).

Questions

What is the inheritance of this condition?
Autosomal dominant inheritance. Myotonic dystrophy type 1 (the more common and typically the more severe of the two major types) is caused by an expanded cytosine–thymine–guanine (CTG) repeat on chromosome 19q13.3 in the 3′-untranslated region of *DMPK*, a gene for a dystrophia myotonica protein kinase (a serine–threonine protein kinase). The condition usually presents in the third and fourth decades. The disease tends to be worse in successive generations (known as anticipation). As a result, the grandparent may merely have cataracts while the grandchild develops a severe progressive form of the disease. Positional cloning has helped to identify the gene for myotonic dystrophy and localized a dynamic mutation with an increase in the number of trinucleotide repeats. The repeat size typically increases from generation to generation, providing a molecular basis for the clinical phenomenon of anticipation.

The less common form of the disease, myotonic dystrophy 2, is caused by an expanded CCTG repeat (with expansions ranging from 80 to 11,000 repeats) in the first intron of *ZNF9*, the gene for zinc finger protein 9.

Transcribed RNA repeats fold into a hairpin, and the RNA is retained in the nucleus, where it alters the ratio of cytosine uracil guanine (CUG) RNA-binding proteins, such as CUG-binding protein 1 (CUG-BP1) and muscleblind-like 1 (MBNL1). Splicing misregulation in myotonic dystrophy results from altered functions of these two RNA-binding proteins, which were identified because they bind CUG repeats in RNA. CUG-BP1 and MBNL1 are direct and antagonistic regulators of alternative splicing events that are normally regulated during development and misregulated in myotonic dystrophy. Increased activity of CUG-BP1 and decreased activity of

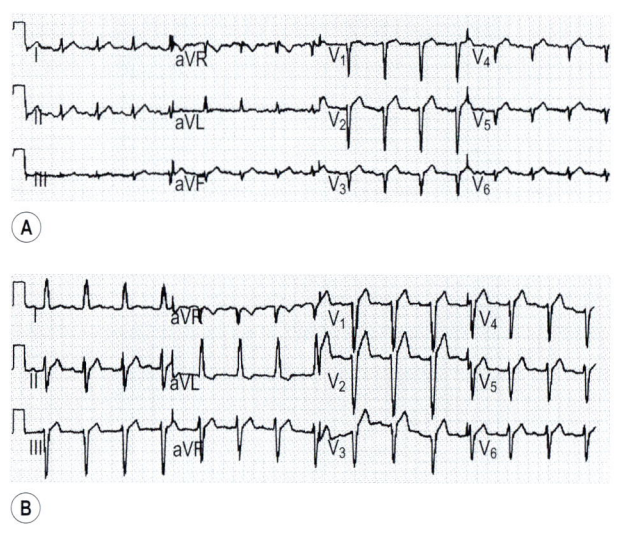

Fig. 189.2 Electrocardiogram in myotonic dystrophy (**A** taken around a year before **B**). There are abnormal Q waves in the precordial leads. The increasing severity of conduction disease is indicated by increasing PR interval and QRS duration in (**B**).

MBNL1 induce 'embryonic pattern' splicing (i.e. isoforms typically expressed in the developing embryo and fetus predominate). The fact that MBNL1 colocalizes with nuclear RNA foci in the cells of patients with myotonic dystrophy suggests that MBNL1 is sequestered by mutant RNAs. Increasing the expression of MBNL1 in a mouse model of myotonic dystrophy restores the adult splicing pattern of the muscle-specific chloride channel (ClC-1) protein and reverses the myotonia associated with ClC-1 misregulated splicing. These data support a primary role of MBNL1 depletion in the pathogenesis of the disease.

What are the other features of this condition?
- Cardiomyopathy and cardiac conduction defects (Fig. 189.2). A severe abnormality on the electrocardiogram (ECG) and a diagnosis of an atrial tachyarrhythmia predict sudden death. An implantable cardioverter defibrillator should be considered in all patients.
- Respiratory infection (low serum immunoglobulin G levels)
- Somnolence
- External ophthalmoplegia (occasionally).

What do you understand by myotonia?
It is continued contraction of the muscle after voluntary contraction ceases, followed by impaired relaxation.

What therapeutic modalities are available?
Mexiletine, acetazolamide, or phenytoin has been used in *disabling* myotonia. No treatment has altered the course of progressive weakness.

What other forms of myotonia do you know?
Myotonia congenita, or Oppenheim disease, is an autosomal dominant condition that presents at birth with feeding difficulties. The myotonia improves with age and there is no dystrophy.

Although this is considered to be a myopathy, changes have been reported in the motor nuclei of the spinal cord and motor cortex.

In which myopathies is distal weakness prominent?
- Myotonic dystrophy
- Welander distal myopathy (more common in Scandinavians).

If this patient requires major surgery, what fact would you keep in mind?
Patients with myotonic dystrophy tend to do poorly after the administration of general anaesthetic (caused by impaired cardiorespiratory malfunction) and will require intensive postoperative observation.

Mention some causes of bilateral ptosis.
- Myasthenia gravis
- Congenital muscular dystrophies
- Ocular myopathy
- Syphilis.

What is the pathognomonic pattern of cataract in myotonic dystrophy?
Stellate or 'Christmas tree' cataract (myotonic dystrophy; Fig. 189.3).

The patient's sister is worried about risks to her offspring. What tests would you do?
- Clinical examination
- Electromyography
- Slit-lamp examination for cataracts.

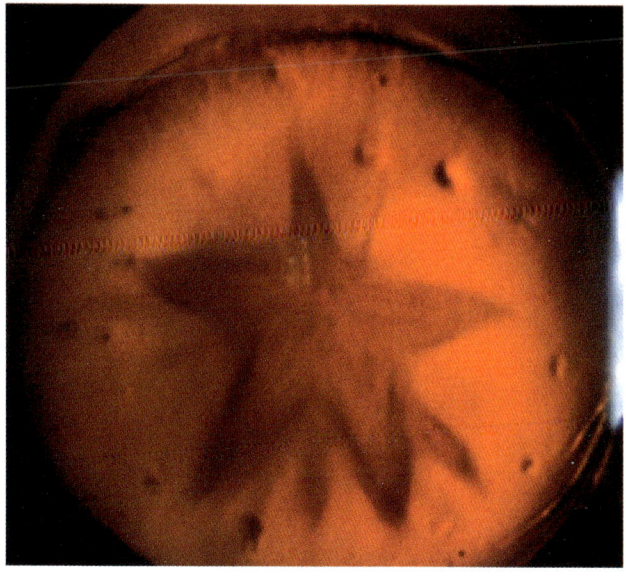

Fig. 189.3 Myotonic dystrophy. (With permission from Kanski, J.J., Bowling, B., 2011. Clinical Ophthalmology: A Systematic Approach, seventh edn. Saunders, London, pp. 269–309.)

Is prenatal diagnosis available?
Yes—in some families. The myotonic dystrophy gene is linked to the *ABH* secretor gene.

Babies born to mothers with myotonic dystrophy are prone to hypotonicity; in most instances, there is a family history of this disease, which is dominantly inherited. The mother may have undiagnosed myotonic dystrophy.

What is the characteristic electromyography finding?
Waxing and waning of the potentials, known as the dive-bomber effect. Electromyography changes are found in almost any muscle.

How would you manage such patients?
- Foot drop is controlled by calipers or moulded-foot orthoses.
- Myotonia when disabling may respond to phenytoin (avoid quinidine and procainamide as they can worsen cardiac conduction).
- Advanced heart block with or without syncope should be considered for pacemaker insertion.

Further Information

Délége, in 1890, first described the association of myotonia with muscular atrophy.
Batten and Gibb (1909) and Steinert (1909) independently described the clinical features of the symptom complex.
Curschmann, in 1912, emphasized the dystrophic symptoms and applied the term dystrophia myotonica.

CHAPTER 190

Parkinson Disease

Instruction
Examine this patient.

Salient Features
HISTORY
- Tremor: usually unilateral at onset; usually starts in upper limbs. This is also seen in the legs (commonly in vascular parkinsonism) and jaw.
- Rigidity: ask about history of falls, poor balance, pain, and muscle stiffness.
- Poverty of movement: ask about drooling of saliva, difficulty in writing (micrographia), difficulty in turning in bed, and change in voice (softness of voice).
- Ask for family history of disease (susceptibility genes include α-synuclein, leucine-rich repeat kinase 2, and glucocerebrosidase).
- Ask for history of smoking (never smokers are twice as likely to develop disease) and caffeine intake (those who take no or very low quantities of daily caffeine are at increased risk, ~25%).
- Ask for history of exposure to manganese dust, carbon disulfide, or carbon monoxide.
- Determine use of 1-methyl-4-phenyl-1,2,3,6-tetrahydropyridine (MPTP) for recreational purposes.
- Elicit a drug history, particularly regarding neuroleptics (reserpine, metoclopramide).
- Ask for history of herbal medications, particularly Pacific sedative kava kava and Indian snake root *Rauwolfia serpentina*.
- Ask for history of severe head injury, encephalitis, hypertension, or cerebrovascular disease.

EXAMINATION
Usually, florid cases are seen in the examination and have striking abnormalities (Fig. 190.1):
- an expressionless or 'mask-like' face (fixed stare, infrequent blinking, and ironed-out wrinkles)
- drooling of saliva
- resting or pill-rolling movement (most common in the distal extremities). Can be exaggerated by distraction.

Proceed as follows:
- Comment on the expressionless face, pill-rolling movement, and drooling of saliva so that the examiner knows that you have observed these abnormalities. Elicit bradykinesia by asking the patient to touch her thumb with each finger in turn.
- Examine the tone, in particular at the wrist for cog-wheel rigidity.

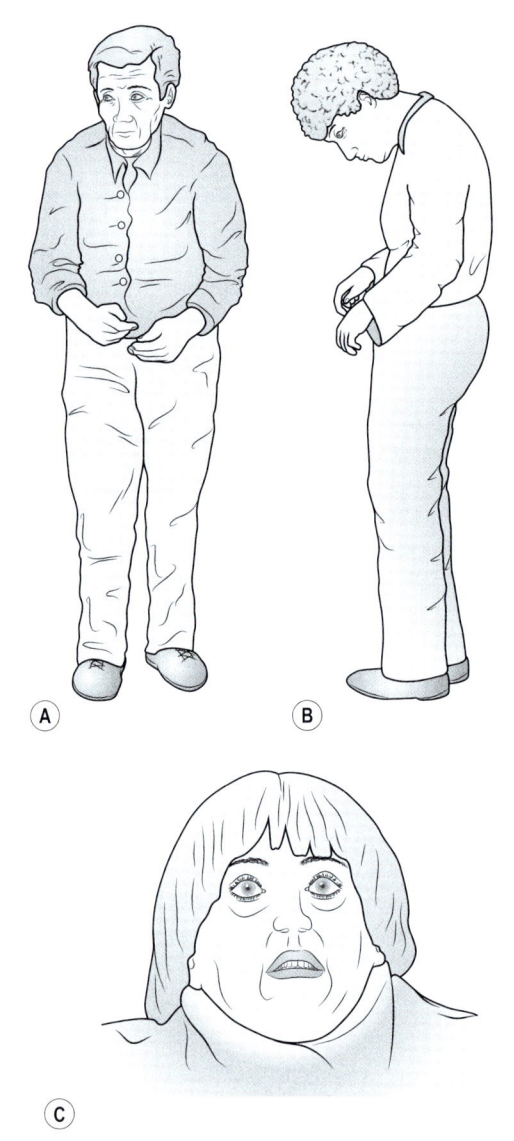

Fig. 190.1 Parkinson disease. **(A)** The slightly anxious frozen face and characteristic flexed posture. **(B)** Development of anterocollis. **(C)** Typical facial expression of a patient with progressive supranuclear palsy, illustrating worried or surprised appearance, with furrowed brow and fixed expression of lower face.

- Proceed to do the glabellar tap; tap the forehead just above the bridge of the nose repeatedly (about twice per s): in normal subjects, the blinking will stop, whereas the patient with Parkinson disease continues to blink: referred to as Myerson's sign. (It must be remembered that this sign is unreliable.)
- Ask the patient to walk and comment on the paucity of movement, including the absence of arm swing and festinating gait (the patient walks with a stooped posture as if trying

to catch up with her centre of gravity). The feet may scrape the floor in taking steps so the patient trips easily (be prepared to prevent the patient from falling when examining the gait).
- Tell the examiner that you would like to:
  - ask the patient a few questions with a view to assessing her speech
  - assess handwriting (tremulous and small, micrographia).

Tell the examiner that you would like to:
- look for postural hypotension
- look for impaired vertical gaze (progressive supranuclear palsy)
- check for anosmia (an early sign)
- look for seborrhoea.

The diagnosis of Parkinson disease is entirely clinical, but the results of certain investigations may help in recognizing alternative causes for parkinsonism.

Diagnosis

This patient has features of Parkinson disease (lesion). Their previous head injury may have contributed to the development (aetiology). The patient is severely disabled by the bradykinesia (functional status).

Questions

What comprises Parkinson disease?
- Upper body dyskinesia must be present; it is a symptom complex containing many of the following features:
- Slowness of movement (bradykinesia)
- Poverty of movement (mask-like facies, diminished arm swing)
- Difficulty in initiating movement
- Diminished amplitude of repetitive alternative movement
- Inordinate difficulty in accomplishing some simultaneous or sequential motor acts
- Rigidity usually but not always present
- Lead-pipe rigidity is where the increase in tone is equal in flexors and extensors of all four limbs but slightly more in flexors, resulting in a part flexed 'simian' posture
- Cog-wheel rigidity is caused by superimposed or underlying tremor
- Postural instability is usually a late feature
- Tremor:
  - Absent in about one-third of patients with Parkinson disease at presentation and throughout its course in some
  - Resting, 3 to 5 Hz pill, pronation and supination rolling tremor of the upper limb
  - Intermittent (can usually be brought about by getting the subject to count backwards with the eyes closed and hands resting on thighs)
  - Intensified by emotion or stress and disappearing during sleep
  - May affect legs, head, and jaw as well; jaw tremor is rare but is most distressing as the teeth may pound together until they become unbearably painful.

What are the pathological changes in Parkinson disease?
The most typical pathological hallmarks of Parkinson disease are:
- neuronal loss with depigmentation of the substantia nigra
- Lewy bodies, which are eosinophilic cytoplasmic inclusions in neurons consisting of α-synuclein.

The following associations have been made with clinical features and pathological changes:

Clinical Deficit	Pathology
Motor symptoms	Degeneration of dopaminergic nigrostriatal pathway
Cognitive defects	Degeneration of dopaminergic mesocortical and mesolimbic pathways
Autonomic dysfunction	Dopamine depletion in the hypothalamus
'Freezing phenomenon'	Degeneration of the noradrenergic locus ceruleus
Dementia	Degeneration of the cholinergic nucleus

What is the mental status of patients with Parkinson disease?
- In the initial stages, intellect and senses are usually preserved. Many patients have some intellectual deterioration—slowness of thought and of memory retrieval (bradyphrenia) and subtle personality changes.
- Global dementia may develop in one-fifth of patients.
- Depression occurs in one-third of patients.
- Delirium can be precipitated by drug therapy.

Note: Parkinson disease must be kept in mind in elderly patients presenting with a history of frequent falls.

What are the causes of Parkinson disease?
True parkinsonism:
- Idiopathic (caused by degeneration of the substantia nigra); also known as Parkinson disease
- Drug induced (chlorpromazine, metoclopramide, prochlorperazine)
- Anoxic brain damage such as cardiac arrest and exposure to manganese and carbon monoxide
- Postencephalitic, as a result of encephalitis lethargica or von Economo disease
- MPTP toxicity, seen in drug abusers
- Familial: mutation of the gene for α-synuclein or linkage to a region on chromosome 2.

Parkinson plus syndromes:
- Multiple system atrophy
- Progressive supranuclear atrophy.

Pseudoparkinsonism:
- Essential tremor
- Atherosclerotic (vascular) pseudoparkinsonism (mention that in the past, atherosclerosis was thought to be a cause of Parkinson disease, but this is no longer accepted as a cause)
- Hemiparkinsonism (presenting feature of a progressive space-occupying lesion).

What differences are seen in rigidity, spasticity, and gegenhalten?
- Rigidity indicates increased tone affecting opposing muscle groups equally and is present throughout the range of passive movement. When smooth, it is called lead-pipe rigidity and when intermittent is termed cog-wheel rigidity. It is common in extrapyramidal syndromes: Wilson disease and Creutzfeldt–Jakob disease.
- Spasticity of the clasp-knife type is characterized by increased tone, which is maximal at the beginning of movement and suddenly decreases as passive movement is continued. It

occurs chiefly in the flexors of the upper limb and extensors of the lower limb (antigravity muscles).
- Gegenhalten, or paratonia, is where the increased muscle tone varies and becomes worse the more the patient tries to relax.

What is the role of protein diets in patients who have episodes of sudden and substantial loss of mobility?

High-protein diets should be avoided in these patients because a large influx of dietary amino acids can interfere with the transport of levodopa into the brain. No more than 0.8 g protein/kg body weight should be consumed per day if taking levodopa.

What do you understand by the term lower half parkinsonism?

It refers to vascular parkinsonism, which usually presents with severe failure to initiate gait, a broad-based shuffling gait, mild bradykinesia, rigidity of the arms, and subtle hypomimia. Risk factors include hypertension and history of transient ischaemic attack. There is often no resting tremor; olfaction is normal and response to levodopa is usually poor.

How is the severity of Parkinson disease graded?

Hoehn–Yahr staging grades Parkinson disease into five stages:
    I: newly diagnosed disease
    II and III: moderately severe disease
    IV and V: advanced disease.

How would you manage a patient with Parkinson disease?

Step I: replacing dopamine neurotransmitter that is lost as the dopamine neurons degenerate is the mainstay of treatment. All drugs are started at low doses and doses are increased slowly to reduce adverse effects (start low, go slow). Withdrawal of therapy also should be done slowly to avoid worsening of parkinsonism or precipitating neuroleptic malignant syndrome:
- First-line dopaminergic agents: carbidopa plus levodopa (immediate release and controlled release), carbidopa plus levodopa plus entacapone, dopamine agonists including nonergot (pramipexole, ropinirole) and ergot (pergolide)
- Second-line alternatives: anticholinergic agents (trihexyphenidyl, benztropine), selective monoamine oxidase B inhibitors (selegiline) and N-methyl-D-aspartate antagonist (amantadine); anticholinergic drugs are more effective in alleviating tremor and rigidity rather than bradykinesia but can worsen cognition.

Step II: transplanting fetal nerve tissue to replace dopamine neurons that have been lost.

Step III: halting neuronal loss altogether with trophic factors; this is in the early stages of clinical testing. At present, there are no neuroprotective therapies, although clinical trials with monoamine oxidase B inhibitors, dopamine agonists, and coenzyme Q_{10} may slow progression. Glial cell line-derived neurotrophic factor is under investigation. Data are still needed to clarify neuroprotective therapies.

In which condition is levodopa absolutely contraindicated?

Melanoma.

What do you know about 'drug holidays' in levodopa therapy?

Drug holidays (i.e. discontinuation of therapy) were previously claimed to enhance the efficacy of treatment when it was resumed; it is now known to be dangerous (deaths have occurred) and of doubtful value.

What do you know about dopamine receptors?
At least four types of receptor have been reported: D_1 and D_2 are the two major families of dopamine receptors. For neurotransmission to occur, a complex consisting of a dopamine receptor and a G protein (guanine nucleotide-binding protein) must be formed. This complex then usually couples with the enzyme adenylate cyclase, which controls the formation of the second messenger cyclic adenosine monophosphate. Alteration of the second messenger leads to a cascade of events that ultimately determines the transfer of information between nerve cells. The D_{2A} receptor is involved in the therapeutic response elicited by dopaminergic agonists in parkinsonism, although the mechanism is not clear at a physiological level. The role of the D_1 family is unclear—whether the activation of these receptors leads to useful effects (i.e. reduction of parkinsonian deficits), undesirable effects (e.g. dyskinesia), or both. Bromocriptine, pergolide, and lisuride all stimulate D_2 receptors, whereas bromocriptine and lisuride are D_1 receptor antagonists and pergolide is a D_1 receptor agonist.

What is the role of stem cells in the potential treatment of Parkinson disease?
Parkinson disease is characterized by loss of the midbrain dopamine neurons that innervate the caudate and putamen. Patients tend to have a reduced response to levodopa after 5 to 20 years of therapy, with 'on–off' fluctuations consisting of dyskinesia alternating with immobility. Animal experiments have suggested that fetal dopaminergic neurons can survive transplantation and restore neurological function. Trials are underway to determine whether stem cell transplantation can improve motor function in patients with Parkinson disease. Despite high expectations for stem cell therapy curing Parkinson disease, work is ongoing to improve safety and efficacy concerns.

What is the role of thalamotomy in the treatment of Parkinson disease?
Thalamotomy used to be the main treatment until 1950, but with the introduction of levodopa, it became less popular. However, there has been a revival of stereotactic surgery prompted by the failure of levodopa in four main aspects: in severe tremor, levodopa-induced dyskinesia, advanced Parkinson disease, and akinetic–rigid syndromes. Three types of stereotactic surgery are practised:
- Thalamotomy is used for intractable tremor and radiofrequency ablation of an area of the ventral intermediate nucleus of the thalamus. It is unsuitable for bilateral tremor as bilateral thalamotomy tends to cause impairment of speech. Trials are ongoing using magnetic resonance imaging-guided ultrasound thalamotomy as a less invasive technique.
- Deep-brain stimulation of the globus pallidus, subthalamic nucleus, or ventral intermediate nucleus of the thalamus may result in striking improvements in tremor and dyskinesia, resulting in large reductions of levodopa dose and, thus, improvements in levodopa-induced dyskinesias. A fine electrode is placed to stimulate the area and a pacemaker placed under the skin on the chest. Sadly, disease progression continues for non-motor and cognitive symptoms.
- Unilateral posteroventral medial pallidotomy ameliorates contralateral parkinsonian symptoms and medication-related dyskinesia and the effect is sustained for up to 5.5 years. Improvements in symptoms are not sustained, and this is now performed less commonly than deep brain stimulation.

Note: Patients with dementia and hallucinations tolerate all surgical procedures poorly, and any benefit in patients with rapidly progressive parkinsonism is likely to be short lived.

What are Parkinson plus syndromes?

Some patients have other neurological deficits in addition to Parkinson disease. Examples of these so-called Parkinson plus syndromes are:
- progressive supranuclear palsy (also known as Steele–Richardson–Olszewski disease) characterized by akinesia, axial rigidity of the neck, bradyphrenia, supranuclear palsy
- multiple system atrophy (also known as Shy–Drager syndrome)
- olivopontocerebellar degeneration
- striatonigral degeneration
- basal ganglia calcification.

What is tardive dyskinesia?

Tardive dyskinesia is seen in patients taking neuroleptics. Its manifestations are orofacial dyskinesia, such as smacking, chewing lip movements, discrete dystonia, or choreiform movements and rarely rocking movements. Withdrawal of the offending drug will improve these symptoms over a period of 3 to 4 years, except in a small minority of patients. Drug-induced parkinsonism is usually bilateral with evident bradykinesia, rigidity, and tremor. Tremor in drug-induced parkinsonism is often postural.

Mention some heredo-degenerative parkinsonian disorders.

- Hallervorden–Spatz disease: autosomal recessive; patients also have dementia, dystonia, choreoathetosis, retinitis pigmentosa. There is increased iron deposition and increased cysteine in the globus pallidus.
- Fahr disease or familial basal ganglia calcification: patients also have chorea, dementia, and palilalia.
- Olivopontocerebellar and spinocerebellar degenerations: autosomal dominant; associated cerebellar ataxia and retinitis pigmentosa.

How would you manage autonomic and psychological symptoms?

- Insomnia: adjust Parkinson disease drugs; use sleep hygiene techniques or clonazepam
- Depression: use serotonin and noradrenergic reuptake inhibitors
- Rapid eye movement behaviour disorders: adjust Parkinson disease drugs or give clonazepam
- Fatigue: give amantadine or selegiline
- Daytime sleepiness: give modafinil
- Psychosis and hallucinations: adjust Parkinson disease drugs or use an antipsychotic (clozapine, quetiapine, or aripiprazole). Quetiapine typically does not worsen motor function and is often used as first-line therapy. Rivastigmine can also be tried
- Constipation: use osmotic laxatives (macrogol)
- Urinary urgency: check drugs; mirabegron for detrusor overactivity. Avoid anticholinergics as they increase the risk of developing Parkinson disease dementia
- Impotence: use sildenafil, tadalafil, and vardenafil
- Pain: often undertreated. Adjust Parkinson disease drugs, treat coexisting conditions such as arthritis
- Restless legs: use dopamine agonists
- Orthostatic hypotension: adjust Parkinson disease drugs; increase water and salt intake; give fludrocortisone, ephedrine, or midodrine
- Drooling: 0.5% atropine eye drops sublingually, scopoderm patch, or botulinum toxin injections into salivary glands
- Excessive sweating: adjust Parkinson disease drugs; give propantheline, propranolol, or topical aluminium creams.

Further Information

James Parkinson (1755–1824) first reported six cases of this syndrome in 1817 (at the age of 62 years).

Jean Martin Charcot (the father of neurology) proposed that this syndrome be called 'maladie de Parkinson'.

J.C. Steele, J.C. Richardson, and J. Olszewski were all US neurologists.

K. von Economo (1876–1931), an Australian neurologist, also wrote on Wilson disease.

Muhammad Ali (or Cassius Clay; 1942–2016), the world heavy-weight boxing champion, was reported to have had premature Parkinson disease, the 'punch drunk' syndrome.

CHAPTER 191

Peripheral Neuropathy

Instruction

Examine this patient's legs.
Carry out a neurological examination of this patient's legs.

Salient Features

HISTORY

- Progressive and symmetrical numbness in the hands and feet that spreads proximally in a glove and stocking distribution
- Distal weakness, which also ascends
- History of diabetes, alcohol, connective tissue disorder, malignancy.

EXAMINATION

- Bilateral symmetrical sensory loss for all modalities with or without motor weakness
- Proceed by looking for evidence of the following (mnemonic: DAD, RUM):
  - **D**iabetes mellitus (diabetic chart, insulin injection sites, insulin pump)
  - **A**lcoholic liver disease (palmar erythema, spider naevi, tender liver)
  - **D**rug history
  - **R**heumatoid arthritis
  - **U**raemia
  - **M**alignancy.
- Palpate for thickened nerves and look for Charcot's joints.
- Tell the examiner that you would like to do the following:
  - Look for anaemia and jaundice (vitamin B_{12} deficiency).
  - Check urine for sugar.
  - Take a history of alcohol consumption and a drug history.

Diagnosis

This patient has symmetrical, bilateral sensory loss for touch and pain (lesion) caused by diabetes mellitus (aetiology).

Questions

How are polyneuropathies classified?

- Polyneuropathies can be classified as demyelinating or axonal
  - Demyelinating: acute inflammatory demyelinating polyradiculoneuropathy (subtype of Guillain–Barré syndrome), diphtheria, chronic inflammatory polyradiculoneuropathy, Charcot–Marie–Tooth disease type 1

687

- Axonal: acute motor axonal neuropathy, acute motor and sensory axonal neuropathy, multifocal motor neuropathy, associated with HIV, diabetes, medications, toxins
- They can also be classified according to the diameter of the affected nerve fibre. Larger fibres are heavily myelinated and, therefore, most subject to processes that damage myelin.
- Most polyneuropathies, including the diabetic type, are axonal.

Mention a few causes of thickened nerves.
- Amyloidosis
- Charcot–Marie–Tooth disease
- Leprosy
- Refsum disease (retinitis pigmentosa, deafness, and cerebellar damage)
- Déjérine–Sottas disease (hypertrophic peripheral neuropathy).

What are the causes of motor neuropathy?
- Guillain–Barré syndrome
- Peroneal muscular atrophy
- Lead toxicity
- Porphyria
- Dapsone toxicity
- Organophosphate poisoning.

What are the causes of mononeuritis multiplex?
Mononeuritis multiplex is a neuropathy affecting several nerves and causes include (mnemonic: WARDS, PLC):
- **W**egener's granulomatosis
- **A**myloidosis
- **R**heumatoid arthritis
- **D**iabetes mellitus
- **S**ystemic lupus erythematosus
- **P**olyarteritis nodosa
- **L**eprosy
- **C**arcinomatosis, Churg–Strauss syndrome.

Mention a few causes of predominantly sensory neuropathy.
- Diabetes mellitus
- Alcoholism
- Deficiency of vitamins B_{12} and B_1
- Chronic renal failure
- Leprosy.

What are the types of neuropathy described in diabetes mellitus?
- Symmetrical, mainly sensory, polyneuropathy
- Asymmetrical, mainly motor, polyneuropathy (diabetic amyotrophy)
- Mononeuropathy
- Autonomic neuropathy.

Be aware that there are different classifications (Fig. 191.1).

What drugs are used for painful peripheral neuropathy of diabetes?
Tricyclic antidepressants, phenytoin, carbamazepine, and topical capsaicin. The National Institute for Health and Clinical Excellence recommends treating neuropathic pain with amitriptyline, duloxetine, pregabalin, or gabapentin.

191 – PERIPHERAL NEUROPATHY

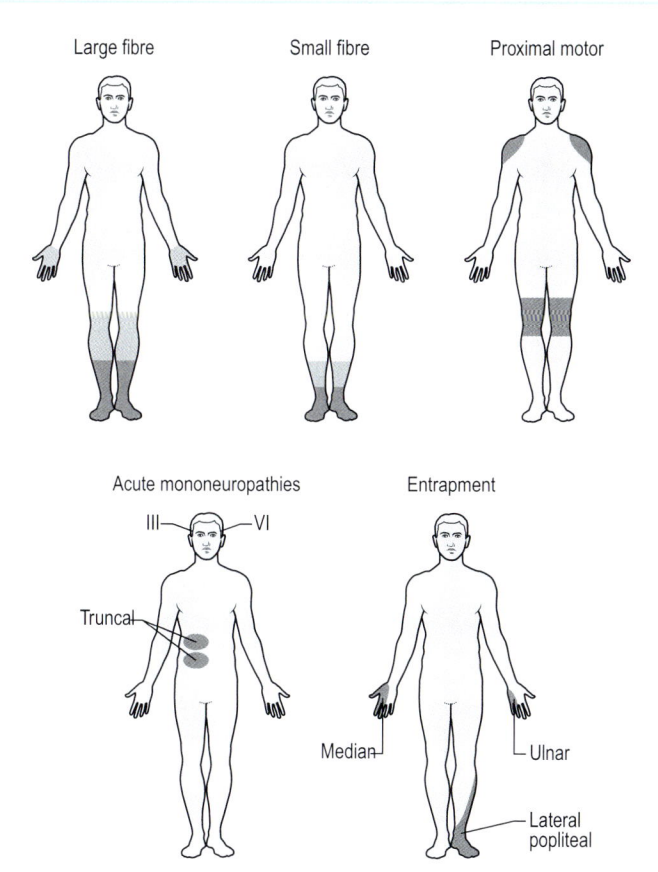

Fig. 191.1 Different clinical presentations of diabetic neuropathies.

What are the other effects of alcohol on the central nervous system?
- Wernicke encephalopathy (ophthalmoplegia, nystagmus, confusion, and neuropathy)
- Korsakoff psychosis (recent memory loss and confabulation)
- Cerebellar degeneration
- Marchiafava–Bignami disease (symmetrical demyelination of corpus callosum)
- Central pontine myelinolysis
- Amblyopia
- Epilepsy
- Myopathy and rhabdomyolysis.

Further Information
K. Wernicke (1848–1904) worked in Poland.
S.S. Korsakoff (1853–1900), a Russian neuropsychiatrist.
Jacob Churg (1910–2005) qualified in Poland and was Professor of Pathology in New York.
Lotte Strauss, a pathologist in New York.

CHAPTER 192

Proximal Myopathy

Instruction
Perform a neurological examination of this patient's arms or legs.

Salient Features
HISTORY
- Weakness of proximal muscles
- Patient has difficulty in standing from the sitting position (getting up from chairs, getting off the commode) or difficulty in combing hair—elicit this history.

EXAMINATION
- Check the gait, looking for waddling gait.
- Look for an underlying cause:
  - Diabetic amyotrophy (asymmetrical, usually in the lower limbs in non-insulin-dependent diabetes mellitus)
  - Cushing syndrome (characteristic facies, history of steroid ingestion)
  - Hypothyroidism (look for goitre, skin changes)
  - Polymyositis (heliotropic rash, tender muscles)
  - Drug history (alcohol, steroids, chloroquine)
  - Carcinomatous neuropathy
  - Osteomalacia (bone pain)
  - Hereditary muscular dystrophy.

Diagnosis
This patient has weakness of the proximal muscles of the lower limbs (lesion) caused by Cushing syndrome (aetiology) and is severely limited by the weakness (functional status).

Questions

What is Gowers' sign?
In severe proximal myopathy of the lower limbs, a patient on rising from the floor uses their hands against the body to climb up to vertical. It has been classically described in Duchenne's muscular dystrophy.

What do you know about diabetic amyotrophy?
It is an asymmetrical motor polyneuropathy that presents with asymmetrical weakness and wasting of the proximal muscles of the lower limbs and sometimes upper limbs, diminished or absent knee jerk, and sensory loss in the thigh. It is usually accompanied by severe pain in the thigh, often

awakening the patient at night. The prognosis is good, and most patients recover over months or years with diabetic control.

What are the causes of proximal myopathy?
- Metabolic and endocrinological causes (Cushing syndrome, hypothyroidism, hypokalaemia, hypocalcaemia, uraemia, disorders of lipid metabolism)
- Autoimmune and rheumatological diseases (vasculitis, lupus, rheumatoid arthritis, inflammatory myositides)
- Drugs and toxins (alcohol, steroids, illicit drugs)
- Inherited myopathies
- Disorders of the neuromuscular junction (myasthenia gravis)
- Infections (viral, parasitic).

What is the difference between type 1 and type 2 muscle fibres?
- Type 1 muscle fibres are high in myoglobin and oxidative enzymes and have many mitochondria. They perform tonic contraction and are involved in weight bearing and movements requiring sustained force. Chloroquine causes vacuolation of myocytes, predominantly type 1 fibres.
- Type 2 muscle fibres are rich in glycolytic enzymes; they perform rapid phasic contractions and are involved in sudden movements and in purposeful motion. In steroid myopathy, the muscle fibre atrophy predominantly affects these fibres.

Further Information

Sir W.R. Gowers (1845–1915), Professor of Medicine at University College Hospital, London, invented a haemoglobinometer, personally illustrated an atlas of ophthalmology, and wrote a book on spinal cord diseases and a manual on the nervous system. He also founded a society of medical stenographers.

Guillaume-Benjamin-Amand Duchenne (1806–1875) was first to describe Duchenne's muscular dystrophy in 1868 in a paper where he described 13 cases of the disease; by 1870, he had seen about 40 cases.

CHAPTER 193

Pseudobulbar Palsy

Instruction
This patient is having difficulty swallowing; please examine his cranial nerves.

Salient Features
HISTORY
- Ask the patient whether there is difficulty in swallowing or nasal regurgitation.
- Ask if there are any changes in speech.
- Look for emotional lability.
- Ask for history of stroke, multiple sclerosis, parkinsonism, or motor neurone disease.

EXAMINATION
- Small, stiff, and spastic tongue
- Donald Duck speech
- Patient emotionally labile (uncontrollable laughter, crying, irritability, or anger)
- Sluggish movements of the palate when the patient is asked to say 'aah'.

Proceed as follows:
- Check the jaw jerk.
- Tell the examiner that you would like to do the following:
  - Check the gag reflex.
  - Look for upper motor neuron signs in the limbs.

Diagnosis
This patient has pseudobulbar palsy (lesion) caused by a stroke (aetiology); he has difficulty in swallowing and emotional lability (functional status).

Questions
What could be the underlying cause?
- Bilateral stroke
- Multiple sclerosis
- Motor neurone disease
- Parkinson disease and Parkinson plus syndromes.

How would you differentiate bulbar palsy from pseudobulbar palsy?

	Pseudobulbar Palsy	*Bulbar Palsy*
Prevalence	Common	Rare
Type of lesion	Upper motor neuron	Lower motor neuron, muscular
Site of lesion	Bilateral, usually in the internal capsule	Medulla oblongata
Tongue	Small, stiff, and spastic	Flaccid, fasciculations
Speech	Slow, thick, and indistinct	Nasal twang
Nasal regurgitation	Not prominent	Prominent
Jaw jerk	Brisk	Normal or absent
Other findings	Upper motor neuron lesions of the limbs	Lower motor neuron lesions of the limbs
Effect	Emotionally labile	Normal effect
Causes	Stroke, multiple sclerosis, motor neurone disease, Creutzfeldt–Jakob disease	Motor neurone disease, poliomyelitis, Guillain–Barré syndrome, myasthenia gravis myopathy

How would you manage the swallowing and speech difficulties?
The patient would initially require assessment by a speech therapist for the difficulty in swallowing and speech deficits. Barium swallow with videofluoroscopy may be required to 'visualize' the swallowing.

Is there any therapy for emotional lability?
A combination of dextromethorphan and quinidine improves symptoms and quality of life in patients with emotional lability and has been used in the short term for those with motor neurone disease and vascular causes.

What do you understand by the term CADASIL?
Cerebral autosomal dominant arteriopathy with subcortical infarcts and leukoencephalopathy (CADASIL) is the most common heritable cause of stroke and vascular dementia in adults. Clinical and neuroimaging features resemble those of sporadic small-artery disease, although patients with CADASIL have an earlier age at onset of stroke events, an increased frequency of migraine with aura, and a slightly variable pattern of ischaemic white matter lesions on brain MRI. *NOTCH3* (Notch homolog 3), the gene involved in CADASIL, encodes a transmembrane receptor primarily expressed in systemic arterial smooth-muscle cells.

Further Information
Charles Darwin described pseudobulbar affect in *The Expression of Emotions in Man and Animals* (1872): 'certain brain diseases, such as hemiplegia, brain wasting and senile decay, have a special tendency to induce weeping'.

CHAPTER 194

Ptosis and Horner Syndrome

Instruction
This patient presents with weight loss. Please examine his cranial nerves.

Salient Features
HISTORY
- Absence of sweating on one side of the face
- History of lung cancer
- History of cervical sympathectomy
- Migraine.

EXAMINATION
In the examination, if you notice **ptosis**, then you must answer the following questions:
- Is ptosis complete or incomplete?
- Is it unilateral or bilateral?
- Is the pupil constricted (Horner syndrome) or dilated (third nerve palsy)?
- Are extraocular movements involved (third nerve palsy or myasthenia gravis)?
- Is there fatiguability (myasthenia gravis)?
- Is the eyeball sunken (enophthalmos)?
- Is the light reflex intact (intact light reflex in Horner syndrome)?

Once Horner syndrome is established, additional questions will guide you to a possible cause:
- Is there heterochromia (congenital Horner syndrome)?
- Is there anhidrosis (preganglionic lesion)?
- Does the pupil dilate after eye drops (preganglionic lesion)?

If you have examined the cranial nerves, including fundoscopy, and the only positive finding is **Horner syndrome**, then proceed as follows:
- Examine the supraclavicular area.
- Percuss the supraclavicular area, looking for dullness from Pancoast tumour.
- Look for scar of cervical sympathectomy (be prepared with indications for cervical sympathectomy).
- Look for enlarged lymph nodes.
- Examine the neck:
  - for carotid and aortic aneurysms
  - for tracheal deviation (Pancoast tumour).

- Examine the hands:
  - for small muscle wasting
  - for pain sensation with a pin
  - for clubbing.

These should help in making a diagnosis of syringomyelia or Pancoast tumour.

If Horner syndrome is not the only clinical finding on cranial nerve examination but there are deficiencies in multiple cranial nerves, then proceed to examine for cerebellar and pyramidal signs to ascertain brainstem vascular disease or demyelination.

Diagnosis

This patient has Horner syndrome (lesion) associated with dullness in the supraclavicular area indicating a Pancoast tumour (aetiology).

Questions

What causes Horner syndrome?
The syndrome is caused by the involvement of the sympathetic pathway. It starts in the sympathetic nucleus and travels through the brainstem and spinal cord to the level of C8/T1/T2 to the sympathetic chain, stellate ganglion, and carotid sympathetic plexus. Its significance requires an understanding of the oculosympathetic pathway 3-neuron chain. The first-order nerve fibres descend from the hypothalamus without decussation to the thoracic spinal cord before synapsing with the second-order neurons (SONs). The SONs exit the spine at the C8, T1, and T2 levels to enter the sympathetic chain and travel over the pleural cap of the lung and loop around the subclavian artery before synapsing near the carotid bifurcation. The final third-order neurons travel along the internal carotid artery to innervate the eyelids and the eye and also along the external carotid artery to innervate facial sweat glands.

What are the features of Horner syndrome?
It is characterized by:
- Miosis (resulting from paralysis of the dilator of the pupil) (Fig. 194.1)
- Partial ptosis or pseudoptosis (caused by paralysis of the upper tarsal muscle)
- Enophthalmos (caused by paralysis of the muscle of Müller)
- Often, slight elevation of the lower lid (because of paralysis of lower tarsal muscles).

What additional feature would you see in congenital Horner syndrome?
There would be heterochromia of the iris: the iris remains grey-blue (Fig. 194.2).

How would you determine the level of the lesion using only history?
The level of the lesion is determined by the distribution of the loss of sweating:
- Central lesion: sweating over the entire half of the head, arm, and upper trunk is lost.
- Lesions of the neck:
  - Proximal to the superior cervical ganglion: diminished sweating on the face
  - Distal to the superior cervical ganglion: sweating is not affected.

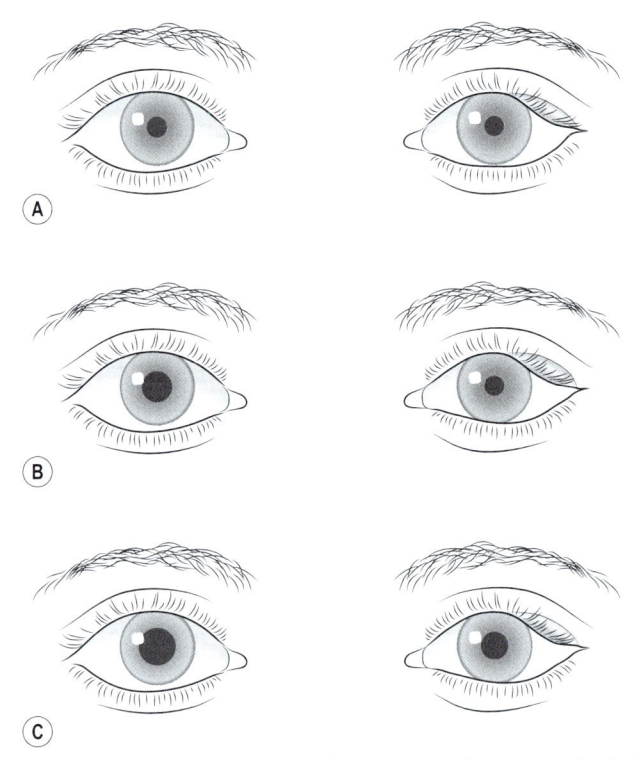

Fig. 194.1 Horner syndrome affecting the left eye. **(A)** Mild upper lid ptosis and miosis in room light. **(B)** Anisocoria is increased at 5 s after the lights are dimmed as a result of dilation lag of the left pupil. **(C)** At 15 s after the lights are dimmed, the left pupil has increased dilation compared to that at 5 s **(B)**.

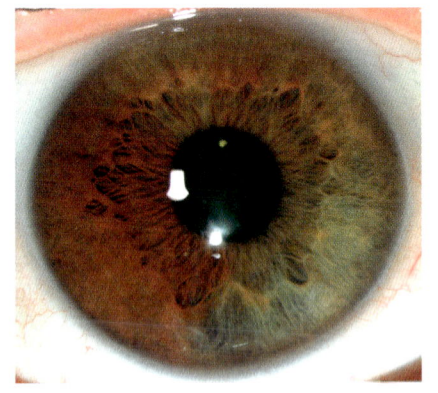

Fig. 194.2 Heterochromia iridis. The iris is bicolored. (With permission from Pineda II, R., Friedman, N.J., Kaiser, P.K., 2021. The Massachusetts Eye and Ear Infirmary Illustrated Manual of Ophthalmology, fifth edn. Elsevier.)

194 — PTOSIS AND HORNER SYNDROME

How would you differentiate whether the lesion is above the superior ganglion (peripheral) or below the superior cervical ganglion (central)?

Test	Above	Below
Sweating	Such lesions may not affect sweating at all as the main outflow to the facial blood vessels is below the superior cervical ganglion	Such lesions affect sweating over the entire, head, neck, and arm upper trunk. Lesions in the lower neck affect sweating over the entire face
Cocaine 4% in both eyes	Dilates the normal pupil, no effect on the affected side	Dilates both pupils
Epinephrine (adrenaline, 1:1000) in both eyes	Dilates affected eye, no effect on normal side	No effect on both sides

Note: In peripheral lesions, there is depletion of amine oxidase as a result of postganglionic denervation. As a result, this sensitizes the pupil to 1:1000 epinephrine (adrenaline), whereas it has no effect on the normal pupil or in central lesions (where the presence of the enzyme rapidly destroys the epinephrine).

Mention one cause of intermittent Horner syndrome.
Migraine.

Mention a few causes of Horner syndrome.
- First-order neuron: stroke, space occupying lesion, and demyelination in the brainstem and hypothalamus. Trauma, spinal tumour, syringomyelia, demyelination, transverse myelitis
- Second-order neuron: Pancoast tumour, thyroid malignancy, iatrogenic causes
- Postganglionic lesions: internal carotid artery dissection, cavernous sinus venous thrombosis, space occupying lesion.

What are the causes of ptosis?
Unilateral:
- Third nerve palsy
- Horner syndrome
- Myasthenia gravis
- Congenital or idiopathic.

Bilateral:
- Myasthenia gravis
- Dystrophia myotonica
- Ocular myopathy or oculopharyngeal dystrophy
- Mitochondrial dystrophy
- Tabes dorsalis
- Congenital
- Bilateral Horner syndrome (as in syringomyelia).

If the patient has Pancoast tumour, what is the most likely underlying pathology?
Squamous cell carcinoma.

What are the causes of Horner syndrome with unilateral headache and what investigations should be performed?

The diagnosis that needs to be thoroughly investigated for a presentation combination of Horner with unilateral headache is aortic dissection. A computed tomography (CT) angiogram should be performed in the first instance to look for aortic dissection, and if the clinical suspicion is still high despite a negative result, magnetic resonance angiography should follow. Another cause for Horner syndrome associated with unilateral headache is Raeder syndrome, or paratrigeminal oculosympathetic syndrome, which can be caused by trauma, middle cranial fossa mass, syphilis, or sinusitis, and a magnetic resonance imaging of the brain should be performed to search for underlying disease.

Further Information

J.F. Horner (1831–1886), Professor of Ophthalmology in Zurich, conceded that Claude Bernard had recognized the syndrome before him.

Henry K. Pancoast (1875–1939) was the first Professor of Radiology in the United States at the University of Pennsylvania.

CHAPTER 195

Radial Nerve Palsy

Instruction

This patient has developed tingling in her arm. Please perform a neurological examination of this patient's arms.

Salient Features

HISTORY

- An intoxicated person sleeping with the head resting in the upper arm, causing compression of the nerve over the middle third of the humerus, known as Saturday night palsy (Fig. 195.1)
- Trauma to the nerve while it courses through the axilla: crutch palsy, shoulder dislocation, fractures of humerus or radius
- History of exposure to lead (lead neuropathy).

EXAMINATION

- There is weakness of extension of the wrist and elbow (wrist flexion is normal).
- The patient is unable to straighten the fingers.
- However, if the wrist is passively extended, the patient is able to straighten the fingers at the interphalangeal joints (caused by the action of interossei and lumbricals) but is unable to extend the metacarpophalangeal joint.
- There appears to be a weakness in abduction and adduction of the fingers, but this is not present when the hand is kept flat on a table and the fingers are extended.

Proceed as follows:
- Test brachioradialis, looking for weakened elbow flexion. When the patient attempts to flex the elbow against resistance, the muscle belly no longer springs up.
- Test the triceps.
- Check sensation over the first dorsal interosseous (Fig. 195.2).

> **Note:**
> - The radial nerve gives off two branches at the elbow:
>   - Superficial radial (entirely sensory)
>   - Posterior interosseous (entirely muscular).
> - If the injury is situated above the junction of the upper and middle thirds of the humerus, the action of triceps is lost.
> - If the lesion is situated in the middle third of the humerus (frequent site of fracture of the humerus), the brachioradialis is spared.

Be prepared to differentiate from high and low radial nerve palsy (later).

Radial Nerve Compression

Compression of nerve in axilla or upper arm in patient sleeping with arm over chair back, edge of bed, etc, or by crutch

Wrist drop

Fig. 195.1 Radial nerve palsy. (With permission from Netter Images, www.netterimages.com. In Wang, L., Nathan, C., Gao, R., Wu, C.K., Wu, H.H., 2019. Gunner Goggles: Medicine; Honors Shelf Review. Elsevier.)

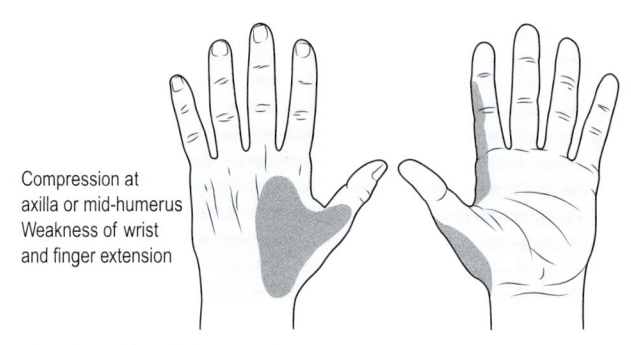

Compression at axilla or mid-humerus Weakness of wrist and finger extension

Fig. 195.2 Sensory impairment in radial nerve palsy.

Diagnosis

This patient has features of radial nerve palsy, with the brachioradialis remaining unaffected (lesion) resulting from a fracture located in the middle third of the humerus (aetiology); she is disabled by the deficits (functional status).

Questions

What are the features of high nerve palsy?
- Motor deficits:
  - Accessory forearm flexion and supination
  - Wrist extension
  - Digital extension
  - Radial abduction of thumb.
- Sensory deficits:
  - Hand dorsum
  - Proximal two-thirds of lateral three and a half fingers.

What are the features of low nerve palsy?
- Motor deficits:
  - Finger extension
  - Thumb extension/abduction.
- Sensory deficits:
  - dorsoradial forearm/hand.
- Functional requirements:
  - Digital extension
  - Radial abduction of thumb.

What is the cutaneous supply of the radial nerve?
Because of overlap in the areas supplied by the median and ulnar nerves, only a small area of skin over the first dorsal interosseous is exclusively supplied by the radial nerve.

What do you know about the origin of the radial nerve?
The radial nerve is the termination of the posterior cord of the brachial plexus and is derived from the fifth, sixth, seventh, and eighth cervical spinal nerves.

What are the branches of the radial nerve in the forearm?
The radial nerve enters the forearm and passes between the two heads of the supinator muscle to become the posterior interosseous nerve.

What muscles are supplied by the radial nerve?
The radial nerve supplies the triceps, anconeus, brachioradialis, and extensor carpi radialis longus and through the posterior interosseous nerve, extensor carpi radialis brevis, supinator, extensor digitorum, extensor digiti minimi, extensor ulnaris, the three extensors of the thumb, and extensor indicis.

What are the management options?
- Most recover spontaneously.
- Splints may be helpful.
- Surgical decompression may be required for nerve entrapment.

CHAPTER 196

Seventh Cranial Nerve Palsy

LOWER MOTOR NEURONE TYPE

Instruction

Look at this patient's face.
Examine the cranial nerves.

Salient Features

HISTORY

- Onset: whether abrupt followed by worsening over the following day (Bell's palsy)
- The face itself feels stiff and pulled to one side.
- Ipsilateral restriction of eye closure
- Difficulty with eating
- Disturbance of taste (caused by chorda tympani fibres)
- Hyperacusis (involvement of stapedius muscle in the inner ear).

EXAMINATION

- Weakness of muscles of one-half of the face; patient unable to screw their eyes tightly shut or move the angle of the mouth on the affected side (Fig. 196.1)
- Loss of facial expression
- Widened palpebral fissure.

Proceed as follows:

- Look for the following when the patient is unaware of being observed:
  - Flatter nasolabial folds on the affected side.
  - Mouth on the affected side droops and participates manifestly less while talking.
  - The eyelid on the affected side closes just after the opposite eyelid.
- Look at the external auditory meatus for herpes zoster (Ramsay Hunt syndrome).
- Look for parotid gland enlargement.
- Examine for taste (loss of taste with the involvement of chorda tympani).
- Check for hearing (for hyperacusis resulting from involvement of the nerve to stapedius muscle).
- Examine tympanic membrane for otitis media.
- Tell the examiner that you would like to test the urine for sugar (diabetes).

Diagnosis

The patient has lower motor neurone seventh cranial nerve palsy (lesion), which is idiopathic (aetiology). She is distressed because the condition causes severe disfigurement while talking and has House–Brackmann grade VI facial palsy (functional status).

196 — SEVENTH CRANIAL NERVE PALSY

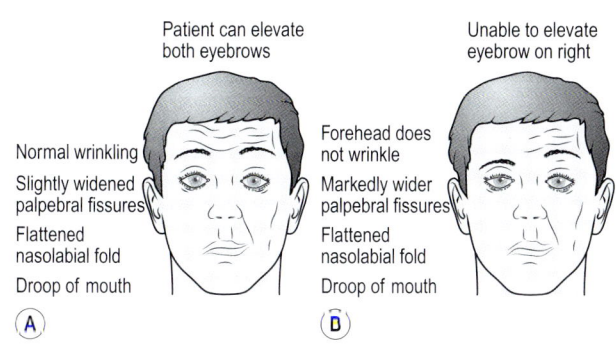

Fig. 196.1 Facial weakness: central (A) and peripheral (B).

Questions

How would you differentiate between upper and lower motor neurone palsy?
In lower motor neurone palsy, the whole half of the face on the affected side is involved. In upper motor neurone palsy, the upper half of the face (the forehead) is spared (Fig. 196.1).

How is facial palsy graded?
House–Brackmann grades:
  I: normal
  II: mild dysfunction, slight weakness, slight synkinesis
  III: moderate dysfunction, obvious weakness, incomplete eye closure, normal symmetry only at rest
  IV: moderately severe dysfunction
  V: severe dysfunction, barely perceptible movement, asymmetry at rest
  VI: total paralysis.

What are the causes of bilateral facial nerve palsy?
- Guillain–Barré syndrome
- Sarcoidosis in the form of uveoparotid fever (Heerfordt disease)
- Facial diplegia (Moebius syndrome)

Melkersson–Rosenthal syndrome, which is a triad of facial palsy, recurrent facial oedema, and plication of the tongue

Myasthenia may mimic bilateral facial nerve palsy.

What are causes of unilateral facial nerve palsy?
Causes can be idiopathic (Bell's palsy; 65%), infective (associated with Bell's palsy), trauma (25%), neoplasms (5%), metabolic, toxic, and other rare causes.
- Lower Motor Neurone

All the muscles of one-half of the face are affected:
  - Bell's palsy. Studies using a polymerase chain reaction have implicated herpes simplex viral infection in Bell's palsy. The incidence of Bell's palsy is 23 per 100,000 individuals per year, or about 1 in 60 to 70 individuals per year. Men or women are affected equally and the peak incidence is between the ages of 10 and 40 years. Both the right and left sides are affected with equal frequency.
  - Herpes zoster
  - Cerebellopontine angle tumours

- Parotid tumours
- Old polio
- Otitis media
- Skull fracture
■ Upper Motor Neurone
The forehead is spared:
- Stroke (hemiplegia).

Is the facial nerve a motor nerve or a sensory nerve?
The facial nerve is predominantly a motor nerve and supplies all muscles concerned with facial expression and the stapedius muscle. Uncommonly, it may have a sensory component, which is small (the nervus intermedius of Wrisberg). It conveys taste sensation from the anterior two-thirds of the tongue and, probably, cutaneous impulses from the anterior wall of the external auditory canal.

What do you know of nervus intermedius?
Nervus intermedius or pars intermedia of Wrisberg is the sensory or the parasympathetic root of the facial nerve and is lateral and inferior to the motor root. Inside the internal auditory meatus, it lies between the motor root and the eighth cranial nerve. The sensory cells are located in the geniculate ganglion (at the bend of the facial nerve in the facial canal), and their nerve fibres enter the pons with the motor root. The geniculate ganglion is continued distally as the chorda tympani, which carries taste and preganglionic parasympathetic fibres. This nerve consists of contributions from three areas:
- Superior salivary nucleus (in the pons) supplies secretory fibres to the glands.
- Gustatory or solitary nucleus (in the medulla) receives taste fibres via the chorda tympani.
- The dorsal part of the trigeminal nerve receives cutaneous sensation from the external auditory meatus and the skin behind the ear (distributed with the facial nerve proper).

How would Bell's palsy present?
Bell's palsy usually presents as an acute mononeuropathy unilaterally. Other nerves are very rarely affected, the syndrome may follow episodes of ear pain or hearing disturbances, and the lesion is easily classified as a lower motor neurone lesion. It is a painless condition and is not associated with any muscle spasms.

How would you manage Bell's palsy?
About 50% to 60% of patients recover spontaneously without deficit; others have considerable improvement, and about 10% have permanent residual deficits. Many physicians tend to initiate steroids in most patients with discernible deficit. Treatment includes:
- Physiotherapy: massage, electrical stimulation, splint to prevent drooping of the lower part of the face
- Protection of the eye with lubricating eye drops and a patch during sleep
- Early treatment (within 72 hours) with prednisolone, which significantly improves the chances of complete recovery at 3 and 9 months
- Acyclovir–prednisolone, which is more effective in improving volitional muscle activity and in preventing partial nerve degeneration than placebo–prednisolone treatment.

What are the branches of the facial nerve?
- Greater superficial petrosal nerve (supplies lacrimal, nasal, and palatine glands)
- Nerve to stapedius muscle

- Chorda tympani (supplies taste to anterior two-thirds of tongue, submaxillary, and sublingual glands)
- Motor branches (exit from the stylomastoid foramen).

How would you localize facial nerve palsy?
- Involvement of the nuclei in the pons: associated ipsilateral sixth nerve palsy
- Cerebellopontine angle lesion: associated fifth and eighth nerve involvement
- Lesion in the bony canal: loss of taste (carried by the lingual nerve) and hyperacusis (caused by involvement of the nerve to stapedius).

Mention reflexes involving the facial nerve.
- Corneal reflex
- Palmomental reflex
- Suck reflex
- Snout reflex
- Orbicularis oculi reflex or glabellar reflex
- Palpebral–oculogyric reflex
- Orbicularis oris reflex.

Mention a few examples of facial synkinesis.
Facial synkinesis means that attempts to move one group of facial muscles result in contraction of associated muscles. It may be seen during anomalous regeneration of facial nerve. For example:
- If fibres originally connected with muscles of the face later innervate the lacrimal gland, anomalous secretion of tears (crocodile tears) may occur while eating.
- If fibres originally connected with the orbicularis oculi innervate the orbicularis oris, closure of the eyelids causes retraction of the mouth.
- Opening of the jaw may cause closure of the eyelids on the corresponding side (jaw-winking).

Have you heard of Moebius syndrome?
It consists of congenital bilateral facial palsy associated with third and sixth nerve palsies and comprises congenital facial diplegia, congenital oculofacial paralysis, and infantile nuclear aplasia.

What is the relationship between diabetes and Bell's palsy?
Diabetes is said to be an important cause in about 10% of cases of Bell's palsy. In one study, Bell's palsy was associated with abnormal glucose tolerance in two-thirds of patients.

What parts of the facial nerve must be imaged when facial nerve palsy is suspected and there is still progression of weakness after 3 weeks of the initial presentation?
Both magnetic resonance imaging and computed tomography of the temporal bone are used when the facial nerve must be examined.
The following anatomic areas must be imaged when the facial nerve is studied:
- The brain and pons (precentral, postcentral, and central gyrus; posterior limb of the internal capsule)
- The cerebellopontine angle
- The internal auditory canal
- The labyrinthine part of the facial nerve canal (VII-1) and geniculate ganglion
- The tympanic part of the facial nerve canal (VII-2)
- The mastoid part of the facial nerve canal (VII-3)
- The stylomastoid foramen and the parotid gland.

Further Information

Sir Charles Bell (1774–1842) was Professor of Surgery in Edinburgh and a founder member of the Middlesex Hospital in London. He discovered that the anterior and posterior spinal nerve roots were motor and sensory, respectively.

James Ramsay Hunt (1874–1937), Professor of Neurology in New York.

P.J. Möbius (1893–1907), a German neurologist.

CHAPTER 197

Sixth Cranial Nerve Palsy

Instruction

Examine this patient's eyes.

Salient Features

HISTORY

- Diplopia in all directions of gaze except away from the affected side
- Patient may rotate the head towards the weak side to produce a single image
- Patient may intentionally close the affected eye to prevent diplopia (pseudoptosis)
- Hearing loss (acoustic neuroma)
- Diabetes or hypertension.

EXAMINATION

- The eye is deviated medially and there is failure of lateral movement.
- The diplopia is maximal when looking towards the affected side. The two images are parallel and separated in the horizontal plane. The outer image comes from the affected eye and disappears when the eye is covered.
- Proceed by telling the examiner that you would like to check the following:
  - Blood pressure and urine sugar
  - Hearing and corneal sensation (early signs of acoustic neuroma).

Diagnosis

This patient has a sixth nerve palsy (lesion) caused by diabetes mellitus (aetiology) and has severe diplopia (functional status).

Questions

What are the causes of sixth nerve palsy?
- Hypertension
- Diabetes
- Raised intracranial pressure (false localizing signs)
- Multiple sclerosis
- Basal meningitis
- Encephalitis
- Acoustic neuroma, nasopharyngeal carcinoma
- Lyme disease.

Where is the nucleus of the sixth nerve located?
In the pons. The nuclei of the first four cranial nerves are situated above the pons and those of the last four cranial nerves are situated below the pons.

What are the structures in close proximity to the sixth nerve nucleus and fascicles?
These include:
- facial and trigeminal nerves
- corticospinal tract
- median longitudinal fasciculus
- parapontine reticular formation.

A combination of clinical findings pointing to the involvement of these structures indicates the presence of an intrapontine lesion.

What you know about the peripheral course of the abducens nerve?
It is lengthy: from the brainstem and base of the skull through the petrous tip and cavernous sinus to the superior orbital fissure and orbit. Lesions at any of these sites may affect the nerve.

Have you heard of Gradenigo syndrome?
Inflammation of the tip of the temporal bone may involve the fifth and sixth cranial nerves as well as the greater superficial petrosal nerve, resulting in unilateral paralysis of the lateral rectus nerve, pain in the distribution of the trigeminal nerve (particularly its first division), and excessive lacrimation.

Do you know any eponymous syndromes where the pons is infarcted and consequently the sixth cranial nerve is involved?
- Raymond syndrome: ipsilateral sixth nerve paralysis and contralateral paresis of the extremities
- Millard–Gubler syndrome, in which there is ipsilateral sixth and seventh nerve palsy with contralateral hemiplegia
- Foville syndrome has all the features of Millard–Gubler paralysis with lateral conjugate gaze palsy.

Mention other syndromes with sixth nerve involvement.
- Duane syndrome: widening of the palpebral fissure on abduction and narrowing on adduction
- Gerhardt syndrome: bilateral abducens palsy
- Möbius syndrome: paralysis of extraocular muscles, especially abducens, with paresis of facial muscles.

What do you know about Tolosa–Hunt syndrome?
It is a syndrome characterized by unilateral recurrent pain in the retroorbital region with palsy of the extraocular muscles resulting from involvement of the third, fourth, fifth, and sixth cranial nerves. It has been attributed to inflammation of the cavernous sinus.

Further Information
C. Gradenigo (1859–1926), an Italian otolaryngologist, described this syndrome in 1904.
E. Tolosa, a Spanish neurosurgeon.
W.E. Hunt, an American neurosurgeon.
A.L.J. Millard (1830–1915), a French physician.
A.M. Gubler (1821–1915), Professor of Therapeutics in France.
A.L.F. Foville (1799–1878), Professor of Physiology at Rouen, described his syndrome in 1848.

CHAPTER 198

Syringomyelia

Instruction
Examine this patient's arms.

Salient Features
HISTORY
- Classically, the patient has a history of painless trauma or burns with cigarettes or hot water.
- The patient may have cuts that never seem to hurt.
- The patient may have a long history of poorly localized unpleasant pain (although pain sensation is impaired, these patients have severe pain).
- The patient may notice scoliosis during childhood.

EXAMINATION
- Wasting and weakness of the small muscles of the hands and forearm (if fasciculation is seen, then the other diagnosis that comes to mind at this stage is motor neurone disease).
- Rarely, patients may have hypertrophy in the limbs, hand, and feet.
- Tone and deep tendon reflexes are diminished.
- Loss of pain and temperature sensation with intact vibration, light touch, and joint position sense: this deficit is the underlying cause for any burns present.
- There may be Charcot's joints of the shoulder and elbow.
- There may be signs of hemihypertrophy of the limbs.

Proceed as follows:
- Examine vibration sense over the fingers, lower end of radius, elbow, and clavicles (note that vibration sense is impaired only at a later stage).
- Look for Horner syndrome.
- Examine the neck posteriorly for scar of previous surgery.
- Ask whether you may examine the following:
    - The lower limbs for pyramidal signs, check gait
    - The face for loss of temperature and pain sensation (starting from the outer part of the face and progressing forward, looking for the 'onion-skin pattern' of sensory loss caused by a lesion in the spinal nucleus of the fifth cranial nerve, which extends from the pons down to the upper cervical cord)
    - For lower cranial nerve palsy
    - For nystagmus and ataxia (caused by involvement of the medial longitudinal bundle from C5 upwards)
    - For kyphoscoliosis (caused by paravertebral muscle involvement).

Diagnosis

This patient has dissociated sensory loss (lesion) caused by syringomyelia (aetiology) and has had severe painless trauma or burns (functional status).

Questions

How common is syringomyelia?
It is a rare disorder affecting both sexes equally; the usual age of onset is the fourth or fifth decade.

How do you explain the clinical features?
- At the level of the syrinx:
  - Anterior horn cell involvement causing a lower motor neuron lesion
  - Involvement of the central decussating fibres of the spinothalamic tract producing dissociated sensory loss and late development of neuropathic arthropathy and other trophic changes.
- Below the level of the syrinx:
  - Involvement of pyramidal corticospinal tracts resulting in spastic paraparesis (sphincter function is usually well preserved)
  - Involvement of cervical sympathetics
  - Horner syndrome (miosis, enophthalmos, ptosis).

What is la main succulente?
In some patients with syringomyelia, the hands have a distinct appearance as a result of trophic and vasomotor disturbances; these commonly result in cold, cyanosed, and swollen fingers and palms.

What are the other causes of dissociated sensory loss?
- Anterior spinal artery occlusion (affecting the dorsal horn and lateral spinothalamic tract)
- Diabetic small-fibre polyneuropathy
- Hereditary amyloidotic polyneuropathy
- Leprosy.

The last three affect small peripheral nerve axons.

What investigations would you do?
Magnetic resonance imaging (MRI) scan (Fig. 198.1). In the past, myelography was performed to confirm the diagnosis but was associated with deterioration of the condition in a large number of patients.

What associated abnormalities may be present?
Arnold–Chiari malformation (Fig. 198.1), spina bifida, bony defects around the foramen magnum, hydrocephalus, spinal cord tumours.

What conditions may present with a similar picture?
- Intramedullary tumours of the spinal cord
- Arachnoiditis around the foramen magnum obstructing the cerebrospinal fluid (CSF) pathway
- Haematomyelia
- Craniovertebral anomalies
- Late sequelae of spinal cord injuries (manifest as a painful ascending myelopathy).

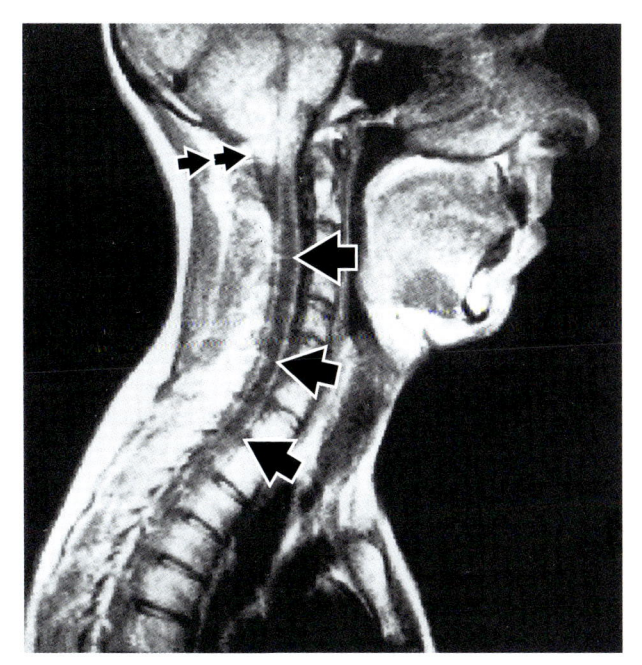

Fig. 198.1 Midsagittal MRI of Arnold–Chiari malformation *(small black arrows)* and syringomyelia *(three large black arrows)*. Note the cerebellar tonsils extending below the posterior rim of the foramen magnum (dark structure immediately above the *black arrow*). The syrinx extends from the medulla well into the thoracic cord. (With permission from Andreoli, T.E., 1997. Cecil Essentials of Medicine, fourth edn. Saunders, Philadelphia, PA.)

What is the difference between hydromyelia and syringomyelia?
Hydromyelia is the expansion of the ependymal-lined central canal of the spinal cord, whereas syringomyelia is the formation of a cleft-like cavity in the inner portion of the cord. Both these lesions are associated with destruction of the white and grey matter and an accompanying reactive gliosis. In syringomyelia, the process generally begins in the cervical cord, and with expansion of the cavity the brainstem and distal cord also become affected.

What are the clinical features of syringobulbia?
- Dissociated sensory loss of the face in an 'onion-skin' pattern (extending from behind forwards, converging on the nose and upper lip)
- Vertigo (common symptom)
- Wasting of the small muscles of the tongue (important physical sign)
- The process may be limited to the medullary region.
- The main cranial nerve nuclei involved are those of the fifth, seventh, ninth, and tenth cranial nerves.

What does the cavity of the syrinx contain?
It contains a fluid similar to CSF but with a higher protein content.

What treatment is available?
- Syringoperitoneal shunting (particularly in patients with basal arachnoiditis and without tonsillar descent)

- Direct drainage of the syrinx into the subarachnoid space (in post-traumatic cavitation)
- When there is an association with Arnold–Chiari malformation, the pressure is relieved by removing the lower central portion of the occipital bone and cervical laminectomy to restore normal CSF dynamics. Emerging evidence suggests that those with mild symptoms do not progress and decompression may not be required for this group.

What other causes of Charcot's joints do you know?
- Diabetes mellitus, especially when the toes and ankles are affected
- Tabes dorsalis, especially when knee and hip joints are affected.

What do you know about Morvan syndrome?
It was initially used to describe painless whitlows on the fingers but was subsequently applied to the progressive loss of pain sensation and its effects (such as ulceration, resorption of the phalanges, and loss of soft tissue) in both hands and feet. These changes are now more commonly seen in leprosy.

Mention some theories of formation of syringomyelia.
Gardner's hydrodynamic theory. This theory posits that syringomyelia is caused by a 'water hammer'-like transmission of pulsatile CSF pressure via a communication between the fourth ventricle and the central canal of the spinal cord through the obex. A blockage of the foramen of Magendie initiates this process.

William's theory. William's theory posits that the development of the syrinx is caused by a differential between intracranial pressure and spinal pressure caused by a valve-like action at the foramen magnum. The increase in subarachnoid fluid pressure from increased venous pressure during Valsalva manoeuvres or coughing is localized to the intracranial compartment. This theory is particularly applicable to patients with Chiari malformation. The malformation of the hindbrain prevents the increased CSF pressure from dissipating caudally. During Valsalva manoeuvre or coughing, a progressive increase in cisterna magna pressure occurs simultaneously with a decrease in spinal subarachnoid pressure. This craniospinal pressure gradient draws CSF caudally into the syrinx.

Oldfield's theory. During dynamic MRI, downward movement of the cerebellar tonsils during systole can be visualized. A piston effect, created by oscillations, in the spinal subarachnoid space that acts on the surface of the spinal cord and forces CSF through the perivascular and interstitial spaces into the syrinx raising intramedullary pressure. The resulting compression of long tracts, neurons, and microcirculation is responsible for the signs and symptoms of neurological dysfunction that appear with distension of the syrinx. Decompression of the syrinx, therefore, potentially reverses the symptoms referable to increased intramedullary pressure.

The intramedullary pulse pressure theory. The intramedullary pulse pressure theory posits that syringomyelia is caused by increased pulse pressure in the spinal cord and that the syrinx consists of extracellular fluid. The distending force in the production of syringomyelia is a relative increase in pulse pressure in the spinal cord compared with that in the nearby subarachnoid space. The syrinx is formed by the accumulation of extracellular fluid in the distended cord.

What do you know about the management of syringomyelia?
- Arnold–Chiari malformation-associated syringomyelia: suboccipital craniectomy and upper cervical laminectomy to decompress the malformation at the foramen magnum
- Intramedullary tumour: surgery with or without radiation therapy
- Posttraumatic syringomyelia: surgery when the neurologic deficits or pain is intolerable.

- The term syringomyelia (from *syrinx*, a pipe or tube) was first used by Ollivier in 1824, in his monograph on diseases of the spinal cord, to denote cavity formation. It denotes the presence of a large fluid-filled cavity in the grey matter of the spinal cord that is in communication with the central canal and contains CSF.

Further Information

J. Arnold (1835–1915), Professor of Pathology at Heidelberg.
H. Chiari (1851–1916), an Austrian pathologist.

CHAPTER 199

Tetraplegia

Instruction
This patient has difficulty walking. Carry out a neurological examination of their lower limbs.

Salient Features

HISTORY
- Ask about bladder symptoms and check sacral sensation.
- Ask about radicular pain.
- Ask whether the weakness was sudden or gradual.
- Ask for history of trauma and multiple sclerosis.

EXAMINATION
- Increased or decreased tone in both lower limbs
- Hyperreflexia
- Ankle clonus
- Weakness in all four limbs
- Wasted hands (cervical spondylosis, motor neurone disease, or syringomyelia).

Remember: The physical examination pertinent to spinal cord dysfunction involves testing in three areas: motor function, sensory function, and reflexes.

Proceed as follows:
- Remember to check the sensory level and examine the spine.
- Tell the examiner that you would like to do the following:
  - Check for cerebellar signs (multiple sclerosis, Friedreich's ataxia).
  - Check blood pressure (BP) (postural hypotension, autonomic dysreflexia).
- Try to localize the level of lesion using the following:
  - Spasticity of all four limbs: lesion above the C4 spinal cord segment
  - Spasticity of the lower limbs with flaccid weakness of some muscles of the upper limb: lesion of cervical cord enlargement (C5–T2)
  - Deep tendon reflexes: an absent biceps jerk with a brisk supinator jerk (inversion of the supinator jerk) or an absent biceps and supinator with a brisk triceps jerk localizes the lesion to C5–C6
  - Radicular pain: useful early in the disease; with time becomes diffuse and ceases to have localizing value
  - Superficial sensation: not good for localizing as the level of sensory loss may vary greatly in different individuals and in different types of lesion.

Note: Be prepared to discuss the Frankel classification (later).

Diagnosis

This patient has weakness in all four limbs (lesion) caused by spinal trauma (aetiology) and is wheelchair bound (functional status).

Questions

What is autonomic dysreflexia?
It is bradycardia, sweating, rhinorrhoea, pounding headaches, and severe paroxysmal hypertension, which presents quickly and can rapidly precipitate seizures and death if not relieved. Precipitating factors include blockage of urinary catheter, visceral distension from full bowel, stimulation of the skin secondary to an irritative pressure sore, and vesicoureteric reflux. Labour in a high-tetraplegic female may also be complicated by it.

What nontraumatic causes are there for spinal cord dysfunction?
- Processes affecting the spinal cord or blood supply directly:
  - Multiple sclerosis
  - Transverse myelitis
  - Spinal arteriovenous malformation/subarachnoid haemorrhage
  - Syringomyelia
  - HIV myelopathy
  - Other myelopathies
  - Spinal cord infarction.
- Compressive lesions affecting the spinal cord:
  - Spinal epidural abscess
  - Spinal epidural haematoma
  - Discitis
  - Neoplasm: metastatic or primary central nervous system.

Does ingestion of food affect BP in tetraplegics?
The ingestion of food causes a small fall in BP, and this exacerbates the postural hypotension in these patients.

How would you manage spasticity in these patients?
- Drugs: diazepam, baclofen
- Surgery: dorsal rhizotomy, neurectomy, myelotomy, orthopaedic procedures that divide and lengthen tendons of spastic muscles

How do you localize the lesion to the fifth cervical root level?
- Muscular weakness: deltoid, supraspinatus, brachioradialis
- Deep tendon reflexes affected: biceps and supinator jerks
- Radicular pain/paraesthesia: neck, top of shoulder, outer aspect of the arm, forearm
- Superficial sensory deficit: outer aspect of the upper arm.

How do you localize the lesion to the sixth cervical root level?
- Muscular weakness: biceps, brachioradialis, extensor carpi radialis longus
- Deep tendon reflexes affected: biceps and supinator jerks
- Radicular pain/paraesthesia: neck, shoulder, outer arm, forearm, thumb, and index finger
- Superficial sensory deficit: thumb and index finger.

How do you localize the lesion to the seventh cervical root level?
- Muscular weakness: triceps and most of the muscles on the dorsum of the forearm
- Deep tendon reflexes affected: triceps jerk
- Radicular pain/paraesthesia: neck, shoulder, arm, forearm to index, and middle finger
- Superficial sensory deficit: mostly middle and index fingers.

How do you localize the lesion to the eighth cervical root level?
- Muscular weakness: flexors of the forearm
- Deep tendon reflexes affected: finger jerk
- Radicular pain/paraesthesia: neck, shoulder, arm, ring, and little fingers
- Superficial sensory deficit: ring and little fingers.

How do you localize the lesion to the first thoracic root level?
- Muscular weakness: small muscles of the hand
- Deep tendon reflexes affected: finger jerk
- Radicular pain/paraesthesia: neck, axilla, medial aspect of the arm and forearm, little and ring finger
- Superficial sensory deficit: medial arm and little finger.

What precautions would you take when transporting patients with acute high-spinal injuries by air?
- Lung function should be stable before transfer.
- Air humidifier and supplemental oxygen should be available.
- Patient should be accompanied by someone trained in manoeuvres to clear airway secretions. Tracheal suction should be done regularly; this may be complicated by reflex bradycardia and cardiac arrest, and so atropine and noradrenaline should be available.

What is the mode of onset in patients with the classic syndrome of foramen magnum?
First, there is weakness of the shoulder and arm, followed by weakness of the ipsilateral leg, then contralateral leg, and finally, contralateral arm. Neoplasms in this region can cause suboccipital pain spreading to the neck and shoulders.

What is Raymond–Cestan syndrome?
Raymond–Cestan syndrome is the result of the obstruction of twigs of the basilar artery causing lesions of the pontine region; it is characterized by tetraplegia, nystagmus, and anaesthesia.

Can you describe Frankel's classification of neurological deficit?
The classification is into five types:
   A: absent motor and sensory function
   B: sensation present, motor function absent
   C: sensation present, motor function active but not useful (grades 2/5 to 3/5)
   D: sensation present, motor function active and useful (grade 4/5)
   E: normal motor and sensory function.

Further Information
Sir Ludwig Guttmann, FRS, fled from Nazi persecution and worked at the National Spinal Injuries Centre in Stoke Mandeville Hospital, Aylesbury. He was entrusted to look after the paraplegics and tetraplegics of the war. He was the first to show that pressure sores can be avoided by 2-hourly turning of patients.

Professor Hans Ludwig Frankel, OBE, National Hospital of Spinal Injuries, Stoke Mandeville Hospital, Aylesbury.

CHAPTER 200

Third Cranial Nerve Palsy

Instruction

Examine this patient's eyes.

Salient Features

HISTORY

- Diplopia in all directions except on lateral gaze to the side of the third nerve lesion (because the lateral rectus muscle supplied by the sixth cranial nerve is intact)
- Painful onset (berry aneurysm or aneurysmal dilatation of the intracavernous part of the carotid artery causing third nerve palsy)
- Headaches (migraine, cranial arteritis)
- Obtain a history of diabetes or hypertension.

EXAMINATION

- Unilateral ptosis (from paralysis of the levator palpebrae superioris)
- Dilated pupil reacting slowly or incompletely to light (paralysis of the constrictor of the pupil)
- Paralysis of accommodation (from involvement of ciliary muscle)
- Squint and diplopia resulting from weakness of muscles supplied by the third cranial nerve (superior, inferior, medial recti, and inferior oblique). The eye will be in the position of abduction (i.e. down and out) if the fourth and sixth nerves are intact.
- Diplopia may not be obvious until the affected eyelid is elevated manually.

Proceed as follows:
- Exclude the associated fourth cranial nerve lesion (supplies the superior oblique) by tilting the head of the patient to the same side—the affected eye will intort if the fourth cranial nerve is intact. Remember superior oblique intorts the eye (SIN). Inferior oblique externally rotates the eye.
- Tell the examiner that you would like to check:
  - the urine for sugar (diabetes mellitus)
  - blood pressure (BP) (hypertension).

Notes:
- Vascular lesions (such as those associated with diabetes and arteritis) that infarct the third nerve may produce a complete oculomotor palsy with pupillary sparing. The pupillomotor fibres are around the periphery of the third nerve. Compression of the mass or aneurysm often involves the pupil.
- Be prepared to discuss the third cranial nerve anatomy.

Diagnosis

This patient has a R/L third nerve palsy (lesion) caused by diabetes mellitus (aetiology).

Questions

What are the common causes of a third nerve palsy?
- Ischaemia is the most common cause of pupil-sparing third nerve palsy, especially in patients with vascular risk factors, like hypertension and diabetes. (The presence of pain is not a good discriminating feature between diabetes and aneurysm, as pain is present in both.) Diabetic third nerve palsy usually recovers within 3 months.
- Multiple sclerosis
- Aneurysms of posterior communicating artery (painful ophthalmoplegia)
- Cavernous sinus thrombosis
- Trauma
- Tumours, collagen, vascular disorder, syphilis
- Ophthalmoplegic migraine
- Encephalitis
- Parasellar neoplasms
- Meningioma at the wing of sphenoid
- Basal meningitis
- Carcinoma at the base of the skull
- Rhinocerebral mucormycosis (in diabetic ketoacidosis, but about half the patients with diabetes who have this infection do not have ketoacidosis).

How would you investigate such a patient?
- Check BP and urine for sugar.
- C-reactive protein (CRP) levels to exclude temporal arteritis (in the elderly)
- Test to exclude myasthenia and thyroid disease
- Computed tomography (CT) or magnetic resonance imaging of the head
- Arteriography, in the form of magnetic resonance angiogram or CT angiography, especially when the pupil is involved and there is severe pain
- Lumbar puncture if infection is suspected.

When would you suspect a lesion of the third nerve nucleus?
- Unilateral third nerve palsy with contralateral superior rectus palsy and bilateral partial ptosis
- Bilateral third nerve palsy (with or without internal ophthalmoplegia associated with spared levator function).

What do you know about the muscles of extraocular movement?
Each eye is moved by three pairs of muscles, and the precise action of these muscles depends on the position of the eye; the actions are as follows:
- Medial and lateral recti (first pair of muscles): adduct and abduct the eye, respectively
- Superior and inferior recti: elevate and depress the abducted eye
- Superior and inferior obliques: depress and elevate the adducted eye.

Note: Superior and Inferior recti act in the abducted position (mnemonic, RAB).

What do you know about the anatomy of the oculomotor nerve?

Midbrain—the third cranial nerve originates in the midbrain and courses through the cavernous sinus and superior orbital fissure into the orbit to innervate four muscles and provide parasympathetic fibres for pupillary constriction.

Cavernous sinus—in the cavernous sinus or at the superior orbital fissure, the third cranial nerve may lie very close to the optic nerve. The third cranial nerve divides into superior and inferior rami within either the anterior portion of the cavernous sinus or the posterior optic canal. The superior rami supply fibres to the levator palpebrae and superior rectus muscles, and the inferior rami supply the extraocular muscles innervated by this nerve and also carry the pupillomotor fibres, which are in the superomedial portion of the nerve.

> **Note:** Ischaemic disease of the oculomotor nerve (e.g. in patients with diabetes mellitus or hypertension) typically spares the pupil, whereas compressive disease results in pupillary enlargement.

Do you know of any eponymous syndromes in which the third cranial nerve is involved?

- Weber syndrome: ipsilateral third nerve palsy with contralateral hemiplegia. The lesion is in the midbrain.
- Benedikt syndrome: ipsilateral third nerve palsy with contralateral involuntary movements such as tremor, chorea, and athetosis. It is caused by a lesion of the red nucleus in the midbrain.
- Claude syndrome: ipsilateral oculomotor paresis with contralateral ataxia and tremor. It is caused by a lesion of the third nerve and red nucleus.
- Nothnagel syndrome: unilateral oculomotor paralysis combined with ipsilateral cerebellar ataxia.

Further Information

M. Benedikt (1835–1920), an Austrian physician, described this syndrome in 1889.
Sir H.D. Weber (1823–1918) qualified in Bonn and worked at Guy's Hospital, London.
Henri Claude (1869–1945), a French psychiatrist.
Carl Wilhelm Nothnagel (1841–1905), an Austrian physician.

CHAPTER 201

Tremor

PATIENT 1

Instruction

Look at this patient's hands.

Salient Features

EXAMINATION

- Coarse resting tremor that is slow (4–6 per second). Asking the patient to place their hand on their knees, close their eyes, and count backwards from 10 can bring this on
- Adduction–abduction of the thumb with flexion–extension of fingers (pill-rolling movement)
- The tremor is halted by purposive movements of the hands
- The upper limb tremor often increases as the patient walks
- Tell the examiner that you would like to do the following:
  - Look for cog-wheel rigidity.
  - Comment on mask-like facies.
  - Check for festinant gait.
  - Ask the patient's relatives whether sleep relieves the tremor and whether emotion makes it worse.
  - Examine the handwriting (Fig. 201.1).

Diagnosis

This patient with resting tremor and mask-like facies (lesion) has Parkinson disease (aetiology) and is severely disabled by the tremor (functional status).

PATIENT 2

Instruction

Look at this patient's hands.

Salient Features

EXAMINATION

- There is a 10-Hz physiological tremor that is brought on when the arms are outstretched. It can be amplified by laying a sheet of paper on the hands
- Tell the examiner that you would like to do the following:
  - Check for thyrotoxicosis.

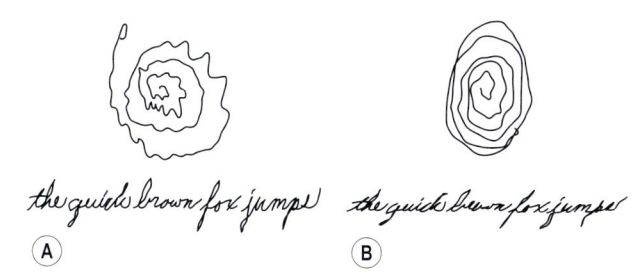

Fig. 201.1 Handwriting and spiral drawing reflects tremor type. **(A)** Large scrawl in essential tremor. **(B)** Cramped, parkinsonian writing and spiral shows little tremor; writing is an action.

- Take a history for alcohol excess.
- Take a drug history (salbutamol, terbutaline, antiepileptics, antipsychotics).
- Take an occupational history for heavy metal exposure (e.g. mad hatter disease).
- Find out whether tremor runs in the family and is relieved by alcohol (benign essential tremor).

Diagnosis

This patient has fine tremor with an enlarged thyroid gland (lesion) caused by Graves disease (aetiology). They are clinically thyrotoxic (functional status).

PATIENT 3

Instruction

Look at this patient's hands.

Salient Features

EXAMINATION

- The patient does not have a resting tremor or a tremor with outstretched hands
- Intention tremor is noted.

Proceed as follows:
- Check the past-pointing: the intention tremor of cerebellar disease.
- Tell the examiner that you would like to check for other cerebellar signs.

Diagnosis

This patient has an intention tremor (lesion) caused by cerebellar syndrome (aetiology).

PATIENT 4

Instruction

Look at this patient's hands.

Salient Features

EXAMINATION

- Unsteadiness when standing still; by contrast, the patient has little or no difficulty while walking, which relieves the symptoms.
- Fine rippling of the muscles of the legs may be seen or felt when the patient attempts to stand still; after a short interval, the patient becomes increasingly unsteady and is forced to take a step to regain balance.

Diagnosis

This patient has primary orthostatic tremor (lesion).

Questions

What are tremors?
Involuntary movements that result from alternating contraction and relaxation of groups of muscles, producing rhythmic oscillations about a joint or a group of joints.

How would you classify tremors?
- Resting tremor, as in Parkinson disease
- Postural tremor (also referred to as action tremor or kinetic tremor). It is brought on when the arms are outstretched and is caused by the following:
  - Exaggerated physiological tremor, caused by anxiety, thyrotoxicosis, alcohol, drugs
  - Brain damage, seen in Wilson disease (look for Kayser–Fleischer rings), syphilis.
- Intention tremor (aggravated by voluntary movements) in cerebellar disease
- Tremor from neuropathy (postural tremor; arms more than legs).

Mention a few involuntary movements.
- Chorea
- Athetosis
- Hemiballismus
- Fasciculation
- Torticollis
- Clonus.

What are the causes of drug-associated tremors?
- Drug-induced tremors: beta-2 agonists (e.g. salbutamol), caffeine, theophylline, lithium, tricyclic antidepressants, serotonin reuptake inhibitors, neuroleptics, sodium valproate, corticosteroids
- Tremors associated with drug withdrawal: alcohol (delirium tremens), benzodiazepines, barbiturates, opiates.

What do you know about the investigation and management of primary orthostatic tremor?
- In primary orthostatic tremor:
  - Electromyography (EMG) shows rhythmic activation of lower limb muscles at a frequency of 4 to 18 Hz.
  - PET shows increased activity in the cerebellum.
- Treatment is supportive and the patient is often relieved to know the diagnosis, especially when a psychiatric cause or Parkinson disease has been suspected previously.

What is the pathophysiology of tremor?
- Physiological tremor has both mechanical and central components.
- Symptomatic palatal tremor is most likely caused by rhythmic activity of the inferior olive.
- Essential tremor is also generated from within the olivocerebellar circuits. The most common action tremor is essential tremor, a tremor of the hands at 4 to 12 Hz.
- Rest tremor of Parkinson disease arises from the basal ganglia loop, and dystonic tremor originates from within the basal ganglia.
- Orthostatic tremor originates from unidentified brainstem nuclei.
- Cerebellar tremor is in part caused by a cerebellar circuit that involves feedforward control of voluntary movements.
- Neuropathic tremor is believed to be caused by abnormally functioning reflex pathways.
- Toxic and drug-induced tremors have many underlying causes.
- Psychogenic tremor is thought to be mediated by reflex mechanisms.

What is the treatment for tremor?
- Avoid stimulants including caffeine.
- Large utensil handles can help, seek advice from occupational therapy.
- Tremor caused by Parkinson disease: levodopa, dopamine agonists. Tremor often responds less well to treatment than rigidity or bradykinesia symptoms and may require additional second-line treatment with clozapine, amantadine. Beta-blockers should be used with caution due to risk of postural hypotension and bradycardia.
- Essential tremor: beta-blockers, primidone, or both; 40% to 70% of these patients have some improvement with this treatment. Second-line treatments include gabapentin and topiramate.
- Cerebellar tremor: no standard treatment; clonazepam is sometimes effective, as is treatment with levodopa, primidone, or clozapine.
- Drug-resistant tremor: thalamic stimulation (continuous deep-brain stimulation) and thalamotomy are equally effective, but thalamic stimulation has fewer adverse effects and results in a greater improvement of function.

Further Information

Mercury poisoning came to be known as 'mad hatter disease' as workers involved in the manufacture of felt hats were exposed to mercury.

CHAPTER 202

Deformity of a Lower Limb

Instruction
Examine the lower limbs of this patient who has had this abnormality since childhood.

Salient Features
HISTORY
- History of trauma to the spine and/or leg
- History of poliomyelitis
- History of weakness and fasciculations
- Bladder and bowel symptoms.

EXAMINATION
- Wasting and deformity of one lower limb (or both with one side being more affected than the other)
- Fasciculations
- Normal tone in both lower limbs
- Loss of sensation (L5 and/or S1 sensory loss in spina bifida)
- Examination of the spine:
  - Kyphoscoliosis (seen in poliomyelitis, indicating involvement of trunk muscles)
  - Tuft of hair in the lower lumbosacral spine (closed spina bifida)
- Bony deformity in the affected leg
- Gait abnormality and Romberg's sign test.

Diagnosis
This patient has unilateral wasting and deformity of the right/left leg (lesion) caused by poliomyelitis in childhood (aetiology) and wears calipers on that leg (functional status).

Questions
What is the differential diagnosis?
- Old poliomyelitis (Fig. 202.1)
- Spina bifida (Fig. 202.2).

What are the causes of lower motor neuron signs in the legs?
- Peripheral neuropathy
- Prolapsed intervertebral disc
- Diabetic amyotrophy
- Poliomyelitis

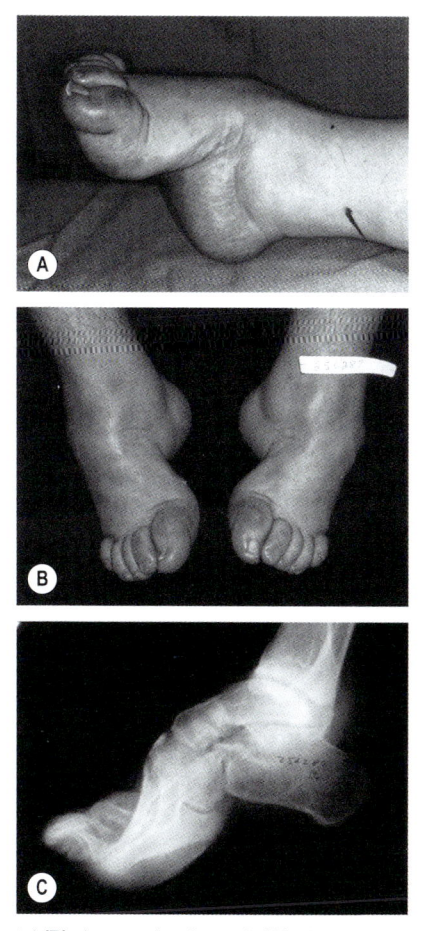

Fig. 202.1 Medial **(A)** and frontal **(B)** views and radiograph **(C)** of severe calcaneocavovarus deformities as sequelae of poliomyelitis. (With permission from Canale, S.T., Beaty, J.H. (eds.), 2007. Campbell's Operative Orthopaedics, eleventh edn. Mosby, Philadelphia, PA.)

- Cauda equina lesions
- Motor neurone disease.

What is the cause of polio?
Polio is caused by a picornavirus of the genus *Enterovirus*; there are three antigenic types: I (Brunhilde), II (Lansing), and III (Leon).

Is the muscular involvement of polio in childhood progressive?
Usually, paralytic polio remains stable after the initial attack. However, in some patients, new muscle weakness and atrophy involving previously affected muscles or even unaffected muscles occur, and this deterioration can occur as long as 30 years after the first attack; this is known as postpoliomyelitis muscular atrophy. The progression of this involvement is slow and is said to be distinct from motor neurone disease. It is not entirely clear why only some patients are affected, but it has been reported that it is more likely to occur in those with widespread paralysis and poor immune status.

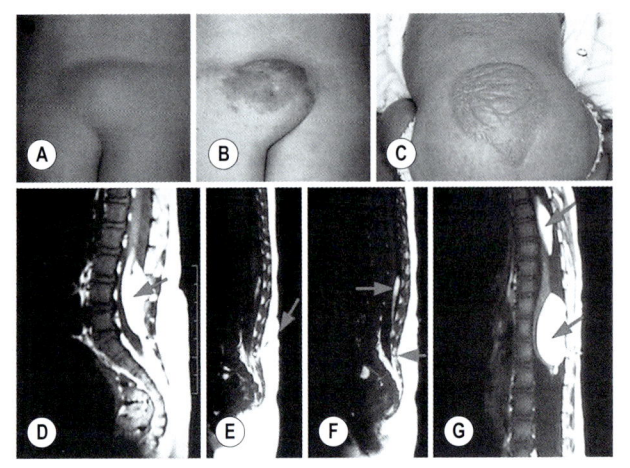

Fig. 202.2 Clinical features and corresponding occult spinal dysraphism detected by sagittal, T_1-weighted magnetic resonance imaging studies of the spinal cord. **(A)** Sacral lipoma and deviated gluteal furrow. **(B)** Lumbar port-wine stain, lipoma, dermal sinus, and deviated gluteal furrow. **(C)** Dorsal and lumbar unclassified hamartomas. **(D)** Lipoma of the conus *(arrow)*. **(E)** Dermal sinus *(arrow)*. **(F)** Top of the lipoma of the filum terminale *(upper arrow)* and fistula *(lower arrow)*. **(G)** Multiple lipomas of the thoracic cord *(upper arrow)* and posterior conus *(lower arrow)*. (With permission from Guggisberg, D., Hadj-Rabia, S., Viney, C., et al., 2004. Skin markers of occult spinal dysraphism. Arch. Dermatol. 140, 1109–1115.)

Is poliomyelitis preventable?
Yes, two types of poliovaccine are available (each containing all three strains of the virus):
- Oral polio vaccine of Sabin consists of live attenuated virus (OPV)
- Killed or inactivated vaccine of Salk (IPV).

With which vaccine is paralytic poliomyelitis associated?
Vaccine-associated paralytic poliomyelitis is associated with oral polio vaccine, particularly in immunodeficient individuals. Such individuals and their household contacts should be given inactivated vaccine.

What do you know about 'provocation poliomyelitis'?
Provocation poliomyelitis is caused by the administration of intramuscular injections during the incubation period of wild-type poliovirus or shortly after exposure to oral poliovaccine (either as a vaccine recipient or through contact with a recent recipient).

What do you understand by the term spina bifida?
Spina bifida means an incomplete closure of the bony vertebral canal and is commonly associated with a similar anomaly of the spinal cord. The commonest site is the lumbosacral region, but the cervical spine can be involved and may be associated with hydrocephalus. It results from failure of fusion of the caudal neural tube and is one of the most common malformations of human structure. The causes include single gene disorders, chromosome abnormalities, and teratogenic exposures. Although the cause is not known in most cases, up to 70% of spina bifida cases can be prevented by maternal periconceptional folic acid supplementation. The mechanism underlying this protective effect is unclear, but it is probably related to genes that regulate folate transport and metabolism. Individuals with spina bifida often require both surgical and medical management. Surgical closure is usually done in the neonatal period. Medical management is a lifelong.

What are the features of closed spina bifida?
- Cutaneous: lumbosacral lipoma, hypertrichosis, sinus or dimple above the sacrum, naevus, or scarring
- Unilateral shortening of one leg and foot with a deficiency of the muscles below the knee. There may be calcaneovalgus or equinovarus deformity. Sensory loss in the fifth lumbar and first sacral dermatome is common.
- Neuropathic bladder, enuresis
- Bony changes on plain radiograph: sacral dysgenesis, scoliosis, laminar fusion of vertebral body, pedicle erosion, and bony spurs.

Is the neurological deficit in closed spina bifida progressive?
This issue is contentious as much of the deficit is fixed antenatally and any progression is a result of growth and posture. However, in some patients, the late appearance of bladder dysfunction indicates that the neurological deficit is progressive in these individuals.

Mention some teratogenic factors responsible for neural canal defects.
- Maternal type 1 diabetes and sacral dysgenesis
- Sodium valproate in pregnancy and neural tube defects.

Mention some prenatal screening tests for spina bifida.
- Amniotic α-fetoprotein levels
- Amniotic acetylcholinesterase estimation
- High-resolution diagnostic ultrasonography.

What is the basic mechanism of muscle atrophy?
Muscle atrophy (associated with disuse, nerve injury, fasting and many diseases including cancer, AIDS, and tuberculosis) has a single basic mechanism: excessive activation of the ubiquitin–proteasome pathway in the muscle. The proteasome is a large protein complex that acts like a cell's garbage disposal by grabbing onto excess and damaged proteins and degrading them; ubiquitin is an enzyme (now called adenosine triphosphate (ATP)–dependent protease) responsible for protein breakdown.

Further Information
M.H. Romberg (1795–1873), German neurologist and Professor of Medicine in Berlin.

The 1952 Nobel Prize was jointly awarded to John F. Enders (1897–1985) and Thomas H. Weller (1915–2008), both of Children's Medical Center and Harvard Medical School, Boston, and Frederick C. Robbins (1916–2003) of Western Reserve University, Cleveland, Ohio, for their discovery of the ability of poliomyelitis viruses to grow in cultures of various types of tissue.

US President Franklin Delano Roosevelt is known for his defiant struggle with his permanent lower-limb paresis (caused by polio). In 1937, Roosevelt announced the formation of a National Foundation for Infantile Paralysis that would 'lead, direct, and unify the fight of every phase of this sickness'. Soon, millions of US citizens were responding to the pleas of the radio personality Eddie Cantor to 'send their dimes directly to the President at the White House' and now this movement is called 'the March of Dimes'.

CHAPTER 203

Ulnar Nerve Palsy

Instruction
Carry out a neurological examination of this patient's upper limbs.

Salient Features
HISTORY
- Repeated trivial trauma to the elbow; the patient feels the 'funny bone'.
- The patient may be immobilized in the orthopaedic ward and use the elbows to shuffle in bed.
- History of fracture of the upper arm in childhood (supracondylar fractures of humerus in childhood have an insidious course and can result in acute ulnar nerve palsy 20–30 years later: tardy-ulnar palsy).

EXAMINATION
- There is generalized wasting of the small muscles of the hand.
- There may be features of ulnar claw hand: hyperextension at the metacarpophalangeal joints and flexion at the interphalangeal joints of the fourth and fifth fingers (Fig. 203.1).
- There is weakness of movement of the fingers, except that of the thenar eminence.
- There is sensory loss over the medial one and half fingers.

Proceed as follows:
- Examine the elbow for scars and signs of osteoarthrosis.
- Comment on the large carrying angle at the elbow, particularly in women (repeated extension and flexion of the arm can result in damage of the olecranon and consequently the ulnar nerve).
- Look for features of rheumatoid arthritis.

Diagnosis
This patient has wasting of the small muscles of the hand, and claw hand with sensory loss over the medial one and half fingers (lesion) caused by ulnar nerve palsy following trauma (aetiology). She is unable to button her clothes (functional status).

Questions

What are the muscles supplied by the ulnar nerve?
The ulnar nerve is derived from the eighth cervical and first thoracic spinal nerves. It gives no branches above the elbow and supplies:
- In the forearm:
  - Flexor carpi ulnaris
  - Medial half of the flexor digitorum profundus.

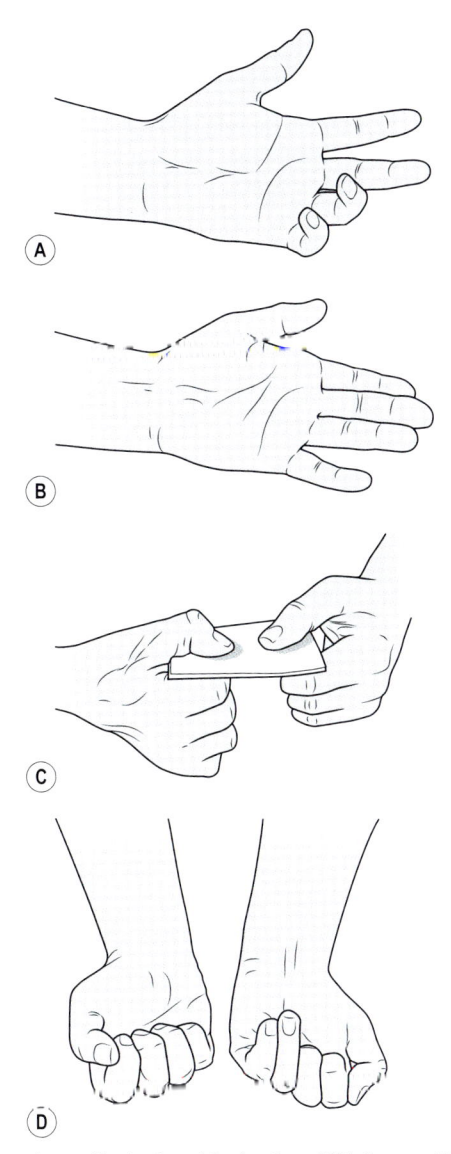

Fig. 203.1 **(A)** Benediction posture, with clawing of the fourth and fifth fingers while the fingers and thumb are held slightly abducted. **(B)** Wartenberg's sign, abduction of the little finger with the hand at rest. **(C)** Froment's sign, seen when using the thumb and index finger to pinch an object. **(D)** Weakness of the ulnar flexor digitorum profundus, inability to completely flex the distal phalanx of the fourth and fifth digits.

- In the hand:
  - Movers of the little finger: abductor digiti minimi, flexor digiti minimi, and opponens digiti minimi
  - Adductor pollicis (oblique and transverse heads)
  - Dorsal and palmar interossei
  - Third and fourth lumbricals

- Palmaris brevis
- Inner head of flexor pollicis brevis.

How would you differentiate between a lesion above the cubital fossa and a lesion at the wrist?
- In lesions above the cubital fossa, the flexor carpi ulnaris is involved.
- In lesions at the wrist, the adductor pollicis is involved.

How would you test the flexor carpi ulnaris?
Ask the patient to keep the hand flat on a table with the palm facing upwards and then to perform flexion and ulnar deviation at the wrist.

How would you test the adductor pollicis?
Ask the patient to grip a folded newspaper between the thumb and index finger of each hand so that the thumbs are uppermost—this causes the adductor to contract. When the muscle is paralyzed, the thumb is incapable of adequate adduction and becomes flexed at the interphalangeal joint caused by contraction of the flexor pollicis longus (innervated by the median nerve). This is known as Froment's sign (Fig. 203.1C).

What is ulnar paradox?
The higher the lesion in the upper limb, the lesser is the deformity. A lesion at or above the elbow causes paralysis of the ulnar half of the flexor digitorum profundus, interossei, and lumbricals. Thus, the action of the paralyzed profundus is not unopposed by the interossei and lumbricals; as a result, the ring and little fingers are not flexed, and hence, there is no claw, whereas a lesion at the wrist causes an ulnar claw hand.

What causes the ulnar claw hand?
A lesion of the ulnar nerve at the wrist. The little and ring fingers are flexed at the interphalangeal joints and hyperextended at the metacarpophalangeal joints. The index and middle fingers are less affected as the first and second lumbricals are supplied by the median nerve.

What are the causes of claw hand?
True claw hand is seen in the following conditions:
- Advanced rheumatoid arthritis
- Lesion of both the median and ulnar nerves, as in leprosy
- Lesions of the medial cord of the brachial plexus
- Anterior poliomyelitis
- Syringomyelia
- Polyneuritis
- Amyotrophic lateral sclerosis
- Klumpke paralysis (lower brachial plexus, C7–8 involvement)
- Severe Volkmann ischaemic contracture.

How can the ulnar nerve be affected at the wrist?
The deep branch of the ulnar nerve is motor and may be compressed in Guyon's canal, which runs between the pisiform and hook of the hamate. This results in wasting and weakness of the interossei, particularly the first and the adductor pollicis, but sensation is spared. The hypothenar muscles are usually spared, although the third and fourth lumbricals may be affected. The nerve may be compressed in Guyon's canal by a ganglion, neuroma, or repeated trauma. Surgical exposure of the nerve may be necessary when there is no history of trauma.

What is the most common cause of an ulnar nerve lesion at the elbow?
It is caused by compression of the nerve by the fibrous arch of the flexor carpi ulnaris (the cubital tunnel), which arises as two heads from the medial epicondyle and the olecranon.

What you understand by 'tardy ulnar nerve palsy'?
This occurs when injuries or arthritic changes at the elbow cause a delayed or slowly progressive involvement of the ulnar nerve.

How would you rapidly exclude an injury to a major nerve in the arm?
- Radial nerve: test for wrist drop
- Ulnar nerve: test for Froment's sign (see earlier)
- Median nerve: Ochsner's clasping test.

Further Information
R. von Volkmann (1830–1889), Professor of Surgery in Halle, Germany.

Augusta Déjérine-Klumpke (1859–1927), a French neurologist, was the first woman to receive the title 'Internes des Hôpitaux' in 1877.

Jules Froment (1876–1946), Professor of Clinical Medicine, Lyons, France.

A.J. Ochsner (1896–1981), a US surgeon, also investigated the role of tobacco in lung cancer.

CHAPTER 204

Wallenberg Syndrome (Lateral Medullary Syndrome)

Instruction

Examine this patient's cranial nerves.

Salient Features

HISTORY

- Severe nausea, vomiting, nystagmus (involvement of the lower vestibular nuclei)
- Limb and/or gait ataxia (involvement of the inferior cerebellar peduncle)
- Intractable hiccups, dysphagia, hoarse voice (ninth and tenth cranial nerve involvement).

EXAMINATION

- Nystagmus
- Ipsilateral involvement of fifth, sixth, seventh, and eighth cranial nerves
- Bulbar palsy: impaired gag, sluggish palatal movements
- Horner syndrome.

Proceed as follows:
Tell the examiner that you would like to check for the following:
- Cerebellar signs on the same side
- Pain and temperature sensory loss on the opposite side (dissociated sensory loss).

> **Remember:**
> - The main features of this syndrome are *ipsilateral* Horner syndrome and *contralateral* loss of pain and temperature sensation.
> - Wallenberg syndrome is an infarction of the lateral portion of the medullary tegmentum. The most common cause is occlusion of the intracranial vertebral artery.
> - Neuroimaging: magnetic resonance imaging (MRI) is preferred because computed tomography provides less complete visualization of the brainstem, owing to artefacts related to the skull. MRI with diffusion-weighted imaging is the most sensitive test available to detect acute infarcts.

Diagnosis

This patient has lateral medullary syndrome (lesion) caused by a stroke (aetiology) and has dysphagia (functional status).

Questions

Which vessel is occluded?
Any of the following five vessels:
- Posterior inferior cerebellar artery
- Vertebral artery
- Superior, middle, or inferior lateral medullary arteries.

How may these patients present?
With sudden onset of vertigo, vomiting, and ipsilateral ataxia, with contralateral loss of pain and temperature sensations.

Where is the lesion in lateral medullary syndrome?
It results from infarction of a wedge-shaped area of the lateral aspect of the medulla and inferior surface of the cerebellum. The deficits are from involvement of one side of the nucleus ambiguus, trigeminal nucleus, vestibular nuclei, cerebellar peduncle, spinothalamic tract, and autonomic fibres.

What is the medial medullary syndrome?
It is caused by occlusion of the lower basilar artery or vertebral artery. Ipsilateral lesions result in paralysis and wasting of the tongue. Contralateral lesions result in hemiplegia and loss of vibration and joint position sense.

Mention a few other eponymous syndromes with crossed hemiplegia.
- Weber syndrome: contralateral hemiplegia with ipsilateral lower motor neuron lesion of the oculomotor nerve. The lesion is in the midbrain.
- Millard–Gubler syndrome: contralateral hemiplegia with lower motor neuron lesion of the abducens nerve. The lesion is in the pons.
- Foville syndrome: as Millard–Gubler syndrome with gaze palsy.

What is Benedikt syndrome?
It causes cerebellar signs on the side opposite of the third nerve palsy (which is produced by damage to the nucleus itself or to the nerve fascicle). It is caused by a midbrain vascular lesion, causing damage to the red nucleus, interrupting the dentatorubrothalamic tract from the opposite cerebellar signs.

Further Information

Achille L.F. Foville (1799–1878), a Parisian neurologist.
Adolf Wallenburg (1862–1949), a German neurologist, described this syndrome in 1895.
Auguste L.J. Millard (1830–1915) and Adolphe Marie Gubler (1821–1879), Parisian physicians.
Savitz and Caplan (2005) wrote a classic article.

CHAPTER 205

Wasting of the Small Muscles of the Hand

Instruction

Examine this patient's hands.
Ask the patient whether her hands are painful.

Salient Features

HISTORY

- Rheumatoid arthritis
- Painful neck movements (cervical spondylosis)
- Fasciculations, weakness (motor neurone disease)
- Associated sensory loss (syringomyelia)
- Family history (Charcot–Marie–Tooth disease)
- Ascending muscle weakness (Guillain–Barré syndrome)
- Trauma to upper limbs (bilateral median and ulnar nerve lesions).

EXAMINATION

- Wasting of thenar and hypothenar eminences and dorsal interossei.

Proceed as follows:
- Look for deformity and swelling.
- Look for fasciculations.
- Check sensation over the hand, especially the index and little fingers.
- Test grip and pincer movements.
- Test for median and ulnar nerve compression.
- Ask the patient to unbutton clothes or to write.
- Palpate for cervical ribs and compare radial pulses.
- Look for Horner syndrome.
- Examine the neck and test neck movements.

Diagnosis

This patient has bilateral wasted hands (lesions) caused by cervical myelopathy (aetiology) and is unable to button her clothes (functional status).

Questions

What are the causes of wasted hands?

Bilateral wasted hands:
- Rheumatoid arthritis
- Old age
- Cervical spondylosis
- Bilateral cervical ribs
- Motor neurone disease (Fig. 205.1)
- Syringomyelia
- Charcot–Marie–Tooth disease
- Guillain–Barré syndrome
- Bilateral median and ulnar nerve lesions.

Unilateral wasting: causes additional to the previously mentioned ones:
- Brachial plexus trauma
- Pancoast tumour
- Cervical cord lesions.
- Malignant infiltration of the brachial plexus
- Thoracic outlet syndrome (Fig. 205.2).

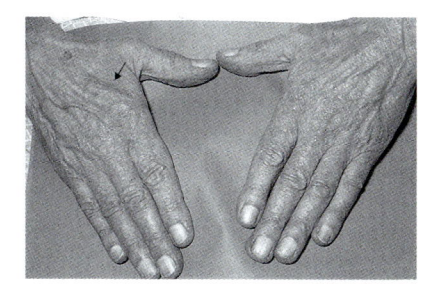

Fig. 205.1 Motor neurone disease. There are fasciculation and wasting of the muscles between the thumb and index finger on the dorsal *(arrow)* and palmar surfaces. (With permission from Goldman, L., Ausiello, D.A., 2007. Cecil Textbook of Medicine, twenty-third edn. Saunders, Philadelphia, PA.)

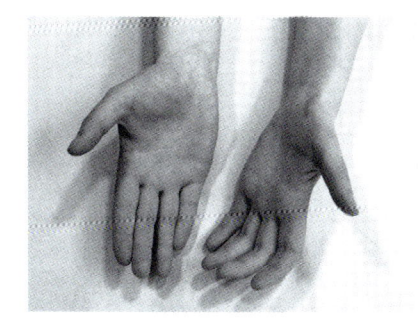

Fig. 205.2 True neurologic thoracic outlet syndrome with wasting of muscles clearly shown in the left hand. (With permission from Frontera, W.R., Silver, J.K., Rizzo, T.D., 2008. Essentials of Physical Medicine and Rehabilitation, second edn. Saunders, Philadelphia, PA.)

In unilateral wasting, what is the level of the lesion?
C8, T1. These muscles are predominantly supplied by the ulnar nerve (the median nerve supplies the thenar eminence), the inner cord of the brachial plexus, the T1 spinal root, and the anterior horn cells. Thus, lesions of these structures may all produce wasting of the small muscles of the hand:
- Lesions of the radial, median, and ulnar nerves (trauma)
- Brachial plexus (trauma, cervical lymph nodes, cervical ribs, tumour of superior sulcus of lung)
- Anterior root (cervical spondylosis)
- Anterior horn cell (motor neurone disease, tumours of spinal cord, syringomyelia, poliomyelitis).

CHAPTER 206

Long Thoracic Neuropathy

Instruction

This patient has difficult brushing their hair. Please inspect their back and proceed.

Salient Features

HISTORY

- Difficulty in raising the arms above the level of the shoulders leading to problems brushing hair and teeth, carrying shopping, and difficulties pushing or pulling objects
- Winging of the scapula
- Pain around scapula.

EXAMINATION

- Winging of the scapula (see Fig. 206.1)
- Difficulty in raising the arms above the horizontal: limited flexion and abduction.

Proceed as follows:

- Check whether the winging is unilateral or bilateral.
- Ask the patient to push the outstretched arm firmly against your hand and check whether or not the winging is more prominent.
- Weakness of the upper arm in a patchy distribution.
- Tell the examiner that you would like to examine the muscles in the arm to rule out muscular dystrophy.

Diagnosis

This patient has winging of the scapula (lesion) caused by palsy of the long thoracic nerve of Bell (aetiology).

Questions

Which nerve lesion is responsible for these signs?
Long thoracic nerve of Bell arising from the anterior rami of C5, C6, and C7. Treatment is conservative with physiotherapy as recovery may be spontaneous.

To what can long thoracic neuropathy be attributed?
Brachial plexus injury, trauma, or repetitive strain.

Which muscle is supplied by this nerve?
Serratus anterior.

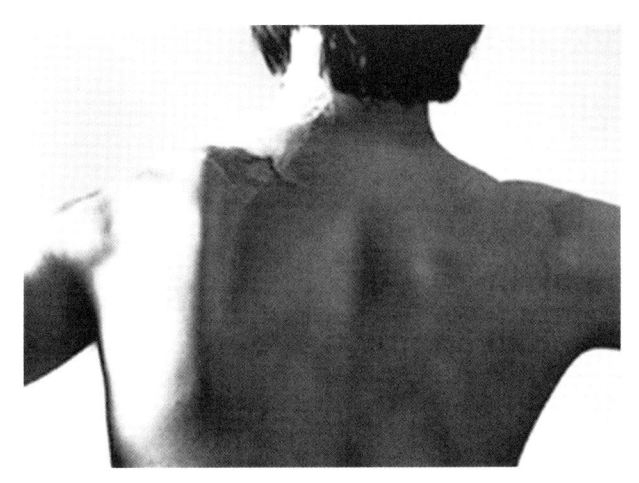

Fig. 206.1 Winging of the scapula.

What is the action of the serratus anterior?
It is responsible for the lateral and forward movement of the scapula, keeping it closely applied to the thorax.

Which other muscle palsies can cause winging of the scapula?
Paralysis of the trapezius—if conservative treatment does not improve symptoms, decompression of the spinal accessory nerve may be required.

Paralysis of the rhomboids—treatment is likewise mostly conservative with decompression of the dorsal scapular nerve an option in those with refractory symptoms.

How would you differentiate winging of the scapula caused by serratus anterior palsy from that of trapezius palsy?
In serratus anterior palsy, abduction of the arm laterally produces little winging of the scapula, whereas winging caused by weakness of the trapezius is intensified by abduction of the arm against resistance.

What do you know about brachial neuritis?
Brachial neuritis (neuralgic amyotrophy, Parsonage–Turner syndrome) often follows an infection or surgery. Diagnosis may be difficult initially when the patients have only pain. Later, the patients have muscular weakness, affecting particularly the deltoid and serratus anterior (winging of the scapula). Atrophy often becomes prominent. In this syndrome, there is often more than one lesion. The white cell count in the cerebrospinal fluid is occasionally raised. Recovery occurs over the next year and may not be complete.

Anxiety

Instruction

This lady presents with chronic anxiety and fatigue. Please examine her, paying particular attention to her mental state.

Salient Features

HISTORY

- Women more likely to be affected than men.
- Family history of mental health illness, especially major depression
- Substance use disorder
- Medically unexplained symptoms
- Chronic pain
- Restlessness
- Irritability and sleep disturbance
- Physical manifestation such as muscle tension, chronic headache, palpitations, abdominal pain, and hyperventilation.

EXAMINATION

- Physical examination to rule out primary endocrine disorder (e.g. thyroid swelling), cardiac disease, neurological disease, and respiratory pathology
- Mental State Examination
- Use *Diagnostic and Statistical Manual of Mental Disorders, Fifth Edition*, criteria to diagnose generalized anxiety disorder (GAD):
  - Excessive worry that is very challenging to control more often than not for at least 6 months

AND at least three of the following:
  - Restlessness
  - Fatigue
  - Impaired concentration
  - Irritability
  - Muscle soreness/ache
  - Sleep disturbance.

Diagnosis

This 37-year-old female presents with fatigue, chronic headache, and anxiety for 2 years (lesions) caused by GAD (aetiology). She is currently experiencing anxiety to the extent that she is unable to work (functional status).

739

Questions

Do you know of any screening tools that can be used in anxiety disorders?
The Generalized Anxiety Disorder seven-item scale can be used in primary care not only as a screening tool but also to track progress and response to treatment.

This scale assesses the incidence and prevalence of symptoms (feeling nervous or anxious, not being able to stop worrying, worrying too much about different things, trouble relaxing, restlessness stopping the patient sitting still, irritability, and feelings of fear/impending doom) over the previous 2 weeks.

The Hospital Anxiety and Depression Scale is a reliable and sensitive test that also quantifies depression risk.

How would you approach treating this patient?
Both pharmacotherapy and psychotherapy are important in treating this chronic disorder. Serotonergic medication including selective serotonin reuptake inhibitors (SSRIs) and serotonin noradrenaline reuptake inhibitors (SNRIs) are generally considered first-line medication for GAD.

Commonly used SSRIs are citalopram, escitalopram, sertraline, and paroxetine, with other SSRIs such as fluoxetine thought to have much the same efficacy. SNRIs include venlafaxine and duloxetine and are similarly effective in the treatment of GAD.

Pregabalin is now licensed for GAD and should be considered when other first-line medications have failed.

Other drugs that act on serotonergic receptors like buspirone are mostly used as adjunctive medication where maximum-dose SSRI medication has failed to adequately control symptoms.

Psychotherapy is mainly based on cognitive-behavioural therapy (CBT) principles but works best for those patients who are self-motivated so that they can actively use the techniques when on their own, without the presence of a trained therapist. Computer-based CBT has been found to be equally effective.

Patients are also taught relaxation techniques by first tensing all muscle groups in the body, then systematically relaxing specific muscle groups in a predefined order.

How would you manage sexual dysfunction in patients taking serotonin reuptake inhibitor medication for generalized anxiety disorder?
Sexual dysfunction is commonly seen with SSRI drugs and effects appear to be dose related.

Switching SSRI medication may help as the response appears to be governed by patients' genetic polymorphisms together with particular drugs.

Adjunctive antidepressant medication in the form of buspirone may help in female patients while male patients are often commenced on phosphodiesterase 5 (PDE5) inhibitors (sildenafil, tadalafil, vardenafil). Gingko biloba has been found to improve sexual symptoms in some patients taking SSRIs.

Exercise has shown benefit in patients with sexual dysfunction secondary to SSRIs.

It is true amongst all the research base for sexual dysfunction that women are less bothered by this side effect than men are, so are less likely to start or complete treatment cycles at the research phase, making statistical analysis challenging in this field of work.

CHAPTER 208

Back Pain

Instruction
Please assess this 56-year-old patient who complains of back pain.

Salient Features

HISTORY
- Trauma/fall—what was the mechanism of injury?
- Presence of rest pain or night pain (nonmechanical pain)
- Rule out red flags:
  - Profound neurological deficit
  - Systemic features—sweats/weight loss/fevers
  - Medication—prolonged steroid use
  - Patient age/frailty
  - History of cancer
  - History of injecting drug use.

EXAMINATION
- Control pain to allow examination.
- Examine the gait if the patient can walk.
- Examine spinal range of movement.
- Is the pain worse with flexion or extension?
- Look for swelling/bruising/bogginess of spine—could there be a fracture underneath?
- Conduct neurological assessment.
- Look for signs of incontinence—catheter/pads.
- Look for signs of arthritis, systemic illness (chronic or acute), and/or frailty.

Proceed as follows:
- Tell the examiner that you would like to complete a full neurological examination.

Diagnosis
This patient has low back pain radiating into the left leg with weakness on the same side (lesions), following a trip and fall at home (aetiology). They are currently unable to bear weight or walk (functional status).

Questions

What are the causes of back pain?
There are any number of conditions that can cause back pain. The task for the doctor is to elicit red-flag signs or symptoms that should prompt further investigation and treatment, sometimes on an emergency basis.

Most back pain is mechanical (97%), made worse by movement and eased by rest. Many cases have no clear aetiology.
- Lumbar sprain/strain—intense pain is caused by tearing of muscle fibres, followed by muscle spasm.
- Degenerative discs/facets—the disc is thought to be the primary pain source but facet joints and the sacroiliac joint are implicated too. Pain worse on flexion is likely discogenic, and pain worsened by extension is likely facet joint related.
- Herniated nucleus pulposus—leg pain (often dermatomal) > back pain. Exacerbated by straight leg raise. Back pain is caused by annulus tear.
- Spondylolisthesis—mainly low back pain that worsens and radiates to the leg with extension. Patients may have an exaggerated lumbar lordosis.
- Compression fracture—can occur in the absence of trauma. The patient workup should include assessment of bone quality and screening for malignancy.
- Spinal stenosis—anatomical narrowing of the spinal canal secondary to osteophytes and facet joint hypertrophy. The pain typically worsens with standing and walking and is accompanied by numbness or weakness of the leg, which settles on sitting.

A small subset of patients will have back pain caused by a systemic problem. These include the following:
- Infection: discitis, epidural abscess, osteomyelitis
- Malignancy
- Connective tissue disorder
- Inflammatory arthropathy: ankylosing spondylitis, psoriatic arthropathy, enteropathic arthritis.

Finally, there are a few patients who present with back pain as the primary symptom but are actually presenting with referred pain to the back. Conditions include the following:
- Genitourinary:
  - Kidney stones
  - Pyelonephritis
  - Pelvic infection.
- Gastrointestinal:
  - Cholecystitis
  - Pancreatitis
  - Peptic ulcer disease
  - Aortic aneurysm.

How common is back pain?

Back pain is one of the most common reasons for patients to consult with a doctor.

It has a prevalence of 30% in the adult population in developed countries, with annual incidence of around 15%. Back pain treatment alone costs the US $88 billion/year, with total burden to the UK economy estimated to be around £12 billion/year.

However, the outlook for most patients is good, with the vast majority of patients making a full recovery.

How would you investigate a patient with mechanical back pain?

The vast majority of patients with mechanical back pain will have nonspecific low back pain likely caused by a lumbar strain or sprain. The history and benign examination should point the clinician to this diagnosis and reassure that no further investigation is necessary. Recent British and American guidance is to avoid any imaging in those with nonspecific back pain.

Where imaging is being considered, this should be performed in a specialist setting. Those with signs suggestive of herniated nucleus pulposus or spinal stenosis should be assessed with magnetic resonance imaging as a first line. Patients with suspected compression fracture, spondylolisthesis, or degenerative discs and facet joint pathology should be assessed with X-rays initially.

Patients presenting with red-flag signs should be discussed with a specialist urgently to assess the need for emergency imaging and intervention.

Do you know of any risk stratification tools for chronic back pain?
The STarT Back Tool is a validated questionnaire used to stratify nonspecific back pain by prognosis and guide targeted intervention to reduce back pain–related disability.

It uses a biopsychosocial approach to identify modifiable risk factors and stratifies patients into three risk categories. Patients at moderate and high risk receive targeted physiotherapy and psychosocial support. This reflects the current evidence supporting nonpharmacological treatment and self-care of low back pain.

CHAPTER **209**

Pruritus

Instruction

This patient has developed an irritating itch; please examine her abdomen.

Salient Features

HISTORY

- Parts of body affected; localized versus generalized pruritus
- Timeline of symptoms; associations with specific environments or allergens
- Associated skin lesions
- Other members of the household affected by the same symptoms
- Presence of systemic symptoms; fevers, night sweats, weight loss
- Detailed medical history, including thyroid, liver, and renal disease
- Social history, including detailed travel history and sexual history
- Allergen exposure history; new environment, new detergents, pets at home, recent changes to medications

Associated symptoms in primary biliary cirrhosis (PBC):
- Fatigue: commonest symptom
- Lethargy and right upper quadrant pain (in 25%)
- Symptoms of hepatic decompensation (in 20%): jaundice, ascites, variceal haemorrhage
- Steatorrhoea.

EXAMINATION

With localized skin lesions: detailed examination of the lesion is appropriate, including skin biopsy if the diagnosis is not clear after history and examination.

In the presence of urticarial lesions or generalized urticarial rash: demonstration of dermographism is helpful.

In the absence of skin lesions: full clinical examination should take place with particular focus on findings of thyroid, liver, or renal disease.

Signs that are associated with PBC:
- Usually occurs in middle-aged women
- Clubbing
- Generalized pigmentation
- Xanthelasma (may occur at any stage but more common in advanced disease)
- Icterus
- Scratch marks
- Hepatosplenomegaly (common in early stages).

Proceed as follows:
- Look for xanthomata over joints, skin folds, and sites of trauma to the skin.
- Examine for clinical features of other autoimmune diseases, such as rheumatoid arthritis, dry mouth of Sjögren syndrome, systemic sclerosis, CREST syndrome, Hashimoto thyroiditis, and dermatomyositis.
- Check for proximal muscle weakness from osteomalacia.
- Examine for peripheral neuropathy.
- Tell the examiner that you would like to test for high serum levels of alkaline phosphatase and antimitochondrial antibodies (AMAs; present in 95% of patients, with M2 antibody being more specific; it is almost always negative in extrahepatic obstruction).

Diagnosis

This middle-aged woman has generalized pigmentation, jaundice, xanthelasmata, and pruritus with hepatosplenomegaly (lesions) caused by PBC (aetiology). She has liver cell failure as evidenced by the hepatic flap (functional status).

Questions

How does primary biliary cirrhosis present?
Classically, it presents with itching in a middle-aged woman. However, in 50% of cases, there may be no liver symptoms. There are four phases:

Asymptomatic with normal liver tests: Antibodies to pyruvate dehydrogenase complex (AMA) are detectable and about three-quarters develop symptoms of PBC in 2 years and 83% develop abnormal liver function tests at a median period of 5 years from first detection of AMA. Most patients have liver histology compatible with, or diagnostic for, PBC.

Asymptomatic with abnormal liver tests: Circulating AMAs are present. More than 50% have established fibrosis at diagnosis. Up to 80% of patients develop symptoms or signs of PBC during the first 5 years of follow-up. The median time from diagnosis to death is 8 to 12 years.

Symptomatic: Lethargy and pruritus are prominent and time to death or transplantation is 5 to 10 years.

Decompensated PBC: Signs include ascites, variceal haemorrhage, or jaundice. The mean time to death or transplantation is 3 to 5 years.

What diseases are associated with primary biliary cirrhosis?
- Common (up to 80%): sicca syndrome
- Frequent (~20%): arthralgia, lung fibrosis, Raynaud syndrome, sclerodactyly, thyroid disease
- Rare (<5%): Addison disease, glomerulonephritis, hypertrophic pulmonary osteoarthropathy, myasthenia gravis, systemic lupus erythematosus, thrombocytopenic purpura, vitiligo.

Is primary biliary cirrhosis associated with cancer?
It is estimated that patients with PBC have up to a nine-fold increased risk of hepatocellular carcinoma. The risk is higher for those who do not respond to ursodeoxycholic acid and those who have developed cirrhosis.

How would you investigate this patient?
- Liver function tests are normal in the presymptomatic stage; characteristically cholestatic pattern (raised alkaline phosphatase, 5-nucleotidase, and γ-glutamyltransferase) may be seen; serum aminotransferases may be slightly raised but rarely exceed five times the upper limit of normal.

- Hepatic synthetic function is well preserved until late stages; a prolonged prothrombin time may indicate malabsorption of vitamin K in cholestasis.
- Serum lipids: hypercholesterolaemia is common, lipoprotein lp(a) is low, high-density lipoprotein cholesterol is increased in the early stages but falls as the disease progresses.
- Immunological tests: immunoglobulin M (IgM) and IgG are elevated; complement activation occurs although C3 levels are normal; several antibodies are elevated but antibodies to components of the nuclear pore complex and AMA are very closely elevated with PBC. AMA is found in 96% of patients with PBC but the E2 subtype is specific to PBC. Autoimmune cholangitis is a variant of PBC that has characteristic histological features of PBC but is negative for AMA in serum. The AMA is directed against the mitochondrial pyruvate dehydrogenase complex.
- Histology identifies nonsuppurative destructive cholangitis or granulomatous cholangitis
- Abdominal ultrasound maybe normal in early stages, but in advanced PBC, features of cirrhosis will be seen.

What are the stages of primary biliary cirrhosis?
PBC is divided into four histologic stages:
1. Inflammation is localized to the portal triads
2. The number of normal bile ducts is reduced and inflammation extends beyond the portal triads into the surrounding parenchyma
3. Fibrous septa link adjacent portal triads
4. End-stage liver disease is characterized by frank cirrhosis with regenerative nodules.

Is liver biopsy necessary to confirm the diagnosis?
Although liver biopsy is routinely used to confirm the diagnosis, the need for this procedure for either diagnosis or prognosis is questionable. The very close association between histology and E2 AMA in PBC means that liver histology is not required unless clinical and serological features are equivocal. The presence of cirrhosis is of very little value in determining the prognosis, and clinically significant portal hypertension (ascites, variceal haemorrhage) may occur during the early histological stages.

What is the mechanism for itching in these patients?
The exact pathogenesis of pruritus in cholestasis is not fully understood. The symptom of pruritus needs specific mediators to be released in order for signal transmission to take place and the symptom to develop. In dermatological conditions, for example in urticaria, histamine can be the mediator. The mediator in cholestasis was traditionally believed to be bile, so the itching used to be ascribed to retention of bile acids with cholestasis. More recent work emphasized the importance of naturally occurring opioid tone, characterized by an increase in the concentration of endogenous opioid receptors and upregulation of opioid receptors. Endogenous serotonin may also be involved. These findings led to the use of opioid antagonists for treatment of pruritus. Autotaxin and lysophosphatidic acid have also been proposed as pruritus mediators.

How do you treat pruritus?
Treatment of pruritus comprises a combination of topical and systemic treatment. In the case of localized disease, topical treatment with emollients and skin moisturizers and topical application of corticosteroids, antihistamines, and capsaicin or calamine lotion are first line. These therapies can be combined with systemic treatments like oral antihistamines. In cholestasis, ursodeoxycholic acid is first-line, cholestyramine and rifampicin are second-line, and naloxone and sertraline are third-line agents used to treat pruritus.

What do you know of phototherapy for controlling pruritus?
Phototherapy has been used in pruritus, with varied results, and is reserved for patients who cannot tolerate medical therapy.

What drugs have been used to treat primary biliary cirrhosis?
Ursodeoxycholic acid should be used, including for those with asymptomatic disease. For those with a suboptimal response, corticosteroids may be tried. Other immunosuppressants and colchicine are no longer recommended.

What is the rationale behind bile salt therapy?
Hepatocytes affected by autoimmune processes are further injured by endogenous bile acids (such as chenodeoxycholic acid and cholic acid), which accumulate as a result of associated cholestasis. Partial replacement of water-soluble bile acids such as ursodeoxycholic acid may reduce pruritus and damage to the liver cell.

Is there a cure for primary biliary cirrhosis?
Liver transplantation is the only known cure. The 5-year survival following transplantation exceeds 80%. It is associated with a rapid resolution of lethargy and itching, and bone loss slows after the first year. Although the quality of life is not normal, it is usually excellent. Disease recurrence has been seen in 18%.

When is liver transplantation indicated?
Indications for liver transplantation are either symptoms (e.g. intractable pruritus, lethargy) or signs and symptoms of end-stage liver disease: increasing jaundice with serum bilirubin >170 μmol/L, estimated survival <1 year, intractable ascites, encephalopathy, fasting serum albumin (<30 g/L), progressive muscle loss, recurrent spontaneous bacterial peritonitis, increasing osteoporosis, hepatopulmonary syndrome, early incidental hepatocellular carcinoma, and unacceptable quality of life.

What factors predict survival after transplantation?
- Serum urea and albumin
- Presence of ascites
- Child's grade and United Network for Organ Sharing status (reflecting whether the patient is at home, general hospital bed or intensive care unit).

What do you understand by secondary biliary cirrhosis?
It occurs secondary to large duct obstruction and is usually caused by extrahepatic obstruction such as bile duct stricture, gallstones and sclerosing cholangitis.

Further Information
Professor Peter Brunt, gastroenterologist and liver physician, Aberdeen Royal Infirmary, was also the personal physician to the Queen and an astute clinician. He was president of the Association of Physicians of Great Britain, a society founded by Osler.

Roger Williams, Professor at King's College, London, and Sir Roy Calne, Professor of Surgery, Cambridge, pioneered liver transplantation in the United Kingdom.

CHAPTER 210

Speech Disturbance

Instruction

This patient's relatives are having trouble understanding his speech. Please assess further.

Salient Features

HISTORY

- Is the difficulty in finding the correct word (dysphasia) or with speaking itself (dysarthria)?
- Take a history of the change in speech. Is it:
  - acute or over months
  - hoarse voice
  - slurred or nasal sounding or 'gurgly'
  - excessively loud or quiet or monotone
  - hesitant?
- Is there difficulty moving the tongue or lips?
- Is there difficulty with swallowing? Is there associated drooling?
- Other neurological symptoms
- History of stroke or neurodegenerative disorders
- How are the difficulties impacting on communication, social interactions? Check for coexisting depression.
- Medication history: sedatives and analgesics, including opiates.

EXAMINATION

- Full neurological examination, looking for evidence of stroke, cerebral palsy, bulbar or pseudobulbar palsy, Parkinson disease, head injury, myasthenia gravis
- Ensure that dentures fit correctly (common cause of dysarthria).
- Ask the person to say:
  - Baby hippopotamus, British constitution, or West Register Street: these can accentuate dysarthria.
- Check for expressive and receptive dysphasia.
- Check for ability to name common objects such as pen and watch.
- In an older person, offer to complete a cognitive assessment.

Diagnosis

This person has a quiet monotone voice due to Parkinson disease (aetiology), which is impacting on his ability to communicate with his friends and family, leading to social isolation (functional status).

Questions

What investigations would you perform?
- Computed tomography or magnetic resonance imaging (MRI) of the head, looking for evidence of infarcts: the most common area of infarct causing dysarthria is in the corona radiata, followed by the pons, internal capsule, cerebellum, middle cerebral artery territory, frontal region, thalamus, and striatocapsular junction.
- In dysphasia, functional MRI remains a primarily research-based tool but may progress to a tool in rehabilitation, particularly as transcranial direct current stimulation is researched as an additional treatment of post-stroke aphasia.
- 18-Fluorodeoxyglucose positron emission tomography can be used to diagnose primary progressive aphasia. Reduced glucose uptake is seen in the language regions, including frontotemporal areas.

What different types of dysarthria do you know about?
- Ataxic: seen in cerebellar conditions
- Flaccid: seen in bulbar palsy; signs include nasal regurgitation, tongue fasciculation, and loss of gag reflex. Caused by bilateral lower motor neuron lesions of cranial nerves IX, X, XII.
- Hyperkinetic: seen in dystonic conditions
- Hypokinetic: seen in parkinsonism
- Spastic: seen in pseudobulbar palsy: signs include nasal speech often known as 'Donald Duck' or 'hot potato' speech, positive jaw jerk and bilateral upper motor neuron signs. Caused by bilateral upper motor neuron lesions, such as stroke.
- Mixed (any combination of the previous types)
- Mechanical causes such as ill-fitting dentures.

What are the different types of dysphasia?
- Expressive dysphasia: failure of speech content and expression, including the inability to name familiar objects such as pen and clock despite knowing what they are. Caused by lesion, usually stroke, in the dominant hemisphere in Broca's area of the frontoparietal lobe.
- Receptive dysphasia: failure of integration of hearing and speech, leading to inability to understand speech. Lesion in Wernicke's area in the dominant hemisphere in the temporoparietal lobe.
- Aphasia: inability to express thoughts through language. Caused by lesions in multiple language areas. Aphasia can improve poststroke but if not can lead to severe disability. Important to note that cognition can be preserved.
- Primary progressive aphasia: slow and progressive impairment of speech and language caused by neurodegenerative conditions such as Alzheimer disease and frontotemporal dementia. Symptoms may start with impaired word finding and progress through non-fluency through to becoming mute.

What is the role of speech and language therapists?
- Aid with diagnosis
- Advise on strategies to improve dysarthria, including slowing speech and increasing volume or clarity
- Support with assistive devices
- Assess swallow and advise on modifications to diet and fluids to reduce aspiration risk.

What communication aids do you know?
- Alphabet board
- Word or picture chart
- Amplifiers
- Computerized voice output system.

If someone has dysarthria, suggest simple ways you can optimize communication on the ward or in clinic.
- Reduce background noise and distractions.
- Look at the person as he or she talks.
- Allow the person plenty of time; the dysarthria may worsen if he or she feels rushed or anxious.
- Don't try and finish their sentences.
- Be honest if you don't understand; seek clarification if necessary using yes/no questions.

CHAPTER 211

Unsteadiness

Instruction

This man presents with feelings of unsteadiness. Take a history and perform a focused examination.

Salient Features

HISTORY

- Distinguish between vertigo and light-headedness. Vertigo is sensation of movement, often the room spinning. Light-headedness relates to a sensation of imbalance or presyncope and may be described as 'wooziness or giddiness'.
- Establish if it is associated with change in position or posture.
- Any associated hearing or visual loss
- Any change in speech or strength in arms, legs, or face
- Any episodes of transient loss of consciousness or falls? Are they related to meals, micturition, coughing?
- Is it acute or chronic?
- Vascular risk factors or known disease.

EXAMINATION

- Cranial nerves, including tests of hearing and vision
- For cerebellar signs, including nystagmus, dysarthria, and ataxia
- Balance
- Check for postural hypotension.
- Cardiovascular system for arrhythmia or aortic stenosis. Consider carotid sinus massage.

Diagnosis

This gentleman presents with acute vestibular neuronitis (lesion) caused by a viral infection (aetiology) and currently needs assistance to stand (functional status).

Questions

What are the common causes of vertigo?
Lesions of the inner ear, eighth nerve, or vestibular system.
- Benign paroxysmal positional vertigo (BPPV): free-floating debris accumulates in the semicircular canals in the labyrinthine structures of the inner ear. This leads to inappropriate activation of the sensory structures within the canals during specific movements such as rolling over in bed or looking up to pull curtains. Symptoms include acute episodes of short-lived spinning sensations, which may be associated with nausea and vomiting.

- Ménière disease: the cause is unknown but may be related to poor drainage of the endolymph system, viral infection, or allergy or head injury. It results in intermittent attacks of vertigo lasting over 20 min associated with unilateral tinnitus and hearing deficit.
- Vestibular neuronitis: viral infection of vestibular pathway causes acute vertigo with nausea, vomiting, and ataxia. Symptoms last a few days to weeks with varying severity.
- Acoustic neuroma (cerebellopontine angle tumours): compression of the eighth cranial nerve leads to unilateral sensorineural hearing loss. There may be associated facial numbness if the trigeminal nerve is also affected. Vertigo may be a late feature. Investigate with magnetic resonance imaging (MRI) and refer to ear, nose, and throat (ENT).
- Brainstem vascular disease: vertigo in isolation is rarely caused by a cerebral vascular event but if associated with neurological signs including dysarthria, nystagmus, ataxia, and possibly sensory or motor signs may be due to a stroke. Vertebrobasilar insufficiency is due to a transient compromise of the anterior cerebral circulation resulting in the aforementioned acute onset symptoms. MRI is usually required to investigate both conditions. After a brainstem stroke, some people can develop a chronic sensation of dizziness unaffected by posture. This is often debilitating with no effective treatment. Vascular risk factors should be managed.

What are the clinical signs in vestibular neuronitis?
- Nystagmus is usually horizontal with the fast phase beating away from the affected side.
- Positive head impulse test
- On examination of gait with closed eyes, the patient may sway towards the affected side.
- Possible hearing loss on the affected side in viral labyrinthitis.

How can clinical examination help you distinguish vestibular neuronitis from a cerebellar cause of vertigo?
Nystagmus originating from the periphery is suppressed with visual fixation. Also, patients with vestibular neuronitis will have a positive head impulse test. Cerebellar events on the other hand will be accompanied by cerebellar signs on examination (dysdiadochokinesia, past-pointing, dysarthria). If clinically the distinction between a cerebellar stroke or a peripheral cause of vertigo is not apparent, the patient should undergo brain imaging to rule out a possible central cause for their symptoms.

Name other causes of unsteadiness.
- Medication:
    - Ototoxic medications can cause vertigo. Common drugs include gentamicin, furosemide, quinine, and nonsteroidal antiinflammatory drugs.
    - Antihypertensives, antidepressants, opiates, and levodopa can cause postural hypotension.
- Anxiety may present with a feeling of dizziness generally not affected by movement.
- Cardiac arrhythmias: brady- and tachy-arrhythmias can cause reduced cerebral perfusion leading to a sensation of 'light-headedness'.
- Any visual problem; vision is required to help maintain awareness of the position of the body.
- Peripheral neuropathy can lead to a disruption in proprioception and consequent postural instability.
- Joint diseases, myopathy, and sarcopenia can lead to instability and, therefore, a feeling of unsteadiness.

In older people, the cause is often multifactorial due to dysfunction in multiple systems. Optimizing each problem may be required.

Occupational therapists can assist in improving home environment to provide grab rails, perching stools, decluttering, etc. Physiotherapists can assist in gait and balance retraining, as well as strength training to improve muscle mass and stability.

How do you diagnose and treat benign paroxysmal positional vertigo?

Diagnosis is through the Dix–Hallpike test, which is 50% to 80% sensitive. Stand behind the patient and firmly hold their head between your hands 45 degrees to the affected side. Smoothly lie them down so the head is 30 degrees below the level of the couch looking down to the floor. Look for nystagmus towards the floor, which stops after less than 30 s and ask about symptoms.

If Dix–Hallpike test is positive, proceed to the Epley manoeuvre, a series of movements that transfer the debris in the semicircular canals into the utricle, away from the sensory hair cells. Up to one-third may recur; these people may benefit from Brandt–Daroff exercises at home or via a specialist physiotherapist.

What medications may be used in the treatment of vertigo?

Any causative medications should be stopped in the first instance. Symptoms of vertigo can be very difficult to treat, but histamine receptor antagonists including cyclizine and betahistine may be useful in the acute situation, although not for BPPV. However, if used long-term, they can paradoxically worsen symptoms. Prochlorperazine or benzodiazepines may also be tried in the short-term.

Some people who develop chronic vestibular neuronitis may benefit from vestibular rehabilitation exercises by physiotherapists or ENT nurses, designed to retrain the vestibular system.

How do you use nystagmus to differentiate lesions?

- Horizontal nystagmus: fast phase in direction away from affected side in labyrinthine lesions
- Vertical nystagmus: vertical with rotatory component in cerebellar lesions
- A peripheral nystagmus can be suppressed by visual fixation.

Further Information

Prosper Ménière (1799–1862), a French doctor, first described the classic triad of symptoms in 1861 after working at the Imperial Institute for Deaf-Mutes where he focused on diseases of the ear. He trained under Dupuytren.

SECTION XI

Acute Internal Medical Cases

SECTION OUTLINE

212 Absent Radial Pulse
213 Confusion
214 Acute Kidney Injury
215 Acute Pancreatitis
216 Anaphylaxis
217 Chest Pain—Angina
218 Cauda Equina Syndrome
219 Cellulitis
220 Coarctation of Aorta
221 Deep Vein Thrombosis
222 Gallop Rhythm
223 Guillain–Barré Syndrome
224 Hyperkalaemia
225 Hypernatraemia
226 Hypokalaemia
227 Hyponatraemia
228 Melaena
229 Paracetamol Overdose
230 Pericardial Rub
231 Pleural Effusion
232 Sepsis
233 Consolidation
234 Pulmonary Embolism
235 Jugular Venous Pulse

236 Seizures
237 Painful Knee Joint
238 Slow Pulse Rate
239 Spontaneous Pneumothorax
240 Subacute Combined Degeneration of the Spinal Cord
241 Subarachnoid Haemorrhage
242 Syncope
243 The Pregnant Patient
244 Central Line Insertion
245 Chest Drain Insertion for Spontaneous (Nontraumatic) Pneumothorax
246 Emergency Synchronized Direct Current Cardioversion
247 Knee Arthrocentesis
248 Lumbar Puncture
249 Therapeutic Abdominal Paracentesis
250 Temporary External Pacing

CHAPTER 212

Absent Radial Pulse

Instruction
Examine this patient's pulses.

Salient Features
HISTORY
- History of insertion of an arterial line for blood gases or arterial pressure monitoring
- Systemic symptoms in the past (Takayasu's arteritis)
- History of cardiac surgery (Blalock–Taussig shunt)
- History of severe heart failure and previous cardiac surgery
- Cervical rib.

EXAMINATION
- Start with left and right radial pulses, examine for delays or differences in volume, and establish that there is indeed a pulse.
- Examine all other pulses (including carotid, brachial, femoral, popliteal, posterior tibial, and dorsalis pedis pulses).
- Check the blood pressure (BP) in both the upper limbs (differences in BP between both arms of >10 mm Hg systolic or 5 mm Hg diastolic are abnormal).

Diagnosis
This patient has an absent radial pulse (lesion) that is caused by a previous Blalock–Taussig shunt (aetiology).

Questions

In which conditions may the pulse rate in one arm differ from that in the other?
Usually, slowing of the pulse on one side occurs distal to an aneurysmal sac. Therefore, an aneurysm of the transverse or descending aortic arch causes a retardation of the left radial pulse. Also, the artery feels smaller and is more easily compressed than usual. An aneurysm of the ascending aorta or common carotid artery may result in similar changes in the right radial pulse.

What are the causes of absent radial pulse?
- Aberrant radial artery or congenital anomaly (check the brachial pulse and BP)
- Tied off at surgery or previous surgical cut-down
- Catheterization of the brachial artery with poor technique
- Following a radial artery line for monitoring of blood gases or arterial pressure
- Subclavian artery stenosis

- Blalock–Taussig shunt on that side (shunt from subclavian to pulmonary artery)
- Embolism into the radial artery (usually caused by atrial fibrillation)
- Takayasu's arteritis (rare).

What are the causes of differences in blood pressure between arms or between the arms and legs?
- Occlusion or stenosis of the artery of any cause
- Coarctation of the aorta
- Dissecting aortic aneurysm
- Patent ductus arteriosus
- Supravalvular aortic stenosis
- Thoracic outlet syndrome.

What is Adson's test?
The clinician palpates the radial pulse and abducts the arm slightly (Fig. 212.1). The clinician asks the patient to hyperextend the neck and turn it to the affected side and inhale deeply. Adson's test is positive if the patient reports paraesthesia or if the pulse fades away. Diminution or obliteration of the pulse is caused by compression of the axillary artery by the anterior scalene muscle. The patient should turn the head to the opposite side (reverse Adson's test) to test the compressive effect of the middle scalene.

What do you know about Takayasu's arteritis?
It tends to affect young women, and most of the cases have been reported in Japan. Prodromal systemic symptoms include fever, night sweats, anorexia, weight loss, malaise, fatigue, arthralgia, and pleuritic pain. It predominantly involves the aorta and is of three types: type I (Shimizu–Sano),

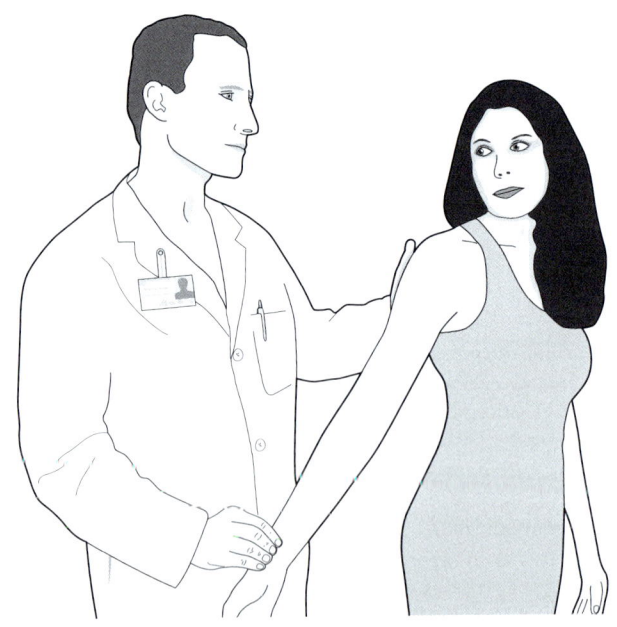

Fig. 212.1 Adson's test. Hold the patient's arm in slight abduction while palpating the radial pulse. Ask the patient to extend the neck and rotate toward the affected side. Adson's test is positive if the patient reports paraesthesia or if the pulse fades away.

212—ABSENT RADIAL PULSE

which involves primarily the aortic arch and brachiocephalic vessels; type II (Kimoto), which affects the thoracoabdominal aorta and particularly the renal arteries; and type III (Inada), which has features of types I and III. Types I and III may be complicated by aortic regurgitation.

What is the Allen test?

The Allen test is used to determine the patency of the radial or ulnar artery (Fig. 212.2). To perform an Allen test, both the radial and the ulnar arteries should be occluded while the patient elevates the hand and makes fist. The patient extends the fingers and blanching of the hand is seen. When the radial artery alone is released, the colour of the hand returns to normal. An abnormal test result occurs when the colour of the hand does not return within 5 to 10 s. In thrombosis of

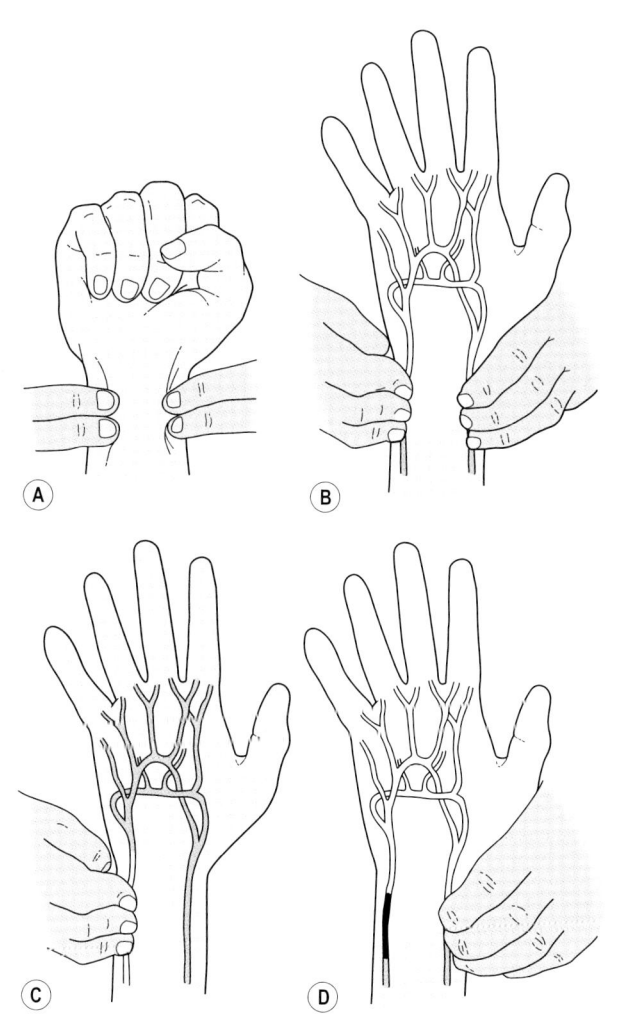

Fig. 212.2 Allen test for patency of radial and ulnar arteries. **(A)** Both the radial and the ulnar arteries are occluded while the patient elevates the hand and makes a fist; **(B)** blanching can be seen with both arteries occluded; **(C)** releasing the radial artery alone returns the hand colour to normal; **(D)** if the ulnar artery alone is released, the hand remains blanched if there is thrombosis of the ulnar artery.

the ulnar artery, the hand remains blanched when this artery alone is released. The Allen test can be used before puncturing the radial artery for cannulation as it is important to identify a competent ulnar artery should injury to the radial artery occur.

What is the cause of absent pulses everywhere in an ambulatory patient as above?
The patient may have a left ventricular assist device, which produces continuous flow and as such does not produce a palpable pulse.

What other physical findings can accompany a patient with a left ventricular assist device?
- Absent pulse
- Small pulse pressure or unrecordable BP
- Non-distinguishable heart sounds
- Continuous hum of the assist device on cardiac auscultation.

Further Information

M. Takayasu (1860–1938), Japanese ophthalmologist.

CHAPTER 213

Confusion

Instruction

This patient was brought by ambulance to the hospital this morning accompanied by her daughter, who feels her mother is 'not quite right'. Please take a history, examine the patient, and advise on further management.

Salient Features

HISTORY

- Acute change in behaviour, cognition, and/or perception
- Hyperactive type: heightened arousal, agitation, aggression, restless, walking with purpose
- Hypoactive type: withdrawn, quiet, reduced oral intake, decreased responsiveness, slowed motor skills
- Mixed type: mix of hyperactive and hypoactive symptoms
- Disturbed sleep–wake cycle
- Delusions and disorientation
- Inappropriate behaviour or emotional lability
- Psychomotor disturbance
- Any new medication
- Presence of pain
- Recent surgery or illness
- Any change in environment.

EXAMINATION

- Older person: much more common in those aged over 65 years
- Glasgow Coma Scale
- Top-to-toe examination to look for potential precipitants or causes, including the following:
  - Evidence of recent surgery
  - Signs of Parkinson disease or previous stroke, which are predisposing factors
  - Presence of indwelling catheter
  - Signs of infection, pain, constipation, malnutrition, urinary retention.
- Look for hearing and vision aids, if absent may be exacerbating symptoms.

Diagnosis

This female aged in her 70s with mild cognitive impairment presents with agitation and aggression (lesion), caused by a urinary tract infection (aetiology). She is currently shouting inappropriately and has had an episode of urinary incontinence (functional status).

Questions

What is delirium?

An acute syndrome characterized by disturbed consciousness, attention, or cognition. It usually develops over days and has a fluctuating course. Also known as 'acute confusional state', it can be considered acute brain failure and should be treated as a medical emergency. It usually affects vulnerable patients with multiple predisposing factors, which interact with exposure to noxious insults or precipitants. These interactions are complex and not fully understood.

Precipitants include physical restraints, urinary catheterization, infection, metabolic disturbance, immobility, malnutrition, surgery, trauma, urgent admission, and drugs, including polypharmacy.

How might people with delirium present?
- Any change in behaviour; the collateral history from family or carers is vital in the diagnosis of delirium.
- Loss of mental clarity, distractibility, hallucinations, often with lack of insight
- Behaviour change is often worse at night.
- Loss of ability to write or speak a second language
- Altered perception of simple shapes or faces.

What investigations would you do?

Initial investigations are based on looking for a precipitating cause:
- Bloods: look for raised inflammatory markers, electrolyte disturbance, acute kidney or liver injury, hypo- or hyperthyroidism, B_{12} deficiency.
- Electrocardiogram: look for signs of acute myocardial infarction and heart block.
- Chest X-ray: look for precipitants.
- Microbiology: cultures for infection based on history and examination.

Younger patients will need brain imaging and electroencephalography. Subsequent investigations will be decided according to history, examination, and the results of the initial tests. Other indications for brain imaging are new focal neurological signs, history of head injury or falls, or evidence of raised intracranial pressure.

What is the management?

The priorities of managing a patient with confusion are:
- Maintaining patient safety by reducing harm
- Identifying and treating precipitants
- Managing symptoms.

Nonpharmacological management techniques include the following:
- Maintaining nutrition and hydration
- Encouraging family involvement such as reassurance, touch, meaningful activities
- Addressing sensory impairment but avoid overstimulation
- Reorientation
- Maintaining safe mobility
- Encouraging self-care
- Regular nonconfrontational communication
- Normalizing sleep–wake cycle
- Quiet, warm, soothing environment: difficult to achieve in hospitals!

If the patient is severely agitated interrupting essential treatment, or displaying severe psychotic symptoms, pharmacological management may be required in the short-term. The principles of starting low and going slow apply to avoid oversedation. Haloperidol or risperidone are first line in these cases (but should be avoided in those with Parkinson disease and Lewy body dementia), under guidance from the mental health team. If the patient requires rapid sedation due to risk of harm to themselves or others, then benzodiazepines such as lorazepam may be used. However, their use may prolong the episode of delirium so should be used with caution.

Recent studies have shown no benefit from cholinesterase inhibitors, which actually increased the duration of confusion and also mortality. There are ongoing studies around use of antiinflammatories and neuroprotective agents in treatment and prevention of delirium.

Why is recognizing delirium important?
Patients who develop delirium have worse outcomes including increased length of stay, increased mortality, and increased hospital-associated harm such as falls and pressure sores. If recognized early and multifactorial interventions started, delirium can be reduced. There is an association between delirium and subsequent dementia. The development of delirium is also associated with increased likelihood of admission to a care home.

Distinguishing between dementia and delirium can be challenging. They can coexist. If there is any doubt, the patient should be treated for delirium in the first instance.

Tools to help confirm the diagnosis include the Confusion Assessment Method. Diagnosis of delirium requires 1 + 2 and either 3 or 4:
1. Acute onset and fluctuating course
2. Inattention: are they easily distractible, e.g. unable to count from 20 to 1?
3. Disorganized thinking
4. Altered level of consciousness: hyperalert (vigilant) or hypoalert (lethargic, sleepy).

How common is delirium?
- On medical wards in hospital, the prevalence of delirium is 20% to 30%.
- Some 10% to 50% of people having surgery develop delirium.
- In long-term care, the prevalence is under 20%.
- Between 30% and 40% is felt to be preventable.

What is the 4AT tool?
The 4AT tool is a quick and simple validated bedside screening tool used to help acute services and clinicians of all levels screen for delirium on a daily basis, highly specific (96%) and highly sensitive (75%) for the diagnosis of delirium. Four elements are assessed [attention, alertness, Abbreviated Mental Test 4 (AMT4), evidence of fluctuation in alertness and cognition].

What is the pathophysiology of delirium?
The exact pathophysiology is unknown, but neuronal networks are interrupted causing disturbance of global cognitive function. Neurotransmitters involved include reduced levels of acetylcholine, with excess dopamine, serotonin, and γ-aminobutyric acid. Melatonin is also disturbed. Proinflammatory markers including interferon α and β; interleukins 6, 8, and 10; tumour necrosis factor α; and prostaglandin E are also implicated. Physiological stressors such as cortisol and hypoxia also have a role.

Does delirium cause dementia?
- The development of delirium can unmask previously unrecognized dementia in someone who may have been compensating for their progressive cognitive decline.
- Delirium is associated with accelerated cognitive decline.
- In most instances, delirium resolves over days to weeks. Occasionally, it can take months. For some, it can result in permanent cognitive impairment. One study found an eight-fold increased risk of this occurring.

What do you know about anticholinergic burden?
The following table shows commonly prescribed drugs with high anticholinergic activity. The list is not exhaustive. Taking these medications regularly increases risk of confusion and is dose dependent. Efforts should be made to reduce the burden and use alternatives with less anticholinergic activity.

Lower	*Moderate*	*Higher*
Haloperidol	Cetirizine	Amitriptyline
Olanzapine	Loratadine	Oxybutynin
Mirtazapine	Loperamide	Chlorpheniramine
Paroxetine	Solifenacin	Hydroxyzine
Trazodone	Tolterodine	Chlorpromazine
Ranitidine	Baclofen	Imipramine
Atenolol	Nortriptyline	
Codeine	Clozapine	
Morphine	Nifedipine	

What do you know of transient global amnesia?
Transient global amnesia is a syndrome affecting mainly older adults with cardiovascular risk factors. Patients present with acute onset of anterograde amnesia with all other cognitive functions being normal. Patients have an otherwise normal neurology and the only sign identified on examination is their inability to form new memories. Characteristically patients will be scared when brought to a hospital as they will be forgetting over and over again why they have changed environment and some may complain of a headache. The symptoms resolve after some hours and patients go back to normal with no recollection of the events during the acute episode. Pharmacological treatment is not needed and no intervention is indicated for this condition.

What is limbic encephalitis?
Limbic encephalitis is a clinical syndrome that presents with acute onset of memory loss, behavioural changes, and cognitive impairment. It is a manifestation of antibodies against the limbic system, more commonly associated with either underlying malignancy or autoimmune encephalitis. Patients are usually brought by family members, with a history of acute change in behaviour over the course of a few days prior to the admission. On examination they are cognitively impaired, with most modalities of cognition being affected. There is no history of psychiatric history or previous episodes. Magnetic resonance imaging (MRI) of the brain often reveals the affected areas, mostly the temporal lobes. Diagnosis is confirmed with detection of the responsible antibodies in the patient's cerebrospinal fluid (CSF). Electroencephalogram (EEG) will show slow activity on the temporal lobes. Treatment consists of immunosuppression.

CHAPTER 214

Acute Kidney Injury

Instruction

This patient presented with deterioration in renal function after running a marathon in hot weather. Please assess further.

Salient Features

HISTORY

- Preceding symptoms to suggest volume loss (diarrhoea, vomiting)
- Muscle pain, weakness, dark urine (the history given can be suspicious for rhabdomyolysis)
- Fever, pain, general deterioration, organ specific enquiry (to look for potential sepsis and source)
- History of diabetes, hypertension, scleroderma, malignancy (all can be complicated with acute kidney injury or hide an underlying cause of acute kidney injury)
- Symptoms related to possible small vessel vasculitis (e.g. skin rash)
- Symptoms of hypercalcaemia in multiple myeloma
- Drug history for nephrotoxic medications or toxins
- History of recent myocardial infarction or scanning for contrast nephropathy.

EXAMINATION

- Pallor from bleeding or haemolysis
- Hypertension in malignant hypertension or renovascular disease
- Neurological signs leading to stupor and coma in severe uraemia, electrolyte abnormalities, diabetic ketoacidosis with severe dehydration or thrombotic thrombocytopenic purpura (TTP)
- Hypotension in hypovolaemia or sepsis or low cardiac output
- Dehydration in hypovolaemia or oedema and ascites and pulmonary oedema in cardiorenal syndrome
- Oliguria or anuria
- Urine dipstick for proteinuria and haematuria.

Diagnosis

This young patient presents with lethargy, reduced urine output and confusion (lesions) caused by prerenal acute kidney injury secondary to hypovolaemia (aetiology). Following aggressive fluid challenge, they have regained a normal level of cognition (functional status).

Questions

How is acute kidney injury staged following the KDIGO (Kidney Disease – Improving Global Outcomes) criteria?
- Stage 1—Increase in serum creatinine 1.5 to 1.9 times baseline or reduction in urine output to <0.5 mL/kg/hour for 6 to 12 hours
- Stage 2—Increase in serum creatinine 2.0 to 2.9 times baseline or reduction in urine output to <0.5 mL/kg/hour for ≥12 hours
- Stage 3—Increase in serum creatinine 3.0 times baseline or reduction in urine output to <0.3 mL/kg/hour for ≥24 hours, or anuria for ≥12 hours, or the initiation of kidney replacement therapy.

How can causes of acute kidney injury be classified?
The causes of acute kidney injury can be divided into:
- Prerenal (hypovolaemia, decreased cardiac output, haemorrhage, diarrhoea and vomiting, burns, dehydration, contrast induced)
- Intrinsic renal (nephrotoxic drugs, interstitial nephritis, acute tubular necrosis, drug related, scleroderma, lupus nephritis, toxins, rhabdomyolysis, tumour lysis syndrome, TTP, haemolytic uraemic syndrome (HUS), atheroembolic disease, small vessel vasculitis)
- Postrenal (renal stones, bladder outflow obstruction from prostate enlargement, bladder and colon malignancy).

What are the indications for renal replacement therapy and haemofiltration in the context of acute kidney injury?
- Pulmonary oedema
- Uraemic pericarditis
- Severe hyperkalaemia refractory to medical treatment
- Severe metabolic acidosis that cannot be corrected with hydration
- Acute overdose of medications that can be cleared by haemofiltration (e.g. aspirin)
- Uraemic coma.

How can acute uraemia be distinguished from chronic uraemia?
History, current and previous blood tests and kidney ultrasound can help distinguish acute from chronic kidney uraemia. An abrupt rise in serum creatinine, for example in the context of a 3-day history of diarrhoea and vomiting, signifies acute kidney injury with a likely prerenal cause. Acute kidney injury is not expected to be accompanied by anaemia, unless it is caused by acute haemolysis or severe haemorrhage. Acute electrolyte disturbances, such as hyponatraemia, hypernatraemia, and hyperkalaemia, are more likely to occur with acute kidney injury. In contrast, chronic renal failure is more associated with hyperphosphataemia. Chronic kidney disease is often associated with a normocytic normochromic anaemia. Signs of renal osteodystrophy are indicative of chronic renal failure. Kidney ultrasound can also guide towards distinction between the two conditions. Small kidneys with increased echogenicity are usually seen in chronic renal failure (with the exception of diabetes and amyloidosis).

How is prerenal acute kidney injury treated?
The initial step is to assess whether the patient needs emergency renal replacement therapy. If this is not the case and the patient is fluid depleted, then rehydration should start as soon as possible with a rate that is appropriate to the patient's clinical condition. Initial resuscitation in hypovolaemic shock should be with aggressive fluid boluses with continuous monitoring of response. Thereafter, patient-specific replacement of fluid should take into account all fluid losses including

insensible loss. All patients should have strict input and output documented with the aim of positive balance and close monitoring of the renal function and electrolytes. A urine dipstick should be obtained and all nephrotoxic medications should be discontinued. If acidosis is severe but the patient does not need urgent renal replacement, therapy sodium bicarbonate should be given. In hypervolaemic patients, for example patients with cardiorenal syndrome, then diuretics may be needed to increase the renal perfusion and reverse the acute kidney injury. If a patient is hypervolemic and not anuric then high doses of intravenous loop diuretics should be used, alone or in combination with thiazide diuretics. Hyperkalaemia should be treated promptly. Nutritional support is extremely important for these acutely unwell patients, as acute kidney injury is associated with a variety of electrolyte imbalances.

How can ischaemic tubular necrosis be prevented?
The first step to prevent acute ischaemic tubular necrosis and subsequent acute kidney injury is to identify patients who are at risk of developing the condition. Once patients are identified (sepsis, hypovolaemic, undergoing major surgery, burns), then optimization of fluid status and avoiding nephrotoxins are the key to preventing acute kidney injury.

Name some factors that play a pathophysiological role in acute tubular necrosis.
- Impaired intrarenal vasodilation and increased vasoconstriction
- Increased leucocyte adhesion to endothelium with obstruction and inflammation
- Tubular cell necrosis or apoptosis due to casts, ischaemia or reperfusion after initial ischaemia, increased intracellular proteases, hypoxia, and increase of nitric oxide
- Back leak of filtrate fluid due to loss of function of the tubular cells
- Obstruction of the tubule by debris
- Glomerular contraction

Further Information

Willem Kolff (1911–2009), a Dutch physician, is credited with the first successful treatment by dialysis in 1945 of a patient who actually survived. Previous attempts some 30 years earlier had ended with the death of all the patients treated, likely due to the use of hirudin as the anticoagulant.

In the UK, dialysis first started at the Hammersmith hospital using one of Kolff's machines. The unit was set up and run by Dr Eric Bywaters (1910–2003) who had initially trained as a histopathologist before becoming interested in renal medicine after seeing multiple renal biopsies of patients affected by crush injuries during the bombing of London in World War II.

CHAPTER 215

Acute Pancreatitis

Instruction

This patient presents to acute medical services with vague generalized abdominal pain. Please assess.

Salient Features

HISTORY

- Abdominal pain—epigastric, upper abdominal pain, generalized abdominal pain, traditionally been described like a band-belt around the abdomen and back—onset can be sudden, as in cholelithiasis, or insidious, as in alcohol-related pancreatitis.
- Nausea and vomiting which preceded or followed the pain but has no direct relation or effect on the pain
- Respiratory symptoms can develop either because of local diaphragmatic inflammation or in severe pancreatitis as part of respiratory failure.

Proceed as follows:
- Focus the history on potential related causes:
    - Alcohol consumption
    - Previous episodes of pancreatitis
    - History of gallstones
    - Medications and remedies taken
    - Prior operations
    - Constitutional symptoms preceding the event.

EXAMINATION

- Vital signs and haemodynamic physiology: patients may be hypotensive, tachycardic, pyrexial, tachypnoeic, and hypoxaemic.
- Abdominal signs can vary from mild localized tenderness on deep palpation to generalized tenderness with normal or diminished bowel sounds. In many cases the pain reported by the patient is out of proportion to the objective clinical findings.
- Expose the abdomen fully to look for Cullen and Grey Turner ecchymoses.
- Extrapancreatic signs may be present (arthritis, migratory erythema, panniculitis, pleural effusions).

Diagnosis

This patient's presentation is consistent with acute pancreatitis (lesion) probably caused by cholelithiasis (aetiology). They need urgent blood tests and imaging.

Questions

How is the diagnosis of acute pancreatitis established?
The diagnosis is based on three elements: clinical presentation and examination findings, typical biochemical results, and radiological findings on imaging (computed tomography (CT), magnetic resonance imaging (MRI), ultrasonography).

What are the biochemical changes that aid the diagnosis of acute pancreatitis?
Haemoconcentration, leucocytosis with predominant neutrophilia, increased inflammatory markers and possible acute kidney injury, hyperglycaemia, and hypocalcaemia.

Raised amylase: amylase is expected to be more than twice or three times the upper limit of normal during an acute attack. However, amylase may not be raised enough to be diagnostic and a raised amylase can be caused by extrapancreatic pathology. In cases with high clinical suspicion of acute pancreatitis, especially when the suspected aetiology is alcohol or in delayed (>24 hours) presentation, lipase levels should be requested simultaneously. Lipase is more sensitive and specific than amylase in diagnosing acute pancreatitis.

What are the findings of acute pancreatitis on the computed tomography of the abdomen?
- Acute inflammation of the pancreatic parenchyma (acute pancreatitis; Fig. 215.1)
- Oedematous pancreas (localized or generalized oedema)
- Pancreatic necrosis evident by lack of parenchymal enhancement by intravenous contrast (acute pancreatitis; Fig. 215.2)
- Peripancreatic fluid collection
- Pancreatic pseudocyst
- Necrotic collections appearing as heterogeneous densities in different locations
- Walled-off necrosis (heterogeneous liquid and nonliquid densities with well-defined encapsulated wall)
- CT may also reveal the underlying cause of acute pancreatitis (pancreatic or biliary cancer, common bile duct stones).

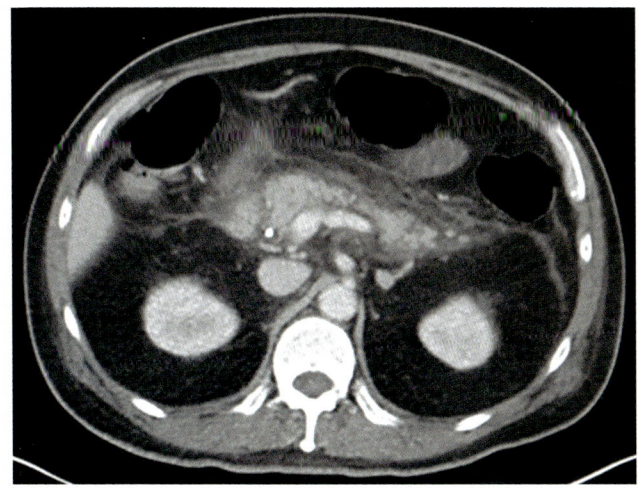

Fig. 215.1 Computed tomography image of acute pancreatitis with visible stranding. (From Arshad, A., Marudanayagam, R., 2016. Upper gastrointestinal emergencies. Surgery 34, 558–562.)

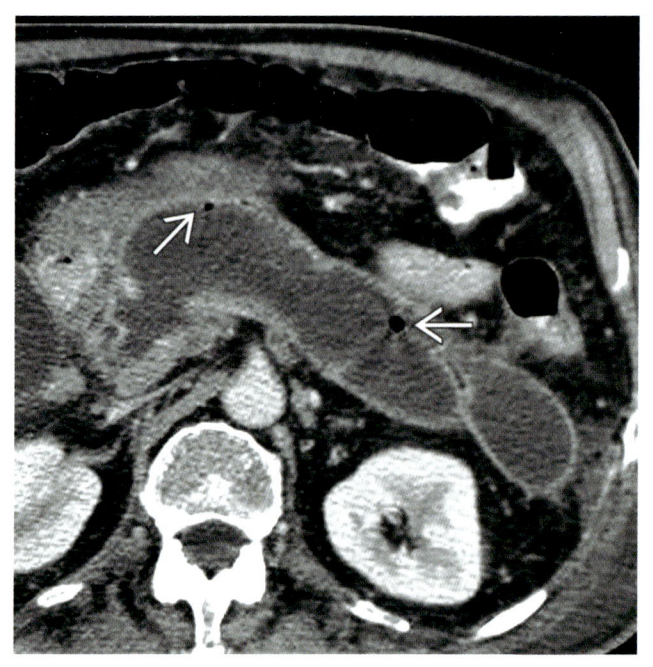

Fig. 215.2 Axial computed tomography shows infected pancreatic necrosis. Note that there is no enhancing parenchyma. The necrotic tissue contains gas bubbles, which indicate infection. (From Zaheer, A., Raman, S.P., 2022. Diagnostic Imaging: Gastrointestinal, fourth edn. Elsevier.)

What are the causes of acute pancreatitis?
- Gallstones
- Alcohol
- Drugs (isoniazid, metronidazole, statins, valproic acid, amiodarone, lamivudine, nelfinavir, azathioprine)
- Hypercalcaemia
- Hereditary pancreatitis
- Trauma
- Idiopathic
- Hypertriglyceridaemia
- Biliary obstruction (Vater's malignancy)
- Iatrogenic (postendoscopic retrograde cholangiopancreatography, intraoperative hypotension)
- Infections (mycoplasma, legionella, viral infections)
- Systemic vasculitis [SMA (superior mesenteric artery) and PAN (polyarteritis nodosa)].

Describe the scoring systems used to predict the severity and the outcome of acute pancreatitis.
There are multiple scoring systems for acute pancreatitis that are designed to predict severity, prognosis and outcome. The most commonly used ones are the Ranson criteria, the Acute Physiology and Chronic Health Examination (APACHE) II score, the Systemic Inflammatory Response Syndrome (SIRS) scoring, and the CT severity index.

Ranson's criteria: Ranson's score is one of the traditional scoring systems used in acute pancreatitis and include clinical and biochemical criteria. It consists of 11 parameters, 5 of which are assessed on presentation and 6 in the next 48 hours, and is used to predict mortality. Mortality is predicted to be less than 3% if the score is less or equal to 3, 15% if the score is 4 or 5, and nearly 50% if the score is more than 6. The five elements taken into account upon presentation are age, white cell count, blood glucose, lactate dehydrogenase (LDH), and aspartate transaminase (AST). The remaining elements assessed are haematocrit, urea, calcium, pO2, base deficit, and fluid sequestration.

APACHE II: widely used intensive care unit prognostic scoring system used to predict outcome in critically ill patients. It takes into account six physiologic parameters (temperature, mean arterial pressure, heart rate, respiratory rate, Glasgow Coma Scale (GCS) score, fraction of inspired oxygen), six biochemical parameters (arterial pH, sodium, potassium, creatinine, haematocrit, white cell count), and patient age.

SIRS score: this can be used to assess daily progress and SIRS existence (temperature, white cell, pulse rate, respiratory rate).

CT severity index (Baltazar score): a scoring system based on radiological findings in acute pancreatitis. It is graded based upon findings on nonenhanced CT (normal pancreas, enlargement of the pancreas, peripancreatic inflammation, fluid collections, and gas collections) and upon findings on contrast-enhanced CT (necrosis and extension of necrosis).

How is a patient with acute pancreatitis managed?

Depending on the disease severity, the patient will need to be hospitalized in a level 1 hospital bed or in intensive care. Patients with multiorgan support will of course need to have organ support in intensive care, but even patients with no established organ failure but with severe disease and high predictive scores will need intensive care monitoring. Initial management consists of supportive care with fluid resuscitation, nutritional support, pain control, and close monitoring. Fluid resuscitation is with continuous crystalloid given at a rate dictated by clinical need. Regardless of the rate of replacement, these patients need close attention for the first 48 hours. Meperidine is preferred as morphine can result in increased pressure in the sphincter of Oddi. Patients should be kept nil by mouth and a feeding tube placed for enteral feeding with early reestablishment of oral feeding when possible.

List some systemic complications of acute pancreatitis.

- Pleural effusions—respiratory failure—pulmonary oedema—acute respiratory distress syndrome (ARDS)
- Acute kidney failure
- Shock
- Vascular leak syndrome
- Sepsis
- New-onset diabetes
- Acute liver failure
- Disseminated intravascular coagulopathy
- Bowel ischaemia
- Paralytic ileus.

CHAPTER 216

Anaphylaxis

Instruction

A patient is brought in by ambulance with respiratory distress having eaten a peanut sauce at a Thai restaurant. He has a known allergy to peanuts. Please assess and treat.

Salient Features

HISTORY

- Sudden and acute onset
- Hives, urticarial rash, pruritus (Fig. 216.1)
- Nausea, vomiting, abdominal pain
- Facial swelling, swollen lips, paraesthesia lips, swollen tongue
- Dyspnoea, wheeze, stridor
- Dizziness, syncope.

EXAMINATION

- Systematic Advanced Life Support (ALS) approach:
  - A (airway), B (breathing), C (circulation), D (disability), E (exposure) assessment.
- Airway compromise, stridor, tongue, uvula, and lip oedema
- Increased respiratory rate, hypoxia, respiratory distress, bronchospasm, wheeze
- Hypotension, tachycardia
- Confusion, coma
- Rash—localized or widespread, periorbital oedema.

Diagnosis

This patient has facial swelling, stridor, and hypotension (lesions). This is secondary to anaphylaxis (diagnosis), which is a medical emergency. He is currently critically ill in the resuscitation room (functional status).

Questions

How do you treat anaphylaxis?
Anaphylaxis is a medical emergency. Immediate help should be sought and patients should be treated promptly with appropriate resuscitation steps.
- Intramuscular (IM) adrenaline 0.5 mL of 1 mg/mL (1:1.000) immediately in the anterolateral thigh. This dose can be repeated every 5 min if the respiratory or cardiovascular compromise persists. If the symptoms persist despite two doses of IM adrenaline, then expert help should be sought for administration of intravenous adrenaline infusion.
- Airway management with early intubation, if indicated, by an experienced clinician

- The patient should be positioned appropriately in the supine position with elevated legs and avoid sudden changes in posture. Semirecumbent position may be more appropriate for patients in respiratory distress and pregnant women should be placed on their left side.
- High-flow oxygen administration
- Fluid resuscitation with crystalloid
- Initiation of noninvasive cardiac monitoring
- Removal of the causative agent if possible
- Adjunctive treatment can be given once resuscitation is complete. Medications used are steroids, antihistamines, and nebulizers. These treatments are not life-saving interventions and they should not delay or interfere with the initial treatment with adrenaline.
- Patients on beta-blockers may need glucagon 1 mg over 5 min followed by an infusion.

How does adrenaline work?

Adrenaline is an $\alpha 1$, $\beta 1$, and $\beta 2$ adrenergic agonist. It causes vasoconstriction, increases peripheral vascular resistant with a positive effect on blood pressure, and reduces mucosal oedema (effect on $\alpha 1$ receptors). It is a positive inotropic and chronotropic agent increasing the blood pressure, heart rate, and stroke volume (effect on $\beta 1$ receptors) and causes bronchodilation easing the effort of breathing ($\beta 2$ agonistic effect).

Once treated, how long does a patient need to be observed in a hospital?

Once a patient has been stabilized and is out of immediate danger, they cannot be discharged from hospital. Rarely, the causative agent may cause a second wave of life-threatening anaphylaxis, called biphasic anaphylaxis. Up to one in five patients will have a second anaphylaxis reaction usually 1 to 12 hours after the first reaction. Theoretically a biphasic reaction can take place up to 72 hours after the initial anaphylaxis, but an occurrence after 12 hours is extremely rare. As such, a patient having been treated for anaphylaxis and with normal physiology and no symptoms should still be monitored in a hospital environment for 1 day. Before discharge the patient should be

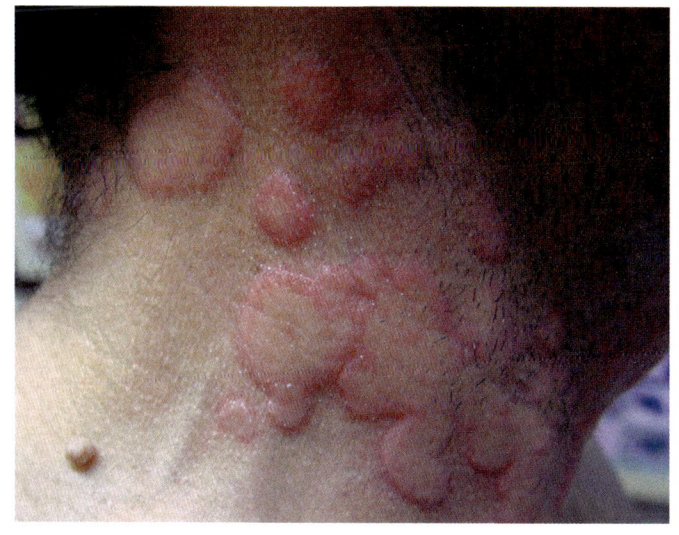

Fig. 216.1 Urticaria—wheal. (Courtesy Rui Tavares Bello.)

trained how to administer IM adrenaline in the event of recurrence, given a supply of adrenaline IM autoinjectors, and referred to an immunology service for further investigation and follow-up.

What is the pathophysiology of anaphylaxis?

The initial assault is exposure to an allergen. The reaction requires previous exposure to the allergen, followed by reexposure. Once absorbed, the allergen binds to an allergen-specific immunoglobulin E (IgE) presented on the surface of mast cells and basophils, and an acute immune-mediated generalized reaction follows. These cells in turn become activated and degranulate, releasing mediators such as histamine and tryptase into the systemic circulation. These mediators cause the reactions seen in anaphylaxis (angioedema, tachycardia, hypotension) and also activate other cells such as eosinophils to release more mediators which can trigger a domino effect which can lead to death if treatment with adrenaline is delayed (Fig. 216.2).

Are there any tests to support the diagnosis of anaphylaxis?

Anaphylaxis is a clinical diagnosis and immediate treatment has to be given on suspicion or recognition of signs. Untreated anaphylaxis can cause death. There are no tests to confirm the diagnosis in the emergency situation and guide treatment, and performing tests during anaphylaxis may delay life-saving treatment. As part of the initial ALS assessment, a blood sample is likely to be drawn and should, amongst other routine blood tests, be sent for plasma tryptase levels. Plasma tryptase levels will be nearly doubled during anaphylaxis, with a peak concentration at 30 to 60 min after the onset of anaphylaxis and would be expected to normalize thereafter with a

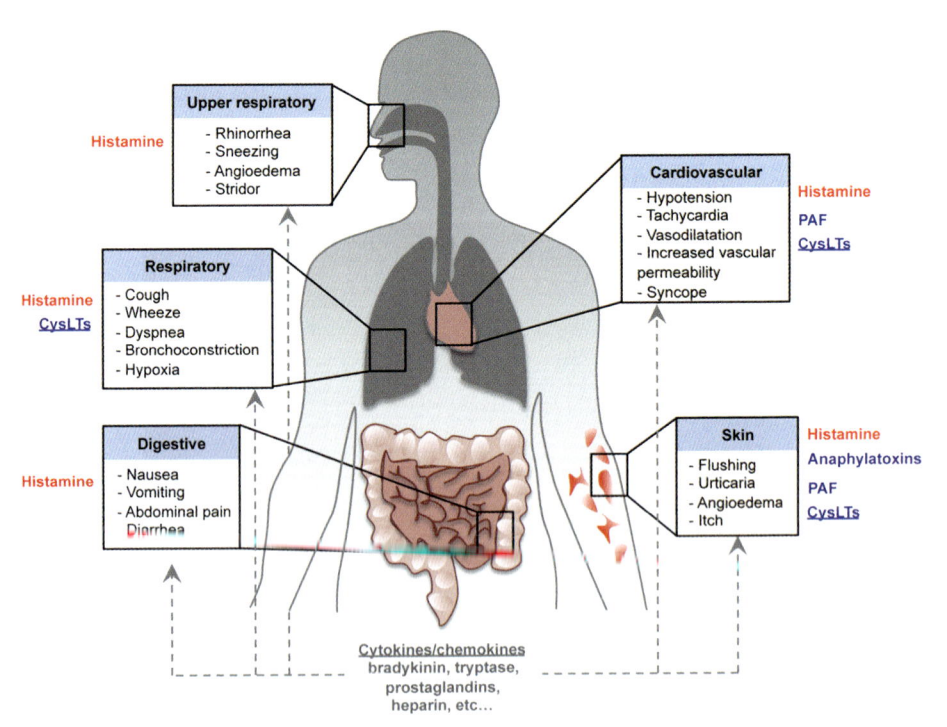

Fig. 216.2 Pathophysiologic changes in anaphylaxis and mediators. (With permission from Reber, L.L., Hernandez, J.D., Galli, S.J., 2017. The pathophysiology of anaphylaxis. J. Allergy Clin. Immunol. 140, 335–348.)

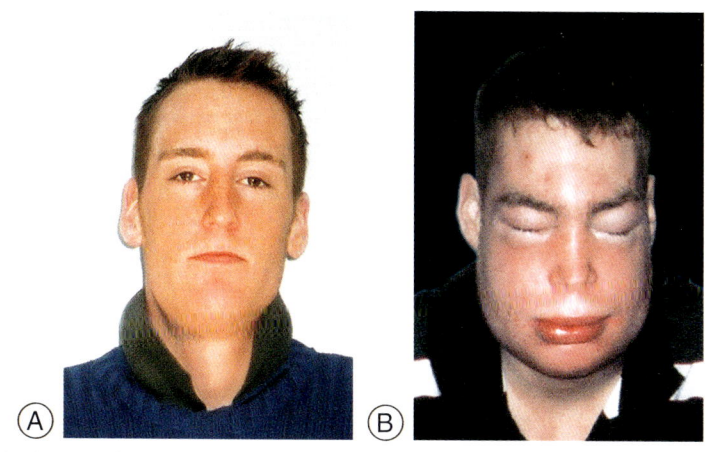

Fig. 216.3 Angioedema. **(A)** Normal appearance. **(B)** During an acute attack. (With permission from Helbert M., 2006. Flesh and Bones of Immunology. Churchill Livingstone, Elsevier Ltd, Edinburgh.)

half-life of 2 hours. Therefore, if samples for plasma tryptase levels are obtained 30 to 60 min into the reaction and 3 hours after the reaction, put immediately on ice, and analysed, the comparison of tryptase levels can give valuable information to the immunology team following the patient up.

How does angioedema differ from anaphylaxis?
Angioedema is subcutaneous swelling of tissues with loose connective tissue (face, genitalia, limbs) (Fig. 216.3). It can be bradykinin or histamine mediated. Bradykinin-mediated angioedema is not accompanied by a rash and it does not cause bronchospasm or allergic symptoms. Histamine-mediated angioedema can be accompanied with skin signs. Causes of angioedema can be medications (angiotensin-converting enzyme inhibitor (ACE-I), nonsteroidal antiinflammatory drugs (NSAIDs)), hereditary angioedema with C1-esterase inhibitor deficiency, or idiopathic. It differs from anaphylaxis in that there is localized tissue swelling without systemic organ failure and it presents more insidiously than anaphylaxis. Angioedema is usually benign and self-terminates within a few hours or days. However, if there is circulatory or respiratory involvement, treatment should not differ from anaphylaxis. If not, then management is directed towards the underlying cause.

What do you know of the term FPIES and how is this related to anaphylaxis?
Food protein enterocolitis syndrome is an adverse reaction to specific foods that starts in infancy. It is characterized by profuse vomiting and dehydration with high fever 2 to 4 hours after ingestion of the causative agent, followed by lethargy. Although FPIES is not an IgE-mediated reaction, 10% of patients diagnosed with FPIES will already have or later develop an IgE immune response to the causative agent, including anaphylaxis.

Is there a role of immunotherapy in preventing anaphylaxis in known allergens?
Immunotherapy has been used in different forms of anaphylaxis as a long-term prevention technique for patients. It has no role in food allergies, and the only preventive method for food-related anaphylaxis is avoidance of the allergen. However, immunotherapy has been used successfully and is recommended in venom anaphylaxis. Immunotherapy should be given by an immunology team and treatment therapies last for years.

Further Information

Charles Richet (1850–1935), a French doctor and Professor of Physiology, coined the term 'anaphylaxis' to describe a lethal reaction to a previously tolerated toxin. The other term that he is credited with inventing is 'ectoplasm' as he was a renowned spiritualist and believer in the paranormal. He was awarded the 1913 Nobel Prize for Medicine for his work on anaphylaxis.

CHAPTER 217

Chest Pain — Angina

Instruction

You are the medical doctor on call in the acute assessment unit. This 40-year-old patient presents with some episodes of chest pain of recent onset. The last one happened a few hours ago, woke the patient up from sleep, and was severe enough for him to call an ambulance on this occasion. Please assess the patient and advise on further investigations and treatment.

Salient Features

HISTORY

- Onset of pain (sudden, insidious, at rest, on exertion)
- Character of pain (pleuritic, sharp, dull ache, squeezing, burning, stabbing, electric shock pain)
- Duration of each episode and frequency of episodes (seconds, minutes, hours, intermittent, constant)
- Exacerbating factors (exertion, movement, breathing, lying flat, sitting up, eating, cold weather)
    - Have you noticed anything that brings on the pain?
    - Have you noticed anything that makes the pain worse?
    - Do you get the pain if you exert yourself?
- Alleviating factors (rest, glyceryl trinitrate spray, antacids, analgesics)
    - Have you noticed anything that helps with the pain?
- Site of pain (central, right sided, left sided, across the chest, epigastric, localized)
    - Can you show me where the pain is when it comes?
- Radiation of pain (jaw, neck, shoulders, arms, back)
    - Does the pain go anywhere else?
- Associated symptoms (dyspnoea, palpitations, diaphoresis, nausea, vomiting, dizziness, cough, sputum, fever, haemoptysis, upper respiratory tract infection symptoms)
    - Have you had any other symptoms when you experienced the pain?
    - How have you been in yourself before these episodes came on?
- Medical history
    - Risk factors for cardiac disease (hypertension, smoking, hypercholesterolaemia, diabetes, obesity, known cardiac disease, family history)
    - History of trauma
    - Medical history (previously diagnosed cardiovascular disease, risk factors for thrombo-embolism, known diagnosis of gastrointestinal disease)
    - Medication history.
- Social history.

EXAMINATION

- Cardiovascular examination (character, volume, rate and rhythm of radial pulse, radioradial or radiofemoral delay, cardiac auscultation looking for murmurs or pericardial rub, palpation for signs of pulmonary hypertension associated with underlying respiratory disease)
- Chest examination (chest wall palpation for localized tenderness, chest auscultation for signs of pneumothorax, consolidation, or effusion)
- Leg examination (looking for signs of venous thromboembolism)
- Back examination (looking for spinal tenderness across the thoracic vertebrae).

Diagnosis

This obese patient with a 40 pack-year history of smoking describes exertional chest pain of recent onset (lesion) that is relieved by rest. His symptoms are explained by angina caused by coronary artery disease (aetiology). He has presented on this occasion with chest pain which is present at rest and he should be treated for an acute coronary syndrome (functional status).

Questions

What is the mechanism of angina pectoris?
It is commonly caused by increased myocardial oxygen demand triggered by physical activity, but can also be caused by transient decreases in oxygen delivery as a result of coronary vasospasm. Unstable angina is caused by nonocclusive intracoronary thrombi.

What changes in resting 12-lead electrocardiogram are consistent with coronary artery disease and suggest ischaemia or previous infarction?
- Pathological Q waves
- Left bundle branch block
- ST-segment and T-wave abnormalities (e.g. flattening or inversion).

What do you understand by the term syndrome X?
- Syndrome X, or microvascular angina, is the presence of classic angina and ST depression on exercise stress testing and a normal coronary angiogram in the absence of any other demonstrable cardiac abnormalities.
- Reaven syndrome, or 'endocrine' syndrome X, is the association of insulin resistance, hypertension, and increased very-low-density lipoprotein and decreased high-density lipoprotein cholesterol concentrations in the plasma.

What is the treatment for stable angina?
- Short-acting nitrates to treat episodes of stable angina
- Angina prevention treatment:
  - Beta blockers
  - Calcium channel blocker if deemed more appropriate or beta-blocker is contraindicated
  - A combination of the previous treatments (if a combination is needed, then a dihydropyridine calcium channel blocker is preferred).
- If both these medications are not enough to manage the symptoms, then second-line treatment should be added, including the following:
  - Long-acting nitrates
  - Ivabradine

217 — CHEST PAIN — ANGINA

- Nicorandil
- Ranolazine.
- A third agent is added only if the symptoms are not controlled with two agents and the patient is either awaiting revascularization or the patient is deemed unsuitable for revascularization.
- Appropriate secondary prevention should be given according to relevant guidance (aspirin, statin, angiotensin-converting enzyme inhibitor, antihypertensives).
- Revascularization therapy with percutaneous coronary intervention (PCI) or coronary artery bypass grafting (CABG) is reserved for patients who remain symptomatic on optimal medical therapy, active patients who cannot tolerate medical therapy will and want a better quality of life, and patients whose angiogram has revealed coronary anatomy where revascularization has a proven survival benefit. CABG is reserved for patients with left main stem or triple-vessel disease, or for patients in whom the best method of revascularization is in doubt after angiography.

What is Levine's sign?
In acute myocardial infarction (MI), the patient often describes the pain by illustrating a clenched fist.

What are the major risk factors for an acute myocardial infarction?
- Smoking
- Dyslipidaemia
- Diabetes
- Hypertension
- Family history of premature coronary artery disease.

How would you use the electrocardiogram to localize ST-elevation myocardial infarction?
- Anterior or anteroseptal—the QRS complexes in leads V_1 and V_2 indicate anteroseptal infarction. A characteristic notching of the QRS complex, often seen with infarcts, is present in lead V_2. The septum is supplied with blood by the left anterior descending (LAD) coronary artery. Septal infarction generally suggests that one of the branches of the LAD is occluded, whereas a strictly anterior infarct generally results from occlusion of the LAD coronary artery.
- Anterolateral—ST segment elevation in leads I, aVL, and V_1 to V_6 with Q waves in V_1 to V_4
- Posterior—tall R waves in leads V_1 and V_2. In most cases of posterior infarction, the infarct extends either to the lateral wall of the left ventricle (LV) resulting in characteristic changes in lead V_6, or to the inferior wall of that ventricle resulting in characteristic changes in leads II, III, and aVF. Because of the overlap between inferior and posterior infarctions, the more general term inferoposterior is used when the electrocardiogram (ECG) shows changes consistent with either inferior or posterior infarction.
- Inferior—ST elevations in leads II, III, and aVF and reciprocal ST depression in leads I and aVL. Inferior wall infarction is generally caused by occlusion of the right coronary artery. Less commonly, it occurs because of a left circumflex coronary obstruction.
- Right ventricular infarction—Q waves and ST-segment elevations in leads II, III, and aVF are accompanied by ST elevations in the right precordial leads.

This classification is not absolute, and infarct types often overlap.

What are the complications of myocardial infarction?
- Extension of infarct and postinfarct ischaemia
- Rhythm disorders: tachycardia, bradycardia, ventricular ectopics, ventricular fibrillation, atrial fibrillation and tachycardia

- Heart failure: acute pulmonary oedema
- Circulatory failure: cardiogenic shock
- Infarction of papillary muscle: mitral regurgitation and acute pulmonary oedema
- Rupture of interventricular septum
- LV aneurysm
- Mural thrombus
- Thromboembolism, cerebral or peripheral
- Venous thrombosis
- Pericarditis
- Dressler syndrome: characterized by persistent pyrexia, pericarditis, pleurisy (first described in 1956 when Dressler recognized that chest pain following MI is not caused by coronary artery insufficiency).

What do you know about right ventricular infarction?
Right ventricular infarction presents with retrosternal chest discomfort, nausea, vomiting, and diaphoresis, unlike LV infarction which presents with dyspnoea. In right ventricular infarction, there is a raised jugular venous pressure with no evidence of pulmonary congestion; the patient often has a low cardiac output with hypotension. The patient typically presents with ST elevation in the inferior leads (II, III, and aVF) and in one or more right-sided lead, particularly V_4. The cornerstones of therapy include restoration of infarct artery patency, intravascular volume expansion, and inotropic support.

What is the single most successful therapy in a patient with ST-elevation myocardial infarction?
Of all interventions and treatments given in a patient with an acute ST-elevation MI, primary PCI is the single most important intervention as it has the smallest number needed to treat (NNT) of all treatments studied (25 for death and 6 for recurrent ischaemia). The NNT is the number of patients you need to treat to prevent one additional bad outcome (death, stroke etc.). For example, if a drug has an NNT of 6, six patients have to be treated with the drug to prevent one additional bad outcome. The ideal NNT is 1, where everyone improves with treatment and no one improves with control. The higher the NNT, the less effective is the treatment.

Treatment	NNT
Nitrates	333
Beta-blocker	33
Aspirin	38
Fibrinolytics	53
Heparin	200
Primary PCI	25

Describe electrocardiographic evidence of acute infarction.
The principal electrocardiographic indicators of acute infarction are shown in Fig. 217.1.

217 — CHEST PAIN — ANGINA

A ST segment elevation (⇒ injury)

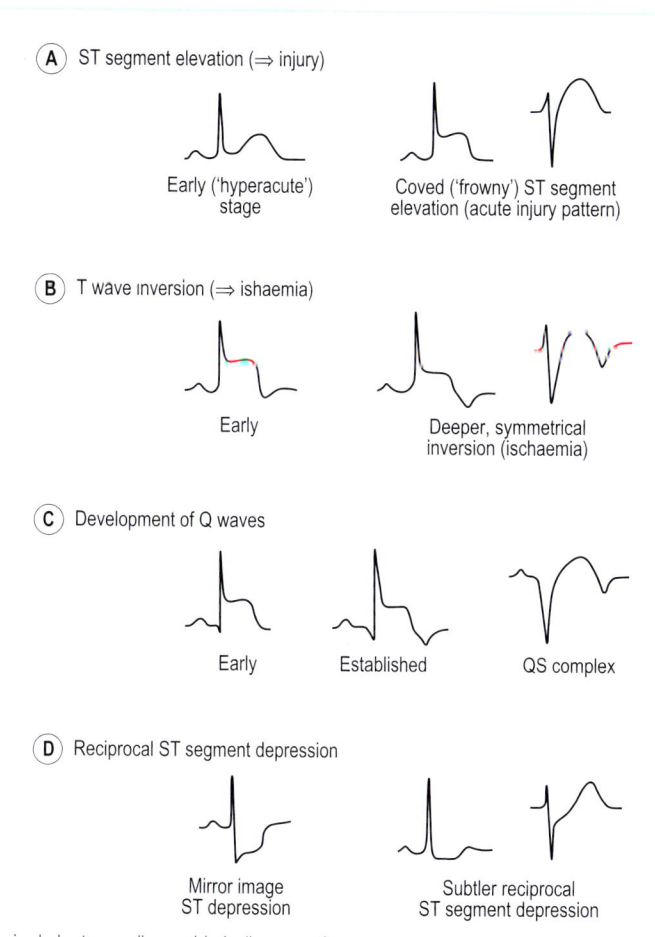

Early ('hyperacute') stage

Coved ('frowny') ST segment elevation (acute injury pattern)

B T wave inversion (⇒ ishaemia)

Early

Deeper, symmetrical inversion (ischaemia)

C Development of Q waves

Early   Established   QS complex

D Reciprocal ST segment depression

Mirror image ST depression

Subtler reciprocal ST segment depression

Fig. 217.1 Principal electrocardiographic indicators of acute infarction.

Further Information

Werner Grossman (1904–1979), a German physician, shared the 1956 Nobel prize for Medicine for his work on cardiac catheterization. He started in 1929 by performing a venous cutdown on himself and inserting a catheter into his own right atrium before walking up to the X-ray department at his hospital and undergoing a chest X-ray to demonstrate its position.

The first balloon angioplasty was performed in Zurich in 1977 by Andreas Gruentzig (1935–1989).

CHAPTER 218

Cauda Equina Syndrome

Instruction
This patient has bowel and bladder dysfunction; examine the lower limbs.

Salient Features
HISTORY
- Presence and localization of pain; pain projected to the perineum and thighs represents root pain in the dermatomes L2 or L3, or S2 or S3, whereas pain in L4, L5, or S1 distribution is commonly attributed to disc disease.
- History of trauma and 'neural claudication' (where the patient develops root pain and leg weakness, usually a foot drop while walking that rapidly recovers with resting)
- Pain in the anterior thigh, wasting of the quadriceps muscle, weakness of the foot invertors (caused by L4 root lesion), and an absent knee jerk
- History of malignancy such as leukaemia or prostatic carcinoma (primaries for bony metastases).

EXAMINATION
- Flaccid, asymmetrical paraparesis
- Knee and ankle jerks diminished or absent
- Saddle distribution of sensory loss up to the L1 level
- Plantars downgoing.

Diagnosis
This patient has flaccid paraparesis with saddle anaesthesia caused by cauda equina syndrome (lesion) due to a compressive lesion (aetiology). They are being prepared for emergency spinal decompression surgery (functional status).

Questions
What is the relationship of the spinal cord to the vertebra?
The spinal cord extends from the foramen magnum to the interspace between the 12th thoracic (dorsal) and 1st lumbar spines, although the thecal membranes may extend down the body of the second sacral vertebra. To determine the spinal segments in relation to the vertebral body:
- For cervical vertebrae, add 1
- For thoracic 1 to 6, add 2
- For thoracic 7 to 9, add 3
- The lumbar segments lie opposite the 10th and 11th thoracic spines and the next interspinal space
- The first lumbar arch overlies the sacral and coccygeal segments.

218 – CAUDA EQUINA SYNDROME

The sacral segments are compressed into the last inch of the cord known as the conus medullaris, which is located behind the T9 to the L1 vertebra.

At which vertebral level is the lesion in cauda equina syndrome?
A lesion in the spinal canal at any level below the T10 (dorsal) vertebra can cause cauda equina syndrome.

How would you differentiate between cauda equina and conus medullaris syndrome?
The cauda equina consists of lower spinal roots (T12 to S5), and hence, a lesion causes lower motor neuron signs, whereas the conus medullaris is the lowest part of the spinal cord and lesions result in upper motor neuron signs. Both conus and cauda lesions result in a mixed picture. In its purest form, conus medullaris syndrome presents with sphincter disturbances, saddle anaesthesia (S3–S5), impotence, and absence of lower extremity abnormalities.

What are the causes of cauda equina syndrome?
- Centrally placed lumbosacral disc or spondylolisthesis at the lumbosacral junction
- Tumours of the cauda equina (ependymoma, neurofibroma).

What are the types of cauda equina syndrome in adults?
- Lateral cauda equina syndrome: pain in the anterior thigh, wasting of the quadriceps muscle, weakness of the foot invertors (caused by L4 root lesion), and an absent knee jerk. Causes include neurofibroma, a high disc lesion
- Midline cauda equina syndrome: bilateral lumbar and sacral root lesions. Causes include disc lesion, primary sacral bone tumours (chordomas), metastatic bone disease (from prostate), and leukaemia.

What is the most important investigation that needs to be performed urgently on this patient?
Magnetic resonance imaging of the lumbar spine.

CHAPTER 219

Cellulitis

Instruction

Look at this patient's leg.

Salient Features

HISTORY

- History of fever and chills
- Diabetes
- Animal (or human) bites
- Exposure to seawater (*Vibrio vulnificus*), fresh water (*Aeromonas hydrophila*), aquacultured fish (*Streptococcus iniae*), warm baths (*Pseudomonas aeruginosa*).

EXAMINATION

- Red, inflamed leg with a definite demarcation of erythematous area (cellulitis; Fig. 219.1)
- Oedema
- Increased temperature
- Crepitus: crepitant cellulitis is produced by either *Clostridia* spp. or non-spore-forming anaerobes (*Bacteroides* spp., peptostreptococci, and peptococci).

Proceed as follows:
- Examine the peripheral pulses.
- Look for varicose veins (varicose eczema should be considered in the differential diagnosis of cellulitis of the leg.
- Look for superficial ulcers.

Note: Cellulitis is a clinical diagnosis; it is a deep, subcutaneous infection characterized by warmth, swelling, tenderness, and erythema and may be accompanied by lymphatic streaking. Pruritus is absent (unlike in contact dermatitis).

Diagnosis

This patient has cellulitis of the leg (lesion) caused by pyogenic bacterial infection (aetiology), and the leg is acutely swollen and painful (functional status).

Questions

How would you manage such a patient?
- Cultures of aspirates and lesions
- Blood cultures: bacteraemia is uncommon in cellulitis but blood cultures are useful in those with lymphoedema.

219 — CELLULITIS

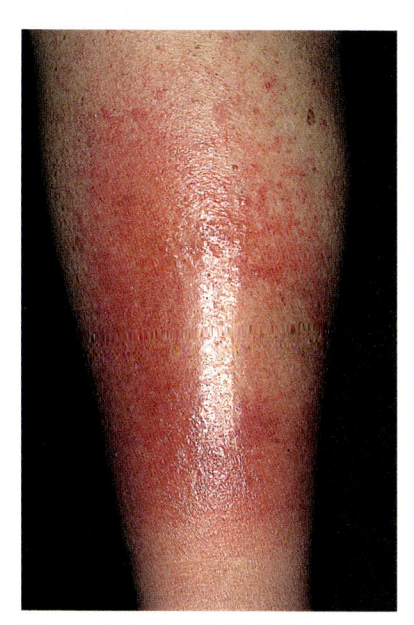

Fig. 219.1 Cellulitis on the leg. (With permission from Habif, T., Campbell Jr., J.L., Dinulos, J.G.H., Chapman, M.S., Zug, K.A., 2011. Skin Disease: Diagnosis and Treatment, third edn. Saunders, St Louis.)

- Radiology: plain film radiography or computed tomography is useful when accompanying osteomyelitis is suspected. Gallium-67 scintigraphy may aid in the detection of cellulitis superimposed on recently increasing chronic lymphoedema of a limb.
- Intravenous antibiotics: because most cases of cellulitis are caused by streptococci and *Staphylococcus aureus*, beta-lactam antibiotics with activity against penicillinase-producing *S. aureus* are the usual drugs of choice. Flucloxacillin can be used until the microbe is identified.
- Pain relief
- Surgical referral
- Experimental: granulocyte-colony stimulating factor, particularly in patients with diabetes.

What are the causes of bilateral swollen legs?
- Cardiac failure
- Renal failure
- Hypoproteinaemia (from cirrhosis or nephrotic syndrome).

What are the causes of an acutely swollen leg?
- Deep vein thrombosis (DVT)
- Cellulitis
- Arterial occlusion
- Trauma
- Arthritis.

What are the causes of a chronically swollen leg?
- Vascular causes: varicose veins, postphlebitic limb
- Lymphoedema: Milroy disease, filariasis (in the tropics)
- Congenital.

When would you admit a patient with cellulitis to hospital for intravenous antibiotics?
Uncomplicated limb cellulitis can be managed at home with oral antibiotics or in an ambulatory care setting. However, signs that warrant medical admission for close observations and intravenous antibiotics are:
- Signs of sepsis or systemic inflammatory response with fever, tachycardia, tachypnoea, hypotension
- Signs of organ hypoperfusion; oliguria, confusion, generalized malaise, dizziness
- Failure of oral treatment; progression of the erythema and the swelling despite 24 to 48 hours of oral antibiotics
- Inability to weight bear on cellulitis of lower limb
- Close proximity of the lesion to an indwelling medical device
- Immunocompromised patients.

The patient described earlier is admitted to hospital for intravenous antibiotics because he was febrile and tachycardic on initial presentation. The nursing staff looking after him report rapid deterioration with blue discolouration of the initial rash. What is the underlying diagnosis and what is the treatment for it?
The condition described is possible necrotizing fasciitis or necrotizing cellulitis. The patient needs urgent review, if signs of necrotizing infection are present, he needs urgent surgical exploration. Clinical signs of necrotizing fasciitis are grey-blue-purple discolouration of the skin, crepitus on palpation, systemic signs of sepsis, excruciating pain before paraesthesia of the affected limb, necrosis of the skin.

What is the most common microorganism causing cellulitis?
The most common bacteria causing cellulitis are staphylococcus responding to beta-lactam antibiotics. Under the microscope staphylococci appear like berries that form clusters resembling a bunch of grapes. *Staphyli* is the Greek name for grape.

Further Information

W.F. Milroy (1855–1942) described familial lymphoedema of the legs in 1892.

CHAPTER 220

Coarctation of Aorta

Instruction
This patient presented with severe hypertension. Please examine their cardiovascular system.

Salient Features
HISTORY
- Asymptomatic usually
- Symptoms often those of hypertension: headache, epistaxis, dizziness, and palpitations
- Claudication (caused by diminished blood flow to the legs)
- Patients sometimes seek medical attention because they have symptoms of heart failure or aortic dissection. Women with coarctation are at particularly high risk for aortic dissection during pregnancy.

EXAMINATION
- The upper torso is better developed than the lower part (as the lower body has chronic low systolic blood pressure (BP) compared to the upper part).
- The systolic arterial pressure is higher in the arms than in the legs, but the diastolic pressures are similar; therefore, a widened pulse pressure is present in the arms. (Note: this condition results in hypertension in the arms. Less commonly, the coarctation is immediately proximal to the left subclavian artery, in which case a difference in arterial pressure is noted between the arms.)
- Radial pulse on the left side may be less prominent.
- The femoral arterial pulses are weak and delayed (simultaneous palpation of the brachial and femoral arteries using the thumbs is the most convenient method of comparing pulsations in the upper and lower limbs).
- A systolic thrill may be palpable in the suprasternal notch.
- There is heaving apex caused by left ventricular enlargement.
- A systolic ejection click (caused by a bicuspid aortic valve which occurs in 50% of cases) is frequently present, and the second heart sound is accentuated.
- A harsh systolic ejection murmur may be identified along the left sternal border and in the back, particularly over the coarctation.
- Scapular collaterals are visible (listen over these collaterals for murmur).
- A systolic murmur, caused by flow through collateral vessels, may be heard in the back.
- In about 30% of patients with aortic coarctation, a systolic murmur indicating an associated bicuspid aortic valve is audible at the base.

Tell the examiner you would like to look for:
- Turner syndrome (female, webbing of the neck, increased carrying angle)
- Berry aneurysms (extraocular movements impaired caused by third cranial nerve involvement).

Diagnosis

This patient has coarctation of the aorta (lesion) with left ventricular failure (functional status).

Questions

What are the types of aortic coarctation?
Common:
- Infantile or preductal where the aorta between the left subclavian artery and patent ductus arteriosus is narrowed. It manifests in infancy with heart failure. Associated lesions include patent ductus arteriosus, aortic arch anomalies, transposition of the great arteries, ventricular septal defect.
- Adult type: the coarctation in the descending aorta is juxtaductal or slightly postductal. It may be associated with bicuspid aortic valve or patent ductus arteriosus. It commonly presents between the ages of 15 and 30 years.

Rare:
- Localized juxtaductal coarctation
- Coarctation of the ascending thoracic aorta
- Coarctation of the distal descending thoracic aorta
- Coarctation of the abdominal aorta
- Pseudocoarctation is of no haemodynamic significance and is a 'kinked' appearance of the aorta in the juxtaductal region without stenosis.

Is aortic coarctation commoner in men or women?
This condition is more common in males than females.

What conditions are associated with coarctation of aorta?
It may occur in conjunction with gonadal dysgenesis (e.g. Turner syndrome), bicuspid aortic valve, ventricular septal defect, patent ductus arteriosus, mitral stenosis or regurgitation, or aneurysms of the circle of Willis.

How would you investigate this patient?
- Electrocardiogram in adults usually shows left ventricular hypertrophy (Fig. 220.1).
- Chest radiograph shows symmetric rib notching. The coarctation may be visualized as the characteristic '3' sign on a chest radiograph (Fig. 220.2). The upper bulge is formed by dilatation of the left subclavian artery high on the left mediastinal border; the sharp indentation is the site of the coarctation, and the lower bulge is called the poststenotic dilatation of the aorta.
- Echocardiography may visualize the coarctation; Doppler examination makes possible an estimate of the transcoarctation pressure gradient.
- Computed tomography, magnetic resonance imaging, and contrast aortography are useful to determine the precise anatomy regarding the location and length of the coarctation; in addition, aortography permits the visualization of the collateral circulation.

What do you understand by the term pseudocoarctation?
It refers to buckling or kinking of the aortic arch without the presence of a significant gradient.

What causes rib notching?
Collateral flow through dilated, tortuous, and pulsatile posterior intercostal arteries typically causes notching on the undersurfaces of the posterior portions of the ribs. The anterior parts of the

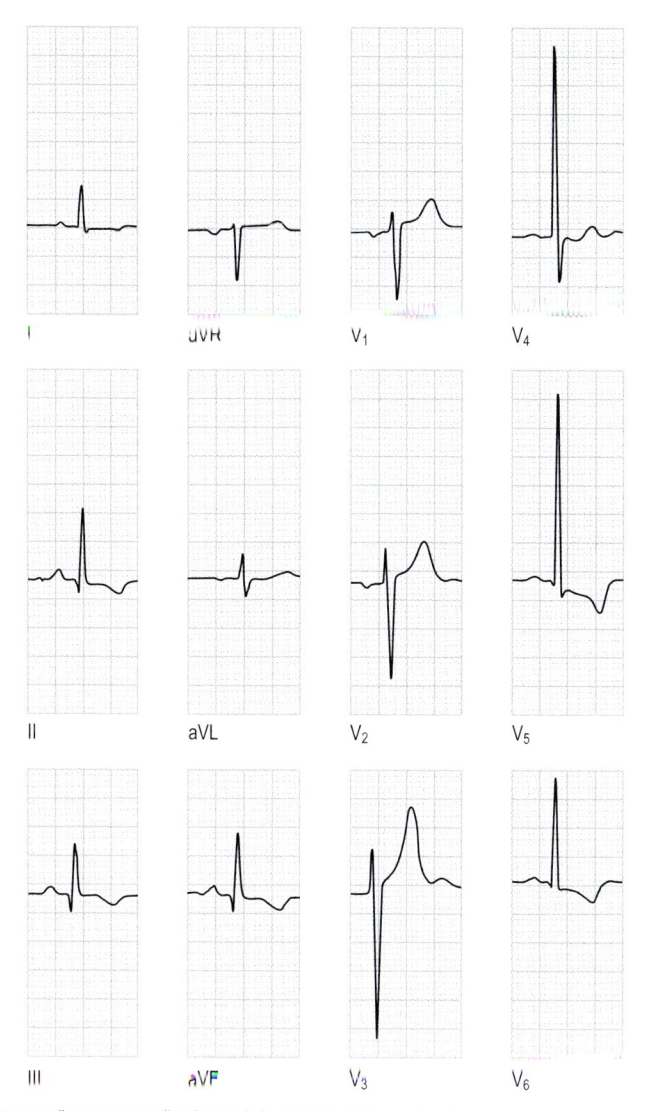

Fig. 220.1 Electrocardiogram usually shows left ventricular hypertrophy.

ribs are spared because the anterior intercostal arteries do not run in the costal grooves. Notching is seldom found above the third or below the ninth rib and rarely appears before the age of 6 years.

Mention a few conditions in which rib notching is seen.
- Coarctation of aorta
- Pulmonary oligaemia
- Blalock–Taussig shunt
- Subclavian artery obstruction
- Superior vena cava syndrome
- Neurofibromatosis
- Arteriovenous malformations of the lung or chest wall.

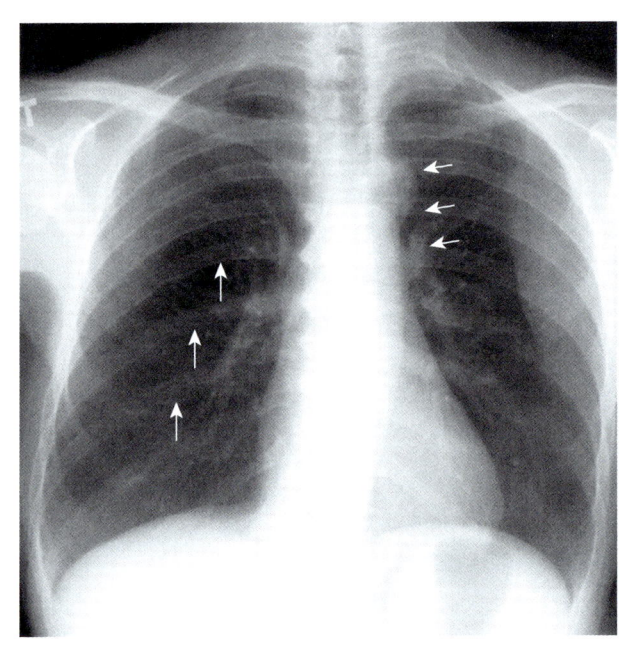

Fig. 220.2 Chest radiograph shows the 'number 3' sign *(short arrows)* and rib notching *(long arrows)* is seen on the inferior portion of the posterior ribs (ribs 3 to 9). (With permission from Carey, W.D., 2010. Current Clinical Medicine, second edn. Saunders, Philadelphia, PA.)

What are the complications of aortic coarctation?
- Severe hypertension and resulting complications:
  - Stroke
  - Premature coronary artery disease
  - Left ventricular failure (two-thirds of patients aged >40 years who have uncorrected aortic coarctation have symptoms of heart failure)
  - Rupture of aorta.
- Infective endocarditis endarteritis (at the site of the coarctation or on a congenitally bicuspid aortic valve)
- Intracranial haemorrhage (combination of hypertension and ruptured berry aneurysm)
- Death occurs in 75% of patients by the age of 50 years, if left untreated.

What are the fundal findings in coarctation of aorta?
Hypertension caused by coarctation of aorta causes retinal arteries to be tortuous with frequent 'U' turns; curiously, the classic signs of hypertensive retinopathy are rarely seen (coarctation; Fig. 220.1).

What are the indications for treatment of coarctation?
- Patients with proximal hypertension with a noninvasive pressure difference of more than 20 mm Hg between the upper and lower limbs, pathological BP response during exercise, or left ventricular hypertrophy should undergo intervention.
- Patients with more than 50% aortic narrowing, irrespective of pressure gradient or proximal hypertension, may also be considered for intervention.

- As the condition can be associated with other cardiac structural pathology (i.e. aortic valve stenosis or regurgitation), all lesions have to be taken into account when it comes to decisions regarding surgical intervention.

What are the different types of intervention for such patients?
- Balloon angioplasty with stent insertion
- Corrective surgery (resection and end-to-end anastomosis may be needed, although a tubular graft may be required if the narrowed segment is too long).

What are the postoperative complications?
- Recurrent coarctation
- Persistent hypertension
- Possible sequelae of a bicuspid aortic valve.

What happens to the hypertension after surgery?
Despite surgery, some patients may continue to have residual or recurrent hypertension and will require monitoring for hypertension and premature coronary artery disease. The incidence of persistent or recurrent hypertension is influenced by the patient's age at the time of surgery:
- Among patients who undergo surgery during childhood, 90% are normotensive 5 years later, 50% are normotensive 20 years later, and 25% are normotensive 25 years later.
- Among those who undergo surgery after the age of 40 years, half have persistent hypertension, and many of those with a normal resting BP after successful repair have a hypertensive response to exercise.

Is survival improved by surgery?
Survival after repair of aortic coarctation is influenced by the age of the patient at the time of surgery:
- Repair during childhood: 89% of patients are alive 15 years later and 83% are alive 25 years later.
- Repair between ages of 20 and 40 years: 25-year survival is 75%.
- Repair in patients >40 years of age: the 15-year survival is only 50%.

CHAPTER 221

Deep Vein Thrombosis

Instruction
This patient presented with a swollen leg. Please examine them.

Salient Features

HISTORY
- Recent history of immobilization including recent surgery, stroke, myocardial infarction
- Onset: acute vs. chronic
- Pain
- Personal and family history of thromboses including deep vein thrombosis (DVT), pulmonary embolism
- Drug history: oral contraceptives
- Air travel; the evidence is circumstantial.
- Symptoms that may signify pulmonary embolism such as chest pains, palpitations, dizziness, or dyspnoea.

EXAMINATION
- Painful calf
- Erythema
- Engorged superficial veins
- Unilateral swollen leg with pitting oedema
- Pain on the calf on dorsiflexion of the foot: Homans' sign (not diagnostic).

Proceed as follows:
- Check for pitting oedema on both sides (look at the patient's eyes while eliciting this sign to ensure that you are not causing pain).
- Compare the temperature of both the legs (use the dorsum of your fingers to elicit this sign).
- Check the arterial pulses in the leg.

Diagnosis
This patient has unilateral leg oedema and tenderness (lesion) caused probably by deep venous thrombosis (aetiology). He displays no signs or symptoms of pulmonary embolism and I cannot identify any signs of malignancy.

Questions

How would you estimate the clinical probability of a deep vein thrombosis episode?
The most commonly used validated score in clinical practice is the modified Well's score.

221 — DEEP VEIN THROMBOSIS

The Well's score takes into account and assigns 1 point for each of the following present conditions:
- Active cancer
- Paralysis, paresis, or recent immobilization of the lower limbs
- Major surgery within the last 12 weeks
- Localized tenderness along the deep veins
- Entire leg swelling
- Unilateral calf swelling at least 3 cm more than the other side
- Pitting oedema to the symptomatic leg
- Collateral superficial veins and
- Previous history of DVT.

If clinically an alternative diagnosis is equally or more likely than DVT, then 2 points are subtracted from the total Well's score.

The final score gives the total clinical probability of DVT existence. In the United Kingdom, the two-level Well's score is used, where 2 points deems DVT likely, whereas 1 point and lower deems DVT unlikely.

What are the predisposing factors for venous thrombosis?
- Surgery (particularly of leg or pelvis, or after prostatectomy)
- Following cerebrovascular accident (about half of the patients develop DVT)
- Following myocardial infarction (one-third of patients have DVT)
- Obesity
- Malignancy
- Varicose veins
- Oral contraceptives
- Older age (exponential increase above the age of 50 years)
- Immobilization (paralyzed limbs in stroke, paraplegia)
- Previous DVT (risk increases two- to three-fold)
- Pregnancy (risk increased in postpartum period)
- Hypercoagulable states: antithrombin III deficiency, protein C deficiency, protein S deficiency, antiphospholipid syndrome, excessive plasminogen activator inhibitor, polycythaemia rubra vera, erythrocytosis
- Tissue trauma.

How would you investigate a possible deep vein thrombosis?
After focused history and clinical examination, the order of the investigations that need to take place will be guided by the clinical probability of a suspected DVT as determined by the Well's score.
- If clinical probability of DVT is high (≥2 points on the two-level Well's score):
  - Doppler ultrasound of the affected leg should be obtained. If the Doppler identifies a thrombus within the deep vein system, this is diagnostic of DVT. If the Doppler does not demonstrate thrombus, but the clinical probability was calculated as high, then blood for D-dimer assay should be taken. If raised patients would have a repeat ultrasound Doppler of the affected leg in a week's time.
- If clinical probability is low (≤1 point on the two-level Well's score):
  - D-dimers assay should be performed. If D-dimer levels are within normal limits, then a diagnosis of DVT can be safely excluded. If D-dimer levels are expected to be raised due to a coexisting condition (like recent surgery), then there is no point in performing the test. In this case, Doppler ultrasonography of the affected leg would still be the next most appropriate step in diagnosing DVT. A Doppler ultrasound should also be performed in this category patients if the D-dimers are raised. A negative Doppler excludes the diagnosis, whereas a thrombus seen on Doppler confirms the diagnosis of a DVT.

What is the standard treatment for a deep vein thrombosis?
Proximal DVT (iliac, femoral, or popliteal vein) is treated with a direct oral anticoagulant (DOAC) for 3 months with review of anticoagulation at 3 months. Patients with uncomplicated DVT by a reversible risk factor or first unprovoked DVT would stop anticoagulation after 3 months. Patients with DVT provoked by an irreversible risk factor such as active cancer would continue for a further 3-month period with a subsequent review at month 6.

Exception to the general rule can be specific patient populations, where vitamin K antagonists (VKAs) or heparin are more appropriate options (renal failure, antiphospholipid syndrome).

What are the challenges in diagnosing a recurrent deep vein thrombosis?
The recommendations regarding clinical probability scoring, the use of D-dimers, and ultrasonography remain the same regardless of whether the episode is recurrent or first DVT. However, there is additional difficulty in interpreting the presentation and the results when it comes to recurrent episodes.

Clinical presentation of a postthrombotic syndrome which occurs months after a first episode of DVT can share symptoms with a possible recurrent DVT, mainly pain, oedema, and vein dilation. D-dimers are highly sensitive in both first and recurrent episodes, but they lose specificity in recurrent episodes. As such, although a D-dimer test is equally helpful in excluding a recurrent DVT episode, its usefulness declines for diagnostic purposes in suspected recurrent DVT.

A positive Doppler ultrasound is equal to the identification of the thrombus. Given that once a thrombus formation has already occurred in a vein it does not completely resolve with treatment, it is hard for the operator to distinguish between an old and a recurrent DVT.

What is phlegmasia cerulea dolens?
It is a clinical condition secondary to massive thrombus burden within the iliac and femoral veins causing blood flow occlusion within the venous system leading to presentation with a picture resembling acute ischaemia. This condition often needs unfractionated heparin and vascular intervention.

When would you consider long-term anticoagulation for a patient with a deep vein thrombosis?
Extending anticoagulation beyond the initial 3- or 6-month period is a difficult clinical decision and it has to involve the patient, their risk of recurrence, their risk of bleeding, and their overall preference. The risk of recurrence of a DVT as studied to date is around 5% for the first year for a provoked episode and 10% for an unprovoked episode, and it is cumulative thereafter increasing year on year. When deciding on long-term anticoagulation, one has to take into account persistent risk factor for recurrence such as malignancy, thrombophilia, nephrotic syndrome, inflammatory bowel disease, obesity, and autoimmune disease. The other important factor to consider is bleeding risk in the individual, as a recurrent venous thromboembolism (VTE) does not carry a similar risk of fatality compared to a major bleed. Since the introduction of DOACs, bleeding rates have been reduced compared to warfarin use, however, bleeding risk should still be calculated and taken into account as it remains around 1% to 1.5% per year overall.

What is Virchow triad?
VTE is a result of three major abnormalities—stasis or pooling of blood, vascular endothelial injury, and hypercoagulable states. Most patients with a documented DVT will have one, two, or all three of the these triad present.

What are the complications of deep vein thrombosis?
- Pulmonary embolism
- Postthrombotic syndrome

- Venous gangrene
- Pain, particularly in iliofemoral thrombosis.

What is the risk of pulmonary embolism in patients with below-knee thrombi?

The risk in such cases is low (almost half the risk of proximal DVT), and many physicians refrain from prescribing anticoagulation to these patients. If anticoagulation is considered, treatment should only be continued for a maximum of 6 weeks.

How is bleeding risk from anticoagulation calculated?

The two most commonly used scores for assessing bleeding risks are the HEMORR$_2$HAGES and HAS-BLED.

The HEMORR$_2$HAGES score is computed by adding 1 point for each bleeding risk factor:
- Hepatic or renal disease
- Ethanol abuse
- Malignancy
- Older (age >75 years)
- Reduced platelet count (<75 × 10^9/l) or function
- Rebleeding risk (2 points for major bleed and 1 point for minor bleed)
- Hypertension (uncontrolled), systolic blood pressure >160 mm Hg
- Anaemia (hematocrit <30%)
- Genetic factors
- Excessive fall risk
- Stroke

The risk of bleeding is then predicted by the following table:

HEMORR$_2$HAGES Score	Bleeds per 100 Patient-Years Warfarin
0	1.9 (0.6–4.4)
1	2.5 (1.3–4.3)
2	5.3 (3.4–8.1)
3	8.4 (4.9–13.6)
4	10.4 (5.1–18.9)
≥5	12.3 (5.8–23.1)

HAS-BLED also is calculated with 1 point for each of the factors:

Hypertension, Abnormal renal function, Abnormal liver function, Stroke, Bleeding tendency, Liable INRs (for patients on warfarin), Elderly (>75), Drugs or alcohol excess.

HAS-BLED Score	Bleeds per 100 Patient-Years Warfarin
0–1	1.1
2	1.88
3	3.74
4	8.7
>5	Insufficient data

What are causes of recurrent venous thrombosis?
- Pregnancy, surgery, trauma, oral contraceptives
- Abnormalities in antithrombin III, protein C, protein S, fibrinogen, or factor V
- Acquired conditions such as antiphospholipid antibody syndrome, occult cancer, myeloproliferative disorders, some vasculitides
- Potential abnormalities, including thrombomodulin, tissue factor pathway inhibitor, vitronectin associated with heparin and antithrombin III, and fibrinolytic receptors.

Further Information

J. Homans (1877–1954) was an American surgeon who worked at Johns Hopkins Hospital with Cushing, initially on experimental hypophysectomy and later on vascular disease. He first reported venous thrombosis related to air travel in a 54-year-old physician who developed DVT after a 14-h flight (Homans, 1954).

G.R.V. Hughes, contemporary London physician, Raynes Institute, St Thomas' Hospital, first described the antiphospholipid antibody syndrome (Khamashta et al., 1995).

Rudolph Virchow (1821–1902) was a German doctor, amongst many other talents, known to his peers at 'the Pope of Medicine'.

Phil Wells is a Professor of Medicine in Ottawa, Canada.

CHAPTER 222

Gallop Rhythm

Instruction

Listen to the precordium.
Examine this patient's heart.

Salient Features

HISTORY

- Dyspnoea
- Determine New York Heart Association class
- Paroxysmal nocturnal dyspnoea
- Swelling of the feet.

EXAMINATION

- Presence of an abnormal third or fourth heart sound (Fig. 222.1) with tachycardia. (The presence of a normal third or fourth heart sound does not connote a gallop rhythm unless there is associated tachycardia.)
- Auscultate with the bell as third and fourth heart sounds are low pitched.
- Gallop rhythm as a result of third heart sound seems to sound like 'Kentucky', whereas that because of the fourth heart sound sounds like 'Tennessee'.

> **Notes:**
> - A left ventricular third heart sound is best heard at the apex, whereas the right ventricular third heart sound is best heard along the left sternal border.
> - The left ventricular third heart sound is heard over the left ventricular impulse, especially when the impulse is brought closer to the chest wall by placing the patient in a partial left lateral decubitus position.
> - In emphysematous patients, the gallop is better heard when listening over the xiphoid or epigastric area.

Diagnosis

This patient has gallop rhythm (lesion), which indicates that he is in cardiac failure (functional status).

Questions

What is the expression used when both the third and fourth heart sounds are heard with tachycardia?
This is known as the summation gallop. It can sometimes be confused for a diastolic rumbling murmur.

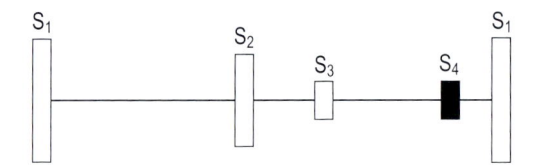

Fig. 222.1 Heart sounds, with the abnormal fourth sound.

What is the mechanism of production of the third heart sound?
It is caused by rapid ventricular filling in early diastole.

What is the mechanism of production of the fourth heart sound?
It is caused by vigorous contraction of the atria (atrial systole) and is hence heard towards the end of diastole.

How do you differentiate between the fourth heart sound, a split first heart sound and an ejection click?
The fourth heart sound is not heard when pressure is applied on the chest piece of the stethoscope, but pressure does not eliminate the ejection sound or the splitting of the first heart sound.

What are the causes of a third heart sound?
- Physiological: in normal children and young adults
- Pathological:
    - Heart failure (third heart sound gallop is relatively specific for elevated left ventricular end-diastolic pressure and left ventricular dysfunction)
    - Left ventricular dilatation without failure: mitral regurgitation, ventricular septal defect, patent ductus arteriosus
    - Right ventricular third heart sound in right ventricular failure, tricuspid regurgitation.

What are the implications of a third heart sound in patients with valvular heart disease?
- In patients with mitral regurgitation, they are common but do not necessarily reflect ventricular systolic dysfunction or increased filling pressure.
- In patients with aortic stenosis, third heart sounds are uncommon but usually indicate the presence of systolic dysfunction and raised filling pressure.

What are the causes of a fourth heart sound?
- Normal: in the elderly
- Pathological:
    - Acute myocardial infarction
    - Aortic stenosis (the presence of a fourth heart sound in individuals <40 years of age indicates significant obstruction)
    - Hypertension (it is a constant finding in hypertension)
    - Hypertrophic cardiomyopathy
    - Pulmonary stenosis.

Note: The fourth heart sound does not denote heart failure, unlike the third heart sound gallop.

Further Information

Potain credited Jean Baptiste Bouillaud (1786–1881), Professor of Medicine in Paris, as being the first person to describe gallop rhythm (Potain, 1931).

Pierre Carl Edouard Potain (1825–1901), Parisian physician, was the first to distinguish between various types of gallop in a short account titled Théorie du Bruit de Gallop, in 1885.

CHAPTER 223

Guillain–Barré Syndrome

Instruction
This patient presented with bilateral leg weakness. Please examine their peripheral nervous system.

Salient Features

HISTORY
- Weakness: difficulty in rising up from seated position or climbing stairs; legs usually affected before upper limbs
- Dyspnoea: late in the course suggesting diaphragmatic and intercostal muscle weakness
- Cranial nerve involvement: diplopia, drooling of saliva, regurgitation of food
- Paraesthesia
- Urinary symptoms
- Systemic symptoms: fatigue
- Ascertain whether the onset was preceded by a trivial viral illness.

EXAMINATION
- Weakness of distal limb muscles
- Distal numbness
- Areflexia
- Reduced forced vital capacity (respiratory failure)
- Labile blood pressure (BP) (autonomic dysfunction).

Polyneuropathies can be classified as demyelinating or axonal. They can also be classified according to the diameter of the affected nerve fibre. Larger fibres are heavily myelinated and therefore most subject to processes that damage myelin. Most polyneuropathies, including the diabetic type, are axonal.

Diagnosis
This patient has Guillain–Barré syndrome (GBS) (lesion) and is currently experiencing weakness of the distal limb muscles (functional status).

Questions

What features are required for diagnosis?
- Progressive weakness in both arms and legs (might start with weakness only in the legs)
- Areflexia (or decreased tendon reflexes).

What features strongly support diagnosis?
- Progression of symptoms over days to 4 weeks
- Relative symmetry of symptoms
- Mild sensory symptoms or signs
- Cranial nerve involvement, especially bilateral weakness of facial muscles
- Autonomic dysfunction
- Pain (often present)
- High concentration of protein in the cerebrospinal fluid (CSF)
- Typical electrodiagnostic features.

What features should raise doubt about the diagnosis?
- Severe pulmonary dysfunction with limited limb weakness at onset
- Severe sensory signs with limited weakness at onset
- Bladder or bowel dysfunction at onset
- Fever at onset
- Sharp sensory level
- Slow progression with limited weakness without respiratory involvement (consider subacute inflammatory demyelinating polyneuropathy or chronic inflammatory demyelinating polyradiculoneuropathy (CIDP))
- Marked persistent asymmetry of weakness
- Persistent bladder or bowel dysfunction
- Increased number of mononuclear cells in CSF (>50 × 10^6/L)
- Polymorphonuclear cells in CSF.

What is the pathology of Guillain–Barré syndrome?
It is an acute inflammatory demyelinating neuropathy. Infections (e.g. with *Campylobacter jejuni*) or other events (e.g. vaccination) might induce an immune response that attacks the peripheral myelin of the Schwann cells and ultimately leads to GBS. The immune response depends on certain antigenic factors, such as the specificity of lipooligosaccharide, and on patient-related (host) factors. Genetic polymorphisms in the patients might partially determine the severity of GBS. Antibodies to lipooligosaccharides can cross-react with specific nerve gangliosides and can activate complement. The extent of nerve damage depends on several factors. Nerve dysfunction leads to weakness and might cause sensory disturbances.

How is the diagnosis confirmed?
The diagnosis is a combination of clinical and laboratory criteria. Required criteria are progressive weakness and areflexia or hyporeflexia in the affected limbs. Supportive but not essential criteria are symmetrical symptoms, pain in the trunk or limbs, cranial nerve involvement, autonomic dysfunction, sensory dysfunction, apyrexia, and relevant findings in nerve conduction studies and CSF analysis. Nerve conduction studies demonstrate slowing of conduction or conduction block. CSF shows albumino-cytological dissociation; a normal cell count but raised protein concentration (in approximately 65% of patients). Antibodies do not help in diagnosis (except for the GQ1b in the Miller-Fisher variant and antiganglioside antibodies in the axonal variants). Magnetic resonance imaging (MRI) of the brain and spine is not part of the diagnostic evaluation of the disease, but it is usually obtained to exclude other differentials. If performed, spinal MRI may reveal enhancement of spinal nerve roots.

What is Miller–Fisher syndrome?
A rare proximal variant of GBS that initially affects the ocular muscles and in which ataxia is prominent.

What other variants of Guillain–Barré syndrome are you aware of?
Alongside Miller–Fisher syndrome (with ataxia and ophthalmoplegia), there are several other variants with atypical presentation recognized to date, but the most common ones are acute motor axonal neuropathy, acute motor and sensory axonal neuropathy, and Bickerstaff brainstem encephalitis.

What is the differential diagnosis?
Poliomyelitis, botulism, primary muscle disease, or other neuropathy (porphyric, diphtheric, heavy metal, and organophosphate poisoning).

How would you treat such patients?
- High-dose intravenous immunoglobulin (IVIG) during the acute phase to reduce the severity and duration of symptoms. This is equivalent to plasma exchange in effectiveness in reducing disability, but the combination of intravenous immunoglobulin and plasma exchange offers no significant additional advantage.
- Ventilatory support if respiratory muscles are affected
- Physiotherapy and occupational therapy for muscle weakness
- Close monitoring for autonomic dysfunction, paralytic ileus, bladder dysfunction, and arrhythmias.

What is the prognosis?
Despite medical therapy, this syndrome often remains a severe disease: 3% to 10% of patients die and 20% are still unable to walk after 6 months. In addition, many patients have pain and fatigue that can persist for months or years. Outcome in patients with GBS can be determined with the Erasmus GBS Outcome Scale (EGOS). Using EGOS, the chance of walking unaided after 6 months can be calculated on the basis of the age of the patient, the presence of diarrhoea, and the severity of weakness in the first weeks. Despite treatment with intravenous immunoglobulin, many patients only partially recover and have residual weakness, pain, and fatigue.

What do you know about chronic inflammatory demyelinating polyradiculoneuropathy?
- This is the most common demyelinating neuropathy.
- It is an idiopathic multifocal inflammation of the nerves that can occur at any age in the form of a subacute sensorimotor polyneuropathy.
- It is diagnosed by the findings of electrical conduction block (segmental demyelination at areas of inflammation, as seen on nerve-conduction studies) and by a high level of protein in the CSF.
- CIDP is usually idiopathic but also can occur as a feature of some connective tissue diseases.
- Corticosteroids, intravenous immunoglobulin, and plasma exchange are usually effective therapies; when these are not effective, immunosuppressive drugs are often added.
- CIDP is clinically similar to GBS, except for the differing time course, and was at one time called chronic GBS.

What do you know about POEMS syndrome?
The acronym POEMS (polyneuropathy, organomegaly, endocrinopathy, M protein, and skin changes) was introduced by Bardwick and team. Polyneuropathy and polyclonal plasma cell proliferation are present in all patients. In the POEMS syndrome, a clonal expansion of plasma cells occurs in association with sclerotic bone lesions (osteosclerotic myeloma). The syndrome may also involve lymph nodes in the form of angiofollicular hyperplasia, also known as Castleman disease. A moderately increased level of CSF protein in this patient is typical of the POEMS syndrome but does not distinguish it from CIDP. A low level of monoclonal immunoglobulin G

with lambda light chain is also characteristic of the POEMS syndrome, whereas kappa light chain predominates in monoclonal gammopathy of unknown significance. However, in contrast to multiple myeloma, the levels of other immunoglobulin subclasses are not reduced in the POEMS syndrome.

Further Information

C. Guillain (1876–1961), Professor of Medicine in Paris.
J.A. Barré (1880–1967), Professor of Neurology in Strasbourg, trained in Paris.

CHAPTER 224

Hyperkalaemia

Instruction

This patient was found to have hyperkalaemia on routine blood tests. He was sent to hospital. Please assess.

Salient Features

HISTORY

- Most patients are asymptomatic.
- Symptoms are not reliable in hyperkalaemia.
- Cardiac arrest due to hyperkalaemia can happen suddenly in an asymptomatic patient.

EXAMINATION

- Muscle weakness, paralysis
- Cardiac arrhythmias.

Proceed as follows:

Tell the examiner that you would like to obtain an urgent 12-lead electrocardiogram (ECG) and repeat the blood test to confirm hyperkalaemia.

Diagnosis

This patient is hyperkalaemic probably due to prescribed medication use. I would like to obtain a 12 lead ECG and start treatment for hyperkalaemia.

Questions

What do you know about potassium adaptation?
Potassium is the main intracellular cation with cells containing 30 times more potassium than the blood. This balance, maintained by the Na-K-ATPase located on the cell membrane, is important for the function of myocytes and neurons.

Potassium adaptation refers to the body's ability to maintain normal potassium levels despite increased potassium intake by food. With normal physiology, increased potassium intake should not lead to hyperkalaemia. Potassium taken orally is absorbed in the jejunum, with the majority taken up by liver and muscle cells with the help of the membrane-bound Na-K-ATPase, and the rest remaining in the plasma stimulating aldosterone secretion and increased potassium excretion in the urine.

What is the first step in treating this patient?
The initial step is confirming that the reported hyperkalaemia is a true finding. Poor venepuncture technique, delay in processing the blood sample, or the centrifugation process can all potentially give rise to false hyperkalaemia. The first thing to be done when this patient arrives to hospital is to repeat the blood tests to confirm the hyperkalaemia.

Name some causes of hyperkalaemia.
- Acute kidney injury
- Chronic kidney disease
- Renal tubular acidosis type 4
- Addison disease
- Intensive exercise
- Burns, trauma
- Metabolic acidosis states
- Drug related (potassium supplements, angiotensin-converting enzyme inhibitor (ACE-I), angiotensin receptor blockers (ARBs), potassium sparing diuretics, aldosterone antagonists, digitalis toxicity).

Name some foods that patients with chronic kidney disease and hyperkalaemia should avoid.
- Fruit: bananas, oranges, mangoes, avocados, pomegranates, prunes, dried figs, raisins
- Vegetables: spinach, Brussel sprouts, artichokes, tomatoes, broccoli, carrots, potatoes
- Red meat
- Dairy: milk, yoghurt
- Foods with salt substitutes
- Liquorice
- Cola.

How are such patients advised to consume root vegetables?
Leaching is a process that helps reduce the potassium content of vegetables. Patients are advised to peel and soak the vegetables in cold water, slice them 3 mm thick, rinse them with warm water and soak them in warm water for hours, rinse them again with warm water, and cook them in lots of water.

What are the electrocardiographic changes associated with hyperkalaemia?
- Tall and tented T waves
- Shortened QT interval
- Prolongation of PR
- Widening of QRS
- Flattened P waves
- Ventricular tachycardia.

What is the emergency treatment of hyperkalaemia?
Patients with severe hyperkalaemia with a potassium more than 6.5 mmol/L or patients with mild or moderate hyperkalaemia that have ECG changes consistent with hyperkalaemia should receive emergency treatment with continuous cardiac monitoring. Calcium gluconate is given if there are ECG changes as this works by protecting myocardium and conduction tissue against hyperkalaemia. Dextrose and insulin infusion is the immediate treatment as insulin increases potassium uptake into cells whilst glucose limits the hypoglycaemic effect of insulin. Use of intravenous (IV) sodium bicarbonate should be limited to cases of severe metabolic acidosis. Potassium binders can also be considered such as calcium resonium, patiromere, and sodium zirconium. Urgent haemofiltration or haemodialysis may be required.

What are the nonemergency options of treating hyperkalaemia?
If hyperkalaemia is due to end-stage renal failure, then discussions regarding haemodialysis should take place. If the hyperkalaemia is not associated with chronic kidney disease, resins and cation exchangers are options alongside dietary modification and withholding medications that could cause or worsen hyperkalaemia.

CHAPTER 225

Hypernatraemia

Instruction

This elderly patient from a nursing home with known dementia is admitted to hospital with worsening confusion and lethargy. Please examine.

Salient Features

HISTORY

- Social and past medical history are crucial in identifying hypernatraemia.
- True hypernatraemia is almost always caused by dehydration. Adults respond to water loss with increased thirst and drinking water. Hypernatraemia is most often caused by water loss in patients who do not have access to water or cannot express their thirst because of an intellectual disability. These patients are usually patients with learning difficulties, elderly patients with dementia, and nursing home residents with confusion.
- History of excessive water loss—diarrhoea and vomiting; polyuria in an otherwise independent and alert patient can be a marker of impaired thirst mechanism in an underlying hypothalamic lesion, so focused history should be sought; polyuria; nocturia; head trauma; coexistent autoimmune conditions; pituitary surgery.
- Drug history—medications that can cause diabetes insipidus (DI) (lithium), abuse of laxatives that cause osmotic diarrhoea
- Neurological complaints caused by hypernatraemia—lethargy, generalized weakness, seizures, coma.

EXAMINATION

- Signs of dehydration—reduced skin turgor, dry mucous membranes, prolonged capillary refill time, tachycardia, hypotension, reduced urine output
- Neurological examination—confusion, twitches, seizures, coma.

Diagnosis

This elderly patient has severe hypernatraemia (lesion) due to deprivation of water (aetiology). She is bedbound with a Glasgow Coma Scale (GCS) score of 10/15 (functional status).

Questions

How would you approach this patient?
The initial step in evaluation of hypernatraemia is to take a careful history of the patient's symptoms and living conditions. Hypernatraemia commonly occurs in confused patients who do not have access to water, but if the patient is an otherwise alert and independent person with access to water, then hypothalamic lesions should be suspected and excluded, and essential DI (adipsic)

should be suspected. If polyuria is identified as a new symptom, then water consumption should be quantified. When the human body loses water, the plasma tonicity increases leading to the secretion of antidiuretic hormone and thirst. As a result, retention of water and further water intake will help return sodium levels back to normal. Patients who do not have an intact thirst reflex or who do not have access to water will eventually become hypernatraemic.

Clinical examination is the next step in evaluating the patient with hypernatraemia. Most patients will be hypovolaemic and dehydrated. In the rare event that patients are euvolaemic, this indicates excess sodium influx (oral intake of sodium or potassium or intravenous hypertonic saline) without water loss.

History and clinical examination should be enough to establish an underlying aetiology. Routine biochemical profile will also help exclude osmotic hypernatraemia caused by hyperglycaemia and azotaemia. If clinical evaluation and biochemistry are not enough to establish the underlying aetiology, then urine osmolality should be obtained.

If urine osmolality is appropriately high, then this translates to appropriate urine concentration, or in other words the patient is water depleted. If the urine osmolality is lower than plasma osmolality, then DI is suspected and repeat osmolality with monitoring urine volume after antidiuretic hormone secretion (ADH) administration should help differentiate further.

The aforementioned patient weighs 64 kg. Her measured sodium is 160. History consists of a few episodes of diarrhoea a few days ago that have now resolved and clinical examination only shows dehydration but her vital signs are normal. How would you treat her?

The initial step in water replacement is to establish the total water deficit for this patient. The water deficit is calculated by multiplying the patient's total body water which is half their body weight by measured Na/140 − 1.

Total water deficit = Total body water * (Na/140 − 1) = 3.2 L

Hypernatraemia in this elderly patient is chronic (more than 48 hours of minimum duration). Rarely does hypernatraemia establish itself acutely in less than 48 hours. In chronic hypernatraemia, sodium level should not be corrected by more than 10 to 12 mEq/L in 24 hours.

Roughly 3 mL/kg of dextrose 5% will raise the Na by 1 mEq/L. That means that in this patient, an infusion of around 1920 mL should be given within the first 24 hours.

The rate is initiated at 80 mL/hour and plasma sodium should be closely monitored every 4 to 6 hours with appropriate adjustment of infusion rate.

How is blood volume and sodium concentration regulated and balanced?

Water constitutes around 50% of our lean body weight. This is distributed in two different compartments: intracellular (70%) and extracellular including plasma (30%).

The determinant of water distribution between the two compartments is mainly the oncotic pressure which in turn is dependent on osmotically active solutes, sodium (Na), potassium (K), and plasma proteins.

The cell membrane is the 'wall' between the intracellular and extracellular spaces and is not permeable to Na and K, as the membrane Na/K ATPase prevents K exiting the cell and Na entering the cell.

The capillary wall is the 'wall' between extracellular-interstitial space and plasma. Na crosses the capillary wall with water following across an osmolality gradient.

Total body sodium stores are the main determinant of extracellular fluid volume and tissue perfusion. As a general rule water follows sodium.

Sodium balance in the body and extracellular fluid volume is maintained by hormonal feedback mechanisms. When circulatory volume diminishes, the renin–angiotensin–aldosterone system and the sympathetic system are activated, and sodium is retained in the body. In contrast, when circulatory volume expands, natriuretic peptide promotes sodium excretion.

If Na increases the Na will initially be in the extracellular fluid increasing the tonicity of the extracellular fluid and attracting water from the cells. Water moving from the cells to the extracellular compartment will lead to extracellular volume expansion. This expansion leads to release of natriuretic peptides by the atria and the ventricles increasing sodium excretion.

In contrast, when Na is reduced there is volume contraction. Volume contraction will be detected by vasoreceptors in the juxtaglomerular cells in the afferent glomerular arteriole and the carotid sinus, and renin–angiotensin–aldosterone will be activated. This results in sodium retention, vasoconstriction, and volume expansion with increased blood pressure.

This is how blood volume is regulated in response to increased or decreased sodium content in the blood. When there is water loss, however, the body has to have a mechanism to increase the effective blood volume.

When blood volume is lost, usually because of water loss, then plasma tonicity increases. This increment is sensed by the osmoreceptors in hypothalamus which responds to this change by the release of ADH. ADH in turn promotes thirst and water reabsorption by the kidneys. Increased water intake as a response to thirst and water retention as a result of water reabsorption will prevent hypernatraemia from water loss.

What do you know about diabetes insipidus?

DI is caused either by reduced secretion of ADH (central DI) or ADH resistance (nephrogenic DI). Both conditions are associated with reduced ADH action in the kidneys resulting in polyuria and polydipsia. The biochemical profile of these patients will be characterized by high plasma sodium, and high plasma with low urine osmolality. Low urine osmolality is characteristic to both types of DI. Central DI will respond with concentration of urine on administration of desmopressin, whereas nephrogenic DI will not respond to desmopressin. Central DI can be idiopathic, familiar or secondary to brain trauma, surgery, or tumours, and rarely in Sheehan syndrome and Langerhan's histiocytosis. Nephrogenic DI can also be either inherited or secondary to drugs (lithium) or electrolyte abnormalities. Treatment consists of desmopressin in ADH deficiency or partial resistance and dietary and water intake modifications in nephrogenic aetiology.

CHAPTER 226

Hypokalaemia

Instruction

This 70-year-old patient has been admitted with diarrhoea and vomiting for the last week with reduced appetite and oral intake. Her symptoms have now resolved but she was found to have low potassium on a follow-up blood test. Please assess.

Salient Features

HISTORY

- Nonspecific symptoms like fatigue, generalized weakness, anorexia, and nausea can occur with hypokalaemia.
- Muscle cramps—muscle cramps can be caused by potassium deficiency or magnesium deficiency.
- Muscle weakness—leg weakness precedes trunk and arm weakness, but this feature is rarely seen as in order for muscle weakness to occur, the potassium has to be extremely low.
- Constipation. Severe hypokalaemia can also give rise to paralytic ileus.
- History of diarrhoea and vomiting
- Drug history (laxatives or diuretic abuse)
- Repeated episodes of temporary paralysis that self resolves point towards periodic paralysis.

EXAMINATION

- Cardiac arrhythmias
- Reduced power with no specific pattern
- Hypertension
- Dehydration.

Diagnosis

This patient has severe hypokalaemia (diagnosis) because of gastrointestinal electrolyte losses (aetiology). She is haemodynamically stable with a normal neurological examination and normal electrocardiogram (ECG) and is only complaining of fatigue (functional status).

Questions

What abnormalities are you expecting to see in the electrocardiogram of a person with hypokalaemia?
Hypokalaemia can produce a series of abnormalities on ECG trace and a series of arrhythmias. Some of the most commonly seen abnormalities are:
- ST depression (hypokalaemia; Fig. 226.1)
- Flat T waves

809

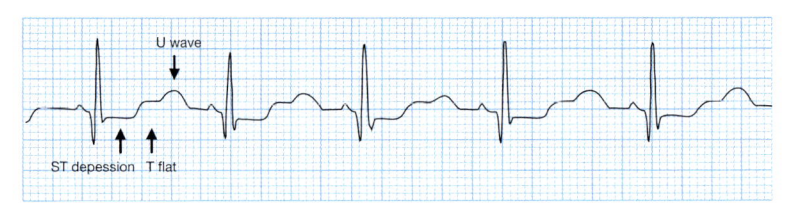

Fig. 226.1 Electrocardiogram manifestations of hypokalaemia. (Courtesy Tor Ercleve, in Brown, A.F.T., Cadogan, M., Celenza, A., Brown, A., 2017. Marshall Ruedy's On Call: Principles and Protocols, third edn. Elsevier.)

- U waves
- Atrial ectopics
- Ventricular ectopics
- Atrioventricular block
- Widened QRS, ventricular tachycardia.

What are the major life-threatening complications of hypokalaemia?
Respiratory failure, cardiac arrhythmias and cardiac arrest, rhabdomyolysis, and acute paralysis.

What are the causes of hypokalaemia?
There are six main causes of hypokalaemia. Identifying the culprit amongst this list of six is important to guide management:
- Potassium loss
- Reduced potassium intake
- Dialysis
- Hypomagnesaemia
- Redistribution of potassium with increased entering into the cells
- Iatrogenic (flucloxacillin, gentamycin, amphotericin, insulin, steroids).

Potassium loss is the most commonly occurring one, and it can be due to gastrointestinal losses (diarrhoea, vomiting, increased stoma output, laxative abuse) or urinary losses (diuretics, polyuria, renal tubular acidosis type 1 and 2, salt-wasting tubulopathies). Redistribution of potassium is rare and it occurs in increased insulin availability situations, in beta-agonist administration, in hypokalaemic periodic paralysis, and in severe alkalosis.

What do you know of hypokalaemic periodic paralysis?
It is an inherited autosomal dominant disorder characterized by recurrent episodes of sudden painless generalized paralysis, precipitated usually by exercise, meals, or stress. Patients have hypokalaemia during the attacks as the cause of the condition is movement of potassium into cells. The attacks last for a few hours and patients are normal between attacks, as is the potassium in their blood. The onset of the disease is usually in young adults, and they eventually develop some proximal myopathy by middle age.

What is the relevance of hypokalaemia in digoxin administration?
Hypokalaemia can increase the toxicity of digoxin and it is one of the most common causes for chronic digoxin toxicity. Hypokalaemia in the context of digitalis toxicity is clinically relevant as if it is not corrected promptly it can worsen during the treatment of digoxin toxicity.

When is intravenous administration of potassium indicated?
- In severe hypokalaemia (less than 2.5)
- In symptomatic hypokalaemia
- When hypokalaemia is associated with ECG changes
- In hypokalaemic patients who are not tolerating oral feed or are nil by mouth.

How would you treat this patient?
This patient needs potassium replacement. Potassium can be replaced orally or intravenously. In severe hypokalaemia or in hypokalaemia associated with severe arrhythmia, where potassium needs to be replaced intravenously at high rates, intensive care admission with continuous cardiac monitoring and potassium chloride through central line is indicated. In this specific scenario, a combination of oral and intravenous replacement of potassium in a normal ward would suffice. As a rough guide, an adult needs 1 mmol/kg/day of potassium, and a drop in 1 mmol/L represents a total loss of minimum 100 mmol of potassium from body stores. Oral potassium tablets usually contain 12 to 18 mmol of potassium per tablet. Magnesium levels should be requested and concurrent hypomagnesaemia should be treated accordingly as if there is a concurrent hypomagnesaemia the potassium will not correct easily.

Name the most commonly known salt-wasting nephropathies.
Bartter syndrome and Gitelman syndrome. They are inherited disorders of the kidney, characterized by secondary hyperaldosteronism, metabolic alkalosis with hypokalaemia, muscle cramps, and chronic fatigue with a low or normal blood pressure.

How can acid–base balance and blood pressure of a patient inform a case of hypokalaemia?
- Primary hyperaldosteronism (including Conn disease), Liddle syndrome, and Cushing syndrome are associated with metabolic alkalosis and hypertension.
- Secondary hyperaldosteronism due to salt-wasting nephropathies, gastrointestinal loss due to vomiting, and overdiuresis due to diuretic abuse are associated with metabolic alkalosis but low or normal blood pressure.
- Renal tubular acidosis and severe gastrointestinal losses due to laxative abuse or villous adenoma are associated with metabolic acidosis.

Further Information
Frederic Bartter (1914–1983), an American endocrinologist, first described syndrome of inappropriate ADH secretion (SIADH).
Hillel Gitelman (1932–2015), an American nephrologist.
William Withering (1741–1799) first described the use of digitalis (foxglove) for medical conditions.

CHAPTER **227**

Hyponatraemia

Instruction

This patient was found to have an incidental sodium of 124 mmol/L. She has been complaining of fatigue. Please examine her.

Salient Features

HISTORY

- History of chronic kidney disease or liver disease
- Social, dietary, and drug history, including medication list, alcohol intake, and low-sodium, low-protein diets
- Recent past medical history for recent intracranial pathology, neurosurgical intervention, or urological surgery
- Recent fluid loss and dehydration—vomiting, diarrhoea, blood loss
- Symptoms suggestive of congestive cardiac failure—peripheral oedema, orthopnoea, paroxysmal nocturnal dyspnoea, fatigue, reduced exercise tolerance, dyspnoea on exertion
- Symptoms suggestive of adrenal or thyroid disease—postural hypotension, low energy, lethargy, abdominal pains, constipation, cold intolerance, weight loss, or weight gain
- Symptoms consistent with malignancy—night sweats, weight loss, and organ-specific symptoms for lung or intra-abdominal malignancy.

Note: Symptoms consistent with multiple myeloma should be sought, as evident paraprotein in the serum can cause pseudohyponatraemia.

Tell the examiner you would like to look at previous blood test results to establish previous electrolyte results and determine if the hyponatraemia is chronic.

EXAMINATION

- Assess the patient to establish their volume status.
- Oedematous patients may have additional sings of congestive cardiac failure, liver failure, or chronic kidney disease.
- Hypovolaemic patients may have signs of haemorrhage.
- Full system examination for physical findings suggesting an underlying cause, such as lung malignancy, adrenal insufficiency, thyroid disease, or pituitary disease
- Neurological examination.

Diagnosis

This patient has an incidental finding of hyponatraemia (lesion), probably due to medication use (cause). She is euvolaemic and asymptomatic (functional status).

Questions

How is hyponatraemia classified?
Measured osmolality less than 275 mOsm/kg always indicates a hypotonic hyponatraemia as the effective osmolality will never be higher than the measured one.
Depending on patient's extracellular fluid status, hypotonic hyponatraemia can be classified into three categories.
Hypotonic hyponatraemia in dehydrated patients:
- Gastrointestinal sodium loss (diarrhoea, vomiting)
- Transdermal sodium loss (cystic fibrosis, extensive burns)
- Renal sodium loss (thiazide diuretics, adrenal insufficiency, cerebral salt wasting syndrome (CSW), kidney disease)
- Capillary leaking syndromes (severe sepsis, pancreatitis, trauma, burns)
- Primary adrenal insufficiency with low aldosterone.

Hypotonic hyponatraemia in euvolaemic patients:
- Hypothyroidism
- Secondary adrenal insufficiency with low cortisol
- Syndrome of inappropriate antidiuretic hormone secretion (SIADH)
- Polydipsia.

Hypotonic hyponatraemia in oedematous patients:
- Heart failure
- Liver failure
- Nephrotic syndrome.

Hyponatraemia can be classified as mild, moderate, and severe and as acute (<48 hours) and chronic (>48 hours). It may be asymptomatic, moderately symptomatic, or severely symptomatic.

How are the symptoms of hyponatraemia related to the sodium level?
Symptoms of hyponatraemia are mainly neurological. They vary from mild symptoms such as fatigue, headache, nausea, vomiting, confusion, and unsteady gait to seizures and coma. Neurological complications such as seizures and coma are very rare in chronic hyponatraemia, but very common in acute hyponatraemia. Even for severe hyponatraemia with sodium levels less than 120 mmol/L, if it is chronic, the risk of seizures is less than 3%. In contrast, 30% of cases with acute severe hyponatraemia that has established within 48 hours are expected to be complicated by seizures.

Name some medications that have been associated with the syndrome of inappropriate antidiuretic hormone secretion.
Antipsychotic drugs, cyclophosphamide, methotrexate, pentostatin, vasopressin analogues, interferon, proton pump inhibitors, amiodarone, linezolid, monoclonal antibodies, lamotrigine, carbamazepine, sodium valproate, venlafaxine, selective serotonin reuptake inhibitors (SSRIs).

What are the essential criteria for diagnosing syndrome of inappropriate antidiuretic hormone secretion?
SIADH remains a diagnosis of exclusion such that other causes of euvolaemic hyponatraemia must be excluded (thyroid, pituitary, adrenal, or renal disease). The patient should not be on diuretic therapy. Effective serum osmolality should be low (<275 mOsm/kg) with inappropriately normal or raised urine osmolality (>100 mOsm/kg) and urinary sodium concentration >30 mmol/L.

What is cerebral salt wasting syndrome?
CSW is caused by inappropriate sodium excretion in the urine in patients with central nervous disease. As SIADH can also accompany central nervous disease and laboratory findings are

similar in both conditions, the only finding that differentiates the two is the patient's volume status. Patients with CSW are by definition dehydrated with low central venous pressures and low arterial pressures or orthostatic hypotension. Patients with SIADH are euvolaemic, so central venous pressures and arterial pressures will be normal. Although many clinicians have doubted the existence of CSW, it is important to distinguish between the two, as the treatment would differ. Hyponatraemia of CSW should correct with isotonic saline. In contrast SIADH is treated with fluid restriction. Fluid restriction can be dangerous for hyponatraemic patients post neurosurgical intervention or subarachnoid haemorrhage, as it can cause infarction.

What do you understand of the terms hypotonic hyponatraemia and hypertonic hyponatraemia?
Most cases of hyponatraemia will be hypotonic, where reduction of sodium in the bloodstream results in reduced effective osmolality. However, in some cases the existence of other osmoles increases the effective osmolality of the serum and reduces the serum concentration of sodium by shifting more water into the vessels. This is sometimes called pseudohyponatraemia and can be isotonic or hypertonic.

Examples of isotonic hyponatraemia are hyperglycaemia in patients with diabetic ketoacidosis, hypertriglyceridaemia in patients with pancreatitis, and iatrogenic hyponatraemia after urological surgery due to irrigation fluids.

What is effective osmolality?
Serum osmolality ranges between 275 and 290 mOsm/kg. Effective osmolality may differ from the measured plasma osmolality and determines the transcellular distribution of water. Effective osmolality cannot be measured directly but can be calculated by taking into account sodium, potassium, and plasma glucose levels. The difference between measured and effective osmolality is that measured osmolality takes into account most osmoles, whereas effective osmolality only takes into account those involved in water distribution. The ineffective osmoles are ones that move freely between membranes at a cellular level and as such do not have an impact on transcellular water distribution.

Effective osmolality only includes osmoles that are restricted to extracellular fluid volume.

Depending on the effective osmolality, hyponatraemia can be classified into hypotonic, isotonic, or hypertonic. Effective osmoles that can lead to isotonic or hypertonic hyponatraemia are glucose, mannitol, urea, alcohol, ethylene glycol, triglycerides and cholesterol, paraproteins.

How would you treat hypotonic hyponatraemia?
- Depends on the severity, duration, and symptoms at the time of presentation
- Chronic mild asymptomatic hyponatraemia will not need correction but should prompt investigation and monitoring.
- All other forms of hyponatraemia will need correction. Acute moderate hyponatraemia, severe hyponatraemia, and symptomatic hyponatraemia all need hospitalization for inpatient correction of sodium.
- Severe symptomatic hyponatraemia requires intravenous administration of hypertonic saline with close monitoring of serum sodium hourly, with an aim of rapid correction of around 5 mmol/L. Boluses of 100 mL of hypertonic saline 3% are given guided by symptom improvement.
- After the initial emergency correction, sodium correction should not exceed 8 mmol/L/24 hours to avoid overcorrection and risk of osmotic demyelination syndrome.

Moderate asymptomatic hyponatraemia and mild acute hyponatraemia can be investigated and treated accordingly. Low urine osmolality is usually a result of primary polydipsia. Normal or increased urine osmolality should trigger additional testing. In these patients, high sodium concentration in the urine could be due to kidney disease or diuretic use. If kidney disease is excluded and diuretics are stopped, then the patient should be assessed for fluid volume status. Dehydrated patients would need intravenous fluid replacement; euvolaemic patients would need investigation for thyroid and adrenal disease. Patients with SIADH are treated with fluid restriction; oedematous patients may need diuresis.

How do you treat hyponatraemia after urological operations involving bladder irrigation?

The treatment of hypertonic or isotonic hyponatraemia after urology surgery depends on the patient's symptoms.

- Asymptomatic patients will not need any treatment.
- Symptomatic euvolaemic patients with low osmolality can have hypertonic saline for rapid correction of their hyponatraemia.
- Symptomatic euvolaemic patients with increased osmolality benefit from haemofiltration.
- Dehydration should be treated accordingly with crystalloid fluids.
- Symptomatic oedematous and overloaded patients can be treated with loop diuretics.

Further Information

Frederic Bartter (1914–1983), an American endocrinologist, independently described SIADH as well as the primary kidney disorder which still carries his name.

William Schwartz (1922–2009) was an American nephrologist who also described SIADH and pioneered the science behind the use of diuretic drugs.

CHAPTER 228

Melaena

Instruction
This patient presents with black stools. Please take a history and examine their abdomen.

Salient Features

HISTORY
- Presence of melaena: black, tarry stools with a characteristic offensive smell
- Onset, duration, number of episodes
- Associated haematemesis or fresh rectal bleeding
- Epigastric pain or reflux symptoms
- Syncope or postural hypotension symptoms (may be a guide to expected blood loss)
- Features of liver disease, which may suggest a variceal bleed, including jaundice, abdominal distension (ascites) and/or peripheral oedema, pruritus, encephalopathy
- History of alcohol use disorder, hepatitis B or C, intravenous blood products, intravenous drug use disorder, Wilson disease
- Previous gastrointestinal (GI) bleed
- Medications precipitating bleeding or ulceration: antiplatelets, anticoagulants, corticosteroids, nonsteroidal antiinflammatory drugs (NSAIDs), antidepressants, bisphosphonates, nicorandil, calcium channel blockers
- Any gastroprotective medications: proton pump inhibitors (PPIs), H_2 antagonists
- Other causes of black stools: ingestion of iron tablets or food or drink high in iron such as Guinness; ingestion of liquorice, charcoal, bismuth
- Previous gastroscopy and treatment required.

EXAMINATION
- Pulse and blood pressure for signs of haemodynamic compromise
- Hands for evidence of liver disease: clubbing, leukonychia, Dupuytren contracture (Fig. 228.1), palmar erythema, spider naevi (in distribution of superior vena cava), tattoos, hepatic flap, pallor, scratch marks, generalized pigmentation. Also, evidence of rheumatological disease suggesting use of corticosteroids or NSAIDs
- Eyes and face for signs of liver disease: icterus, cyanosis, parotid enlargement, xanthomas
- Chest for other signs of liver disease: spider naevi, loss of axillary hair, gynaecomastia (can be unilateral)
- Abdomen for epigastric tenderness, hepatomegaly (particularly in alcoholic liver disease), splenomegaly (seldom >5 cm below the costal margin): a sign of portal hypertension suggesting that varices are probable
- Ascites
- Obesity: can be a sign of fatty liver or a risk factor for hiatus hernia
- Offer rectal examination to confirm the presence of melaena.

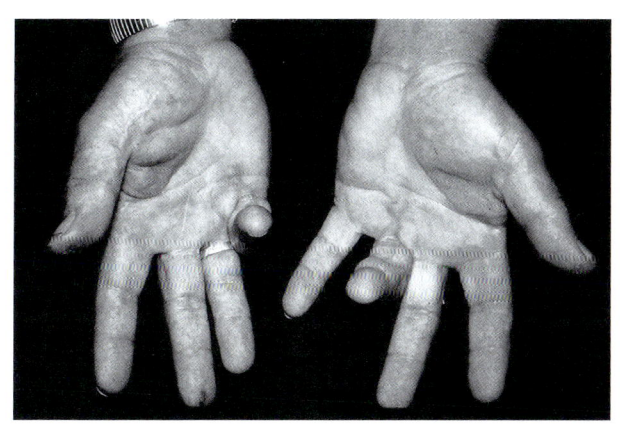

Fig. 228.1 Dupuytren's contracture.

Diagnosis

This patient has acute-onset melaena probably from a bleeding GI ulcer caused by steroids taken for rheumatoid arthritis (aetiology). They are currently haemodynamically stable (functional status).

Questions

What are the common causes of acute upper gastrointestinal bleeding?
- Gastric ulcers are responsible for around 25% of acute upper GI bleeds. Bleeding is caused by erosion of an underlying artery. There may be little or no preceding dyspepsia. Particularly significant haemorrhage can occur from posterior duodenal ulcers eroding the gastroduodenal artery, as well as lesser curve gastric ulcers eroding the left gastric artery.
- Oesophagitis is becoming a more common underlying cause for upper GI bleeding. Common in elderly people. Treatment is supportive and with PPIs.
- Gastritis, duodenitis, or gastric erosions: causes include *Helicobacter pylori* infection and NSAID use. Stop the offending medication and eradicate *H. pylori*.
- Oesophageal varices have a high index of suspicion if there are other features of decompensated liver disease. Bleeding is often high volume.
- Mallory–Weiss tear: review cause of initial vomiting such as medications, alcohol excess, malignancy. The bleeding often stops spontaneously and may not require endoscopic treatment.
- Vascular causes include the following:
  - Arteriovenous malformations in elderly are often idiopathic and in younger people can be due to hereditary haemorrhagic telangiectasia.
  - Gastric antral vascular ectasia or 'watermelon stomach': an uncommon vascular anomaly seen in endoscopy as red streaks radiating from pylori into the gastric antrum. They readily bleed. It is associated with autoimmune conditions. Treatment is with endoscopic thermoablation, including argon plasma coagulation and cryotherapy, or band ligation. Repeat treatment is often required, as well as regular blood transfusions. Curative treatment is with surgical resection, but this has high morbidity and mortality.
  - Portal hypertensive gastropathy: portal hypertension results in venous congestion of the gastric mucosa.

- Dieulafoy lesion: a dilated submucosal vessel that erodes the overlying lining but not associated with a peptic ulcer. The cause is unknown. Treatment is with endoscopic ablation.
- Aortoduodenal fistula: bleeding in duodenum occurs after aortic graft. Can result in massive haemorrhage.
- Oesophagogastric tumours: these rarely cause acute bleeding but can occur.
- Rarely melaena can be caused by small bowel or right-sided colonic diseases.

How would you manage a patient presenting with an upper gastrointestinal bleed?
- Use an 'airway, breathing, circulation' approach.
- Ensure that adequate intravenous access is available, ideally with a large cannula in an antecubital fossa. Use crystalloids initially to stabilize blood pressure. Transfuse packed red cells to those with shock and actively bleeding, although do not delay treatment of the underlying cause. Aim to maintain haemoglobin concentration above 80 g/L.
- Platelet transfusion for those with platelets $<50 \times 10^9$/L
- Vitamin K for those with coagulopathy
- Fresh frozen plasma (FFP) for those with prothrombin time more than 1.5 times normal. If fibrinogen level is less than 1.5 g/L despite FFP, also give cryoprecipitate.
- For those receiving warfarin and are actively bleeding, give prothrombin complex concentrate. Seek advice for those taking other anticoagulants. Advice should be sought if the patient has a metallic valve or high risk for thromboembolism.
- Closely monitor; this may require a high dependency environment.
- Once the patient is resuscitated, proceed to endoscopy for a diagnosis and potential treatment. Ideally, endoscopy should be performed within 24 hours of presentation. At endoscopy treatments, use combination therapy to stop active bleeding; this can be adrenaline injection plus thermal coagulation or fibrin or thrombin. This stops active bleeding in 90% of cases. Clipping of a bleeding vessel with 'endoclips' with or without adrenaline can also be used.
- PPIs: Use of intravenous infusion of PPI in those who have major stigmata of recent haemorrhage at endoscopy acts to stabilize clots due to neutralization of gastric acid. This leads to a reduction in the rate of rebleeding.
- Prophylactic antibiotics should be given to those with a history of cirrhosis prior to endoscopy as their risk of infection is up to 50%.
- If rebleeding occurs, endoscopy should be repeated. If this fails to treat the bleeding, an angiogram and embolization may be required. If interventional radiology is not available refer for surgery.

How would you manage variceal bleeding in cirrhosis?
- Blood transfusion to maintain haemoglobin at 70 to 80 g/dL in haemodynamically stable patients
- Aim for systolic blood pressure 90 to 100 mm Hg.
- Give terlipressin as soon as variceal bleeding is suspected and continue until haemostasis is achieved or for to up to 5 days.
- Early endoscopy to find the bleeding site
- For gastric varices:
  - Inject with cyanoacrylate.
  - Offer transjugular intrahepatic portosystemic shunts (TIPS) if bleeding is not controlled.
- For oesophageal varices:
  - Band ligation via endoscopy. Repeat may be required at 2 to 4 weekly intervals until the varices are eradicated. Band ligation has been shown to reduce mortality and rebleeding compared with sclerotherapy.

- Consider TIPS if bleeding is not controlled by banding. In the interim, Sengstaken–Blakemore tube may be required. Specialist help should be sought.
- For primary and secondary prevention, use noncardioselective beta-blockers such as propranolol.
- Several interventional radiology procedures are effective for variceal bleeding: coil embolization, balloon-occluded retrograde transvenous obliteration (BRTO), gelatin sponge.

What risk assessment tools do you know of for acute upper gastrointestinal bleeding?

- The Rockall score includes endoscopic findings and is a good predictor of mortality.

Variable	Score 0	Score 1	Score 2	Score 3
Age (y)	<60	60–79	>80	–
Shock	None	Pulse >100 beats/min Normal blood pressure (BP)	Pulse >100 beats/min Systolic BP <100 mm Hg	–
Comorbidity	None	–	Cardiac Gastrointestinal cancer Other major comorbidity	Renal failure Liver failure Disseminated malignancy
Diagnosis	Mallory–Weiss tear No lesion No stigmata of recent haemorrhage	All other diagnoses	Malignancy of upper GI tract	–
Major stigmata of recent haemorrhage	None or dark spots		Blood in the upper GI tract Adherent blood clot Visible or spurting vessel	–

- A score of 0 to 2 has 0.2% mortality, score 3 to 5 has 3% to 11% mortality, score 6 has 17% mortality, score 7 has 27% mortality, and score >8 has a 41% mortality.
- The Blatchford score can be used prior to endoscopy and can be used to predict the likelihood of requiring interventions such as blood transfusion or endoscopic intervention. It therefore can be used to aid decisions regarding those who could be safely discharged with urgent outpatient endoscopy versus those requiring inpatient endoscopy and monitoring. Those with a score of less than 1 can be considered for outpatient management.

Admission Variable	Score 1	Score 2	Score 3	Score 4	Score 6
Blood urea (mmol/dL)		>6.4 to <8	>8 to <10	>10 to <25	>25
Haemoglobin (g/L)	Men: >120 to <130 Women: >100 to <120		Men: >100 to <120		Men: <100 Women: <100
Systolic BP (mm Hg)	>99 to <109	>90 to <99	<90		

Admission Variable	Score 1	Score 2	Score 3	Score 4	Score 6
Others	Pulse > 99 beats/min	Presentation with syncope			
	Presentation with melaena	Hepatic disease			
		Heart failure			

- Both Blatchford and Rockall scores have a low predictive accuracy for re-bleeding risk.

Further Information

Professor Tim Rockall, contemporary professor of colorectal surgery at the University of Surrey.
Dr Oliver Blatchford, retired public health consultant in Glasgow.

CHAPTER 229

Paracetamol Overdose

Instruction

This patient presented with intentional paracetamol overdose. Please assess.

Salient Features

HISTORY

- Time of ingestion—time of ingestion and duration of ingestion are crucial as these will inform further management.
- Exact quantity—calculation of the total dose ingested and dividing that with the patient's weight (or ideal weight for patients more than 110 kg) will give the clinician a rough guide to hepatotoxicity risk.
- Drug history (risk of hepatotoxicity increases in coingestion of P450 enzyme inducers)
- Previous overdoses and history of self-harm
- History of glutathione deficiency
- Nausea and vomiting—these are early features of severe hepatocellular necrosis and they usually last for the first 24 hours and self-settle afterwards.
- Abdominal pain—tenderness may indicate hepatic necrosis.

EXAMINATION

- Jaundice
- Confusion
- Coma
- Encephalopathy
- Spontaneous bleeding (coagulopathy)
- Abdominal tenderness
- Signs of previous self-harm
- Vital signs

Diagnosis

This young female with a history of mental health problems has arrived confused and complaining of abdominal pain (lesions). This is due to an intentional overdose of paracetamol (aetiology). She has an acute liver injury (functional status).

Questions

What is the maximum oral recommended therapeutic dose of paracetamol?
4 g in 24 hours.

821

How do you define paracetamol overdose?
- Acute paracetamol overdose—excessive amounts of paracetamol ingested within a 1-hour period
- Staggered paracetamol overdose—excessive amounts of paracetamol ingested over longer than 1-hour period.

In what quantities of paracetamol is toxicity usually seen in acute overdose?
Toxicity usually occurs in doses that exceed 75 mg/kg/24 hours.

What is the antidote for paracetamol overdose?
N-acetylcysteine (NAC).

When is N-acetylcysteine infusion indicated in acute paracetamol overdose?
- For patients who present after 4 hours of acute ingestion, NAC is started when the paracetamol plasma levels are above treatment line on the modified Rumack–Matthew nomogram (paracetamol overdose, Fig. 229.1).
- For patients who present after 8 hours of acute ingestion, NAC infusion is started if they have ingested more than 150 mg/kg.
- For patients who present more than 24 hours after the acute ingestion, NAC should be started if there are signs of liver injury such as liver tenderness, acutely deranged liver function tests (LFTs) with increased alanine transaminase (ALT), acutely deranged coagulation with an international normalized ratio (INR) of more than 1.3.

When is N-acetylcysteine infusion indicated in staggered overdose?
All patients who have ingested a staggered overdose should be treated with NAC. However, significant hepatotoxicity is unlikely if the last ingestion was more than 4 hours prior to hospital presentation, the patient has no symptoms suggesting liver damage, the paracetamol concentration is less than 10 mg/L, their ALT is within the normal range, and their INR is 1.3 or less.

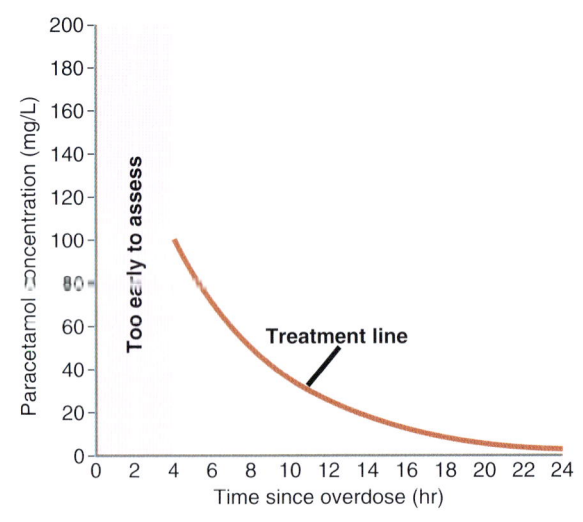

Fig. 229.1 Paracetamol treatment nomogram.

What are the main side effects of N-acetylcysteine?
One-third of patients may develop nausea or vomiting.

One in ten patients will experience an anaphylactoid reaction. Treatment for anaphylaxis should be readily at hand but, as this reaction is not immunoglobulin E (IgE) mediated, it tends to be mild to moderate and disappears as infusion is restarted at a lower rate.

What are the King's College Criteria for liver transplant in patients presenting with paracetamol overdose?
- An arterial pH of less than 7.30, irrespective of grade of encephalopathy **or**
- Grade III or IV encephalopathy and a prothrombin time (PT) greater than 100 s and a serum creatinine concentration greater than 301 micromol/L.

What is the most common N-acetylcysteine infusion regime used in clinical practice?
The most common regime is the 21-hour NAC infusion which consists of three bags of NAC infusion. The first bag consists of 150 mg/kg in 200 mL of dextrose 5% given over the first hour. The second bag consists of 50 mg/kg NAC in 500 mL of dextrose 5% given over 4 hours, and the third bag consists of 100 mg/kg NAC in 500 mL of dextrose 5% given over 16 hours.

CHAPTER 230

Pericardial Rub

Instruction
Please examine this patient's cardiovascular system.

Salient Features
HISTORY
- Precordial pain changing with posture (worse on lying down and relieved by sitting forward)
- Myocardial infarction
- Viral infection (coxsackie A and B viruses)
- Chronic renal failure
- Trauma
- Tuberculosis.

EXAMINATION
Scratching and grating sound heard best with the diaphragm at the left sternal border, with the patient leaning forward and the breath held in expiration.
- A pericardial rub usually disappears when a pericardial effusion develops.
- The pericardial rub sounds similar to the sound that our feet or shoes make when walking into soft snow.

Diagnosis
This patient has a pericardial rub (lesion) caused by pericarditis secondary to an upper respiratory viral infection (aetiology) and is not in pain (functional status).

Questions

What are the characteristic features of a pericardial friction rub?
It typically consists of three components:
- A presystolic rub during atrial contraction
- A ventricular systolic rub, which is almost always present and usually the loudest component
- A diastolic rub, which follows the second heart sound (during rapid ventricular filling).

What are the characteristic electrocardiographic findings in pericarditis?
The most common electrocardiogram (ECG) changes in acute pericarditis are (Fig. 230.1):
- ST elevation in most ECG leads with the concavity upwards
- T-wave inversion occurs after the ST segment returns to baseline (unlike in acute myocardial infarction, where the ST segment is concave downwards like a cat's back and there is some amount of T-wave inversion accompanying the ST elevation)
- PR-segment depression (caused by inflammation of the atrial wall).

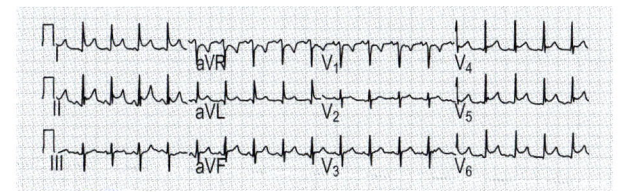

Fig. 230.1 Pericarditis with sinus tachycardia, diffuse, concave upward ST-segment elevation, PR segment depression (lead II), and PR segment elevation (lead aVR).

How common is pericardial rub in constrictive pericarditis?
It is not heard in constrictive pericarditis.

What is the treatment for acute pericarditis?
- Combination of colchicine and nonsteroidal antiinflammatory drugs (NSAIDs) (e.g. indomethacin)
- Steroids considered only when the pain does not respond to a combination of NSAIDs
- Treatment of the underlying cause
- Treatment is tapered down slowly to prevent recurrences and the total duration of colchicine is usually around 3 months for an initial episode.
- Rarely, pericardiectomy may be required for pain even in the setting of no haemodynamic impairment.
- Abstinence from strenuous activity until inflammation subsides.

What do you know about the transient constrictive phase of acute pericarditis?
About 10% of patients with acute pericarditis have a transient constrictive phase, which may last 2 to 3 months before it gradually resolves either spontaneously or with treatment with antiinflammatory drugs. These patients usually have a moderate amount of pericardial effusion, and as the effusion resolves, the pericardium remains thickened, inflamed, and noncompliant, resulting in constrictive haemodynamics. Clinical features include shortness of breath, raised jugular venous pressure, peripheral oedema, and ascites. Constrictive haemodynamics can be documented by Doppler echocardiography, and resolution of constrictive physiology can be serially followed with this technique.

What are the indications for admission to hospital?
Evidence of damage to the myocardium with raised cardiac enzymes, fever, haemodynamic compromise with evidence of tamponade, immunosuppressed patients, suspicion of haemopericardium, such as history of trauma or anticoagulant use.

What are the indications for drainage of pericardial fluid?
- Overt clinical tamponade, in those with suspicion of purulent pericarditis and in patients with idiopathic chronic large pericardial effusion
- Tamponade, either unresolved or relapsing after pericardiocentesis, and persistent active illness 3 weeks after hospital admission.

Pericardial drainage is not indicated in the initial management of patients with large pericardial effusions without clinical tamponade because of its low diagnostic yield and poor influence on the evolution of pericardial effusion (Fig. 230.2). Even the presence of right chamber collapse (suggesting raised intrapericardial pressure) on echocardiography does not by itself warrant pericardial drainage because most of these patients do not evolve to overt tamponade.

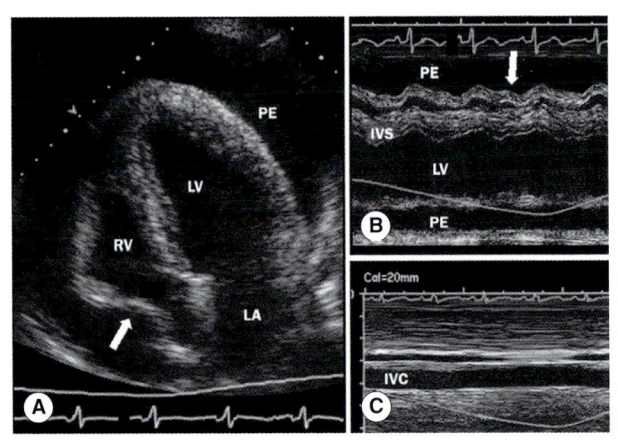

Fig. 230.2 Echocardiographic images of large pericardial effusion *(PE)* with features of tamponade. **(A)** Apical four-chamber view showing large PE with diastolic right-atrial collapse *(arrow)*. **(B)** M-mode image in parasternal long axis showing circumferential PE with diastolic collapse of RV free wall *(arrow)* during expiration. **(C)** M-mode image from subcostal window showing inferior vena cava *(IVC)* plethora without inspiratory collapse. *LA*, Left atrium; *LV*, left ventricle; *RV*, right ventricle. (With permission from Troughton, R.W., Asher, C.R., Klein, A.L., 2004. Pericarditis. Lancet 363, 717–727.)

What is Dressler syndrome?

It is characterized by persistent pyrexia, pericarditis, and pleurisy. It was first described in 1956 when Dressler recognized that post–myocardial infarction chest pain is not caused by coronary artery insufficiency. It usually occurs 2 to 3 weeks after myocardial infarction and is considered to be of autoimmune aetiology; it responds to NSAIDs.

What do you know about postcardiotomy syndrome?

It occurs in about 5% of patients who have cardiac surgery and with symptoms of pericarditis from 3 weeks to 6 months after surgery. It is initially treated with NSAIDs, and with systemic steroids if refractory. Pericardiectomy is rarely required. It is said to be the result of autoimmune response and is most likely to be related to surgical trauma and irritation of blood products in the mediastinum and pericardium.

What are the functions of the pericardium?

- The pericardium protects and lubricates the heart.
- It contributes to the diastolic coupling of the left ventricle and right ventricle (RV): an effect that is important in cardiac tamponade and constrictive pericarditis.

Further Information

W. Dressler (1890–1969), a US physician educated in Vienna. He worked at the Maimonides Hospital, Brooklyn, New York.

CHAPTER 231

Pleural Effusion

Instruction
Examine this patient's chest.

Salient Features
HISTORY
- Fever
- Pleuritic pain (made worse on coughing or deep breathing)
- Cough (pneumonia, tuberculosis (TB))
- Haemoptysis (associated parenchymal involvement in bronchogenic carcinoma or TB)
- Shortness of breath (large effusions, cardiac failure)
- Exposure to asbestos (mesothelioma)
- Nephrotic syndrome
- Drugs (methotrexate, amiodarone, phenytoin).

EXAMINATION
- Decreased chest movement on the affected side
- Stony dull note on the affected side
- Decreased vocal resonance and diminished breath sounds on the affected side
- Tracheal deviation to the opposite side.

Proceed as follows:
- Comment on evidence of pleural aspiration.
- Percuss for the upper level of effusion in the axilla.
- Listen for bronchial breath sounds.
- Listen for aegophony at the upper level of the effusion.
- It is important to elicit any evidence of an underlying cause, such as clubbing, tar staining, lymph nodes, radiation burns and mastectomy, raised jugular venous pressure, rheumatoid hands, or butterfly rash.

> **Remember:**
> For clinical detection, 500 mL of pleural fluid should be present.
> There are five major types of pleural effusion: exudate, transudate, empyema, haemorrhagic pleural effusion/haemothorax, and chylous effusion.
> The most common causes of pleural effusion in the Western world are congestive heart failure, pneumonia, and malignancy.
> The first step in developing a differential diagnosis of a pleural effusion is to establish whether the effusion is a transudate or an exudate by analysis of fluid obtained at thoracocentesis.

Diagnosis

This patient has a pleural effusion (lesion) probably caused by bronchogenic carcinoma (aetiology) and is short of breath at rest (functional status).

Questions

How would you investigate this patient?
- Chest radiography (plain posteroanterior chest film is abnormal in the presence of 200 mL of pleural fluid. Obliteration of costophrenic angle to hemithorax suggests fluid. Subpulmonic effusion can simulate an elevated diaphragm) (Fig. 231.1).
- Blood tests.

For bilateral effusions, or suspected/confirmed transudates:
- Pro-B-type natriuretic peptide, thyroid function, biochemical profile.

For confirmed exudates:
- Serum tumour markers, autoimmune screen
- Abdominal and chest axial imaging/ultrasound
- Cytology

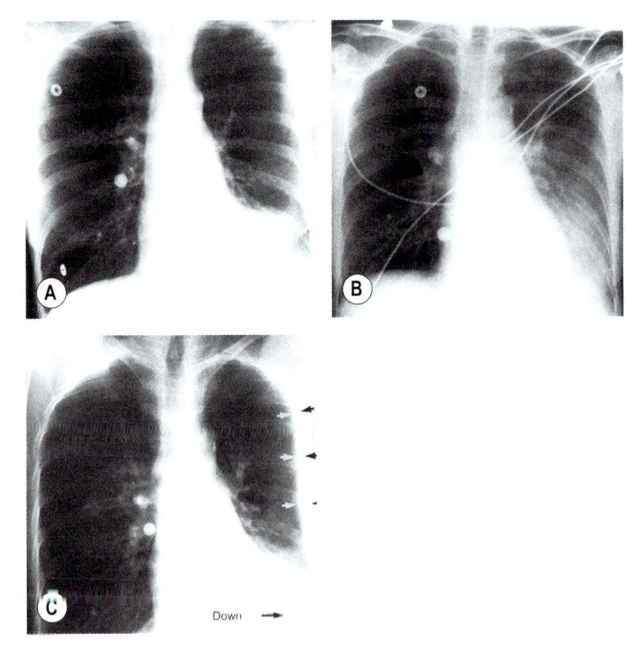

Fig. 231.1 The appearance of pleural effusions in chest radiography depends on patient position. **(A)** Upright posteroanterior: a large left pleural effusion obscures the left hemidiaphragm, the left costophrenic angle, and the left cardiac border. **(B)** Supine anteroposterior view: fluid runs posteriorly, causing a diffuse opacity over the lower two-thirds of the left lung, the left hemidiaphragm remaining obscured (this can easily mimic left lower lobe infiltrate or left lower lobe atelectasis). **(C)** Left lateral decubitus view: pleural effusion can be seen to be freely moving and layering *(arrows)* along the lateral chest wall. (With permission from Mettler, F.A., 2004. Essentials of Radiology, second edn. Saunders-Elsevier, Philadelphia, PA.)

- Pleural tap: Pleural fluid for determination of the levels of protein, albumin, lactate dehydrogenase (LDH), glucose, Gram stain microscopy, culture, and cytology.

Note: Simultaneous blood sample should be obtained for estimation of glucose, protein, albumin, and LDH.

- When empyema is suspected or seen or in nonpurulent effusions when pleural infection is suspected, pleural fluid pH should be obtained.
- When TB is suspected, pleural fluid adenosine deaminase, Ziehl–Neelsen stain, and pleural fluid mycobacterial cultures should be obtained.
- Pleural fluid amylase levels should be estimated when malignancy, pancreatic disease, or oesophageal rupture is suspected.
- The appearance of the pleural fluid or any odour should be recorded.

Fluid	*Suspected Disease*
Putrid odour	Anaerobic empyema
Food particles	Oesophageal rupture
Bile stained	Chylothorax (biliary fistula)
Milky	Chylothorax/pseudochylothorax
Anchovy sauce-like fluid	Ruptured amoebic abscess

- Pleural biopsy: the biopsy specimen is sent for histopathological examination and mycobacterial culture.

What are the causes of dullness at a lung base?
- Pleural effusion
- Pleural thickening
- Consolidation and collapse of the lung
- Raised hemidiaphragm.

How would you differentiate?
- Pleural effusion: stony dull note; the trachea may be deviated to the opposite side in large effusions.
- Pleural thickening: the trachea is not deviated; breath sounds will be heard.
- Consolidation: vocal resonance is increased; bronchial breath sounds and associated crackles are present.
- Collapse: lung volume is reduced, the trachea is deviated to the affected side, and breath sounds are absent.

What criteria could you use to differentiate between an exudate and a transudate?
The protein content of an exudate is more than 3 g/L. However, if this criterion alone is applied, about 10% of exudates and 15% of transudates will be wrongly classified. A more accurate diagnosis is made when Light's criteria for an exudate are applied:
- The ratio of the pleural fluid to serum protein is greater than 0.5.
- The ratio of pleural fluid to serum LDH is greater than 0.6.
- Pleural fluid LDH is greater than two-thirds the upper normal limit for blood LDH.

Light's criteria have been shown to have a sensitivity of 100% but a low specificity of 72%. This was because many patients with effusion caused by chronic cardiac failure have protein values in the exudate range, particularly when on chronic diuretic therapy. Serum–effusion albumin gradient (i.e. serum albumin minus pleural fluid albumin) was 95% sensitive but a more specific (100%) marker of exudative effusion. A gradient of less than 12 g/L indicates an exudative effusion whereas a gradient more than 12 g/L indicates a transudative effusion. Measuring the difference between the serum and the pleural-fluid albumin levels is useful in patients with heart failure who are taking diuretics because a difference more than 12 g/L is consistent with a transudative effusion, even though other Light's criteria for an exudative effusion have been met. The level of protein elevation is sometimes helpful itself to point towards a more specific cause of an exudate. For example, very high concentrations of protein in an exudative pleural effusion can be seen in paraproteinaemias.

Mention a few causes for an exudate and a transudate.
Exudate:
- Malignancy (lung, mesothelioma)
- Secondaries in the pleura (lung, breast, ovary, and pancreas)
- Parapneumonic effusions
- TB
- Pulmonary infarction
- Rheumatoid arthritis and other autoimmune diseases
- Lymphoma
- Benign asbestos effusion
- Pancreatitis
- Post–myocardial infarction/post–coronary artery bypass graft
- Drugs
- Yellow nail syndrome.

Transudate:
- Left ventricular failure
- Liver cirrhosis
- Nephrotic syndrome
- Hypoalbuminaemia
- Peritoneal dialysis
- Hypothyroidism
- Mitral stenosis
- Constrictive pericarditis
- Urinothorax
- Meigs syndrome.

Mention a few conditions in which the pleural fluid pH and glucose levels are low but lactate dehydrogenase is raised.
Empyema, malignancy, TB, rheumatoid arthritis, systemic lupus erythematosus, and oesophageal rupture.

What is the value of measuring pleural fluid pH and glucose concentrations in malignant effusions?
It is of value in determining the prognosis. Patients with a low pleural fluid pH (<7.3) or low glucose concentration (<600 mg/L) have a shorter life expectancy than those with higher values: 2.1 months versus 9.8 months. The low-pH group tends to have more extensive pleural involvement as determined by thoracoscopy and a higher failure rate for chemical pleurodesis.

What further investigations would you do to determine the underlying cause of the pleural effusion?
- Computed tomography chest scan
- Bronchoscopy (haemoptysis or clinical or radiographic features suggestive of bronchial obstruction)
- Pleural biopsy.

What is the role of pleural fluid cytology in the diagnosis of pleural effusion?
- Pleural fluid usually contains about 1.5×10^9 cells/L (predominantly mononuclear cells). Counts above 50×10^9 cells/L are seen in parapneumonic effusions, whereas transudates usually have counts of $<1 \times 10^9$ cells/L.
- Pleural fluid eosinophilia (i.e. >10%) suggests air or blood in the pleural cavity, and common causes are parapneumonic effusions, drug-induced pleurisy, benign asbestos pleural effusion, Churg–Strauss syndrome, lymphoma, pulmonary infarction, parasitic disease, or malignancy.
- Pleural fluid lymphocytosis usually correlates with long-standing pleural effusion, and common causes include malignancy, TB, cardiac failure, lymphoma, collagen vascular diseases, and sarcoidosis.

What characteristics of the pleural fluid in a parapneumonic effusion indicate a need for closed-tube drainage?
Presence of pus, positive stain for microorganisms, positive pleural fluid cultures, a pleural fluid glucose concentration of less than 60 mg/dL, or a pH less than 7.2 indicates the need for closed-tube drainage.

What does a pleural fluid triglyceride level greater than 110 mg/dL suggest?
It suggests chylothorax and is seen most often in patients with thoracic injuries, thoracic surgery (e.g. oesophagectomy), neoplasm (lymphomas, metastatic carcinoma), disorders of lymphatics (lymphangioleiomyomatosis), TB, cirrhosis, obstruction of central veins, chyloascites.

Pseudochylothorax is defined by a level of cholesterol over 200 mg/dL and low triglycerides and the most common causes are rheumatoid pleurisy and TB.

What is the significance of pleural fluid amylase levels?
A pleural fluid amylase level greater than the serum amylase concentration is seen in patients with acute pancreatitis, pancreatic pseudocyst, rupture of the oesophagus, ruptured ectopic pregnancy, and malignancy (especially adenocarcinoma), and pleural fluid isoamylase determination can be useful; the finding of a pleural effusion rich in salivary isoamylase should prompt an evaluation for carcinoma (particularly a lung primary) but may also be seen in oesophageal rupture.

What are the causes of an exudate with negative cytology findings and pleural fluid lymphocytosis?
Possible causes include TB, cardiac failure, collagen vascular diseases, and tumours, including lymphoma, chylothorax, yellow nail syndrome.

In such patients, what other tests could you perform on the pleural fluid to determine the underlying cause?
- Pleural fluid adenosine deaminase concentration (an enzyme involved in purine metabolism and found in T lymphocytes) is markedly raised in tuberculous and rheumatoid effusions and in empyema compared with malignant effusions. The ADA2 isoenzyme is more specific for TB effusions.
- Combined use of these two tests yields a sensitivity and specificity of 100% for tuberculous effusions if empyema is excluded.
- Gamma-interferon levels are also raised in tuberculous effusions compared with malignant effusions.
- Estimation of pleural fluid rheumatoid factor and antinuclear antibodies should not be measured routinely as it reflects the serum level and is therefore usually unhelpful.

In which conditions is the pleural fluid bloody?
Haemorrhagic fluid is seen in malignancy, pulmonary embolus, TB, post–cardiac injury syndrome (Dressler syndrome), asbestos exposure, and trauma to the chest.

Haemothorax should be considered to be present when the haematocrit of the pleural fluid is more than half that of the peripheral blood.

What are the earliest radiological signs of pleural fluid?
The earliest radiological signs are blunting of the costophrenic angle on the anterior–posterior view or loss of clear definition of the diaphragm posteriorly on the lateral view (Fig. 231.1).

When in doubt of a small effusion, how would you confirm your suspicions?
Either by a lateral decubitus view (which shows a layering of the fluid along the dependent chest wall unless the fluid is loculated) or by ultrasonography.

What are the other uses of ultrasonography in the diagnosis of pleural effusion?
Ultrasonography is also useful for loculated effusions, guided thoracocentesis, closed pleural biopsy or insertion of a chest drain, and differentiation of pleural fluid from pleural thickening.

What is a pseudotumour?
It is the accumulation of fluid between the major or minor fissure or along the lateral chest wall, which can be mistaken for a tumour on the radiograph. Such loculated effusions can be confirmed with ultrasonography.

What do you know about pleural disease in rheumatoid arthritis?
About 70% of patients with rheumatoid arthritis have pleural inflammation at postmortem and about 5% have radiological evidence of pleural inflammation at some time. Pleural involvement is associated with male sex, rheumatoid factor in serum, the presence of nodules, and other systemic manifestations. The effusion is thought to develop as an inflammatory response to the presence of multiple subpleural nodules. For reasons that are entirely unclear, the left side is the more common site of unilateral rheumatoid pleural effusions. The pleural fluid glucose level is characteristically low and is said to be caused by an 'entrance block', in which glucose is unable to enter the pleural space, unlike in empyema and malignant effusions, where the low pleural fluid glucose concentration is attributed to the increased use of glucose by cells. Cytological appearances of slender and elongated macrophages, round giant multinucleated macrophages, presence of very few mesothelial cells, and necrotic background material are thought to be pathognomonic of rheumatoid pleuritis.

What are the complications of thoracocentesis?
Pneumothorax, haemothorax, organ puncture, intravascular collapse, and unilateral pulmonary oedema (the last after withdrawal of large quantities of fluid).

What do you know about Meigs syndrome?
Meigs syndrome comprises pleural effusion (usually right sided and a transudate) and ovarian tumour (usually benign ovarian fibroma).

Mention some causes of drug-induced pleural effusion.
Procainamide (associated with a lupus-like reaction), nitrofurantoin, dantrolene, methysergide, procarbazine, methotrexate, bromocriptine, practolol, amiodarone, mitomycin, bleomycin, and minoxidil.

The patient used to be a shipbuilder: what diagnosis would you consider?

It is most likely that this patient has malignant mesothelioma because he was exposed to asbestos (amphibole asbestos confers a higher risk of mesothelioma (dose for dose) than the more commonly used chrysotile or white asbestos, although the latter is as potent at causing lung carcinoma). If the diagnosis is confirmed, he should be advised to apply for industrial injuries benefit.

What are the mechanisms for abnormal accumulation of pleural fluid?

There are three main mechanisms:
- An abnormality of the pleura itself, such as neoplasm or inflammatory process, usually associated with increased permeability (e.g. increased vascular permeability in pneumonia)
- Disruption of the integrity of a fluid-containing structure within the pleural cavity, such as the thoracic duct, oesophagus, major blood vessels, or tracheobronchial tree, with leakage of the contents into the pleural space (e.g. decreased lymphatic drainage as in mediastinal carcinomatosis)
- Abnormal hydrostatic or osmotic forces operating on an otherwise normal pleural surface and producing a transudate (e.g. increased hydrostatic pressure in heart failure, decreased osmotic pressure in nephrotic syndrome, increased intrapleural pressure as in atelectasis).

Further Information

There is a classic article by Light (2002).

CHAPTER 232

Sepsis

Instruction
This patient presented with pyrexia and abdominal pain. Please assess.

Salient Features

HISTORY
Symptoms from infective source:
- Cough, chest pain, sputum production (pneumonia)
- Sore throat, painful swallowing (tonsillitis)
- Eye erythema, eyelid swelling, visual problems (periorbital cellulitis)
- Joint pain and swelling (septic arthritis)
- Headache, photophobia, neck stiffness, rash (meningitis)
- Abdominal pain (intraabdominal collection)
- Vaginal discharge and pain (endometritis)
- Rash with erythema, subcutaneous oedema (cellulitis)
- Bone pain (bone abscess)
- Peripheral emboli (endocarditis)
- Pain at the site of recent surgery (infection of foreign body or infection of site wound).

Symptoms suggesting systemic response, regardless of the source
- Fever
- Nausea and vomiting
- Dizziness
- Lethargy
- Generally unwell
- Fatigue.

EXAMINATION
Abnormal vital signs
- Tachycardia
- Tachypnoea
- Pyrexia or hypothermia
- Hypotension.

Signs signifying infectious process of any source:
- Bounding pulse
- Flushed skin.

Late signs of organ hypoperfusion in shocked patients:
- Diminished bowel sounds or ileus
- Oliguria
- Reduced consciousness level

834

- Mottled skin
- Prolonged capillary refill
- Cyanosis.

Proceed as follows:
Examine all systems for source identification.
Perform the sepsis six care bundle.
Declare this as a medical emergency.

Diagnosis

This patient has sepsis (lesion), likely from an indwelling urinary catheter (aetiology). He is hypotensive and tachycardic (functional status) and needs resuscitation.

Questions

When is the term 'septic shock' used?
When a patient is identified as having sepsis, immediate resuscitation with intravenous fluid to maintain vital organ perfusion is initiated. Patients who, despite adequate fluid resuscitation, have an elevated lactate (>2 mmol/L) or need vasopressor support to maintain a mean arterial pressure >65 mm Hg are defined as being in septic shock.

What groups of patients are at increased risk for sepsis?
- Inpatients in hospital wards and intensive care units. Hospitalization is a risk factor for hospital-acquired infection, and as such patients in hospital are at increased risk for sepsis. Half of admissions to an intensive care unit will be complicated by a hospital-acquired infection.
- Patients with metabolic disorders. Patients with an increased body mass index or patients who suffer from diabetes are not only more prone to infections, but at higher risk of sepsis if they develop an infection.
- Immunocompromised patients. Those with active malignancy, on chemotherapy or immunosuppressants, or who have a congenital or acquired immunodeficiency are at increased risk of becoming septic should they contract an infection.
- Patients with severe acute respiratory distress from viral infections, including SARS-CoV-2 infection, are at increased risk of deteriorating should they develop a secondary bacterial infection, probably because of the temporarily immunocompromised state they are in because of the initial viral infection.

What are the 2021 guidelines for Surviving Sepsis Campaign?
These are international guidelines issued for the treatment of sepsis and septic shock. According to these guidelines, sepsis and septic shock require immediate action and resuscitation.

Assessment and treatment should be based on the systematic approach using 'ABCDE' as in any medical emergency (A for airway, B for breathing, C for circulation, D for disability, and E for environment and everything else).

- Airway—assessment of the airway followed by securing of the airway if indicated
- Breathing—supplemental oxygen should be given to patients with sepsis who have an indication for it, with a target for most patients to maintain their oxygen saturation levels above 90%. Continuous pulse oximetry should be applied to all patients so that target oxygenation levels are monitored at all times.
- Circulation—venous access should be established as soon as possible; blood should be taken for venous gas, blood cultures, procalcitonin, full blood count, full biochemical profile, and

coagulation screen. In patients with hypoperfusion or frank shock, aggressive fluid resuscitation (30 mL/kg) should be commenced immediately using crystalloid fluids (unless the patient is in established pulmonary oedema) and be completed within the first 3 hours of presentation. Fluid therapy should be in the form of fluid boluses (0.5 L per bolus) with continuous monitoring of clinical response after every bolus.
- Disability—mental state of patient should be established and blood sugar be measured and corrected if indicated with insulin with an aim to maintain blood sugar levels less than 10 mmol/L.
- Everything else—clinical examination and relevant additional imaging should focus on identification of the potential source. Antibiotics should be administered within the first hour of presentation using local antibiotic protocols. Even if a primary source is not identified on presentation, administration of antibiotics should not be delayed. Instead, broad-spectrum antibiotics covering Gram-positive and negative bacteria have to be administered as soon as possible, with the addition of antifungal agents in patients who have neutropenic sepsis. Patients with sepsis are acutely unwell and need pharmacological thromboprophylaxis.

Continuous monitoring of vital signs, neuro-observations, and urine output of the patient should take place. Lack of clinical improvement should trigger escalation of treatment to an intensive care environment with vasopressor support and organ support as appropriate. Adults with septic shock and ongoing requirement for vasopressor therapy will need intravenous corticosteroids.

Certain empirical treatments used historically are currently advised against. These include the use of sodium bicarbonate for the treatment of acidaemia within the context of sepsis, the use of vitamin C, and the use of mechanical prophylaxis for deep vein thrombus prevention.

In terms of screening tools, the international guidelines recommend against the use of the quick sequential organ failure assessment (qSOFA) compared with systematic inflammatory response syndrome (SIRS) and early warning scores (NEWS, or MEWS) as a single screening tool for sepsis.

Upon admission to an intensive care unit, international guidelines have specific recommendations for organ support in patients with sepsis. Additionally, the guidelines have included recommendations on family support during admission to hospital and psychosocial patient support following discharge for sepsis survivors.

What is neutropenic sepsis?

Neutropenic sepsis is the term to describe sepsis in a patient with an absolute neutrophil count of less than 0.5×10^9/L. It is a life-threatening condition and, as with all cases of sepsis, is a clinical emergency. It can be complicated by septic shock, coagulopathy, and organ dysfunction as all sepsis cases can be, but is often due to extremely invasive and atypical infective organisms. Neutropenic sepsis should be suspected in any individual who demonstrates even mild symptoms of infection or sepsis and is known to have neutropenia or has risk factors for neutropenia. Risk factors for neutropenia include recent chemotherapy, immunosuppression with cytotoxic drugs, stem cell transplantation, and bone marrow disorders. Treatment remains based on the application of the sepsis care bundle with added attention paid to the likely need to cover for atypical and fungal infections.

What is the long-term prognosis of sepsis?

Sepsis carries a high mortality rate, with around 60% to 90% of the patients who have suffered from sepsis making it to discharge. In survivors of sepsis, morbidity is increased compared to the general population. Quality of life is compromised, and sepsis survivors run not only an increased risk of death within the first 6 months post discharge but also increased risk of rehospitalization, mainly with decompensated chronic preexisting conditions such as heart failure or chronic obstructive pulmonary disease or another infection.

Further Information

The Surviving Sepsis Campaign was initiated in 2002 and has provided international consensus guidelines for the management of sepsis and septic shock.

CHAPTER 233

Consolidation

Instruction
Examine this patient's chest.

Salient Features

HISTORY
- Cough with/without purulent sputum
- Fever with sweating or rigors
- Pleuritic chest pain
- Shortness of breath
- Haemoptysis
- Nausea, vomiting, diarrhoea (consider *Legionella* infection)
- Mental status changes (especially in the elderly)
- Fatigue
- Dyspnoea developing a week after a prodromal with new continuous dry cough, myalgias, headache, possible anosmia, dysgeusia, or gastrointestinal symptoms such as nausea and diarrhoea (consider COVID-19 pneumonia)
- Persistent cough for more than 2 weeks with whoop (Bordetella pertussis)
- Exposure to specific microorganisms (e.g. bird keeping—consider chlamydia pneumonia; recent stay in a hotel with air-conditioning in a warm country—consider Legionella; flu season with preceding upper respiratory symptoms—consider influenza, exposure to contacts with known infection like SARS-CoV-2)
- Vaccination status against SARS-CoV-2.

EXAMINATION
- Purulent sputum
- Tachypnoea
- Reduced movement of the affected side
- Trachea central
- Impaired percussion note
- Bronchial breath sounds over areas of pulmonary consolidation
- Crackles (the distribution may point towards the underlying aetiology)
- Extrapulmonary findings (for example pernio like toes in COVID 19 infection, maculopapular rash in mycoplasma infection).

Diagnosis

This patient has left lower lobe consolidation with purulent sputum (lesion) indicating a bacterial pneumonia (aetiology) and her CURB65 score is 0 (functional status).

233 – CONSOLIDATION

Questions

What is the aetiology?
- Bacterial pneumonia
- Bronchogenic carcinoma
- Pulmonary infarct.

How would you investigate suspected bacterial pneumonia?
- Full blood count, serum urea, electrolytes, and liver function tests
- Sputum and blood cultures
- Arterial blood gases
- Chest radiography (Fig. 233.1)
- Do not routinely offer atypical microbiological tests to patients with low-severity community-acquired pneumonia. However, for patients with moderate- or high-severity community-acquired pneumonia, or for bilateral pneumonia, or pneumonia with atypical features, in addition to blood and sputum cultures, atypical pneumonia screen (pneumococcus and *Legionella*) and HIV test should also be arranged.

In the context of the recent pandemic, all patients presenting with respiratory symptoms would be tested for SARS-CoV-2 infection. However, SARS-CoV-2 would not present with lobar pneumonia and localized consolidation, but with bilateral infiltrates causing acute respiratory distress syndrome (ARDS).

How do you determine the severity of community-acquired pneumonia?
Using the CURB65 severity score, 1 point for each feature present:
- Confusion
- Urea >7 mmol/L

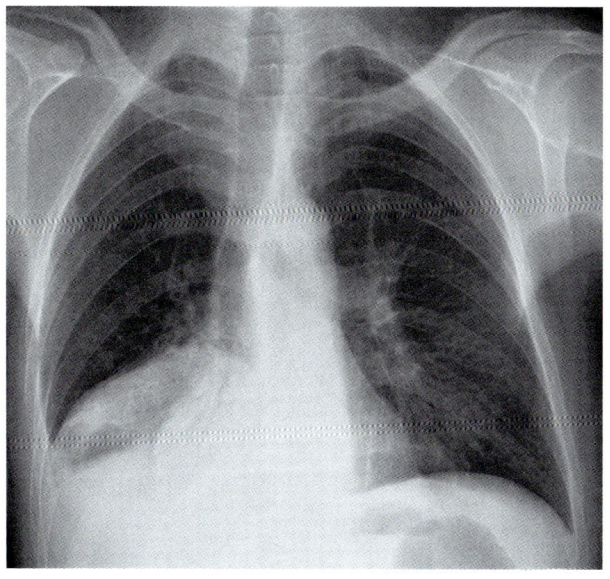

Fig. 233.1 Air bronchograms in a collapsed and consolidated right lower lobe. (With permission from Adam, A., Dixon, A.K., Grainger, R.G., Allison, D.J., 2008. Grainger and Allison's Diagnostic Radiology, fifth edn. Churchill Livingstone, Edinburgh.)

- **R**espiratory rate ≥30/min
- **B**lood pressure (BP) (systolic <90 mm Hg or diastolic ≤60 mm Hg)
- **A**ge ≥**65** years.

The prognosis based on CURB65 score:
- 4 or 5: assess with specific consideration to the need for transfer to a critical care unit
- ≥3: high mortality risk (>15%); consider intensive care assessment, high risk of death
- ≥2: consider hospital-based care
- 0 or 1: low risk (less than 3% mortality risk); may be suitable for ambulatory care.

The CURB65 severity score should be interpreted in context of the overall clinical picture.

What are the causes of a poorly resolving or recurrent pneumonia?
- Carcinoma of the lung
- Aspiration of a foreign body
- Empyema or lung abscess
- Inappropriate antibiotic therapy
- Tuberculosis
- Sequestration (rare; suspect if left lower lobe is involved)
- Other diagnosis: pulmonary embolism, vasculitis, drug reaction, eosinophilic pneumonia.

What do you know about atypical pneumonias?
The atypical bacterial pathogens *Mycoplasma pneumoniae*, *Chlamydia pneumoniae*, and *Legionella pneumophila* are often considered together as 'atypical' pathogens because of their inability to grow on routine bacterial culture media. The clinical characteristic of an atypical pneumonia is the prominence of nonproductive cough, the presence of constitutional symptoms, and the response to macrolide therapy.

What do you know about mycoplasma pneumonia?
M. pneumoniae is an important cause of atypical pneumonia and epidemics are seen every 4 years or so. Its incubation is 2 to 3 weeks and it is usually seen in children and young adults. Reinfection can occur in older patients with detectable *M. pneumoniae* antibody. Like all other pneumonias, mycoplasma pneumonia is common in winter months.

What are the extrapulmonary manifestations of mycoplasma pneumonia?
- Arthralgia and arthritis
- Autoimmune haemolytic anaemia
- Neurological manifestations involving both central and peripheral systems
- Pericarditis, myocarditis
- Hepatitis, glomerulonephritis
- Nonspecific rash, erythema multiforme, and Stevens–Johnson syndrome
- Bullous myringitis or meningoencephalitis
- Disseminated intravascular coagulation.

What are the complications of pneumonia?
- Septicaemia
- Lung abscess
- Empyema
- Adult respiratory distress syndrome
- Multiorgan failure
- Renal failure
- Haemolytic syndrome
- Death.

Which antibiotics would you use in a patient with community-acquired pneumonia where the pathogen is not known?

Recommendations for antibiotic therapy are as follows:

Low-severity community-acquired pneumonia:
> Consider amoxicillin in preference to a macrolide or a tetracycline for patients with low-severity community-acquired pneumonia. Consider a macrolide or a tetracycline for patients who are allergic to penicillin (offer a 5-day therapy course).

Moderate- and high-severity community-acquired pneumonia:
> Consider dual antibiotic therapy with amoxicillin and a macrolide for patients with moderate-severity community-acquired pneumonia (offer a 7–10-day course of antibiotic therapy).

Name some poor prognostic factors in patients with community-acquired pneumonia.

- Age >65 years
- Coexisting conditions such as cardiac failure, renal failure, ischaemic heart disease, severe chronic obstructive pulmonary disease, malignancy, splenectomy, alcoholism, immunosuppressive therapy
- Clinical features: respiratory rate >30 breaths/min, hypotension (systolic BP <90 mm Hg or diastolic BP <60 mm Hg), temperature >38.3°C or hypothermia, impaired mental status (stupor, lethargy, disorientation or coma), extrapulmonary infection (e.g. septic arthritis, meningitis)
- Investigations: haematocrit <30%, white cell count <4 or >30 × 10^6 cells/L, azotaemia, arterial blood gas <60 mm Hg or PO_2 >48 mm Hg while breathing room air, albumin <30 g/L, chest radiograph showing multiple lobe involvement, or rapid spread or pleural effusion
- Microbial pathogens: *Streptococcus* and *Legionella* spp., *Streptococcus pneumoniae*, *Pseudomonas aeruginosa*, or *Staphylococcus aureus*.

What do you know about Panton–Valentine leukocidin-producing *Staphylococcus aureus*?

Panton–Valentine leukocidin-producing *S. aureus* (PVL-SA) infection causes very severe pneumonia, resulting in rapid lung cavitation and multiorgan failure. Affected patients often require admission to the critical care unit. In patients with suspected necrotizing pneumonia, the antibiotic regimen should include a combination of intravenous linezolid 600 mg twice daily, intravenous clindamycin 1.2 g four times a day, and intravenous rifampicin 600 mg twice daily in addition to the initial empirical antibiotic regimen. As soon as PVL-SA infection is either confirmed or excluded, antibiotic therapy should be narrowed accordingly.

What do you know about pulmonary eosinophilic disorders?

The pulmonary eosinophilic disorders are a heterogeneous group of disorders characterized by varying degrees of pulmonary parenchymal or blood eosinophilia. The diagnosis is made with demonstration of either lung eosinophilia on bronchoalveolar lavage (BAL) or lung tissue biopsy, or the combination of abnormal lung pathology on noninvasive imaging combined with peripheral blood eosinophilia. Different classifications of these disorders exist depending on the underlying cause or the eosinophilic count found on BAL, but some of the commonest are:

> Löffler syndrome: This is characterized by transient pulmonary infiltrates and peripheral eosinophilia. It is associated with parasitic infections, drug allergies, and exposure to inorganic chemicals such as nickel carbonyl. The course is benign and respiratory failure is almost unknown.

> Eosinophilia in asthmatics: The most common cause is allergic bronchopulmonary aspergillosis. This condition is benign but chronic.

Tropical eosinophilia: This is secondary to filarial infection (Wuchereria bancrofti or Brugia malayi).

Churg–Strauss syndrome: Diagnosis requires four of the following features: asthma; eosinophilia >10%; mononeuropathy, or polyneuropathy; paranasal sinus abnormality; nonfixed pulmonary infiltrates visible on chest radiographs; and blood vessels with extravascular eosinophils found on biopsy.

Chronic eosinophilic pneumonia: This chronic debilitating illness is characterized by malaise, fever, weight loss, and dyspnoea. The chest radiograph shows a peripheral alveolar filling infiltrate predominantly in the upper lobes (the 'photographic negative' of pulmonary oedema).

What do you know about bronchopulmonary sequestration?
It is an uncommon congenital lesion in which a portion of nonfunctioning lung tissue is detached from the normal lung and supplied by an anomalous systemic artery, usually arising from the aorta or one of its branches. The tissue has no communication with the bronchopulmonary tree. Two types of sequestration have been described: extralobar and intralobar. An extralobar sequestration has its own pleural lining, which separates it from the remaining lung tissue, and the intralobar type shares its pleura with the adjacent normal lung. Patients usually present in childhood with cough and recurrent pneumonia, and occasionally present with haemoptysis.

What is the pathogenesis of ventilator-acquired pneumonia?
Hospital-acquired pneumonia: Micro-aspiration is the primary route of bacterial entry into the lower respiratory tract. Risk factors include sedation, intubation for operative procedures, vomiting, and impaired swallowing.

Ventilator-associated pneumonia: Leakage of bacteria and oral secretions around the endotracheal cuff, inhalation of contaminated aerosols, or reflux of contaminated ventilator tubing condensate are the primary routes of bacterial entry into the lower respiratory tract. Promising biomarkers of early disease include procalcitonin and C-reactive protein.

Outcomes: The 'battlefield' between the pathogens entering the lower respiratory tract and the host defences determines possible outcomes: colonization, tracheobronchitis, or hospital/ventilation-acquired pneumonia.

Name a few medications that have shown survival benefit on hospitalized patients with COVID-19 pneumonia requiring supplemental oxygen.
- Dexamethasone
- Remdesivir
- Baricitinib (JAK inhibitor)
- Tocilizumab (IL-6 inhibitor).

What do you understand by the term healthcare-associated pneumonia?
Pneumonia acquired in the community by patients who have had direct or indirect contact with a healthcare or long-term care facility and are subsequently hospitalized. These patients are more likely to have a coexisting illness and to receive ineffective empirical antibiotic therapy and are at greater risk for mortality than patients who have true community-acquired pneumonia. Therefore, a broader spectrum of antibiotics (especially against *P. aeruginosa*, other multidrug-resistant Gram-negative bacilli, and drug-resistant *S. aureus*) may be needed.

CHAPTER 234

Pulmonary Embolism

Instruction
This patient presented with pleuritic chest pain and difficulty breathing. Please assess.

Salient Features
HISTORY
- Sudden onset of symptoms
- Pleuritic chest pain on one hemithorax
- Palpitations
- Cough
- Haemoptysis
- Ortner syndrome extremely rare in the context of pulmonary embolism (PE)
- Dizziness and presyncopal episode in massive PE
- Preceding symptoms of deep venous thrombosis with oedema and tenderness on one calf
- Recent major operation, trauma, immobility, hospitalization, dehydration, COVID-19 infection
- Recent plane flight
- Previous diagnosed thromboembolic disease
- Underlying known condition that would predispose to thromboembolic disease, malignancy, coagulation disorder, systemic lupus erythematosus (SLE)
- Pregnancy history—pregnant women and women at the postpartum period are at increased risk of developing thromboembolic disease. Recurrent miscarriages in combination with a diagnosis of PE will warrant investigation for antiphospholipid syndrome.
- Use of anticoagulation and full drug history.

EXAMINATION
- Tachycardia
- Tachypnoea
- Oxygen levels, desaturation at rest or desaturation on exercise
- Low blood pressure—hypotension and haemodynamic instability are signs of massive PE that requires thrombolysis.
- Low-grade pyrexia
- Decreased breath sounds with crackles on the affected side
- Signs of acute right ventricular failure—raised jugular venous pressure (JVP), loud P2 component of the second heart sound, right parasternal heave
- Signs of lower limb deep vein thrombosis, rarely signs of upper limb deep vein thrombosis

Tell the examiner you would like to explore possible contraindications to thrombolysis, in anticipation of a clinical deterioration.

Diagnosis

This young lady presents with pleuritic chest pain and breathlessness(lesions). This is due to a PE likely due to oral contraceptive use (aetiology). She is breathless and requires supplementary oxygen (functional status).

Questions

How is massive pulmonary embolism defined?
Massive PE is defined as haemodynamically unstable PE or PE with shock. A systolic blood pressure under 90 mm Hg and a big drop in the patient's previous stable blood pressure are signs of a massive PE. Signs of right ventricular strain clinically or on imaging, raised cardiac enzymes and tachycardia without hypotension comprises another group of patients with submassive PE, not massive PE.

What is the gold standard investigation for diagnosing PE?
Computed tomography pulmonary angiography (CTPA).

What is the use of ventilation/perfusion scan (V/Q)?
Ventilation perfusion scan is used in patients in whom CTPA cannot be performed provided that the patient has had a normal chest X-ray (CXR). The problem with the V/Q scan is that instead of establishing a definite diagnosis, it gives the clinician a probability of a PE episode based on the mismatch of ventilation/perfusion. As this mismatch is not only seen in PE, coexistent lung conditions will make the scan results difficult to interpret.

What does the chest X-ray show?
A CXR in PE can be normal or have nonspecific signs. Atelectasis and small unilateral pleural effusions can be present. Pathognomonic signs on CXR for PE exist, but are not commonly seen.

Hampton's sign is a triangular opacity at the periphery of the lung most commonly associated with a pulmonary infarct.

Westermark's sign is unilateral oligaemia with clear lung fields and reduced pulmonary markings in the periphery, caused by lung hypoperfusion

What will the electrocardiogram show?
The pathognomonic sign of $S_1Q_3T_3$ is very rare (PE, Fig. 234.1). Arrhythmias are not uncommon, with sinus tachycardia being the most commonly detected abnormality in the electrocardiogram (ECG). Other findings are new onset of atrial fibrillation, and signs of right heart strain like right bundle branch block and anterior ST/T changes.

What do you know of D-dimers and age-adjusted D-dimers?
D-dimers are products of fibrin lysis and are expected to be elevated in PE. They are very sensitive but not specific and their real use in PE is their negative predictive value in patients with low clinical or intermediate clinical suspicion of PE. Here are a few different cases that explain the role of D-dimers in clinical practice.

In a patient with low clinical suspicion and low 2-level Well's score, a negative D-dimer is very helpful as it can safely exclude a diagnosis of PE and further investigations are not needed.

In a patient with high clinical probability of PE with a high 2-level Well's score, D-dimers have no diagnostic role as this patient will need imaging regardless of the D-dimer level.

The difficulty in interpreting D-dimer level comes in the group of people whose clinical probability is low, the 2-level Well's score is low, but the D-dimers are slightly elevated. In these

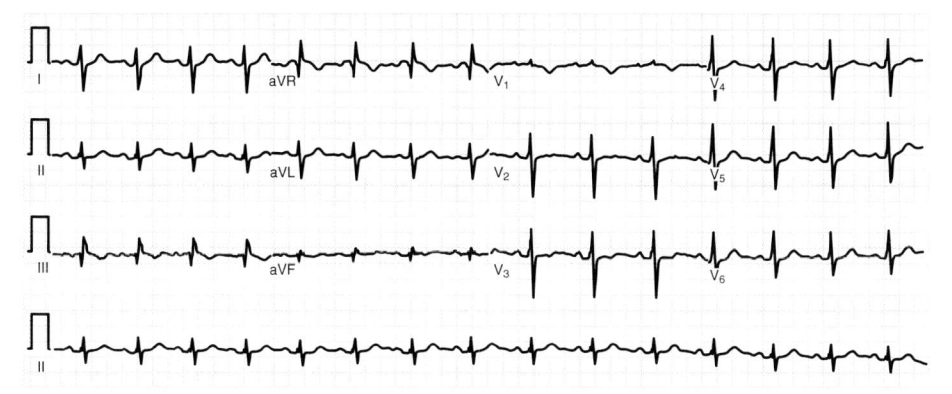

Fig. 234.1 Pulmonary embolism. (With permission from Braunwald, E., Bonow, R.O., Mann, D.L., et al., 2019. Braunwald's Heart Disease: A Textbook of Cardiovascular Medicine, eleventh edn. Elsevier.)

cases, clinician decision making will differ. Some clinicians will proceed to CTPA as an investigation for exclusion rather than diagnosis. Evidence, however, suggests that the use of age-adjusted D-dimers can help in avoiding unnecessary investigation in patients whose D-dimers are above a general cut-off but appropriately raised for their age group.

What are the indications of thrombolysis?

Systemic thrombolysis is definitely indicated in massive PE as defined earlier. Patients who are haemodynamically unstable with hypotension, periarrest, or arrested should be thrombolysed. The debate has been for years regarding thrombolysing patients with submassive PE. Clinicians will differ in their approach, with some clinicians only thrombolysing massive PE and other clinicians assessing the risk of deterioration of patients with submassive PE and choosing to thrombolyse individual cases in this group.

Absolute contraindications to thrombolysis are recent brain surgery, spinal surgery, haemorrhagic stroke, active severe bleeding disorder, nonhaemorrhagic stroke within the last 3 months, and intracranial tumours.

Are there any options for patients with massive or submasssive PE with high risk of deterioration if systemic thrombolysis is absolutely contraindicated?

Interventional techniques such as thrombectomy or catheter-directed thrombolysis can be utilized if available in patients with massive PE with an absolute contraindication to systemic thrombolysis.

How long is anticoagulation recommended for after a first episode of unprovoked PE?

Anticoagulation is recommended for a minimum of 3 months for the first unprovoked episode, extending to 6 months or even 1 year for individual cases. However, a discussion and detailed assessment and risk stratification have to take place prior to stopping anticoagulation with a view to continuing formal anticoagulation for life. Patients who have already had an episode of PE will run a lifelong risk of recurrence no matter what the circumstances. This risk is about 3% to 10% for the first year, increasing cumulatively in consecutive years. Not all patients will need to be anticoagulated indefinitely but some will benefit more than others. For instance, a patient with no bleeding risk factors but with high risk of recurrent thrombosis of 10% for the first year and around 30% in year 5 should be advised to continue anticoagulation.

CHAPTER 235

Jugular Venous Pulse

Instruction

Examine this patient's neck.
Examine this patient's cardiovascular system.

Salient Features

HISTORY

- Shortness of breath
- Symptoms of right heart failure (leg oedema, ascites).

EXAMINATION

- The jugular venous pressure (JVP) is measured in cm above the angle of Louis (manubriosternal angle). Remember that the distance between the angle of Louis and the mid-right atrium can be varied and the JVP may be measured as high as at the level of the ear lobes.
- Comment on the waveform (timing it with the carotid pulse):
  - 'v' waves of tricuspid regurgitation
  - Cannon waves of heart block
  - Absent 'a' waves in atrial fibrillation (irregular carotid pulse)
  - Large 'a' waves of pulmonary hypertension, pulmonary stenosis, tricuspid stenosis.
- Check the hepatojugular reflex.
- Tell the examiner that you would like to look for other signs of heart failure:
  - Basal crackles and pleural effusion
  - Dependent oedema (ankle and sacral oedema)
  - Tender hepatomegaly.

Diagnosis

This patient has raised jugular venous pulse with 'v' waves (lesion) caused by tricuspid regurgitation (aetiology) and is in heart failure (functional status).

Questions

What are the causes of a raised jugular venous pulse?
- Congestive cardiac failure
- Cor pulmonale
- Tricuspid regurgitation (prominent 'v' waves)
- Tricuspid stenosis (prominent 'a' waves)
- Complete heart block (cannon waves)
- Nonpulsatile neck veins seen in superior venal caval obstruction.

235 — JUGULAR VENOUS PULSE

How do you differentiate jugular venous pulsations from carotid artery pulsations?

Unlike the arterial pulse, the venous pulse has a definite upper level, which falls during inspiration and changes with posture. The venous pulse is seen to have a dominant inward motion, towards the midline (the 'y' descent), whereas the arterial pulse exhibits a dominant outward wave. The venous pulse is better seen than felt, whereas the arterial pulse is readily felt by very slight pressure of the clinician's finger.

What do you know about the hepatojugular reflux?

A positive hepatojugular (abdominojugular) reflux is a feature of constrictive pericarditis, acute right heart failure, and left ventricular systolic failure with secondary pulmonary hypertension. It is not pathognomonic of any of these conditions. The reflux means that the right heart cannot accommodate an increase in venous return. It is elicited by upper abdominal compression for more than 10 s and an abnormal response is one where there is an increase that persists throughout the pressure application. The hepatojugular manoeuvre is often useful in eliciting venous pulsations when not readily visible.

What do you know about the waveforms in the jugular pulse?

There are two outward moving waves ('a' and 'v' wave) and two inward moving waves (the 'x' and 'y' descent) (Fig. 235.1):
- The 'a' wave is caused by atrial contraction and is presystolic. It can be identified by simultaneous auscultation of the heart and the examination of the jugular venous pulse.
- The 'a' wave occurs at about the first heart sound.
- The 'c' wave is caused by closure of the tricuspid valve and is not readily visible.
- The 'v' wave is caused by venous return to the right heart (*not* from ventricular contraction) and occurs nearer the second heart sound.

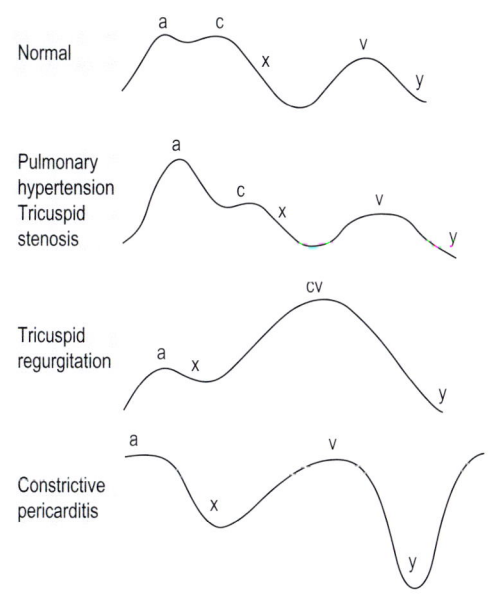

Fig. 235.1 Normal jugular venous pulse.

- The 'x' descent is caused by atrial relaxation (sometimes referred to as systolic collapse).
- The 'y' descent is produced by opening of the tricuspid valve and rapid inflow of blood into the right ventricle (RV).

What is Kussmaul's sign?
Normally, there is an inspiratory decrease in JVP. In constrictive pericarditis, there is an inspiratory increase in JVP. Kussmaul's sign is also seen in severe right heart failure regardless of aetiology. It is caused by the inability of the heart to accept the increase in RV volume without a marked increase in the filling pressure.

What is the prognostic value of raised jugular venous pressure in heart failure?
Raised JVP and third heart sounds are associated with adverse outcomes, including subsequent hospitalization for heart failure, progression of heart failure as defined by death from pump failure, and by the composite end-point of death or hospitalization for heart failure and death from all causes.

What is the mechanism of anaemia in heart failure?
The aetiology and pathophysiology of anaemia in heart failure are also multifactorial and are caused by a complex interaction between cardiac function, renal dysfunction, neurohormonal and inflammatory responses, haemodilution, iron deficiency, impaired ability to utilize available iron stores, bone marrow suppression caused by cytokines (e.g. tumour necrosis factor α (TNF-α), interleukin (IL)-1, IL-6, and C-reactive protein), blunted bone marrow responsiveness to erythropoietin, impaired iron mobilization, and effects of medications. Aspirin and angiotensin-converting enzyme inhibitors contribute to the anaemia potentially through the actions of haematopoiesis inhibitor *N*-acetyl-seryl-aspartyl-lysyl-proline. IL-6 stimulates the production of hepcidin in the hepatic cells, which blocks the absorption of iron in the duodenum and downregulates ferroprotein expression; this, in turn, prevents release of iron from total body stores. TNF-α (and IL-6) inhibits erythropoietin production in the kidney by activating the GATA-binding protein GATA2 and nuclear factor-κB and also inhibits the proliferation of bone marrow erythroid progenitor cells.

Further Information

Pasteur was the first to describe the sign of hepatojugular reflux in 1885 and that was in a patient with tricuspid regurgitation.

Adolf Kussmaul (1822–1902) was Professor of Medicine successively at Heidelberg, Erlangen, Freiburg, and Strasbourg and coined the term polyarteritis nodosa (Kussmaul, 1873). Kussmaul breathing is deep sighing respiration seen when the arterial pH is low.

In 1867, Potain described the waveforms of the internal jugular vein.

In 1902, James Mackenzie championed that the jugular venous pulse is an essential part of the cardiovascular physical examination.

In 1928, Carl Wiggers wrote that the jugular venous pulse might have utility in the interpretation of dynamic events in the heart.

In 1956, Paul Wood wrote, 'Precise analysis of the cervical venous pulse and measurement of the height of each individual wave with reference to the sternal angle is not only possible at the bedside but highly desirable'.

CHAPTER 236

Seizures

Instruction

This patient is referred to your medical outpatient clinic with an episode of loss of consciousness with witnessed seizure activity.

Salient Features

HISTORY

Detailed description of the event, from the patient's recollection and any possible witnesses:
- Symptoms or witnessed behaviour prior to the event (aura, jerky movements, déjà vu, groaning, any symptomatology that the patient noticed immediately prior)
- General health or medical issues in the period preceding the event (symptoms of infection, history of trauma)
- Description of the event (detailed history from witnesses, including loss of bladder/bowel control, seizure type activity, duration, injuries)
- Duration of the event
- Postictal period (immediately regained consciousness, postictal phase of mild confusion, patient fell asleep, Todd's paresis)
- Possible triggers
- Cardiac history
- Medication history and substances
- Previous events, identical or similar
- Family history of epilepsy.

EXAMINATION

Complete neurological and cardiovascular examination is required.

Diagnosis

This patient has had a seizure (lesion), the history of which suggests a generalized tonic–clonic seizure, which appears to have been unprovoked (aetiology). There is no neurological deficit on examination (functional status).

Questions

How do you classify seizures?

Seizures are classified depending on the underlying aetiology into unprovoked or acute symptomatic.

Seizures are also classified depending on where the abnormal electrical activity is within the brain.

- Generalized-onset seizures are characterized by abnormal activity that involves both hemispheres simultaneously. Patients are always unconscious during a generalized seizure. They are further categorized into motor or absence seizures depending on whether they present with increased motor activity. Motor seizures include tonic–clonic, clonic, tonic, myoclonic, atonic, and spasms. Absence seizures include typical, atypical, and myoclonic.
- Focal-onset seizures are characterized by abnormal electrical activity within discrete areas of the brain. During a focal seizure, the patient can be conscious or unconscious during the seizure activity (simple partial or complex partial seizure). They are further categorized into motor and absence seizures. Motor seizures include atonic, clonic, automatisms, hyperkinetic, spasms, myoclonic, and tonic forms. Absence seizures include autonomic, cognitive, emotional, and sensory.

Name some causes that can give rise to a seizure in a patient without epilepsy.
- Intracranial structural pathology (subdural haematoma, subarachnoid haemorrhage, traumatic brain injury, stroke, space occupying lesion)
- Infection of the central nervous system (meningitis, encephalitis, brain abscess)
- Metabolic causes (hypoxic brain injury, hypoglycaemia, acute severe hyponatraemia, hypocalcaemia, hypomagnesaemia, drug intoxication or withdrawal, alcohol intoxications or withdrawal).

How would you investigate this patient?
12-lead electrocardiogram is mandatory in the acute setting, as any cardiac arrhythmia can give rise to hypoxic brain injury and seizure activity.

Routine bloods, including electrolytes and infection screen, are also relevant in the acute setting, as well as urine toxicology if relevant to the clinical situation. Prolactin levels are not recommended as part of routine testing.

Pregnancy test in women of child-bearing age is important as it will have an impact on further management decisions.

Neuroimaging needs to be performed, preferably in the form of magnetic resonance imaging (MRI). The timing of neuroimaging will differ from case to case.

An electroencephalogram (EEG) should also be arranged for evaluation of any first seizure, but again, the timing will differ from case to case. Further investigations will depend on the underlying clinical suspicion (e.g. lumbar puncture if subarachnoid haemorrhage or brain infection is suspected).

What are the first-line antiepileptic drugs depending on the type of seizure?

Seizure Type	*First-Line Antiepileptic Drug (AED)*
Tonic–clonic	Carbamazepine, lamotrigine, sodium valproate
Tonic/atonic	Sodium valproate
Absence	Sodium valproate, lamotrigine, ethosuximide
Myoclonic	Sodium valproate, levetiracetam
Focal	Carbamazepine, lamotrigine

Please select the most appropriate choice of antiepileptic medication in the following scenarios.
Scenario 1:

A 27-year-old male has had two episodes during the last year where he was witnessed to mutter to himself, followed by a loss of consciousness, falling to the floor, and jerking movements for less than a minute. Both episodes were similar. The patient takes no regular medication, has no medical history of note, and has undergone an MRI of the brain, which has revealed normal brain structure, and an EEG soon after the second episode, which reveals focal epileptiform activity. A decision is made to start AEDs.

Which is a suitable option for him?
This is a focal-onset epilepsy. First-line treatment would be carbamazepine or lamotrigine.
   Scenario 2:
   A 22-year-old male medical student is brought to the emergency department after having sustained a tonic–clonic seizure witnessed by his paramedic friend, while studying together. He was brought in the hospital in status epilepticus, which was controlled with two doses of lorazepam intravenously. Routine bloods and brain imaging are normal. He is on no regular medication and has no medical history of note. He does not smoke, drink alcohol, or abuse drugs. He is kept in hospital for observations and has an inpatient neurology review. A decision is made to start antiepileptics.

Which is a suitable option for him?
This is a case of generalized epilepsy, and sodium valproate would be a suitable choice.
   Scenario 3:
   A 22-year-old female nurse is brought to the emergency department after having sustained a tonic–clonic seizure, witnessed by her paramedic friend while studying together. The patient was brought to the hospital in status epilepticus, which was controlled with two doses of lorazepam intravenously. Routine bloods and brain imaging are normal. She is on no regular medications and has no medical history of note. She does not smoke, drink alcohol, or abuse drugs. She is kept in the hospital for observations and has an inpatient neurology review. A decision is made to start antiepileptics.

Is sodium valproate a suitable first-line option for her?
Although this scenario is clinically identical to the previous one and valproate is a first-line treatment option for generalized epilepsy, the problem here is that the patient is a female of childbearing age and sodium valproate has the highest risk of teratogenicity. She should be counselled about the risks and benefits of treatment options and a less teratogenic medication should be offered first. Options include carbamazepine or lamotrigine and the patient should be started on high-dose folic acid.
   Scenario 4:
   A 19-year-old man presents with an episode of generalized seizure while he was sleeping, which was witnessed by his girlfriend. On further questioning, the patient admits that he has frequently experienced jerks in his arms while watching television, but he has never lost consciousness and he has never sought medical attention for that. A decision to start AEDs is taken.

Which antiepileptic medication should be avoided in this case?
Given that myoclonic jerks is the most likely type of epilepsy in this case, carbamazepine should be avoided as it can exacerbate the problem.

Select one of the following options to complete the following sentence.
Status epilepticus is generalized seizures of more than_____duration.
   a. Half an hour
   b. 1 hour
   c. 5 min
   d. 15 min
   Answer: The correct answer is c: 5 min.

How would you treat status epilepticus in hospital?
- Secure airway, resuscitate, administer oxygen, assess cardiorespiratory function, obtain intravenous access.
- Give intravenous antiepileptics (AED) as per local protocol. The standard treatment is lorazepam intravenously as a first-line drug given twice in early status with escalation to intravenous phenytoin with appropriate cardiac monitoring in established status. Recently, some experts advocate the use of other second-line intravenous AEDs.
- Phenytoin used to be the single second-line agent, but now other antiepileptics are used intravenously as they are considered to have a better safety profile. Those are valproate, phosphenytoin, and levetiracetam.
- Refractory status should be treated with general anaesthesia under expert supervision.
- Administer glucose 50 mL of 50% and/or intravenous thiamine in malnourished patients or suspected alcohol use disorder.
- Treat severe acidosis.
- Aim to establish aetiology to target further treatment throughout the process of treating status epilepticus.

CHAPTER 237

Painful Knee Joint

Instruction

Examine this patient's leg.
Examine this patient's knee joint.

Salient Features

HISTORY

- Painful knee joint
- History of trauma and fever
- History of rheumatoid arthritis, gout, or haemophilia.

EXAMINATION

- Pain on movement of the joint (take care not to hurt the patient)
- Swelling of the joint (you must demonstrate fluid in the joint)
- Erythema and warmth of the affected knee
- Check both active and passive movements.
- Look for disuse atrophy of the muscles around the joint.

Tell the examiner that you would like to:
- Examine other joints.
- Radiograph the knee (anteroposterior and lateral views).
- Analyse the joint fluid for cells, sugar, protein, and culture.

Diagnosis

This patient has a painful knee joint with restricted movement (lesion and functional status) following trauma while playing tennis. Clinical examination is consistent with septic arthritis (aetiology) which is a medical emergency.

Questions

What are the common causes of a painful knee joint?
- Rheumatoid arthritis
- Osteoarthritis
- Trauma
- Septic arthritis (will require emergency removal of the pus to prevent joint damage)
- Viral infection
- Gout
- Pseudogout
- Haemophilia.

What is palindromic rheumatoid arthritis?
Palindromic onset of rheumatoid arthritis refers to acute recurrent arthritis, usually affecting one joint, with symptom-free intervals of days to months between attacks. This term was introduced by P.S. Hench and E.F. Rosenberg.

A patient with a painful knee joint and a unilateral facial nerve palsy is seen by you in the outpatient department. Six weeks before this, she developed an annular rash after a camping trip in Europe. What is your diagnosis and what confirmatory test would you carry out?
The diagnosis is Lyme disease and the confirmatory test is an antibody titre against *Borrelia burgdorferi*. The disease was first recognized in Lyme, Connecticut, USA.

What are the causes of acute monoarticular arthritis?
Causes of acute-onset monoarticular or pauciarticular arthritis include bacterial infections (e.g. with *Staphylococcus aureus*, *Neisseria gonorrhoeae*, and *Streptococcus pneumoniae*), reactive arthritis, sarcoidosis, fracture, haemarthrosis, gout, pseudogout, and monoarticular rheumatoid arthritis.

What are the causes of acute polyarticular arthritis?
The causes of acute polyarticular arthritis (involvement of more than just a few joints) include endocarditis, serum sickness, acute hepatitis B infection, HIV infection, parvovirus infection, rheumatic fever, rheumatoid arthritis, and systemic lupus erythematosus.

Name some risk factors for septic arthritis.
- Foreign body
- Age
- Diabetes
- Pre-existing arthropathy
- Immunocompromised patients
- Intravenous drug use.

Which is the most common causative agent of septic arthritis?
S. aureus.

What are the three most important steps in treating septic arthritis of the knee?
- Resuscitate the patient and apply Sepsis Six.
- Knee aspiration under aseptic technique for fluid analysis (Synovial fluid is sent for direct microscopy, where leucocytes are expected to be high >50,000 cells/mL and Gram stain.)
- Antibiotics and joint drainage (As staph is the most common pathogen identified, empirical treatment with intravenous vancomycin should start as soon as synovial fluid is obtained. Following Gram stain and cultures the choice of antibiotics may change. Antibiotics are not enough, as septic arthritis is behaving as a closed abscess. Joint drainage must be performed and may need to be repeated during the in hospital stay.)

CHAPTER 238

Slow Pulse Rate

Instruction

This patient has presented to the general medical clinic after noticing that his pulse was very slow on his smartwatch. Please examine the patient.

Salient Features

HISTORY

- Drug history: beta-blockers, digoxin, verapamil
- Fitness level of patient; slow resting pulse rate is normal in athletes.
- Nonspecific symptoms and symptoms signifying low cardiac output (e.g. dizziness, fatigue, weakness, heart failure)
- History of cardiovascular disease and recent myocardial infarction
- Precipitating factors and associated symptoms or signs
- Presence of nocturnal bradycardia (a feature of obstructive sleep apnoea).

EXAMINATION

- Pulse rate is <60 beats/min.
- Pulse rate may be either regular or irregular.
- If the pulse is irregular, the clinician can count the rate with the patient lying and the patient to standing (in complete heart block there is no increase in rate).
- Jugular venous pulse for cannon 'a' waves
- Auscultation of the heart for cannon first heart sound
- Signs of hypothyroidism particularly in the elderly.

Diagnosis

This patient has a complete heart block (lesion) probably caused by ischaemic heart disease (aetiology) and is disabled by syncopal attacks (functional status).

Questions

What are the causes of bradycardia?
- Physical fitness in athletes
- Idiopathic degeneration (aging)
- Acute myocardial infarction
- Drugs (beta-blockers, digitalis, calcium channel blockers)
- Hypothyroidism
- Obstructive jaundice

- Increased intracranial pressure
- Hypothermia
- Hyperkalaemia.

How would you investigate this patient?
- Electrocardiogram (ECG):
  - 12-lead assessment to confirm bradycardia
  - 24- to 48-hour ambulatory recording in patients with frequent or continuous symptoms.
- Blood tests to exclude other medical conditions causing a bradyarrhythmia (electrolytes, thyroid tests).

What are the indications for temporary cardiac pacing in bradyarrhythmia?
- Symptomatic second- or third-degree heart block caused by transient drug intoxication or electrolyte disturbance (Fig. 238.1A,B)
- Complete heart block, Mobitz II (Fig. 238.1D) or bifascicular (Fig. 238.2) in the setting of an acute myocardial infarct
- Symptomatic sinus bradycardia, atrial fibrillation with slow ventricular response.

What are the indications for permanent pacing in bradyarrhythmia?
- Symptomatic congenital heart block

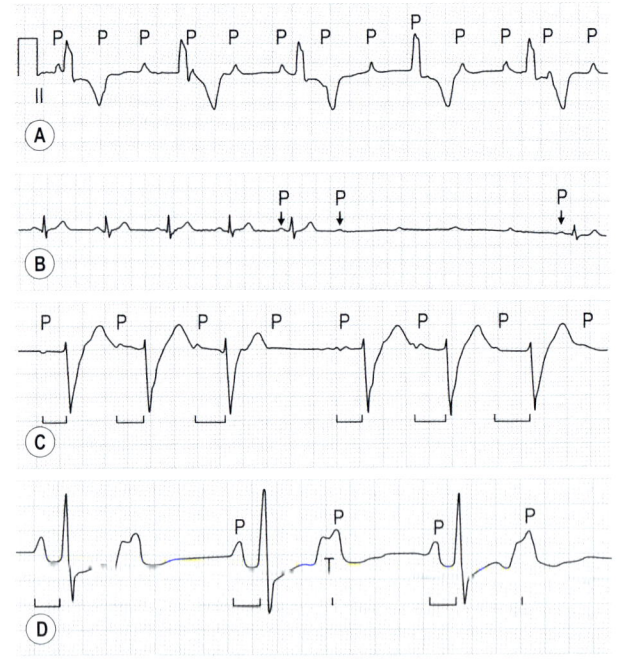

Fig. 238.1 Electrocardiogram showing heart block. **(A)** Complete atrioventricular (AV) block: P waves bear no relationship to the QRS complexes, which are regular and wide; **(B)** intermittent complete heart block: sinus rhythm with normal PR intervals and normal QRS complexes followed by sudden absence of AV conduction; **(C)** Mobitz type I second-degree heart block with progressive lengthening of the PR interval and eventual failure of the P wave to generate a QRS complex; and **(D)** Mobitz type II second-degree heart block, with failure to produce a QRS complex on every second P wave.

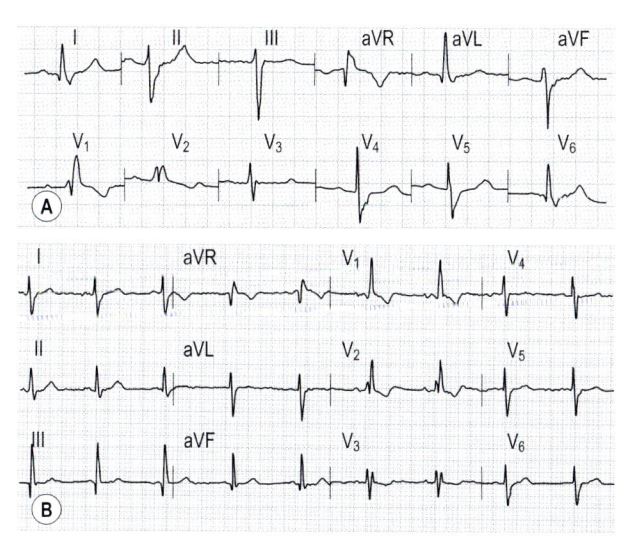

Fig. 238.2 Bifascicular right bundle branch block. **(A)** Left anterior fascicle block; **(B)** left posterior fascicle block.

- Symptomatic sinus node dysfunction (chronotropic incompetence, symptomatic sinus bradycardia)
- Symptomatic second- or third-degree heart block.

What modes of pacemakers used for bradyarrhythmia do you know of?

Pacemakers consist of the generator and the leads. They are named after a three- or four-letter system, of which the three first letters are in use clinically to understand their mode and function:

Letter I: indicates which chamber is paced ('V' for ventricle, 'A' for atrium, and 'D' for both (dual)

Letter II: indicates which chamber is sensed

Letter III: reflects the response of the pacemaker to a sensed event ('I' for inhibition of next pacing, 'T' for triggered response, and 'D' for both)

Letter IV: 'R' presence in the fourth position of this code system means that the pacemaker has rate modulation signifying that the pacemaker will adjust the heart rate in response to patient's activity.

Some examples of these are:

- AAI: senses and paces the atrium, and a sensed event results in inhibition of the next output pulse.
- VVI: senses and paces the ventricle, and a sensed event results in inhibition of the next output pulse.
- DDD: senses and paces both chambers, and a sensed event in the atrium results in inhibition of the next output pulse in the atrium but triggers a ventricular output pulse.

What is the pacemaker syndrome?

It is seen in individuals with a single-chamber pacemaker who experience symptoms of low cardiac output (dizziness, etc.) when standing; it is attributed to the lack of atrial kick. Pacemaker syndrome results from haemodynamic changes following inappropriate use of ventricular pacing: it occurs when ventricular pacing is uncoupled from atrial contraction. It is most common when the VVI mode is used in patients with sinus rhythm, but it can occur in any pacing mode when atrioventricular synchrony is lost. Levels of atrial natriuretic factor are high in pacemaker syndrome.

If pacemaker syndrome occurs in a patient with a VVI pacemaker, the only definitive treatment is converting to a DDD. If the patient has occasional runs of bradycardia, then often, symptoms may be ameliorated by programming the pacemaker to a lower limit and programming with hysteresis 'on'. This allows the patient to stay in normal sinus rhythm for longer periods by minimizing the pacing.

Which drug would you use to treat sinus bradycardia seen in the setting of an acute myocardial infarction?
Intravenous atropine.

What do you understand by the term chronotropic incompetence?
Failure to reach a heart rate that is 85% of the age-predicted maximum (220 – age in years) at peak exercise, failure to achieve a heart rate of 100 beats/min, or a maximal heart rate >2 SD below that in a control population.

What you know about Stokes–Adams syndrome?
It refers to syncope or fits occurring during complete heart block.

Further Information

W. Stokes (1804–1878), Regius Professor of Medicine in Dublin, graduated from Edinburgh.
R. Adams (1791–1875), Professor of Surgery in Dublin, was an authority on gout and arthritis.

CHAPTER 239

Spontaneous Pneumothorax

Instruction

Examine this patient's chest.

Salient Features

HISTORY

- Sudden onset or rapidly progressive dyspnoea
- Ipsilateral acute pleuritic pain: either sharp or a steady ache
- A small pneumothorax may be asymptomatic.
- History of asthma, chronic obstructive pulmonary disease (COPD), or other respiratory disease
- History of trauma or operations/procedures
- History of Marfan syndrome
- History of HIV
- History of positive pressure ventilation.

EXAMINATION

- Decreased movement of the affected side
- Increased percussion note
- Trachea may be central (small pneumothorax) or deviated to the affected side (underlying collapse of lung) or the opposite side (large pneumothorax).
- There may be increased vocal resonance with diminished breath sounds.

Proceed as follows:
- Look for clues regarding aetiology:
    - Pleural aspiration site
    - Tall thin patient or phenotypically marfanoid features
    - Inhaler or peak flow meter by the bedside (asthma, COPD).
- Tell the examiner that you would suspect tension pneumothorax when there is tachycardia (>135 beats/min), hypotension, and pulsus paradoxus.

Diagnosis

This patient has diminished breath sounds and hyperresonant note on the R/L side of the chest (lesion) caused by pneumothorax secondary to Marfan syndrome (aetiology) and is not breathless at rest (functional status).

Questions

What do you understand by the term pneumothorax?
Air in the pleural cavity. It derives from two Greek words, 'pneumo' meaning air and 'thorax' meaning chest.

How do you classify spontaneous pneumothorax?
Primary spontaneous pneumothorax occurs in a patient who does not have a history of respiratory disease. Secondary spontaneous pneumothorax occurs in patients who have underlying lung disease and is usually related to or occurs as a complication of the disease.

How would you investigate this patient?
- Chest radiography (CXR): standard erect CXR in inspiration is the current British Thoracic Society (BTS) recommendation.
- In critically ill patients, pneumothorax is suspected when:
  - The costophrenic angle extends more inferiorly than usual because of air: the 'deep sulcus sign' (Fig. 239.1)

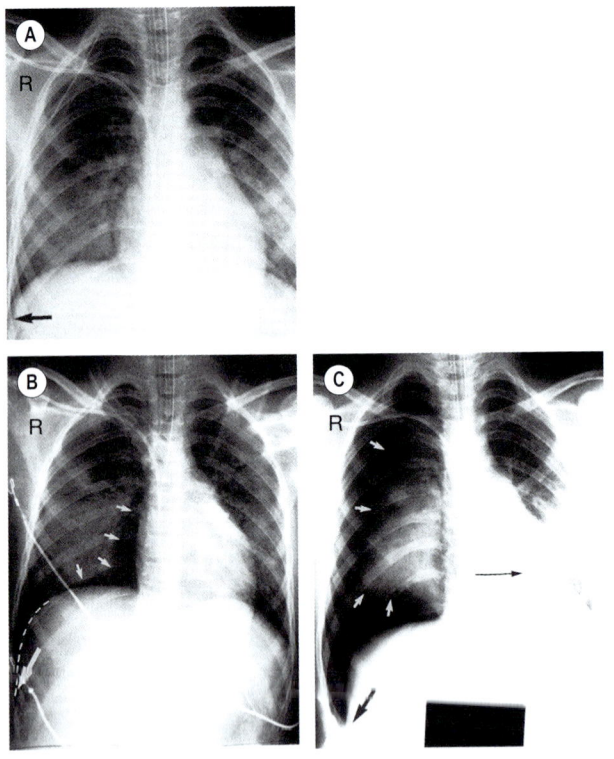

Fig. 239.1 Deep sulcus sign of pneumothorax. **(A)** On posteroanterior chest radiography, the costophrenic angle is normally acute *(arrow)*. In a supine patient, a pneumothorax will often be anterior, medial, and basilar. **(B)** On supine film, the dark area along the right cardiac border and lung base appeared larger *(small arrows)*, and the costophrenic angle much deeper and more acute than normal *(large arrow)*. **(C)** Tension pneumothorax, with an extremely deep costophrenic angle *(large black arrow)*, an almost completely collapsed right lung *(small white arrows)*, and shift of the mediastinum to the left. (With permission from Mettler, F.A., 2004. Essentials of Radiology, second edn. Saunders-Elsevier, Philadelphia, PA.)

- The liver appears more radiolucent and air will outline the medial aspect of the hemidiaphragm under the heart.
- Check blood gases if the patient is breathless: hypoxaemia depending on the shunting, whereas hypercapnia does not develop.
- Computed tomography (CT) scanning is reserved for complex cases or uncertain diagnosis after the initial CXR (for differentiation between pneumothorax and bulla in underlying severe emphysema, detection of small-size pneumothorax not detectable on CXR with continuous clinical suspicion, and identifying other co-existent or underlying lung pathology).

How would you grade the degree of lung collapse?
BTS grading:
- Small: where there is a small rim of air around the lung
- Moderate: when the lung is collapsed towards the heart border
- Complete: airless lung, separate from the diaphragm (aspiration is necessary)
- Tension: any pneumothorax with cardiorespiratory distress (rare and requires immediate drainage).

How do you estimate the size of the pneumothorax?
The classic CXR appearance is that of a thin, visceral pleural line lying parallel to the chest wall, separated by a radiolucent band devoid of lung markings. The average width of this band can be used to estimate the size of the pneumothorax with a fair degree of accuracy. The size of a pneumothorax in a posteroanterior (PA) CXR in inspiration is the distance between the lung margin and the chest wall measured at the level of the hilum. The estimated size of the pneumothorax does not correlate well with the clinical picture of the patient, but the combination of the two can be useful in guiding management decisions. These estimates are used in Europe and the United Kingdom. American guidelines measure the distance between the apex and the cupola. All measurements are done on a CXR or on a CT thorax.

How would you manage this patient?
- The BTS has published guidelines on treatment of both primary and secondary spontaneous pneumothorax, depending on the combination of size of the pneumothorax and its clinical significance.
- Patients with either type of pneumothorax with significant symptomatology, regardless of the size of the pneumothorax, should undergo procedural intervention:
  - In primary spontaneous pneumothorax, aspiration can be initially attempted, and if unsuccessful, a chest drain should be inserted.
  - In secondary spontaneous pneumothorax, a chest drain should be inserted.
- If the patient is asymptomatic, then the size of the pneumothorax should be taken into account.
- In primary spontaneous pneumothorax, if the size is more than 2 cm, then aspiration should be attempted, and if unsuccessful, a chest drain should be inserted; otherwise, the patient can be discharged with follow-up CXR and clinical review in 2 to 4 weeks' time.
- In secondary spontaneous pneumothorax, if the size of the pneumothorax is more than 2 cm, chest drain should be inserted; if the size is between 1 and 2 cm, then aspiration should be attempted; and if the size is less than 1 cm, then patient may not require a procedure/intervention, but they should be admitted for oxygen and observations.
- Once a chest drain has been placed, if repeat radiography in 24 hours shows that the lung remains expanded, the tube can be removed. If the lung has failed to reexpand or there is persistent air leak after 48 hours, then the patient should have further imaging and be

discussed with the cardiothoracic surgeons for surgical pleurodesis, unless their underlying disease deems the pneumothorax inoperable, in which case medical pleurodesis may be more appropriate.

What are the causes of pneumothorax?
- Primary spontaneous pneumothorax
- Iatrogenic
- Trauma
- Bronchial asthma
- COPD: emphysematous bulla
- Carcinoma of the lung
- Cystic fibrosis
- Tuberculosis (TB) (the original descriptions of pneumothorax are commonly associated with TB)
- Mechanical ventilation
- Marfan syndrome, Ehlers–Danlos syndrome
- Infection and HIV
- Catamenial pneumothorax: pneumothorax that occurs in association with menstruation.

How would you do a medical pleurodesis?
By injecting talc into the pleural cavity via the intercostal tube.

In which patients would you avoid doing a pleurodesis?
In patients with underlying cystic fibrosis. Although pleurodesis does not alter the outcome of a subsequent lung transplantation, pleurodesis is associated with an increased rate of recurrence. Patients should instead be referred for partial pleurectomy, which has a success rate of 95%. If the patient is not fit enough to undergo an operation, then pleurodesis is an alternative treatment option.

When would you suspect a tension pneumothorax?
Tension pneumothorax should be suspected in the presence of any of the following:
- Severe progressive dyspnoea
- Severe tachycardia
- Hypotension
- Marked mediastinal shift.

Tension pneumothorax can occur in certain clinical situations, such as ventilated patients (invasive or noninvasive ventilation), trauma, clamped chest drains, and underlying lung diseases. Treatment should be initiated immediately with initial needle decompression with subsequent chest drain insertion.

When should open thoracotomy be considered?
It should be considered if there is one of the following present:
- A third episode of spontaneous pneumothorax
- Any occurrence of bilateral pneumothorax
- Failure of the lung to expand after tube thoracostomy for the first episode.

What do you know about Birt–Hogg–Dubé syndrome?
Birt–Hogg–Dubé syndrome is an autosomal dominant condition that includes skin fibrofolliculomas, pulmonary cysts, spontaneous pneumothorax, and renal cancer. The condition is a result

of germline mutations in the gene *FLCN*, which encodes folliculin; the function of this protein is largely unknown, although FLCN has been linked to the mammalian target of rapamycin pathway. The availability of DNA-based diagnosis has allowed insight into the great variation in expression of *FLCN*, both within and between families.

Further Information

O.K. Williamson (1866–1941), an English physician, described the Williamson sign: BP in the leg is lower than that in the upper limb on the affected side in pneumothorax.

The use of simple aspiration to manage pneumothorax was first reported by O.G. Raja in 1981 when he was a medical registrar (Raja and Lalor, 1981).

Pleurodesis has been performed since 1901 and a huge variety of agents have been tried since the first attempt with hypertonic glucose. Iodized talc pleurodesis was proposed in 1935 by Norman Bethune (1890–1939), a Canadian thoracic surgeon who is revered in China to this day where several statues of him stand and whose name the highest medical honour in China carries.

CHAPTER 240

Subacute Combined Degeneration of the Spinal Cord

Instruction

Carry out a neurological examination of the patient's legs.

Salient Features

HISTORY

- Family history of pernicious anaemia
- History of alcohol consumption and previous gastrectomy
- History of chronic diarrhoea (Crohn's disease, etc.)
- Tingling distal paraesthesia (common presenting symptom)
- Whether the patient is a vegan.

EXAMINATION

- Absent ankle jerks (caused by peripheral neuropathy and motor involvement)
- Brisk knee jerks
- Upgoing plantars (usually first evidence of spinal cord lesion)
- Diminished light touch, vibration, and posterior column signs
- Romberg's sign positive.

Proceed as follows:
- Examine the:
  - mucous membranes for anaemia (pernicious anaemia)
  - abdomen for scars of previous gastrectomy (carcinoma of the stomach)
  - pupils (Argyll Robertson pupil) (because tabes is a differential diagnosis)
  - fundus for optic atrophy, seen in this condition.
- Tell the examiner that you would like to do the following investigations:
  - Mini Mental Status Examination for dementia.
- A 'red tongue and unsteady gait' are seen in the classic condition.

Diagnosis

This patient has absent ankle jerks, brisk knee jerks, and upgoing plantars with posterior column signs (lesion) caused by subacute combined degeneration of the spinal cord (aetiology) and paralysis (functional status).

Questions

Mention a few causes of vitamin B$_{12}$ deficiency.
- Vegan diet
- Impaired absorption:
  - from the stomach: pernicious anaemia, gastrectomy
  - from the small bowel: ileal disease, bacterial overgrowth, coeliac disease
  - from the pancreas: chronic pancreatic disease.
- As a result of fish tapeworm (rare).

What is the pathology of this condition?
There is degeneration of the axons in both the ascending tracts of the posterior columns (sensory) and the descending pyramidal tracts (motor), hence combined degeneration.

How would you investigate such a patient?
- Full blood count and reticulocyte count
- Vitamin B$_{12}$ and folate levels
- Serum ferritin levels (since associated iron deficiency is common)
- Bone marrow examination
- Parietal cell and intrinsic factor antibodies
- Magnetic resonance imaging (MRI) findings are diverse (Fig. 240.1), but vitamin B$_{12}$ deficiency should be considered in differential diagnosis of all spinal cord, peripheral nerve and neuropsychiatric disorders.

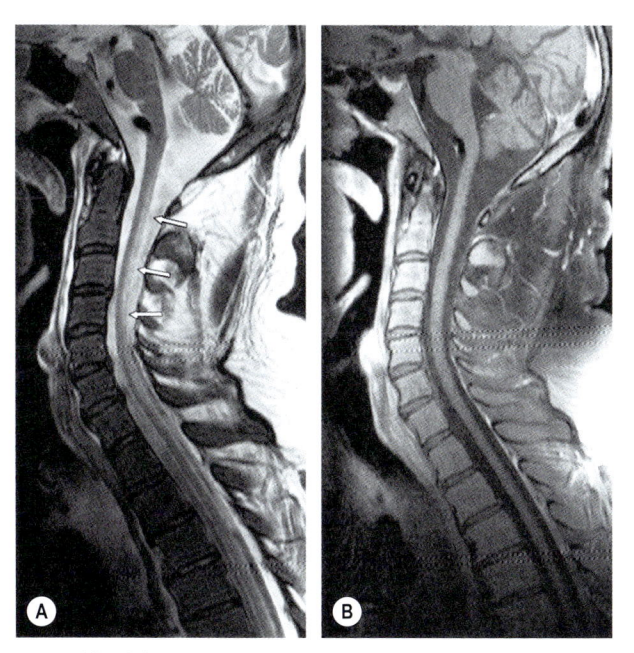

Fig. 240.1 Subacute combined degeneration of the spinal cord in vitamin B$_{12}$ deficiency. **(A)** T$_2$-weighted magnetic resonance image shows abnormal signal intensity of spinal cord extending from C1 to C6 *(arrows)*. **(B)** There is no enhancement after application of gadolinium in the sagittal T$_1$-weighted image. (With permission from Schöllhammer, M., von Rothenburg, T., Schmid, G., Köster, O., Peters, S., 2005. A red tongue and an unsteady gait: MRI in subacute combined degeneration of the spinal cord. Eur. J. Radiol. Extra 54, 77–81.)

If this patient had a haemoglobin level of 6 g/L, how would you treat it?
Avoid giving packed cells before replacing vitamin B_{12} as this may irreversibly exacerbate the neurological manifestations. Furthermore, blood transfusion is reported to precipitate incipient heart failure and death.

What type of anaemia may be seen in such patients?
Macrocytic anaemia.

It can be normocytic anaemia if the cause also results in iron deficiency (e.g. coeliac disease, dietary deficiencies).

Mention a few other causes of macrocytic anaemia.
- With megaloblastic bone marrow: vitamin B_{12} deficiency, folate deficiency
- With normoblastic marrow: haemolytic anaemias, posthaemorrhagic anaemia, severe hypoxia, myxoedema, hypopituitarism, bone marrow infiltration, acute leukaemia, and aplastic anaemia.

What do you know about intrinsic factor antibodies?
Intrinsic factor antibodies are seen in about 50% of patients with pernicious anaemia. About 45% of the patients have no antibody to intrinsic factor. There are two types of antibody:
- Type 1: blocking antibody that prevents vitamin B_{12} from binding to intrinsic factor; occurs in 55% of patients
- Type 2: binding or precipitating antibody, which reacts with intrinsic factor or with vitamin B_{12}–intrinsic factor complex and is seen in 35% of patients.

What is the relationship between pernicious anaemia and gastric carcinoma?
The incidence of gastric carcinoma in patients with pernicious anaemia is increased three-fold compared with that in the general population. The increase is highest in first year after diagnosis of pernicious anaemia.

What gastrointestinal investigations would you do in an asymptomatic patient with pernicious anaemia?
Endoscopy is recommended soon after diagnosis of pernicious anaemia to look for gastric carcinoma.

What do you understand by the term 'combined' degeneration of the cord?
This refers to the combined demyelination of both pyramids (or lateral columns) and posterior columns of the spinal cord.

What is the response of the neurological lesions to treatment with vitamin B_{12}?
The response to vitamin B_{12} therapy is variable: it may improve, remain unchanged, or even deteriorate. Sensory abnormalities improve more than motor abnormalities and peripheral neuropathy responds to treatment better than myelopathy.

Further Information

Subacute combined degeneration is also known as Putnam–Dana syndrome or Lichtheim disease. James Jackson Putnam (1846–1918) and Charles Loomis Dana (1852–1935) were both US neurologists. Ludwig Lichtheim (1845–1928) was a German physician.

Pernicious anaemia was usually fatal, until 1926, when Whipple, Minot, and Murphy described the beneficial effects of feeding liver. The 1934 Nobel Prize in Medicine was awarded jointly to George Whipple (1878–1976) of University of Rochester, New York, to George Minot (1885–1950) and William P. Murphy

(1892–1987) of Harvard Medical School, and to Peter Bent Brigham Hospital, Boston, for their discoveries concerning liver therapy in anaemia. This condition is also known as Addison–Biermer anaemia with reference to Thomas Addison and the German physician Anton Biermer.

William B. Castle first found that oral administration of gastric juice (intrinsic factor) or beef (extrinsic factor, i.e. vitamin B_{12}) alone was not effective in the treatment of pernicious anaemia but that a mixture of both these factors rendered the patient erythropoietically active. Castle worked with Francis Peabody at the Harvard Medical School Unit at Boston City Hospital before he became Professor of Medicine at Harvard.

CHAPTER 241

Subarachnoid Haemorrhage

Instruction

This patient presented to the emergency services with sudden-onset headache. He has a family history of polycystic kidney disease. Please assess.

Salient Features

HISTORY

- Thunderclap headache. This is such a prominent feature of a ruptured aneurysm that every thunderclap headache, regardless of other associated features or accompanying symptoms, must be investigated so as to exclude subarachnoid haemorrhage (SAH) as the cause.
- Very sudden-onset headache. Sudden-onset headache that gradually worsens reaching its maximum intensity within an hour is not a thunderclap headache. The question to ask is 'From the moment you first felt the headache till the time this headache became the worst headache ever how much time do you think elapsed?'
- Maximum intensity is reached within seconds to a minute from onset.
- 'The worst headache of my life.'
- Site of headache—usually SAH causes occipital headache, and this is where the 'as I was hit with a bat on the back of my head' description comes.
- Vomiting
- Neck and back pain
- Preceding similar headache but not as severe a few days or weeks prior to this episode
- Loss of consciousness.

EXAMINATION

- Altered consciousness level
- Preretinal haemorrhages
- Meningism with neck stiffness
- Focal neurological signs and cranial nerve palsies
- High blood pressure
- Sometimes a normal examination.

Diagnosis

This patient gives a history of thunderclap headache (lesion) and needs further evaluation for a possible SAH from a ruptured aneurysm (aetiology) associated with his known autosomal dominant polycystic kidney disease (ADPKD). His Glasgow Coma Scale (GCS) score is 15/15 with no focal neurology (functional status).

Questions

Which inherited conditions are associated with cerebral aneurysms?
- Autosomal dominant polycystic kidney disease
- Bicuspid aortic valve
- Ehlers–Danlos syndrome
- Pseudoxanthoma elasticum
- Familiar hyperaldosteronism type I.

What are the recognized risk factors for an aneurysm rupture?
- Hypertension
- Alcohol consumption
- Smoking
- History of migraine
- Cocaine and amphetamine use
- Aneurysm characteristics for known cerebral aneurysms (large aneurysms, aneurysms in the posterior circulation, previous ruptures)
- Known aneurysms associated with inherited conditions.

How would you investigate a patient with subarachnoid haemorrhage suspicion?
All patients in whom SAH is suspected warrant urgent brain imaging (computed tomography (CT)). A CT scan performed within 6 hours of onset of headache has a sensitivity approaching 100%. If patients present after this 6-hour window, CT sensitivity starts dropping to reach around 90% in the first 12 hours. A negative CT must be followed up with lumbar puncture (LP) performed at least 12 hours after the onset of the headache. LP should include measuring opening pressure and sending cerebrospinal fluid (CSF) samples for cell count, biochemistry, and xanthochromia (oxyhaemoglobin, methaemoglobin, and bilirubin).

Can a computed tomography angiogram replace lumbar puncture as a noninvasive method of investigating a subarachnoid haemorrhage?
Many clinicians advocate the use of noninvasive angiography instead of an LP in the workup of suspected SAH. However, if the patient has presented within the first 10 days of the onset of the headache, an LP will detect any bleeding in the subarachnoid space, and thus confirm a SAH. The role of a CT angiogram is to locate an aneurysm once the diagnosis of a SAH is established. Given that 3% to 5% of the population will have an incidental aneurysm but the prevalence of SAH is around 0.005%, not all aneurysms will cause a SAH. Locating an existing aneurysm in the context of a normal CT and a headache history is not necessarily a confirmation of SAH. Therefore, incidental brain aneurysms pose a conundrum for clinicians treating patients presenting with headache because the only treatment for aneurysms is surgery with all its inherent risks, so the decision to intervene in an incidental finding in this context is a difficult one.

Which other conditions can cause thunderclap headache apart from subarachnoid haemorrhage?
- Pituitary apoplexy
- Meningitis
- Cerebral venous thrombosis
- Reversible cerebral vasoconstriction syndrome
- Posterior reversible leukoencephalopathy syndrome
- Intracerebral haemorrhage.

What is the pharmacological agent that has proven to improve outcome in subarachnoid haemorrhage?
Nimodipine.

Name some complications of subarachnoid haemorrhage.
- Rebleeding
- Cerebral ischaemia
- Hydrocephalus
- Cardiac arrhythmias
- Seizures
- Death.

How is subarachnoid haemorrhage graded?
Multiple severity scoring systems have been developed over the years, taking into account radiological severity of an identified bleed and neurological presentation. The systems currently used are:
- Hunt & Hessle Scale (1968)
- Fisher Scale (1980)
- Glasgow Coma Scale (1974)
- World Federation of Neurological Surgeons Grading (1988).

There are also two systems grading outcome:
- Modified Rankin Scale (1988)
- Glasgow Outcome Scale (1975).

No grading score or scale should be used in isolation to inform a decision regarding intervention but a combination of scales and scores may help multidisciplinary decision making by medical, intensive care, and neurosurgical team.

Hunt & Hessle is based on the clinical presentation:
Grade I—asymptomatic or minimal headache
Grade II—moderate headache, no neurological deficit apart from cranial nerve palsy
Grade III—drowsiness, confusion, moderate neurological deficit
Grade IV—stupor, severe hemiparesis
Grade V—coma, decerebrating rigidity.

Fisher scale is based on CT findings:
Fisher I—no blood detected
Fisher II—diffuse deposition or thin layer with all vertical layers of blood (in interhemispheric fissure, insular cistern, or ambient cistern) less than 1 mm thick
Fisher III—localized clots and/or vertical layers of blood 1 mm or more in thickness
Fisher IV—intracerebral or intraventricular clots with diffuse or no subarachnoid blood.

GCS is widely used in clinical practice and is not specific to SAH. Points are added based on three parameters of neurologic function with a total score between 3 and 15:
Eye opening (spontaneous = 4, response to verbal command = 3, response to pain = 2, no eye opening = 1)
Best verbal response (oriented = 5, confused = 4, inappropriate words = 3, incomprehensible sounds = 2, no verbal response = 1)
Best motor response (obeys commands = 6, localizing response to pain = 5, withdrawal response to pain = 4, flexion to pain = 3, extension to pain = 2, no motor response = 1).

World Federation of Neurological Surgeons Grading
I: GCS score 15, no motor deficit
II: GCS score 13 to 14, no motor deficit
III: GCS score 13 to 14, with motor deficit
IV: GCS score 7 to 12, with or without motor deficit
V: GCS score 3 to 6, with or without motor deficit.

What are the main causes of nonaneurysmal subarachnoid haemorrhage?
Vascular malformations and intracranial artery dissection.

Further Information

Detachable coils for aneurysm coiling (still the treatment of choice for suitable aneurysms today) started in 1989 at Columbia University in New York with S.K. Hilal (1930–2000), an Egyptian radiologist. The technique was refined with engineering breakthroughs at University of California in the ensuing years to design a safe, soft coiling system now in use worldwide.

CHAPTER 242

Syncope

Instruction

This 17-year-old patient presents with an episode of collapse while playing football at school. Please assess him.

Salient Features

HISTORY

A detailed history is crucial in determining the underlying nature of an episode with loss of consciousness. Symptoms that may signify an episode as a syncopal one are as follows:
- Circumstances: episodes occurring on exertion may signify cardiac arrhythmia or structural heart disease, and episodes while in supine position almost always represent an underlying heart disease; episodes occurring from sitting to standing position associated with light-headedness can be because of postural hypotension.
- Preceding symptoms: chest pain, dyspnoea, palpitations, and asymptomatic with no warning are features that can occur in cardiac syncope, while autonomic symptoms such as diaphoresis, dizziness, and nausea can occur in reflex syncope.
- Duration and frequency of episode: syncopal episodes, as opposed to other reasons for loss of consciousness, are usually short-lived (seconds), followed by a rapid recovery. Patients who have had multiple episodes of loss of consciousness over years with no further complications may have a more innocent underlying diagnosis than those with recent onset of recurrent episodes of loss of consciousness with preceding symptoms.
- Triggers: patients should be asked about triggers as situational syncope is part of the differential diagnosis and does not signify possible underlying life-threatening heart disease (after a big meal, after coughing, or urinating). Syncope on pressure over the carotid (tight collar) may signify carotid hypersensitivity, while syncope whilst working with hands over the head may indicate subclavian steal syndrome.
- Medication history and medical history: antihypertensive, diuretic, antiarrhythmic therapy, risk factors for pulmonary embolism
- Family history of sudden cardiac death may signify the presence of structural heart disease or genetic conduction abnormality.

EXAMINATION

Thorough cardiovascular examination and neurological examination.
Proceed as follows:
Obtain a lying and standing blood pressure, blood pressure in both arms, 12-lead electrocardiogram (ECG), and, if possible, a bedside echocardiogram if structural cardiac disease is suspected.

Tell the examiners that you would like to stratify the patient's risk of recurrence or death in order to decide whether further evaluation should follow in an inpatient or outpatient setting.

Diagnosis

This young patient describes an episode of syncope (lesion) and there are elements in the history to signify cardiac syncope (aetiology). The patient is at high risk of recurrent events and thus needs a hospital admission for further cardiac investigations and continuous cardiac monitoring.

Questions

What is the yield of diagnosis from history and clinical examination findings in a patient presenting with syncope?

History and clinical examination including 12-lead ECG will lead to a diagnosis in more than half of patients presenting with syncope and is the most specific and sensitive way to evaluate syncope in the acute setting. These are mandated in the assessment of a patient presenting with a possible syncopal episode to hospital, and they also help with the risk stratification of the patient and the decision for admission or early discharge from hospital with outpatient investigation. Patients are stratified into low, moderate, and high risk (of subsequent mortality and morbidity) and selected patients can be discharged, whereas others will require a period of inpatient monitoring and/or treatment. For instance, patients with exertional syncope, suspicion of structural heart disease, and suspected cardiac arrhythmia leading to syncope or abnormal baseline 12-lead ECG will need inpatient echocardiography and cardiac monitoring. Similarly, elderly patients with polypharmacy and multiple comorbidities will also need hospitalization for further assessment and physical therapies to prevent possible falls and injuries. On the other hand, patients with a convincing history of neurally mediated syncope with normal routine blood tests and normal baseline ECG do not need hospitalization but can be followed up in an outpatient setting if needed.

What are the three main causes of syncope?

As described in the History section, there are three main categories of syncopal episodes:
- Neurally mediated (or reflex syncope)
- Cardiovascular
- Postural hypotension.

What are the neurally mediated syncopal syndromes?
- Neurocardiogenic syncope
- Vasovagal syncope
- Carotid sinus hypersensitivity
- Cough syncope
- Post micturition
- Drug induced.

What is the pathophysiology of neurally mediated syncope?

On standing, blood shifts from the intrathoracic cavity to the lower body under the force of gravity, with a resulting reduction in venous return to the right heart. This is followed by reduced cardiac output.

In normal physiology, reduced cardiac output leads to reduced stimulation of baroreceptors and mechanoreceptors in the carotid sinus and left ventricular wall. The function of these receptors is to inhibit sympathetic neurons in the brainstem, so that reduced stimulation leads to increased sympathetic activity with resulting restoration of blood pressure and heart rate.

In neurocardiogenic syncope, underfilling of the left ventricle leads to forceful contraction with inappropriate stimulation of mechanoreceptors. This stimulation leads to increased inhibition of the sympathetic neurons and resulting relative parasympathetic overactivity with vasodilation (reducing the blood pressure) and bradycardia.

Abnormal overstimulation of receptors inhibiting sympathetic neurons in the brainstem is the common pathway for all types of neurally mediated syncope (e.g. genitourinary receptors in micturition syncope, cardiac C fibres in hypovolaemia, baroreceptors in carotid sinus hypersensitivity, cerebral cortex in emotional syncope).

When would you perform carotid sinus massage?
Carotid sinus syndrome is a cause of syncope but not a common one. Risk factors for sinus hypersensitivity are age or prior neck surgery. The European Society of Cardiology has suggested that carotid sinus massage should be performed when a patient more than 40 years old presents with syncope that is unexplained following initial evaluation. The procedure should be performed by experienced clinicians, within a facility with appropriate resuscitation equipment, and should be avoided if the patient has suffered a stroke or a transient ischaemic attack (TIA) within the last 3 months with no recent carotid Doppler ultrasound to exclude severe stenosis. The procedure is done under continuous cardiac monitoring and repeated blood pressure measurement, and it comprises of 5 to 10 s of neck massage at the angle of the mandible, with the patient in the supine position with the neck extended. If the massage results in sinus pause more than 3 s, drop of blood pressure more than 50 mm Hg, and symptoms of syncope or presyncope then the test is considered positive. Cardiology guidelines recommend performing carotid sinus massage in both supine and head-up positions, as the combination increases the diagnostic yield of the procedure.

Are you aware of any risk stratification scores for discharging or admitting patients who present with collapse with loss of consciousness?
The San Francisco Syncope Rule (SFSR) is one of the clinical decision aids used to identify high-risk patients who should be admitted to hospital for further investigation. The SFSR includes ECG findings, history of heart failure, initial systolic blood pressure, haematocrit measurements, and shortness of breath.

How can hypoglycaemia induce collapse?
Glucose is the obligate metabolic fuel for the brain. When plasma glucose falls below 4.5 mmol/L, insulin secretion falls while simultaneous glucagon secretion is stimulated, followed by adrenaline secretion as blood glucose levels drop below 4 mmol/L. If glucagon secretion fails to prevent a further drop in blood glucose, neuroglycopenic symptoms will occur and the patient will seek to ingest glucose. If the patient either does not ingest glucose or has hypoglycaemia unawareness, blood glucose will continue to fall.

Glucose diffuses into brain cells (as they cannot store or produce glucose) at a rate that depends on the concentration of glucose in the blood. As the blood glucose concentration falls, this diffusion reduces and the brain cells needs outstrip the supply of glucose. As glucose is the sole metabolic fuel for the brain cells, brain failure occurs, with symptoms of cognitive impairment, collapse, and coma.

What is the role of the tilt table test in the evaluation of syncope?
The tilt table test has low sensitivity and specificity and thus is reserved for specific cases where other causes of syncope have been excluded and vasovagal syncope is suspected but the history lacks specific elements to reach the diagnosis with confidence. The test is contraindicated in patients with severe coronary artery or cerebrovascular disease. During the test, the development of syncope on changing position with or without the help of nitroglycerin or isoproterenol in

association with a cardio-inhibitory or vasopressor response indicates a positive tilt table test result. These results must be interpreted in conjunction with the initial evaluation of the patient (history and examination).

What findings on the electrocardiogram of a patient presenting with syncope would alert you?
Red flags on ECG that warrantee further investigations are:
- Heart block and bundle branch block (syncope, Fig. 242.1)
- Sinus pause more than 3 s
- Severe bradycardia (<40 beats/min)
- Bifascicular or trifascicular block (syncope, Fig. 242.2)
- Tachycardias
- Preexcitation (syncope, Fig. 242.3)
- Left ventricular hypertrophy (syncope, Fig. 242.4)
- Brugada syndrome (syncope, Fig. 242.5)
- Any arrhythmia in the context of syncope should prompt further investigations towards cardiogenic syncope.

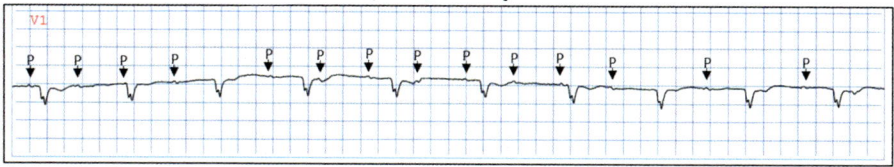

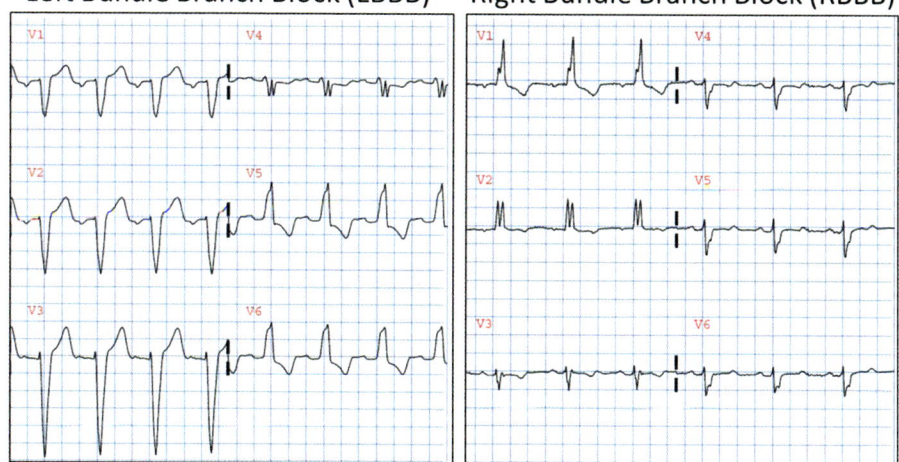

Fig. 242.1 Clinically important conduction disturbances. The upper ECG strip shows a complete heart block with complete dyssynchrony between the P waves *(black arrows)* and the QRS complexes. Atrial rate is higher than the ventricular rate. Bottom strips show the precordial leads of two different cases with conduction disturbance due to a block at the right or left bundle branches. P-QRS synchrony is maintained, but QRS duration and morphology are abnormal. *ECG*, Electrocardiogram. (With permission from El-Baz, A.S., Suri, J. (Eds.), 2022. Cardiovascular and Coronary Artery Imaging. Vol. 1. Academic Press, Elsevier.)

What do you know of Naxos disease?

It is a form of arrhythmogenic dysplasia of the right ventricle. The myocardium is replaced by fatty and fibrous tissue, which gives rise to ventricular arrhythmias. The name may be misleading as the left ventricle may also be involved. Arrhythmogenic dysplasia of the right ventricle can present with cardiac syncope and is one of the main causes of sudden cardiac death. There are two inherited types, an autosomal dominant and an autosomal recessive, known as Naxos disease from the Greek island of Naxos. Patients with Naxos disease share specific phenotypic characteristics; woolly hair and palmar keratomas (syncope, Fig. 242.6)

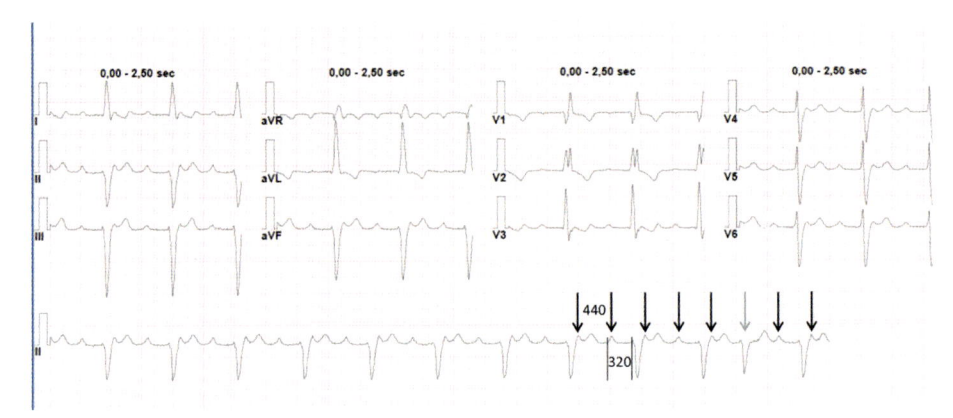

Fig. 242.2 Atrial tachycardia (arrows), A-A interval 440 milliseconds, with 2:1 atrioventricular conduction is present. A complete right bundle branch block and left anterior fascicular block are present (bifascicular block); a long A-V interval should raise suspicion of a more advanced intraventricular block (trifascicular block). (With permission from Savino, K., Bagliani, G., Crusco, F., Padeletti, M., Lombardi, M., 2018. Electrocardiogram and imaging: an integrated approach to arrhythmogenic cardiomyopathies. Card.Electrophysiol. Clin. 10(2), 413–429.)

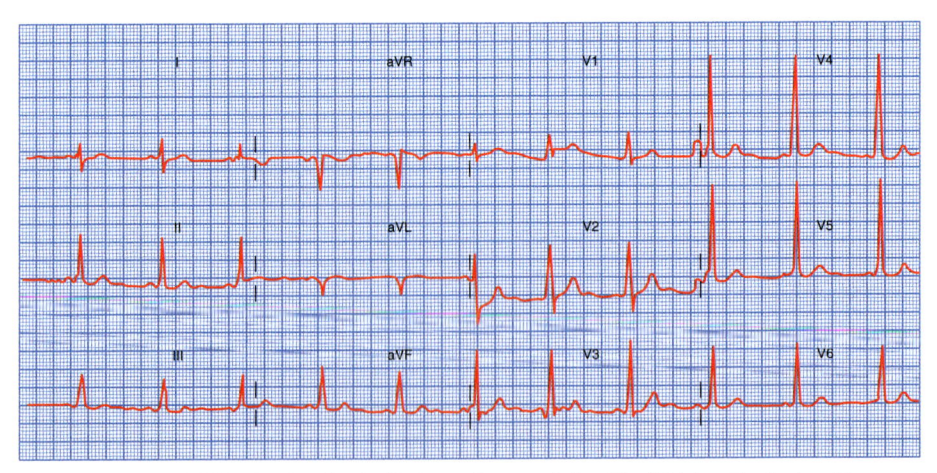

Fig. 242.3 A 12-lead ECG showing classical features of pre-excitation. The PR interval is short and the onset of the QRS complex is characterised by a 'delta wave' or slurred upstroke. *ECG*, electrocardiogram. (With permission from Sharma, S.K., Strachan, M., Grubb, N., Hunter, J.A.A., 2008. Davidson's 100 Clinical Cases. Churchill Livingstone.)

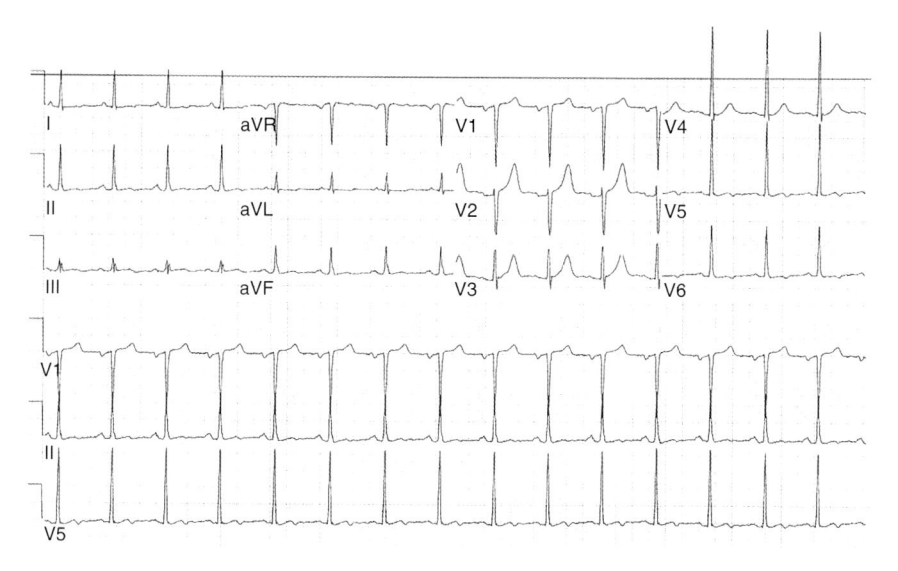

Fig. 242.4 ECG shows sinus rhythm, LVH, and nonspecific repolarization abnormalities. *ECG*, electrocardiogram; *LVH*, left ventricular hypertrophy. (With permission from, Hutchison, S.J., 2009. Aortic Diseases: Clinical Diagnostic Imaging Atlas. Saunders.)

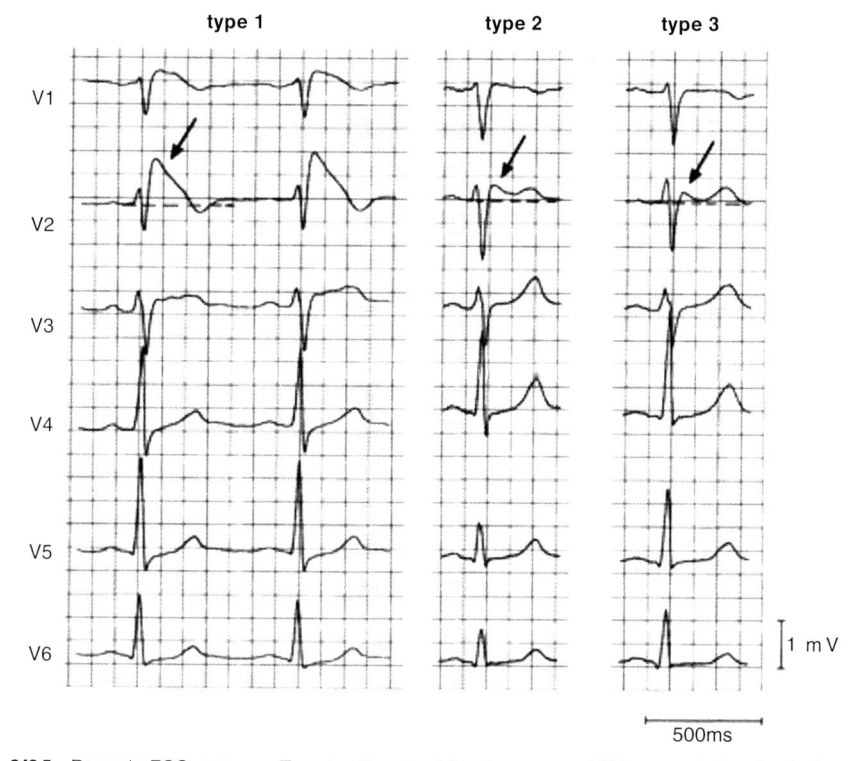

Fig. 242.5 Brugada ECG patterns. Type I pattern is defined as a coved ST-segment elevation in 2 mm in lead V1 or V2. Type II is defined as a saddle-back ST-segment elevation of 1 mm. Type III is defined as an ST-segment elevation 1 mm. Type II and III are suggestive of the diagnosis but only documentation of a Type I pattern is regarded as diagnostic. *ECG*, electrocardiogram. (With permission from Ramachandran, S.V., Sawyer, D.B., (eds.), 2018. Encyclopedia of Cardiovascular Research and Medicine. Elsevier.)

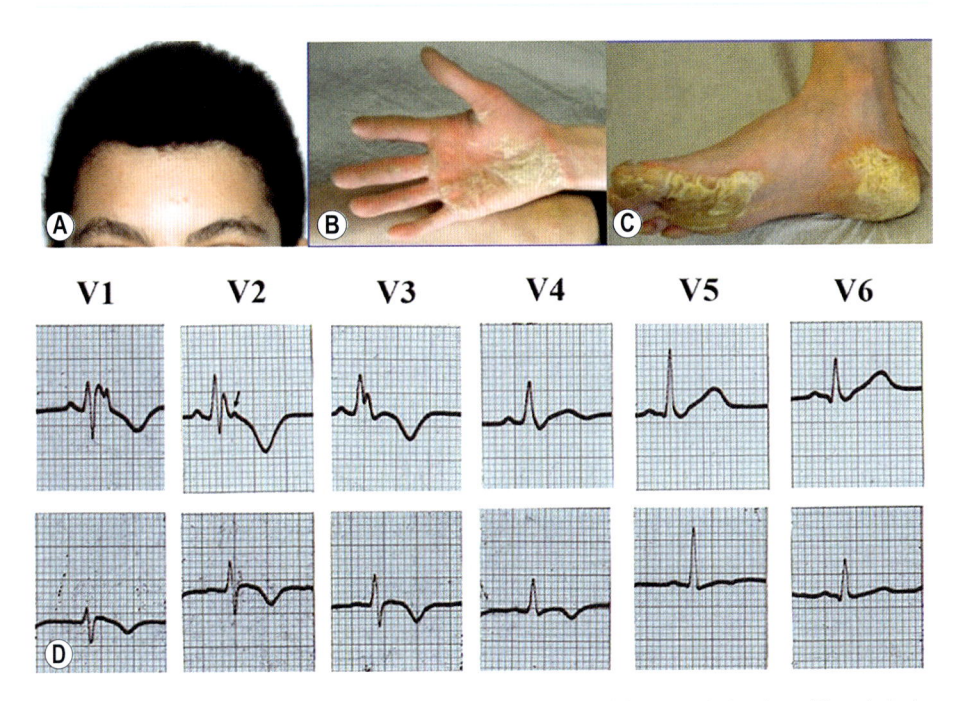

Fig. 242.6 Seventeen-year-old boy with Naxos disease; wooly hair **(A)** and typical palmar **(B)** and plantar **(C)** keratoderma. Precordial lead recordings from his 12-lead resting ECG showing RBBB and epsilon wave in V2 (**D**, *upper*) as compared with the 12-lead resting ECG following excision of an arrhythmogenic focus from right ventricular free wall (**D**, *lower*). Shortened QRS duration and disappearance of epsilon wave can be observed on right precordial leads, corresponding to excised RV myocardial wall segment. *ECG*, electrocardiogram; *RBBB*, right bundle branch block. (With permission from Tsatsopoulou, A., Bossone, E., 2018. Common presentation of rare diseases: arrhythmogenic right ventricular cardiomyopathy and its mimics. Int. J. Cardiol. 257, 371–377.)

What is the role of brain imaging in collapse?
With collapse as the presenting feature, brain imaging is helpful in differentiating the diagnosis. A careful and thorough history of events is crucial to inform further investigation including brain imaging. In the acute setting, computed tomography (CT) of the head should be obtained for:
- Patients with collapse who are on oral anticoagulation
- Patients presenting for the first time with features consistent with a seizure
- Elderly patients for whom a systemic or metabolic reason has not been identified, and the description is not that of mechanical fall
- Those with a report of head injury during collapse
- Those with a history and examination signs consistent with possible stroke or TIA
- Those with a history of headache
- Those with abnormal neurology findings on examination, consistent with intracranial pathology
- Those with reduced, altered or fluctuating level of consciousness.

CHAPTER 243

The Pregnant Patient

Instruction

This patient presented to the ambulatory care unit with sudden-onset right-sided chest pain associated with shortness of breath on exertion. She is 26 weeks pregnant. From initial triage, you know that the patient is clinically stable and looks well. Please review the patient and advise on further investigations and management.

Salient Features

HISTORY

History of presenting symptoms should not differ from the nonpregnant patient, with the addition of further questions.
- Characteristics of the presenting complaint:
  - Site
  - Duration
  - Radiation
  - Intensity
  - Relieving or exacerbating factors
  - Onset
  - Character
  - Associated symptoms of dyspnoea, pre-syncope, syncope, nausea, vomiting, diaphoresis.
- Medical and obstetric history, including:
  - Cardiac disease
  - Hypertension
  - Previous venous thromboembolism (VTE)
  - Previous pregnancies, previous miscarriages
  - Any pregnancy-related complications
  - Diabetes
  - Epilepsy
  - Congenital or ischaemic heart disease.

EXAMINATION

- Cardiovascular and respiratory examination
- Obstetric involvement if more than 20 weeks pregnant
- Observations including blood pressure, urine dip, and blood glucose.

Diagnosis

This patient has features from the history and examination that suggest a possible pulmonary embolus (lesion), as well as signs of deep venous thrombosis (DVT) in the left calf (aetiology).

I would like to investigate further with a chest X-ray (CXR) and a venous Doppler ultrasound scan (USS) of her lower limbs.

Questions

Name some possible differential diagnoses for these symptoms.
Aortic dissection, pulmonary embolism, cardiac event, pneumonia, pneumothorax, musculoskeletal diaphragmatic pain, gastro-oesophageal reflux.

How common is venous thromboembolic disease in pregnancy?
The calculated incidence in the United Kingdom is 1.3 per 10,000 pregnancies. The relative risk for VTE in pregnancy increases four- to six-fold.

What are the main indirect causes of maternal death in the United Kingdom?
- Cardiac disease
- Thrombosis
- Neurological causes
- Non-genital sepsis
- Psychiatric
- Pre-eclampsia.

Who should be considered for prophylaxis of venous thromboembolic disease in pregnancy?
- Previous VTE not related to a single episode of major surgery mandates thromboprophylaxis with low-molecular-weight heparin (LMWH) throughout the antenatal period.
- Patients with any one of the following: hospital admission, VTE related to major surgery, high-risk thrombophilia, high-risk medical comorbidities, acute problems requiring surgery, ovarian hyperstimulation syndrome; should be considered for LMWH throughout the antenatal period.
- The following are also risk factors for VTE: smoker, age >35, body mass index (BMI) >30, gravida >2, varicose veins, multiple pregnancy, prominent varicose veins, pre-eclampsia, reduced mobility, low-risk thrombophilia, in vitro fertilization (IVF) pregnancy, first-degree relative with VTE.
  - Four or more risk factors: LMWH from first trimester
  - Three risk factors: LMWH from 28 weeks
  - Fewer than three risk factors: LMWH not recommended.

How would you investigate suspected nonmassive pulmonary embolism in pregnancy?
- Women used to have a bilateral Doppler leg ultrasound first to identify potential DVT. However, the updated guidelines suggest a Doppler ultrasound only in those cases where there is clinical evidence of DVT. If there is no clinical suspicion or signs of DVT, Doppler ultrasound of the legs should not be performed.
- A negative ultrasound coupled with low clinical suspicion should lead to discontinuation of anticoagulation.
- A negative ultrasound but with high clinical suspicion should prompt repeat Doppler USS at day 3 and day 7.
- An electrocardiogram and CXR should be performed.
- If these investigations are normal, the choice between V/Q scan and computed tomography pulmonary angiography (CTPA) should be discussed with the patient. CTPA is known to increase the chances of future maternal breast cancer (lifetime risk increased by up to 13.6%),

whereas V/Q scanning is associated with increased childhood cancer (1/280,000 versus 1/1,000,000).
- Treatment should be offered at the time of suspicion until investigation has confirmed or rejected the diagnosis.
- There is no role for d-dimers or pretest score probability in pregnancy.

How is venous thromboembolic disease in pregnancy treated?
Treatment of VTE in pregnancy is with LMWH at a dose calculated from the patient's weight at the first antenatal booking appointment, either once daily or in two divided doses. Treatment should continue until at least 6 weeks after delivery and until at least 3 months have passed from diagnosis.

What is the most common medical problem in pregnancy?
The most common is hypertension, either preexisting (chronic) or gestational.
- Mild hypertension is 140–149/90–99 mm Hg
- Moderate hypertension 150–159/100–109 mm Hg
- Severe hypertension >160/110 mm Hg.

How would you manage chronic hypertension in pregnancy?
- Stop angiotensin-converting enzyme inhibitors (ACE-I) and angiotensin receptor blockers (ARBs) if the patient is already taking them and switch to alternative antihypertensives (labetalol is first line in pregnancy, nifedipine is second line, and methyldopa is third line).
- Reduce sodium intake.
- Daily 75 mg aspirin from 12 weeks' gestation.
- Aim for blood pressure under 135/85.
- Close monitoring antenatally and assess regularly for proteinuria.

What are the complications of hypertension in pregnancy?
Hypertension increases the risk of pre-eclampsia. Pre-eclampsia is defined as worsening hypertension with proteinuria and/or organ dysfunction. It is a medical emergency and requires hospital admission for intensive treatment of high blood pressure and monitoring for and treating possible complications: seizures, cerebral bleeding, acute cardiac failure, haemolysis, elevated liver enzymes, low platelets (HELLP) syndrome, acute kidney injury, disseminated intravascular coagulopathy (DIC), and obstetric complications.

How do you classify maternal risk in women with congenital heart disease?
The European Society of Cardiology has adopted the modified World Health Organization classification for maternal risk assessment, according to which women with congenital heart disease are grouped into four categories:
- Class I: not increased risk of maternal mortality and/or mildly increased risk of morbidity
- Class II: small increased risk in mortality and moderate increased risk in morbidity
- Class III: significant increased risk of morbidity and mortality
- Class IV: pregnancy contraindicated.

What do you know of cardiomyopathy in pregnancy?
Peripartum cardiomyopathy is an idiopathic form of cardiomyopathy that develops in pregnancy and has three characteristics:
- Heart failure towards the end of pregnancy (or even postpartum)
- Absence of other cause of heart failure
- Echocardiographic evidence of left ventricular systolic dysfunction with ejection fraction less than 45%.

The cause of the disease is still unknown and is considered multifactorial.

Pregnant women may present with symptomatology of heart failure (dyspnoea, orthopnoea, paroxysmal nocturnal dyspnoea, peripheral oedema). Signs on clinical examination are those of biventricular heart failure (displaced apex, raised jugular venous pressure, pedal oedema, bibasal crackles).

The treatment is also similar to that of heart failure of other causes, with the only difference that specific medications should be avoided in pregnancy due to the known associated risks (ACE-I, ARB, mineralocorticoid receptor antagonist). In postpartum cardiomyopathy, women who are not breastfeeding should be treated identically to heart failure with reduced ejection fraction.

The most common course of the disease is full recovery within months or years of diagnosis. However, it carries an overall mortality of more than 5% in 2 years, and causes of death are progressive heart failure, sudden cardiac death, or thromboembolic episodes.

Women with peripartum cardiomyopathy should receive counselling regarding future pregnancies, as subsequent pregnancies may carry a high risk of complications.

What do you know of gestational diabetes mellitus?

Pregnancy is associated with increased insulin resistance and, when pancreatic insulin secretion fails to keep up with demand, gestational diabetes mellitus (GDM) develops. Patients who are found to have hyperglycaemia in the first trimester likely have undiagnosed pregestational diabetes. There is debate about the role of universal screening for this condition but, if it is performed, it is with oral glucose tolerance test.

Gestational diabetes may lead to acute adverse maternal and foetal outcomes such as foetal macrosomia (with associated peripartum risks), increased risk of stillbirth, pre-eclampsia and neonatal hospital stay, and more long-term problems such as increased risk of persistent maternal type 2 diabetes and increased risk of obesity and type 2 diabetes in the child.

Management includes dietician-led nutritional support, self-monitoring of glucose levels, and drug therapy with metformin and insulin.

CHAPTER 244

Central Line Insertion

Instruction

A 35-year-old patient presents to hospital with severe sepsis. The patient has failed to respond to optimal medical treatment and has been tachycardic, anuric, and hypotensive for the last 12 hours. A decision is made to escalate her treatment to intensive care environment and a central line is needed for inotropic support.

Questions

What are the possible complications after a central line insertion?
- Immediate complications:
  - Puncture of the carotid artery
  - Air embolus
  - Loss of guidewire into the vein
  - Cardiac arrhythmias as the wire proceeds through the tricuspid annulus
  - Pain.
- Early complications:
  - Pneumothorax or haemothorax
  - Cardiac tamponade
  - Extravasation of infusion into subcutaneous tissue.
- Late:
  - Sepsis
  - Vessel thrombosis and stenosis.

List the equipment needed to be ready and checked before proceeding to central line insertion.
- Sterile gown
- Sterile probe cover and gel
- Sterile drapes
- Sterile gauze
- Sterile gloves
- Theatre hat and surgical mask for all staff that will be present and assisting with the procedure
- Appropriate cleaning solution
- 10-mL syringe for aspiration
- 10-mL syringe for saline flush
- 10- to 20-mL syringe for local anaesthetic
- Orange needle (25 G)
- Green needle (18 G)
- Blunt filling needle
- Gallipot for saline
- Ultrasound machine
- Electrocardiogram (ECG) monitor

- Clean trolley
- 1% lidocaine (10–20 mL)
- 0.9% saline (20–30 mL)
- 'Octopus' connectors for each lumen of the line
- 2/0 silk suture on a curved needle
- Transparent dressing.

List the steps you need to take before a central line insertion.
- Check clotting and platelets.
- Check for possible allergies to local anaesthetic or part of equipment.
- Obtain patient consent.
- Place cardiac monitor (three-lead ECG is adequate).
- Position the patient accordingly (for right internal jugular insertion, place patient 'head down' and looking slightly to the left).
- Place disposable pads below the patient's head and on the floor if necessary.
- Check vessels and anatomy with ultrasound.
- Prepare the equipment (during this stage, you may ask the patient to sit up in a comfortable position until you are ready to resume the procedure).

Once you are scrubbed and ready to begin the procedure, list the steps to perform a right internal jugular catheter insertion using the Seldinger technique under ultrasound guidance.
- Prepare the line by flushing every lumen and attaching the bionectors at the end with the exception of the most distal one.
- Remove the cover from the guide wire so that it is ready for use.
- Lay out your equipment in the exact order that you will be needing each piece during the procedure: local anaesthetic, introducer needle with attached syringe, guide wire, scalpel, dilator, catheter. All this equipment should be placed in the nearest convenient sterile place near you, so that you avoid awkward manoeuvres while performing the procedure.
- Prepare the ultrasound probe: ultrasound gel should be placed into the probe cover, which should then be placed over the probe. Once sterilized, you can let go of the ultrasound probe until you next need it but make sure you place the covered part of the probe on the drape to avoid contamination.
- Inject 10 to 20 mL of local anaesthetic into the skin and deeper layers, avoiding vessels.
- Use your sterile probe to visualize the right internal jugular, and for right-handed operators, use your left hand to secure the image of the vein, while you are using your introducer needle with your dominant hand, continuously aspirating at a 45-degree angle, looking at the ultrasound image to ensure positioning. When blood is freely aspirated and your position is easily seen as inside the vein in the screen, detach the syringe and feed the wire through the introducer needle.
- Make sure you do not place the probe anywhere nonsterile as you will need it again to ensure correct placement. As you are now supporting the needle with your left hand and advancing the wire with your right hand, you should instruct your assistant to look at the monitor for any arrhythmia. Once the wire goes through the introducer needle, no matter what stage of the procedure you are at, you must not let go of the guidewire. Ventricular ectopics probably indicate irritation of the tricuspid annulus, so withdraw your wire until they settle.
- Once you are happy with the wire placement, remove the introducer needle and confirm that the wire is intravenous with the ultrasound.
- Make an incision into the skin and dilate with rotational movements using the dilator, in order to create a track between the skin and the vessel for the catheter to pass easily.

- Remove the dilator and place the intravenous catheter. Once the catheter is in place, remove the guidewire and attach the remaining bionector to the distal lumen.
- Check all lumens by aspirating and flushing normal saline and then secure the catheter onto the skin with plastic clips, sutures, and transparent dressings.

How is correct positioning checked once the central line is placed?
A chest X-ray needs to be requested after the central line insertion, firstly to rule out a possible pneumothorax and also for the position of the line to be checked. The tip of the line should be above the right atrium, in the superior vena cava.

Name some clinical indications for central line insertion.
- Infusion of irritant drugs and solutions that cannot be given via a peripheral line (vasopressors, inotropes, high rate potassium infusion, antiarrhythmics)
- Total parenteral nutrition
- Access for extracorporeal blood circuits (haemofiltration, plasma exchange)
- Monitoring (central venous pressure, pulmonary artery pressure, central venous oxygenation, serial blood sampling)
- Transvenous pacing wire insertion.

CHAPTER 245

Chest Drain Insertion for Spontaneous (Nontraumatic) Pneumothorax

Instruction

A 20-year-old nonsmoking male with no medical history of note attended the emergency department with sudden-onset right-sided pleuritic chest pain and dyspnoea for the last couple of hours. The symptoms started suddenly as he was running. Vital signs on admission are as follows: blood pressure 160/70 mm Hg, heart rate 95 beats/min, respiratory rate 20 breaths/min, temperature 36.6°C, and SaO_2 90%. Chest X-ray (CXR) reveals a right-sided pneumothorax, measured as 3.5 cm at the level of the hilum.

Questions

How would you treat the patient?
This patient needs a chest drain insertion. He has a primary spontaneous pneumothorax (young patient with no prerequisite respiratory disease) and is symptomatic (dyspnoeic, tachypnoeic, and hypoxic) with radiological measurement of the pneumothorax more than 2.5 cm.

Where should the drain be inserted?
For any pneumothorax, the preferred site for chest drain insertion is the 'triangle of safety' (Fig. 245.1). The triangle is bordered anteriorly by the lateral edge of pectoralis major, laterally by the lateral edge of latissimus dorsi, inferiorly by the line of the fifth intercostal space, and superiorly by the base of the axilla. Once the safety triangle is located with the patient lying supine with the head of the bed at 45 degrees, and with the arm of the pneumothorax side behind their head, the needle is inserted in the space above the lower rib rather than below the higher rib. This is to avoid damaging the neurovascular bundle running below each rib.

Describe the procedure of chest drain insertion.
- Equipment check:
  Before starting the procedure, check that you have all equipment ready, including the underwater seal tube; check that all equipment is easily accessible to you and an assistant is with you helping you with equipment and the patient.
- Aseptic technique:
  Chest drain insertion is a fully aseptic technique; scrub fully (with gown, hat, sterile gloves and mask), clean the area, and apply the drapes, revealing only the safe triangle.
- Preprocedure analgesia:
  Most clinicians would prepare the patient with intravenous analgesia for the procedure.
- Local anaesthesia:
  Apply local anaesthetic (always aspirate before administering), and after anaesthetizing the skin, go into deeper layers. After the skin, the second most painful sites during your insertion will be the periosteum and the parietal pleura, so make sure you apply anaesthetic

245 — CHEST DRAIN INSERTION FOR SPONTANEOUS (NONTRAUMATIC) PNEUMOTHORAX

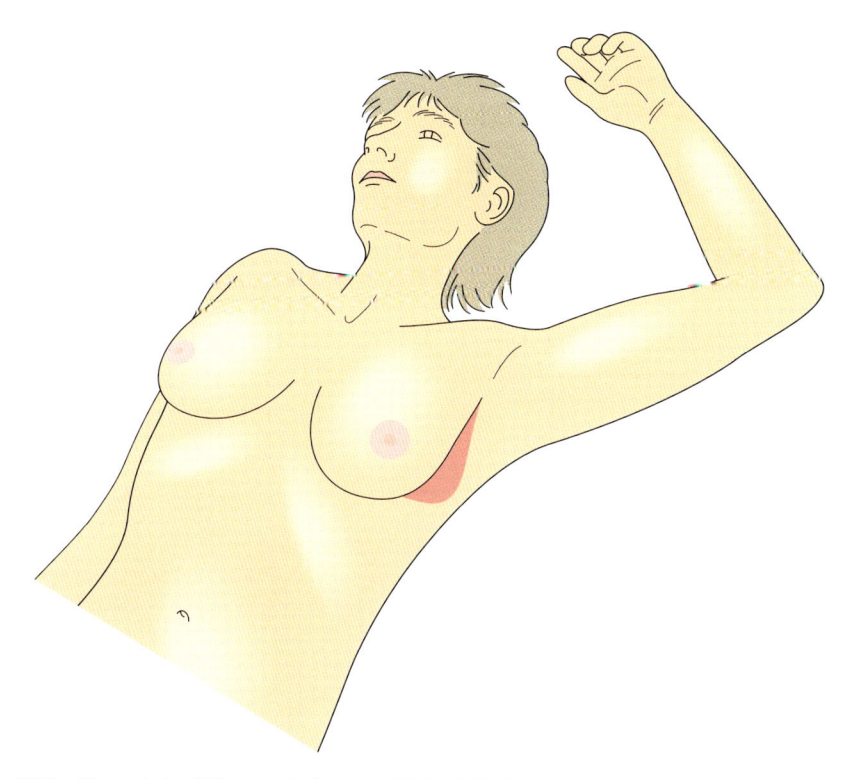

Fig. 245.1 Chest drain. (With permission from Blyth, K.G., Scott, H., Jones, J.B., Scott, H.R., 2009. Davidson's Foundations of Clinical Practice. Elsevier.)

  not inside the pleural cavity but within the parietal pleura. A commonly used local anaesthetic is lidocaine 1% with a maximum dose of 3 mg/kg.
- Size of chest drain:
  Small drains should be preferred to large-bore drains for pneumothoraces; there is no evidence that bigger drains produce better or quicker results, and large-bore drains can be more traumatic and associated with more complications.
- Technique:
  Puncture your site with the introducer needle, to which a 10-mL syringe has been attached to the other end. Once air is freely aspirated, the syringe can be replaced with the guidewire, which should be fed through the introducer needle. There are markings along the guidewire, which should be taken into account during the procedure, as they can alert the clinician if the guidewire has moved. Once the guidewire is deployed, one hand should always hold on to it. While the main operator is concentrating on the procedure, your assistant should continuously monitor the patient and apply supplementary oxygen if needed.

Once the guidewire is advanced (freely with no resistance felt), the introducer needle should be removed without losing hold of the wire. In order to help the dilation, a skin incision of 5 mm can be made caudally to the wire.

Advance the dilator over the guidewire, warning the patient that he or she may feel some pressure, while you push and rotate your dilator. Once you are happy with the dilation, advance the drainage tube over the guidewire.

Connect the drainage tube to a closed underwater seal system. The underwater seal will act as a one-way valve through which air is expelled from the pleural space and prevented from re-entering during the next inspiration. Do not ever raise the sealed bottle above the level of the patient.

Secure the drain to the skin with a suture and clean the area again before applying a transparent dressing.

Inform the patient that the procedure has finished, check the bottle for swinging and water bubbling, perform continuous monitoring of the patient, ask for a check CXR to confirm secure position of the drain, and check for immediate complications.

What are the possible complications of a chest drain insertion for pneumothorax?
- Pain
- Incorrect placement/drain dislodgement
- Recurrent pneumothorax/failure of lung to expand
- Injury to intercostal vessels/bleeding
- Visceral organ damage
- Infection
- Reexpansion pulmonary oedema.

Are there any precautions or contraindications to the procedure?
If not in an emergency setting, then platelets and coagulation should be known and treated if abnormal before a chest drain insertion. Nonurgent chest drains should be avoided in patients who have deranged clotting screen or platelet count, until their international normalized ratio (INR) is in a safe range (INR <1.5) and platelet count more than 50×10^9/L. In an emergency situation, risks and benefits must be assessed before chest drain insertion as it can be a life threatening procedure.

CHAPTER 246

Emergency Synchronized Direct Current Cardioversion

Instruction

A 76-year-old woman with previous aortic valve replacement and known coronary artery disease with previous coronary artery bypass grafting presents with dizziness and chest pain. She has no other medical history of note. She takes aspirin, warfarin, bisoprolol, ramipril, and atorvastatin and has no allergies. On initial assessment, her blood pressure is 90/60 mm Hg, heart rate is 160 beats/min, SaO2 is 95% on room air, and respiratory rate is 16 breaths/min. Her 12-lead electrocardiogram (ECG) reveals regular broad-complex tachycardia at 160 beats/min.

Questions

Is chemical or electrical the most appropriate type of cardioversion in the earlier case?
Electrical cardioversion (synchronized direct current cardioversion (DCCV)). This patient has a regular broad-complex tachycardia (which is ventricular tachycardia until proven otherwise) and is clinically unstable (dizziness, chest pain, low blood pressure). Any broad-complex tachycardia with instability features should be electrically cardioverted. Prior to that, an airway–breathing–circulation (ABC) approach should be followed; apply oxygen if needed, obtain intravenous access, and identify and treat possible reversible causes. A conscious patient, as in the scenario earlier, will require sedation, so an anaesthetist should be present.

What is the appropriate energy to be delivered in this case?
For a broad-complex tachycardia or atrial fibrillation with fast ventricular response, initial energy should be between 120 and 150 joules biphasic, increased in gradual increments if the initial shock fails to restore sinus rhythm.

For atrial flutter and regular narrow-complex tachycardia, then the starting energies can be lower, at a level of 70 to 120 joules biphasic.

What are the possible complications of direct current cardioversion?
- Skin irritation/erythema from the adhesive pads
- Recurrence of the arrhythmia
- Failure of the procedure
- Rare complications (with less than 1% occurrence): underlying heart block may reveal itself necessitating permanent pacing, pulmonary embolism, stroke, acute coronary syndrome.

What are the indications for synchronized cardioversion in an emergency setting?
Any tachyarrhythmia that is associated with adverse features or causes haemodynamic compromise is an indication for emergency cardioversion.

While operating the defibrillator, what steps should you take while delivering the shock during direct current cardioversion?
- Once the patient is consented and sedated, apply the adhesive pads.
- Ensure manual mode is in operation.
- Select the energy according to the patient's underlying rhythm and local protocols.
- Synchronize with the R wave, by pressing the 'synch' button on the defibrillator.
- Charge the defibrillator while verbalizing that you are charging; everybody should step away from the patient and oxygen should be removed—ensure that this has happened before delivering the shock.
- Say 'all clear' loudly and clearly and verbalize that you are about to deliver the shock.
- Deliver the shock and watch the ECG. Once rhythm is restored, follow ABC assessment and obtain a blood pressure and a 12-lead ECG.

A patient with atrial fibrillation is listed for an elective direct current cardioversion. What is the anticoagulation choice and for how long would the patient need to be anticoagulated for prior to the procedure?
For atrial fibrillation of duration more than 48 hours, formal anticoagulation will be needed for 3 to 4 weeks prior to the procedure and continued for at least 4 weeks after successful cardioversion. If the risk of stroke is high, the patient should continue anticoagulation for life, regardless of the success of the procedure. The choice is for direct oral anticoagulants (DOACs) unless contraindicated, where warfarin is given instead.

A patient presents to the emergency unit with palpitations not associated with other symptoms or other adverse features. On examination, vital signs are normal, and three-lead monitor reveals a broad-complex regular tachycardia. Is direct current cardioversion the best course of action?
This is a patient with regular broad-complex tachycardia, which is ventricular tachycardia, unless proven otherwise. A stable patient with broad-complex tachycardia should be given a loading dose of amiodarone. There is no need for emergency DCCV, unless the patient becomes haemodynamically unstable.

List some rhythms that can present with a regular narrow-complex tachycardia on the electrocardiogram.
- Sinus tachycardia
- Atrioventricular (AV) nodal re-entry tachycardia
- AV re-entry tachycardia
- Atrial flutter with 2:1 block.

How do you estimate a patient's annual risk of stroke when a diagnosis of atrial fibrillation is established?
The annual risk of stroke depends on their CHADS-VASC score.

Factor	Point
Cardiac failure	1
Hypertension	1
Age >75 years	2
Age 65–75 years	1
Diabetes	1
Stroke in the past	2
Female sex	1
Vascular disease	1

Depending on the CHADS-VASC score the annual risk of stroke is as follows:

Score	Risk
0	0.2%
1	0.6%
2	2.2%
3	3.2%
4	4.8%
5	7.2%

In patients treated with oral anticoagulation, the earlier risks are reduced by two-thirds.

CHAPTER 247

Knee Arthrocentesis

Instruction

A 45-year-old patient presents with an acutely swollen painful knee. On examination, there is evident effusion in the knee joint, and a decision is taken to aspirate the effusion.

Questions

What are the indications for a joint aspiration?
A joint aspiration can be performed either for diagnostic or for therapeutic purposes:
- Suspected septic arthritis (gonococcal/nongonococcal/tuberculous/fungal)
- Undiagnosed effusion (inflammatory/crystal arthropathy/haemarthrosis/osteoarthritis)
- Therapeutic (effusion drainage for symptom control, with or without intra-articular drug injection).

What are the contraindications in performing joint aspiration?
- Local active infection (skin infection at the site of needle entry, infected psoriasis at the site of insertion, cellulitis, or overlying ulcers on the affected limb)
- Prosthetic joint
- Tumour/mass at the site of entry
- Coagulopathy and patients using anticoagulants (consider use of reversal agents).

What equipment is needed to perform knee aspiration?
- Sterile gloves
- Nonsterile disposable apron
- Dressing pack
- Antiseptic skin cleansing solution
- Lignocaine 1% 10 mL
- Needles (2 × green 21 G and 1 × orange 25 G)
- Syringe (1 × 10 mL and 1 × 20 mL)
- Dressing (adhesive or with adhesive tape)
- Universal sample pots × 3
- Blood culture bottles × 1 set aerobic and anaerobic.

Describe the procedure using the landmark technique.
After explaining the procedure and obtaining written informed consent, place the patient supine with the knee flexed at an angle of 15 to 20 degrees. It is very important that the patient is in a comfortable position in case the procedure takes longer than expected. The patient should be able to relax the leg, so that the muscles at the site of injection are not tensed. The technique should be fully aseptic. During your preparation, you should identify and prepare all sterile equipment, wash hands thoroughly, and then identify your landmarks by palpation. The knee can be approached from the medial or lateral sides. Palpation will help you decide which side is easier in each case. Mark the injection site and after cleaning the area, infiltrate the skin and deeper tissues with local anaesthetic

in the direction of the anticipated trajectory of the needle. Direct the needle behind the patella and slightly superiorly towards the suprapatellar pouch, aiming for the space between the patella and the femur approximately between the upper one-third and lower two-thirds of the patella. Once the space is reached, the resistance in advancing the needle is reduced and fluid appears in the syringe while aspirating the plunger and advancing the needle. Once aspiration is complete, remove the needle, clean the skin, and cover the area with a simple dressing or plaster, which should remain until the following day.

Which tests would you send the synovial fluid for?
Depending on the clinical suspicion, the synovial fluid can be sent for:
- Gram stain (in all cases of monoarthritis)
- Crystal analysis
- Culture
- Cell count and differential
- Cytology (for suspected malignant effusions).

What will the aspirated synovial fluid look like macroscopically?
The macroscopic appearance of the fluid depends on the cause of the effusion:
- Normal appearance: clear and viscous fluid that does not form clots
- Inflammatory fluid: lightly coloured fluid or slightly blood stained
- Infected fluid: thick and creamy, yellow or green
- Haemarthrosis: uniformly blood stained.

What are the possible complications of a knee aspiration?
Knee arthrocentesis is a relatively safe procedure.
- Iatrogenic introduction of infection in the joint space (This is a rare but serious complication, and it is estimated that it occurs in 1 case per 78,000 aspirations.)
- Failure of the procedure (also called dry tap, and aspiration from a different site can be reattempted if the patient agrees)
- Pain during injection
- Reaccumulation of fluid, depending on the underlying cause of the effusion.

For the following scenarios, guess the most likely result of the synovial fluid aspirated from each patient's right knee.
Scenario 1:

A 70-year-old lady presents with a painful right knee. She has been suffering from knee and hip pain, mostly during and after activity, for the past year. However, on this occasion, the pain has resulted in limitation of her daily activities. On examination of her right knee, there is deformity and limitation in range of movement.
- The fluid would probably show increased white cell count with rhomboid shape crystals. The underlying diagnosis is likely osteoarthritis with calcium pyrophosphate crystal deposition, which is one of the commonest forms of pseudogout. Around 20% of patients with osteoarthritis are estimated to have calcium pyrophosphate crystals in the affected joints, some being symptomatic with acute crystal arthropathy and some not.

Scenario 2:

A 60-year-old man presents with acute onset of excruciating pain in his left knee. The pain woke him up at 6 o'clock in the morning. He cannot recall any trauma to the knee as he was out drinking all night the night before, but on examination, there are no signs of trauma or injury. The joint looks inflamed with localized tenderness, erythema, and oedema. He suffers from hypertension, for which he takes losartan and bendroflumethiazide.

- The fluid would probably show increased white cells with needle-shaped crystals. This is probably gout as the patient appears to have risk factors (alcohol binge, thiazide diuretics) as well as features typical of gout presentation (sudden onset early hours of the morning, monoarthritis).

Scenario 3:

A 30-year-old man is admitted to hospital with sepsis. On clinical examination, he is pyrexial but haemodynamically stable. There are no stigmata of infective endocarditis, chest and heart sounds are normal, his abdomen is soft and nontender, and the only positive finding is an inflamed right knee; the knee is tender and hot to touch with evidence of effusion, overlying skin erythema, and localized swelling. He suffers from type 1 diabetes and is a current intravenous drug user.

- This is septic arthritis, so the fluid would demonstrate neutrophilia with Gram-positive cocci. The most common organism in this scenario is *Staphylococcus aureus*, which will be seen as a Gram-positive coccus under the microscope.

CHAPTER 248

Lumbar Puncture

Instruction

A 32-year-old female patient has been sent to the medical unit by the ophthalmologist. During a routine eye check, she was noticed to have bilateral papilloedema. She denies any symptoms apart from an ongoing headache for the last 2 weeks. Her vision is normal, and her neurological examination is normal, apart from bilateral grade 1 papilloedema. She is on the oral contraceptive pill and has no medical history of note. A subsequent computed tomography (CT) of the head and CT venogram are normal.

Questions

What is the next appropriate management step?
Lumbar puncture (LP) should be performed in this case, both as a diagnostic tool and as therapeutic intervention. Bilateral papilloedema with normal neuroimaging in a young female patient raises clinical suspicion for idiopathic intracranial hypertension. Confirmation will come from measuring the opening pressures of the cerebrospinal fluid (CSF) during LP.

What are the possible complications of lumbar puncture you should advise her of?
- Post-LP headache is the most common complication, occurring in 10% to 30% of patients.
- Rarer complications of the procedure are infection, bleeding/haematoma, failure of procedure, nerve damage with paraesthesia, or paralysis of the lower limbs.

The patient has had an epidural before when she gave birth to her child. She mentions that she prefers to have the lumbar puncture procedure sitting up, as that was the most comfortable position for her when she had the epidural. Is this an option?
LP can be performed with the patient either in the lateral recumbent position or sitting upright. However, in cases where opening pressure is measured, as in this case, the lateral recumbent position is the position of choice as it gives a more accurate measurement of the opening pressure.

Describe the procedure.
After explaining the procedure to the patient, and obtaining written consent, try and identify the anatomical landmarks. The iliac crests should be palpated. The line connecting the two iliac crests usually passes through the body of the fourth lumbar vertebra. Having identified the L4 body, the spinous processes of L3/L4/L5 can be palpated.

The patient should be positioned in the fetal position (flexed neck, back, hips, and knees). Once you are happy with the position of the patient and the palpation of the lumbar vertebra interspaces, you can start the procedure; equipment should be ready and sterile on a sterile trolley, the skin should be cleaned, drapes applied, and lidocaine should be used to anaesthetize the skin and deeper tissue layers.

A spinal needle can be inserted into the spaces L3/4 or L4/5. Quincke or Sprotte needles can be used, following local policy. Once CSF appears into the needle and the stylet is withdrawn, opening pressure is measured with a manometer and fluid is collected for analysis.

What are some contraindications to the procedure?
Raised intracranial pressure in the context of intracranial pathology, suspected epidural abscess, overlying skin cellulitis at the site of insertion, and bleeding disorders.

How do you interpret the cerebrospinal fluid results?
Normal CSF is acellular, clear, and colourless, with a protein concentration less than 0.40 g/dL and a glucose concentration more than 60% of the plasma glucose concentration. Typically, in subarachnoid haemorrhage, CSF will be pink and xanthochromia positive. In most pathological conditions, protein will be raised. In infections, white cells will be raised with usually a lymphocyte predominance in viral infections and polymorphonuclear-predominance in bacterial infections. CSF glucose will be less than 50% of the plasma glucose concentration in bacterial infections.

What is the normal cerebrospinal fluid pressure?
The normal CSF pressure is around 150 mm Hg or 17 cm H_2O.

A patient presents to the emergency medical unit with a thunderclap headache that started 2 hours ago. When should a lumbar puncture be performed?
Xanthochromia starts being detectable 2 to 4 hours after the red cells enter the subarachnoid space, but the sensitivity improves with time, reaching more than 90% after 12 hours of headache onset. This patient should have a CT of the head as soon as possible and if that fails to demonstrate a haemorrhage, an LP should be performed after 10 hours (which is 12 hours after the onset of the headache).

What is the normal white cell count of a cerebrospinal fluid sample (per µL)?
Finding up to 5 white blood cell (WBC)/µL in the CSF sample is considered normal. Anything more than that is considered abnormal. In a traumatic LP, when the white cell count (WCC) is neither very high to diagnose pathology nor very low to be considered normal, then the number of WBC has to be corrected against the number of the red blood cells (RBCs) measured in the CSF sample, roughly subtracting 1 WBC for every 500 RBCs measured.

A 19-year-old girl is brought to the emergency department by ambulance, after her mother found her confused at home. On examination, the patient was tachycardic, tachypnoeic, and pyrexial at 39°C. Otherwise, cardiovascular, respiratory, and abdominal examinations are noncontributory. She has neck stiffness and a petechial nonblanching rash spread over her right elbow, and her Glasgow Coma Scale score is 13/15. Is an emergency lumbar puncture indicated to establish the diagnosis of bacterial meningitis?
This patient has high clinical suspicion of bacterial meningitis and has clinical features that are associated with high mortality or adverse outcome in bacterial meningitis. With altered mental state, she will need a CT of the head prior to performing an LP, and as such, performing an LP to confirm the organism will delay the treatment. Blood cultures should be obtained alongside other blood tests, and delay in LP should not delay the treatment. LP can be performed after the initial dose of antibiotics. It may reduce the diagnostic yield of Gram stain and culture, but the pathogen can be isolated up to several hours after the initial dose of antibiotics.

CHAPTER 249

Therapeutic Abdominal Paracentesis

Instruction

A 45-year-old male with known alcoholic liver disease, complicated with portal hypertension, has recurrent ascites refractory to diuretics. He is admitted to hospital with tense ascites. A decision is taken for therapeutic abdominal paracentesis.

Questions

When fluid is obtained from ascites of known origin, what investigations should the fluid be sent for?

If the cause of the ascites is known, then simple microscopy for cells to exclude spontaneous bacterial peritonitis is enough. Cell count differential is the most useful test for the ascitic fluid as it can help detect and treat infections early. A white cell count more than $250/mm^3$ on initial microscopy signifies spontaneous bacterial peritonitis and antibiotics should be started pending cultures.

When fluid is obtained from ascites of unknown origin, except for cell count, what other investigations should the fluid be sent for?

If the cause of the ascites is not known, then fluid analysis can help determine the cause of the ascites. Calculation of the serum to ascites albumin gradient (SAAG) helps determine if the ascites has developed due to portal hypertension. Portal hypertension will usually give a gradient of more than 11 g/L, whereas a calculated gradient less than 11 g/L means that the patient does not have portal hypertension. SAAG calculation cannot distinguish cirrhotic from noncirrhotic portal hypertension. Aside from cirrhosis of any cause, causes of a high albumin gradient are heart failure, constrictive pericarditis, veno-occlusive disease, alcoholic hepatitis, and hepatic metastasis. Low albumin causes are peritoneal carcinomatosis, pancreatitis, and nephrotic syndrome.

Other investigations that would help differentiate intra-abdominal pathologies are sent depending on the underlying clinical suspicion: glucose, lactate dehydrogenase, amylase, pro-B-type natriuretic peptide, and cultures.

Describe the procedure.
 Preparation:
 1. Know your patient (allergies, clotting, and platelets) and the indications for abdominal paracentesis (usually therapeutic drainage, as well as diagnostic testing at the same time).
 2. Obtain formal consent if the patient is able, explaining the procedure and possible complications.
 3. Identify the presence of ascites: confirm the presence of ascites as if you cannot confirm the ascites clinically, you cannot proceed to performing the procedure and the patient needs to undergo ultrasound-guided marking.

4. Identify your site: place the patient supine, with the bed head raised 30 degrees, and identify either left or right lower quadrant of the abdomen. Although both quadrants can be used, as an enlarged liver expands towards the right lower quadrant, palpation should take place to ensure no hepatomegaly is going to complicate the procedure. Mark your site, which has to be horizontal to the umbilicus, and roughly 3 cm lateral to the anterior rectus border, or 15 cm lateral to the umbilicus. The inferior epigastric artery runs superiorly through the rectus sheath, so going too far medially can risk damaging the epigastric artery.
5. If the drain is for ascites due to chronic liver disease (cirrhosis), make sure you preorder human albumin solution (HAS) 20% that will be needed during the drainage. The recommended dose of albumin is 8 g per 1 L of ascites drained. This equates to a 100 mL bottle of 20% HAS, infused 'stat' for every 2.5 L of ascites drained, and several bottles should be prescribed on a fluid chart after drain insertion.

Equipment check:
Identify your equipment, and check that everything is working properly before starting the procedure.

The procedure:
- Sterile gloves and apron are sufficient and should be used.
- Clean the skin and apply lidocaine under the skin and into deeper tissue layers. Use a 25 G orange needle to infiltrate 1% lidocaine subcutaneously, swapping to a green 21 G needle to infiltrate deeper. Ensure that ascites can be withdrawn with the green needle to confirm correct position, prior to insertion of the drain.
- Sometimes, a small incision of the skin over the anaesthetized area of 3 to 4 mm is needed.
- Insert the introducer needle, already preconnected to the drain, which has multiple holes at the end. As you are advancing the needle 90 degrees to the skin, keep aspirating until ascitic fluid is freely withdrawn into the needle. Once flashback is seen, or ascites starts to drain, advance a further 1 cm before feeding the drain over the introducer needle. Slowly withdraw the needle. Connect the catheter to a drainage collector (can be a catheter bag) and apply the transparent dressing, which usually comes with the ascitic drain kit.

What are the possible complications?
- Bleeding or localized abdominal wall haematoma
- Dry tap
- Puncture of internal organs (haemoperitoneum/bowel perforation)
- Infection.

Are there any contraindications to the procedure?
There are no absolute contraindications, but there are a few points to consider before proceeding with abdominal paracentesis:
- Coagulopathy: coagulopathy is common among patients with chronic liver disease, but not a contraindication in itself. There are no specific recommendations on what represents a safe prothrombin time/international normalized ratio, and no evidence to support the routine use of fresh frozen plasma or other clotting products, although caution should be exercised with severe coagulopathy. Vitamin K may help if the patient is deficient, although abnormal coagulation is often due to insufficient production of clotting factors by the liver rather than deficiency of vitamin K.
- Platelets: most clinicians would consider it appropriate to offer platelet transfusion for a platelet count below 50×10^9/L.

- Malignant ascites or loculated ascites: most patients that require ascites drainage have developed ascites secondary to cirrhosis/portal hypertension and the procedure is straightforward. Rarely, however, ascites will be minimal, loculated, or due to peritoneal metastasis, where ultrasound should be used for safety purposes and to reduce the risk of complications.

Further Information

European Association for the Study of the Liver (EASL): http://www.easl.eu
British Society of Gastroenterology (BSG): http://www.bsg.org.uk

CHAPTER 250

Temporary External Pacing

Instruction

An 87-year-old woman with a long list of medications including digoxin and bisoprolol is admitted to hospital with acute confusion. She was diagnosed with a urinary tract infection prior to the admission and was prescribed oral antibiotics. She deteriorated in the community and was admitted for further management. On examination she is dehydrated, with low blood pressure and reduced urine output, she is confused with a Glasgow Coma Scale (GCS) score of 14/15, and her heart rate is 35 beats/min. Her electrolytes are normal and a 12-lead electrocardiogram (ECG) reveals junctional rhythm with a rate of 40 beats/min. Digitalis toxicity is suspected and temporary pacing is deemed appropriate until further treatment is given.

Questions

Describe the steps of external pacing.
- The pads are placed ideally in the anterior-posterior position.
- ECG leads must be connected at the same time.
- The defibrillator should be turned to manual with the pacer mode on.
- The pacing rate should be set around 70 to 80 beats/min, or around 30 beats/min above the patient's intrinsic rhythm to maintain adequate output.
- Current should be gradually increased until electrical capture is consistent on the monitor, which practically means that every spike is followed by a QRS. Once consistent electrical capture is evident on the monitor, then current should be set around 5 to 10 mA above that threshold.
- Electrical capture should be confirmed with mechanical capture by palpating patients femoral pulses while looking at the monitor.

What are the indications for temporary pacing?
Temporary pacing is indicated in symptomatic bradycardia until an underlying reversible condition is treated (for example electrolyte abnormalities, myocardial infarction, digitalis toxicity). This mode of pacing is a bridge to a temporary intravenous pacing wire.

Patients who have an irreversible arrhythmia that warrantees a permanent system may also need some form of temporary pacing in an emergency until the permanent system is established.

Bradycardias that may require external pacing are:
- Severe bradycardia
- Bradycardia that does not respond to atropine
- Second degree Mobitz II heart block, complete heart block, recent asystole, ventricular pauses more than 3 s.

Override pacing for tachycardias in specific scenarios can be an indication for external pacing once all other options have failed. In these cases, transvenous pacing wire is indicated.

List the potential complications of external pacing.
- Cutaneous burns
- Painful muscle contractions
- Capture failure—failure to pace.

BIBLIOGRAPHY

Aithal, G.P., Palaniyappan, N., China, L., et al., 2021. Guidelines on the management of ascites in cirrhosis. Gut. 70, 9–29.

Anders, H., Keller, C., 1997. Pemberton's maneuver – a clinical test for latent superior vena cava syndrome caused by a substernal mass. Eur. J. Med. Res. 2, 488–490.

Apitz, C., Webb, G.D., Reddington, A.N., 2009. Tetralogy of Fallot. Lancet 374, 1469–1471.

Argyll Robertson, D., 1869. Four cases of spinal myosis; with remarks on the action of light on the pupil. Edinburgh Med. J. 15, 487.

Armstrong, P.W., Pieske, B., Anstrom, K.J., et al., 2020. Vericiguat in patients with heart failure and reduced ejection fraction. N. Engl. J. Med. 382(20), 1883–1893. https://doi.org/10.1056/NEJMoa1915928

Barlow, J.B., Bosman, C.K., Pocock, W.A., Marchand, P., 1968. Late systolic murmurs and non-ejection (mid late) clicks. An analysis of 90 patients. Br. Heart J. 30, 203–218.

Barlow, J.B., Pocock, W.A., 1985. Billowing, floppy, prolapsed or flail mitral valves? Am. J. Cardiol. 55(4), 501–502.

Batten, F.E., Gibb, H.P., 1909. Myotonia atrophica. Brain 32, 187.

Bourneville, D.M., 1880. Sclerose tubereuse des circonvolutions cerebrales: idiotie et epilepsie hemiplegique. Paris. Arch. Neurol. 1, 81–91.

Brock, R., 1957. Functional obstruction of the left ventricle; acquired aortic subvalvar stenosis. Guy's Hosp. Rep. 106(4), 221–238.

Bruns, D.L.A., 1959. A general theory of the causes of murmurs in the cardiovascular system. Am. J. Med. 27, 360.

Brunsting, L.A., Goeckerman, W.H., O'Leary, P.A., 1930. Pyoderma (echthyma) gangrenosum: Clinical and experimental observations in five cases occurring in adults. Arch. Dermatol. Syphiol. 22, 655–680.

Carpentier, A., 1983. Cardiac valve surgery – the 'French correction'. J. Thorac. Cardiovasc. Surg. 86, 323–237.

Cirrhosis in over 16 s: assessment and management: NICE guideline [NG50].

Crail, H.W., 1949. Multiple primary malignancies arising in the rectum, brain and thyroid. U.S. Naval. Medical. Bull. 49, 123–128.

Criley, J.M., Lewis, K.B., Humphries, J.O., et al., 1966. Prolapse of the mitral valve: clinical and cine-angiocardiographic findings. Br. Heart J. 28, 488–496.

Crohn, B.B., Ginzburg, L., Gordon, D.O., 1932. Regional ileitis: a pathologic and clinical entity. JAMA, 99(16), 1323–1329.

Cushing, H., 1932. The basophil adenomas of the pituitary body and their clinical manifestations. Bull. Johns Hopkins Hosp. 1, 137.

Dalakas, M.C., 1993. Polymyositis, dermatomyositis, and inclusion-body myositis. N. Engl. J. Med. 325, 1487.

Debré, R., Semölaigne, G., 1935. Syndrome of diffuse hypertrophy in infants causing athletic appearance. Its connection with congenital myxoedema. Am. J. Dis. Child. 50, 1351–1361.

Denton, C.P., Hughes, M., Gak, N., et al., 2016. BSR and BHPR guideline for the treatment of systemic sclerosis. Rheumatology 55(10), 1906–1910.

Dicke, W.K., 1950. Coeliac disease: investigation of the harmful effects of certain types of cereal on patients with coeliac disease. Doctoral thesis, University of Utrecht, the Netherlands; N. Engl. J. Med. 333, 1075–1076.

Diskin, C.J., Stokes, T.J., Dansby, L.M., Carter, T.B., Radcliff, L., Thomas, S.G., 1999. Towards an understanding of oedema. BMJ. 318, 1610–1613.

Dooley, J.S., Lok, A.S., Garcia-Tsao, G., Pinzani, M. (Eds.), 2018. Sherlock's diseases of the liver and biliary system. John Wiley & Sons.

Emery, A.E.H., Emery, M.L.H., 1995. The History of a Genetic Disease: Duchenne Muscular Dystrophy or Meryon's Disease. Royal Society of Medicine Press, London.

Espinel, C.H., 1997. A medical examination of Rembrandt. His self-portrait; ageing, disease and the language of the skin. Lancet. 350, 1835–1837.

Espinel, C.H., 1999. Michelangelo's gout in a fresco by Raphael. Lancet 354, 2149–2152.

European Association for the Study of the Liver, 2010. EASL clinical practice guidelines on the management of ascites, spontaneous bacterial peritonitis, and hepatorenal syndrome in cirrhosis. J. Hepatol. 53, 397–417.

Fallot, E.L.A., 1888. Contribution a l'anatomie pathologique de la maladie bleue. Marseille Méd 25, 418–420.
Forbes, J., 1824. Original Cases with Dissections and Observations Illustrating the Use of the Stethoscope and Percussion in the Diagnosis of the Diseases of the Chest. T. and G. Underwood, London.
Freeman, A.R., Levine, S.A., 1933. The clinical significance of the systolic murmur: a study of 1,000 consecutive 'non-cardiac' cases. Ann. Intern. Med. 6, 1371.
Furdell, E.L., 2007. Eponymous, anonymous: Queen Anne's sign and the misnaming of a symptom. J. Med. Biogr. 15, 97–101.
Gee, S., 1888. On the coeliac affection. St. Barth Hosp. Rep. 24, 17–20.
Graves, R.J., 1835. Clinical lectures. London Med. Surg. J. 7, 516.
Greenspan, D., Conant, M., Silverman Jr., S., et al., 1984. Oral 'hairy' leukoplakia in male homosexuals: evidence of association with both papillomavirus and a herpes-group virus. Lancet 2, 831–834.
Gross, J., Pitt-Rivers, R., 1952. The identification of 3:5:3'-L-triiodothyronine in human plasma. Lancet 1, 439–441.
Gull, W.W., 1873. On a cretinoid state supervening in adult life in women. Trans. Clin. Soc. London 7, 180–188.
Gunn, R.M., 1892. Ophthalmoscopic evidence of (1) arterial changes associated with chronic renal diseases and (2) of increased arterial tension. Trans. Ophthalmol. Soc. U. K. 12, 124–125.
Harrington, C.R., Barger, G., 1927. Chemistry of thyroxine: constitution and synthesis of thyroxine, Biochem. J. 21, 169–183.
Hench, P.S., 1953. A reminiscence of certain events before, during and after the discovery of cortisone. Minnesota Med. 36, 705–710.
Holmes, G., 1939. The cerebellum of man. Brain 62, 1–30.
Homans, J., 1954. Thrombosis of the deep leg veins due to prolonged sitting. N. Engl. J. Med. 250, 148–159.
Hoppe, H.H., 1892. Beitrag zur Kenntniss der Bulbär-Paralyse. Berl. Klin. Wochenschr. 29, 332–336.
Jeghers, H.J., McKusick, V.A., Katz, K.H., 1949. Generalized intestinal polyposis and melanin spots of the oral mucosa, lips and digits; a syndrome of diagnostic significance. N. Engl. J. Med. 241, 993.
Jolly, F., 1895. Über Myastenia gravis pseudoparalytica. Berl. Klin. Wochenschr. 32, 1–7.
Katznelson, L., Laws Jr, E.R., Melmed, S., et al., 2014. Acromegaly: an endocrine society clinical practice guideline. J. Clin. Endocrinol. Metab. 99(11), 3933–3951.
Keat, A., 1995. Spondyloparthopathies. Brit. Med. J. 310, 1321–1324. (classic review).
Keith, N.M., Wagener, H.P., Barker, N.W., 1939. Some different types of essential hypertension: their course and prognosis. Am. J. Med. Sci. 197, 332–343.
Kendall, E., 1915. The isolation in crystalline form of the compound containing iodin, which occurs in the thyroid. JAMA 64, 2042–2043.
Khamashta, M.A., Cuadrado, M.J., Mujic, F., et al., 1995. The management of thrombosis in the antiphospholipid-antibody syndrome. N. Engl. J. Med. 332, 993–997.
Khan, F., Tritschler, T., Kimpton, M., et al., 2021. Long-term risk for major bleeding during extended oral anticoagulant therapy for first unprovoked venous thromboembolism: a systematic review and meta-analysis. Ann. Intern. Med. 174, 1420–1429.
Kowal-Bielecka, O., Fransen, J., Avouac, J., et al., 2017. Update of EULAR recommendations for the treatment of systemic sclerosis. Ann. Rheum. Dis. 76(8), 1327–1339.
Kussmaul, A., 1873. Über schwielige Mediastino-Perikarditis und den paradoxen Puls. Berl Klin Wochnschr 10, 433–435.
Leksell, L., 1971. A note on the treatment of acoustic tumours. Acta. Chir. Scand. 137, 763–765.
Light, R.W., 2002. Pleural effusion. N. Engl. J. Med. 346, 1971–1977.
Lisch, K., 1937. Ueber Beteiligung der Augen, insbesondere das Vorkommen von Irisknotchen bei der Neurofibromatose, Recklinghausen. Z Augenheilkd 93, 137–143.
London, N.J.M., Donnelly, R., 2000. ABC of arterial and venous disease: ulcerated lower limb. BMJ. 320, 1589–1591. (review)
Maiden, N., McLaren, J.S., 2000. Rhumatology: problem, promise and pitfalls. Proc. R. Coll. Phys. Edinb. 30, 191–198.
Marie, P., 1886. Sur deux cas d'acromégalie; hypertrophie singulière non congénitale des extrémités supérieures, inférieures et céphalique. Rev. Med. Liège 6, 297–333.
Marie, P., de Souza-Leite, J.D., 1891. Essays on Acromegaly. New Sydenham Society, London.

McDonagh, T., Metra, M., Adamo, M., et al., 2021. 2021 ESC Guidelines for the diagnosis and treatment of acute and chronic heart failure: developed by the Task Force for the diagnosis and treatment of acute and chronic heart failure of the European Society of Cardiology (ESC). Eur. Heart J. 42(36), 3599–3726. https://doi.org/10.1093/eurheartj/ehab368

McDonald, W.I., 1963. The effects of experimental demyelination on conduction in peripheral nerve: a histological and electrophysiological study. I. Clinical and histological observations. Brain 86, 481–500.

Minkowski, O., 1887. Ueber einen Fall von Akromegalie. Berl Klin Wochenschr 24, 371–374.

Morrison, P.J., Nevin, N.C., 1993. Peutz–Jeghers syndrome. N. Engl. J. Med. 329, 774.

Murray, J.E., Merrill, J.P., Harrison, J.H., Wilson, R.E., Dammin, G.J., 1963. Prolonged survival of human-kidney homografts by immunosuppressive drug therapy. N. Engl. J. Med. 268(24), 1315–1323.

Naldi, L., Rebora, A., 2009. Seborrheic dermatitis. N. Engl. J. Med. 360, 387–396.

NICE, July 2010. Delirium: prevention, diagnosis and management. Clinical Guideline, 103.

Ord, W.M., 1878. On myxoedema, a term proposed to be applied to an essential condition in the "cretinoid" affection occasionally observed in middle-aged women. Med. Chir. Trans. 61, 57.

Pemberton, H.S., 1946. Sign of submerged goitre. Lancet 251, 509.

Potain, P.C.E., 1931. Proc. R. Soc. Med. 24, 1253–1931.

Prins, M.H., Büller, H.R., 1999. Deep-vein thrombosis [review]. Lancet 353, 479–485.

Pyeritz, R.E., 2000. Ehlers–Danlos syndrome. N. Engl. J. Med. 342, 730.

Raja, O.G., Lalor, A.J., 1981. Simple aspiration of spontaneous pneumothorax. Br. J. Dis. Chest 75, 207–208.

Raju, T.N., 1990. The Nobel chronicles, 1950: Edward Calvin Kendall (1886–1972); Philip Showalter Hench (1896–1965); and Tadeus Reichstein (1897–1996). Lancet 353, 1370. https://doi.org/10.1016/S0140-6736(05)74374-9

Ramalho, P.S., Hill, D.W., Dollery, C.T., Paterson, J.W., Henkind, P., Ashton, N., et al., 1965. Retinal microemboli: experimental production of 'cotton-wool' spots. Lancet 7399, 1303–1305.

Raynaud, M., 1888. Selected monographs. Barlow, T. (Ed.),. In: On Local and Symmetrical Gangrene of the Extremities, vol. 121. New Sydenham Society, London.

Russell, B., 1950. Lepra, psoriasis, or the Willan–Plumbe syndrome. Br. J. Dermatol. Syph. 62, 359–361..

Savitz, S.I., Caplan, L.R., 2005. Vertebrobasilar disease. N. Engl. J. Med. 352, 2618.

Schwartz, R., Dameshek, W., 1959. Drug-induced immunological tolerance. Nature, 183(4676), 1682–1683.

Sjoerdsma, A., Weissbach, H., Udenfriend, S., 1956. A clinical, physiologic and biochemical study of patients with malignant carcinoid (argentaffinoma). Am. J. Med. 20, 520–532.

Smith, R.D., 1982. Paganini's hand. Arthritis. Rheum. 25, 1385–1386.

Spalton, D.J., Saunders, M.D., 1981. Fundus changes in histologically confirmed sarcoidosis. Br. J. Ophthalmol. 65, 348–358.

Steinert, H., 1909. Myopathologische Beiträge. Über das klinische und anatomische Bild des Muskelschwundes der Myo-toniker. Dtsch. Z. Nervenheilkd. 37, 58.

Stevens, A.M., Johnson, F.C., 1922. A new eruptive fever associated with stomatitis and ophthalmia: Report of two cases in children. Am. J. Dis. Child. 24, 526–533.

Sumpio, B.E., 2000. Foot ulcers. N. Engl. J. Med. 343, 787–793.

Taussig, H., Blalock, A., 1945. The surgical treatment of malformations of the heart in which there is pulmonary stenosis or pulmonary atresia. JAMA 128, 189–202.

Teare, D., 1958. Asymmetrical hypertrophy of the heart in young adults. Br. Heart J. 20, 1–8.

Terasaki, P.I., Vredevoe, D.L., Mickey, M.R., Porter, K.A., Marchioro, T.L., Faris, T.D., Starzl, T.E., 1966. Sterotyping for homotransplantation: VII; selection of kidney donors for thirty-two recipients. Ann. N Y Acad. Sci. 129(1), 500–520.

Trousseau, A., 1872. Phlegmasia albia dolens Lectures on Clinical Medicine, delivered at the Hôtel-Dieu, Paris. New Wydenham Society, London.281–295.

von Recklinghausen, F.D., 1889. Tageblatt Versamml Dtsch Naturforsch Artze Heidelberg 62, 324–325.

Wallace, M.R., 1994. Elephant man's disease (letter). Science 264, 188.

Wilson, S.A.K., 1912. Progressive lenticular degeneration: a familial nervous disease associated with cirrhosis of the liver. Brain 34, 295.

Wood, P., 1958. The Eisenmenger syndrome: I. British Medical Journal, 2(5098), 701.

INDEX

Note: Page numbers followed by '*f*' indicate figures, '*t*' indicate tables, and '*b*' indicate boxes.

A

ABCC6 gene, 516
ABCD2 scoring system, 639
Abdomen
  auscultation of, 147
  eponymous signs, 148
  examination of, 146–148
    cirrhosis of liver and, 166
    in COPD, 22
  inspection of, 146–147
  palpation of, 147
  percussion of, 147
  skin features of, 147*f*
Abdominal aorta, aneurysm of, 159
Abdominal case, 146
Abdominal distension
  ascites and, 161, 162*f*
  causes of, 161
Abdominal mass, 159
Abdominal paracentesis, therapeutic, 897
  complications of, 898
  contraindications s to, 898–899
  procedure for, 897–898
Abdominal venous hum, portal venous hypertension and, 174
Abdominojugular reflux, 847
Abducens nerve, 610–611. *See also* Sixth cranial nerve
  peripheral course of, 708
Abetalipoproteinaemia, 403
Absent ankle jerk, 621
Absent radial pulse, 757
  causes of, 757–758
    in ambulatory patient, 760
Acanthosis nigricans, 411
  associated conditions of, 412
  histology of, 412
  malignant, 412
  therapy for, 412
  types of, 411
Accessory nerve. *See* Eleventh cranial nerve
Accommodation, paralysis of, 717
Accommodation reflex, 587
ACE inhibitors. *See* Angiotensin-converting enzyme (ACE) inhibitors
Acetylcholine receptor antibodies, in myasthenia gravis, 669
Achalasia, 151
Achilles tendinitis, 248
Aciclovir, 704
  for erythema multiforme, 444
  for hairy leukoplakia, 453

Acne
  classification of, 414*f*
  conglobata, 415
  factors exacerbating, 414
  fulminans, 415
  management of, 414–415
  pathogenesis of, 413
  rosacea *vs.*, 531
  severity of, 413–414
  vulgaris, 413, 414*f*
Acoustic neurofibroma, histology of, 611
Acoustic neuroma, 752. *See also* Vestibular schwannomas
  in cerebellopontine angle tumour, 610
Acquired immunodeficiency syndrome (AIDS). *See* HIV infection/AIDS
Acquired lipodystrophy, 476
Acrochordons, 411
Acrokeratosis paraneoplastica (Bazex syndrome), 412
Acromegaly, 296
  causes of death, 299
  complications of, 297–298
  indicators of disease activity, 298
  investigations of, 298–299
  suspected diagnosis of, initial screening test for, 298
  symptoms of, 297
  therapeutic options for, 299
Acupuncture, for tension headache, 575
Acute gout
  diagnostic criteria for, 260
  treatment of, 259
Acute infarction, electrocardiographic evidence of, 780
Acute ischaemic stroke
  anticoagulants in, 637
  blood pressure reduction in, 636–637
  prognosis of, 638
Acute kidney injury
  causes of, 766
  diagnosis of, 765
  examination, 765
  features of, 765
  history of, 765
  prerenal, 766–767
Acute leukaemia, 231
  in adults, 232–234
  bleeding and bruising, 234
  diagnosis of, 231
  examination, 231
  features of, 231
  history of, 231

908 INDEX

Acute lymphoblastic leukaemia (ALL)
    in adults, 233
    cytogenetics of, 233
Acutely swollen leg, causes of, 785
Acute monoarticular arthritis, 854
Acute myeloid leukaemia (AML)
    diagnosis of, 232
    life-threatening complications, 233
    pathognomonic cell, 232
    types of, 234
Acute myocardial infarction, risk factors for, 779
Acute pancreatitis, 509, 768
    biochemical changes, 769
    causes of, 770
    CT findings of abdomen, 769–770
    diagnosis of, 769
    examination, 768
    features of, 768
    history of, 768
    patient management, 771
    scoring systems, 770–771
    systemic complications, 771
    with visible stranding, 769f
Acute physiology and chronic health examination (APACHE) II score, 770–771
Acute polyarticular arthritis, 854
Acute promyelocytic leukaemia (APML), 232
Acute respiratory failure, treatment for, 25
Acute stroke, tools for, 637
Acute tubular necrosis, pathophysiological role, 767
Acute uraemia, chronic uraemia *vs.*, 766
Adams, R., 858
Addison disease, 331, 745
    associated conditions with, 332
    autoimmune, aetiology, 333
    investigation of, 332–333
Addisonian crisis, 333*b*
Addison, Thomas, 333
Adductor pollicis, 730
Adenoma sebaceum, 539, 540*f*, 541
Adenomatous polyposis, familial, 612
Adenosine deaminase, pleural fluid, 829, 831
Adrenalectomy, Nelson syndrome after, 337
Adrenaline, 773
Adrenal tumours, 337
Adrenocorticotrophic hormone (ACTH)
    deficiency, 301
    in inferior petrosal sinus, 336–337
    plasma, 333, 336
Adrian, Lord Adrian Douglas, 626
Adson's test, 758, 758*f*
Age-adjusted D-dimers, 844–845
Age-related macular degeneration, 366, 367*f*
    in central scotoma, 604
    dry, 367
    risk factors for, 368–369
    treatment of, 369
    types of, 367
    wet, 367
Aggrecan, 265

Agnosia
    description of, 625
    types of, 625–626
Agrammatism, 624
Air bronchograms, 839*f*
Airflow obstruction, in COPD, 21, 23
Air transport, acute high-spinal injuries, 716
Albright, Fuller, 299
Albumin gradient, serum:ascites, 163
Albumin, serum
    corrected total calcium, 326
    low concentration, 166
    pleural effusion gradient and, 829–830
Albuminuria, 199
Alcohol
    in central nervous system, 689
    consumption, cataracts and, 371
Alcoholic cerebellar degeneration, 606
Alcoholism
    hepatomegaly and, 173
    pseudo-Cushing syndrome and, 337
Aldosterone receptor antagonists, for symptomatic heart failure, 134
Alemtuzumab, 227, 662
Alkaline phosphatase, liver disease and, 745
Allen, E. V., 424
Allen test, 422, 759–760, 759*f*
Allergic bronchopulmonary aspergillosis, 41, 841
Allgrove syndrome, 332
Allopurinol, 260
Alopecia. *See also* Hair loss
    drug-induced, 417
    totalis, 417
    universalis, 417
Alopecia areata, 416, 417*f*
    associated disorders of, 416–417
    signs of, 416
    treatment for, 417
5-Alpha reductase inhibitors, for benign prostatic hypertrophy, 582
Alpha-blockers
    for benign prostatic hypertrophy, 582
    for blood pressure, 206
Alzheimer's disease
    Alois, 580
    genetic predisposition to, 580
    treatment options for, 578–579
Amantadine, 662
Amaurosis, 375
Amaurosis fugax, 375
Amblyopia, 375
American College of Rheumatology/European League Against Rheumatism criteria, 272–273
γ-Aminobutyric acid analogues, 36
Aminoglycosides
    for bacterial endocarditis, 142
    for myasthenia gravis, 670
5-Aminosalicylate (5-ASA), for Crohn's disease, 157
Aminotransferases, serum, 745
Amiodarone, 813, 890
    induced hyperthyroidism, 309

INDEX

Amitriptyline, for migraine, 575
Ammonia, serum, measurement of in patients with altered mental status, 167
Ampicillin, maculopapular rash and, 484f
Amylase, pleural fluid, 829, 831
Amyloid light chain (AL) amyloidosis, 221
Amyotrophic lateral sclerosis (ALS), 653, 730. See also Motor neuron disease
   animal model for, 655
   diagnosis of, 654
   heredity of, 654
   magnetic cortical stimulation in, 655
Anacrotic pulse, 63, 64f
Anaemia, 210
   autoimmune haemolytic, 212
   of chronic disease, 271
   in chronic lymphocytic leukaemia, 225–226
   diagnosis of, 211
   examination of, 210–211
   features of, 210–211
   haemolysis, 212, 213f
   haemolytic anaemia, 211
   heart failure and, 848
   hereditary haemorrhagic telangiectasia and, 460
   history of, 210
   iron replacement, 212–213
   macrocytic, 866
   prosthetic heart valve-related, 91
   in rheumatoid arthritis, 270–271
   in scleroderma, 281
   in subacute combined degeneration of spinal cord, 866
Analgesia, for tension-type headache, 575
Anaphylactoid purpura, 454–455. See also Henoch–Schönlein purpura
Anaphylaxis
   angioedema vs., 775
   diagnosis of, 772, 774–775
   examination, 772
   feature of, 772
   history of, 772
   immunotherapy, 775
   pathophysiology of, 774, 774f
   patient observation, 773–774
   treatment, 772–773
ANCA associated small-vessel vasculitis, 292–293
Aneurysms
   of abdominal aorta, 159
   aortic, absent radial pulse and, 758
   berry
      aortic coarctation and, 787
      polycystic kidney disease and, 193, 195
   intracranial
      heritable connective tissue disorders, 516
      polycystic kidney disease and, 194
Angina, 777. See also Chest Pain
   chest pain and, 778
   stable, 778–779
Angina pectoris, 778. See also Coronary artery disease
   aortic regurgitation and, 58
Angiodysplasia, of colon, 65

Angioedema, 775, 775f
Angiofibromas
   facial (adenoma sebaceum), 539, 540f, 541
   subungual, 493, 539, 541f
Angiography, ventricular septal defects, 108
Angioid streaks, 515–516
   Groenblad–Strandberg syndrome, 516
   pseudoxanthoma elasticum, 514–516, 514f
Angiomyolipomas, tuberous sclerosis, 539, 541
Angioplasties, carotid, for carotid transient ischaemic attack, 640
Angiotensin-converting enzyme (ACE), serum, 480
Angiotensin-converting enzyme (ACE) inhibitors
   for diabetes mellitus, 356
   hypertension and, 205
   for polycystic kidney disease, 196
   for symptomatic heart failure, 133
Angiotensin receptor blockers
   for polycystic kidney disease, 196
   for symptomatic heart failure, 133
Angiotensin receptor-neprilysin inhibitor, for symptomatic heart failure, 134
Anisocoria, 587
Ankle clonus, 569
Ankle jerk, 570
   in common peroneal nerve palsy, 621
   hypothyroidism, 321
   normal, 621
Ankylosing spondylitis, 247, 249f, 742
   diagnostic criteria for, 248
   extra-articular manifestations of, 247
   four A's of, 248
   natural history of, 249
Anomia, 624
Anosmia, 681
Anosognosia, 626
Anterior carotid artery, deficits supplied by, 640
Anterior interosseous nerve entrapment, 602
Anterocollis, 680f
Antibiotics
   for cellulitis, 785
   for community-acquired pneumonia, 841
   for COPD exacerbation, 24
   for Crohn's disease, 157
   for Felty syndrome, 188
   for pyogenic bacterial infection, 785
Anticholinergic activity, of prescribed drugs, 764
Anticholinergic agent, for COPD, 24
Anticoagulation
   for acute ischaemic stroke, 637
   bleeding risk from, 795
   mitral stenosis, 80
Antidiuretic hormone secretion
   essential criteria for diagnosis, 813
   medications, 813
Antiepileptic drugs, 850
Antifungals
   for hairy leukoplakia, 453
   seborrhoeic dermatitis, 533

Antihistamines
    oral, for pruritus, 746
    for systemic mastocytosis, 548
    urticaria, 545
Anti-histone antibodies, 287
Antihypertensives, for hypertension, 207
Antimalarials, erythema multiforme from, 443
Anti-mitochondrial antibodies (AMA), 745
Antimuscarinic antagonist, long-acting (LAMA), for COPD, 24
Anti-nuclear antibodies (ANA), 287, 831
    diagnostic value, 287
Anti-phospholipid antibody syndrome, 525
Antiplatelet therapy, for diabetes mellitus, 356
Antipsychotic drugs, 813
Antiretroviral therapy, for patient with tuberculosis and HIV infection, 65
Antiretroviral therapy, tuberculosis, 52
Antisense-mediated exon skipping, 590
Antisynthetase syndrome, 278
Antithyroid drugs, 307
    for multinodular goitre, 317
Anti-TNF treatment, for ankylosing spondylitis, 250
α_1-Antitrypsin, deficiency of, 26
Antituberculous treatment, 52
Antitussives, 36
Anti-Yo antibodies, 609
Anxiety, 739
    diagnosis, 739
    screening tools for, 740
    treatment approach for, 740
    unsteadiness and, 752
Aorta
    coarctation of, 787
        associated conditions, 788
        commoner in men or women, 788
        complications of, 790
        fundal findings in, 790
        intervention for, different types of, 791
        investigations of, 788
        postoperative complications of, 791
        survival improved by surgery, 791
        treatment of, 790–791
        types of, 791
    dissection, 787
    pseudocoarctation of, 791
Aortic aneurysm, absent radial pulse and, 204
Aortic regurgitation, 58
    acute, causes of, 61
    aortic stenosis with, 70
    chronic
        causes of, 59–60
        natural history of, 61
    clinical signs of severity, 61
    follow-up, 62
    investigations of, 60
    mild, 61
    mitral regurgitation with, 89
    mitral stenosis with, 89
    moderate, 61
    surgical intervention, indications for, 62

ventricular septal defect, 106
wide pulse pressure, 60
Aortic sclerosis, 65
Aortic stenosis, 63
    aortic regurgitation with, 70
    aortic sclerosis vs., 65
    asymptomatic, 68
    causes of, 65
    complications of, 66–68
    degree of, 66
    haemolytic anaemia with, 68
    hypertrophic obstructive cardiomyopathy vs., 65
    investigations of, 66
    mechanism of angina in, 66
    medical management in, 68
    mitral regurgitation with, 89
    mitral stenosis with, 88–89
    prevalence in elderly, 65
    rectal bleeding with, 68
    severity of, 68
    signs and symptoms of, 68
    supravalvular, 68
    symptomatic, 68
    third heart sound in, 64
    treatment of, 68
    von Willebrand factor defects, 68–69
Aortic valve
    bicuspid, 64, 66, 67f
    calcification, 66, 67f
    prostheses, 90
Aortic valve disease
    mitral valve disease with, 88
    mixed, 70
Aortic valve replacement
    in aortic stenosis, 66
    choice of prosthesis, 91
Aortoduodenal fistula, 818
Apex beat
    in aortic regurgitation, 58
    aortic stenosis and, 63
    in constrictive pericarditis, 136
    mitral regurgitation, 72
    mixed aortic valve disease, 70
    mixed mitral valve disease, 86
Aphasia, 749
    primary progressive, 624
Apnoea Hypopnoea Index (AHI), 44
Apnoeas, 44
Appendicular abscess, 160
Apraxia, 626
    of speech, childhood, 624
    types of, 626
Argon laser photocoagulation therapy, 370
Argyll Robertson, Douglas MCL, 587
Argyll Robertson pupil, 586
    causes, 586–587
    reversed, 587
    site of lesion, 587
    tabes dorsalis, 586
Armanni–Ebstein nephropathy, 115
Armanni, L., 115

INDEX
911

Arnold–Chiari malformation, syringomyelia, 710, 711f
Arnold, J., 713
Arrhythmias, in aortic stenosis, 67
Arterial blood gas, 8b
Arterial leg ulcers, 420f
　diagnosis of, 419
　management of, 420
Arteriolar sclerosis, in Scheie classification, 385
Arteriovenous crossing sheathotomy, 401
Arteriovenous fistula, 422, 423f
　haemodialysis and, 192, 422
　management of, 422–423
　prosthetic grafts vs., 423
Arteriovenous haemodialysis-access grafts, prosthetic, 423–424, 423f
Arteriovenous malformations, in gastrointestinal bleeding, 817
Arteriovenous nipping, 383, 384f
Arthralgia, 745
Arthritis. See also Osteoarthrosis; Rheumatoid arthritis
　acute monoarticular, 854
　acute polyarticular, 854
　gouty, 259
　psoriatic, 248, 266, 267f, 268f, 517
　　pathogenesis and therapy of, 268
　　patterns of joint involvement, 266–267
　　prognosis of, 267
　septic, 854, 894
　　causative agent, 854
　　risk factors for, 854
　　steps in treating, 854
Arthritis mutilans, 243f, 267f, 268f
Arthrocentesis, knee, 892
Arthroscopic surgery, of osteoarthritis, 265
Articulation, dysarthria, 625
Articulation, of speech, 625
　testing, 608
Asbestos, exposure to, 833
Ascites, 161
　causes of, 161–162
　chronic liver disease and, 162–163
　cirrhosis and
　　formation of, 162
　　management of patient with, 161–163
　complications of, 161
　diuretic-resistant, 163
　investigations for, 162
　of known origin, fluid in, 897
　loculated, 899
　malignant, 899
　tense, 163
　of unknown origin, fluid in, 897–898
Ascitic fluid, uncommon causes for, 164
Aseptic technique, in chest drain insertion, 886
Ash-leaf patches, 539–540, 540f
Ashworth scale, in muscle tone, 658
Aspergillosis, allergic bronchopulmonary, 41, 841
Aspiration, for pneumothorax, 861
Aspirin, for stroke, during hyperacute phase, 636

Asplenia, 187
　dextrocardia with, 121
　infections susceptible to, 187–188
　precautions for, 188
Astasia abasia, 584
Astereognosis, 625–626
Asteroid hyalitis, 408
Asthma, 6
　acute
　　life-threatening indicators in, 8
　　management of, 7–8
　　severe, 8
　beta-receptor polymorphisms in, 9
　chronic, steroids for, 7
　definition of, 7
　diagnosis of, 7
　eosinophilia in, 841–842
　examination for, 6
　extrinsic, 7
　history of, 6
　intrinsic, 7
　obstructive pattern, spirometry, 5
　pulsus paradoxus and, 8
　severe brittle, 9
　trigger factors of, 6–7
　very severe, life-threatening attack of, 8
Asymmetrical scapular winging, 628f
Ataxia
　cerebellar, 607
　sensory, 583, 607t
Ataxic hemiparesis, 641
Atherosclerotic (vascular) pseudoparkinsonism, 682
Atopic dermatitis (eczema), 425, 426f
　criteria for diagnosis of, 425–426
　genetic aspects of, 427
　natural history of, 426–427
　potential complications of, 426
　proposed mechanisms of, 427
　stages (and patterns) of, 425
　treatment of, 426
ATP7B gene, 184
Atrial fibrillation (AF)
　atrial septal defects and, 104
　Graves' disease, 307, 308
　hyperthyroidism, 315, 312
　hypertrophic cardiomyopathy, 129
　mitral stenosis with, 76, 80
　mitral valve replacement, 91
Atrial septal defects (ASD), 100
　complications of, 104
　investigations of, 102–104
　management of, 104
　ostium primum, 101, 104
　ostium secundum, 101, 101f
　pregnancy and, 104
　shunt reversal, 102
　sinus venosus, 101, 101f, 102f
Atrophie blanche (white atrophy), 549
Atropine, sinus bradycardia, 858
4AT tool, 763
Atypical naevi, 485, 486f

Atypical pneumonias, 840
Auditory nerve, 610–611
Auer rod, 232*f*
Auscultation
　of abdomen, in COPD, 33
　of chest, 4
Auspitz, Heinrich, 283
Auspitz's sign, 518
Austin-Flint murmur, 58, 61
Auto-antibody screen, for Crohn's disease, 156
Autoimmune haemolytic anaemias, 212
Autoimmune hepatitis, type 1, 288
Autonomic dysfunction
　in multiple system atrophy, 664
　of Parkinson's disease, 685–686
Autonomic dysreflexia, 714
Autonomic failure, pure, 665
Autosomal dominant polycystic kidney disease (ADPKD). *See* Polycystic kidney disease
Axillary lymphadenopathy, 236
Axonotmesis, 622
Azathioprine, for rheumatoid arthritis, 271–272
Azoospermia, obstructive, 13

B

Babinski, J. J., 572
Babinski response, 569*f*, 570
Bacille Calmette–Guerin (BCG) vaccine, 51
Background retinopathy, 376, 377*f*
Back pain, 741
　ankylosing spondylitis and, 247
　causes of, 741–742
　chronic, risk stratification tools for, 743
　Cushing syndrome and, 334
　inflammatory, criteria for, 250
　mechanical, investigation for, 742–743
　polycystic kidney disease and, 194
　prevalence of, 742
Bacterial endocarditis, 141–142
　management of, 142
　manifestations of, 141–142
Bacterial pneumonia
　aetiology of, 838
　chest radiography of, 839*f*
　CURB65 severity score for, 838
　poorly resolving or recurrent, 840
　suspected, investigation of, 839
Bacteroides spp., 784
'Bag of worms' tongue, 617
Bailey, Charles, 82
Baldness, male pattern, 418
Ballet's sign, 313
Bamboo spine, 248
Bannayan–Ruvalcaba–Riley syndrome, 507
Bannister, Sir Roger, 651
Banting, Fredrick, 478
Barbiturates, erythema multiforme from, 443
Barger, G., 303, 324
Bariatric surgery, 349
Barium swallow, in swallowing difficulties, 150

Barlow, John, 85
Barlow syndrome. *See* Mitral valve prolapse
Barnard, Christiaan, 19, 135
Barré, J. A., 803
Barrett's oesophagus, 150
Barthel index, for acute stroke, 637
Bartter, Frederic, 811, 815
Bartter syndrome, 811
Basal ganglia calcification, familial, 685
Baseline viral screen, for weight loss, 141
Basilar artery, 608–609
Bassen, F. A., 404
Bassen–Kornzweig syndrome, 403, 615
　with spinocerebellar degeneration, 632
Bazex syndrome, 412, 520
Beau's lines, 491, 493*f*
Beck, C. S., 138
Becker muscular dystrophy, 588, 589*f*
Becker myotonia, 673
Becker, P. E., 590
Beck's triad, 137
Beevor, Charles Edward, 629
Beevor sign, 627
BE FEVER mnemonic, for bacterial endocarditis, 141–142
Beighton's nine-point scoring, joint hypermobility, 257
Bell, Sir Charles, 706
Bell's palsy, 703–704
　diabetes and, 705
　management of, 704
Below-knee thrombi, treatment of, 795
Bence-Jones, H., 445
Bendamustine, 227
Benediction posture, 729*f*
Benedikt, M., 719
Benedikt syndrome, 719, 733
Benign paroxysmal positional vertigo, 751
　diagnosis and treatment of, 753
Benign prostatic hypertrophy, 582
Benson's disease, 408
Bergmeister's papilla, 394
Berry aneurysms
　aortic coarctation and, 787
　polycystic kidney disease and, 192, 195
Beta2-adrenergic agonists
　for asthma, 24
　for COPD, 24
　long-acting (LABA), 8–9, 24
Beta-blockers
　for hypertension, 206
　for symptomatic heart failure, 133
Beta-receptor polymorphisms, in asthma, 9
Bethune, Norman, 863
Bevacizumab
　for age-related macular degeneration, 369
　for bronchogenic carcinoma, 48
Bhattacharya, Shoumo, 135
Biceps jerk, 567
Bilateral leg oedema, 56
Bilateral papilloedema warrant, 394–395
Bilateral ptosis, causes of, 677

INDEX

Bilateral pyramidal lesions, in lower limbs, 658–659
Bilateral swollen leg, causes of, 785
Bile salt therapy, 747
Bile salt therapy, for primary biliary cirrhosis, 747
Biliopancreatic diversion procedures, 349
Bilirubin, 148
  serum, for jaundice, 171
Binet staging, chronic lymphocytic leukaemia, 226
Bing reflex, 571
Biologics, for Crohn's disease, 157
Bioprosthetic heart valves, 90–91
  selection, 90
Biopsy, wedge, of erythema nodosum, 446
Biot breathing, 3f
Birt–Hogg–Dubé syndrome, 862–863
Bisphosphonates, for osteogenesis imperfecta, 391
Bitemporal hemianopia, 596
Bladder dysfunction, in multiple sclerosis, 662
Blalock–Taussig shunt, 117
  absent radial pulse and, 757
  in adults, 117
  modified, 118
  signs indicating, 116
Blatchford, Oliver, 820
Blatchford score, 819–820
Blau syndrome, 481
Bleeding risk, anticoagulation, 795
Blindness. See Visual loss
Blisters (bullae), 429
Blood, 148
Blood cultures
  for cellulitis, 784
  for pyogenic bacterial infection, 784
  for weight loss, 141
Blood film, of ankylosing spondylitis, 250
Blood gases, in interstitial pneumonia, 30
Blood pressure (BP). See also Hypertension
  ambulatory, 205
  aortic coarctation and, 787
  discrepancy in, 204, 758
  recording, 204
  reduction
    in acute ischaemic stroke, 636–637
    lifestyle modifications for, 206
  tetraplegia, effects of food ingestion, 715
Blood tests
  in congestive cardiac failure, 134
  for interstitial pneumonia, 30
  in stroke, during hyperacute phase, 636
  for weight loss, 141
Blood transfusion
  before renal transplantation, 201
  in subacute combined degeneration of spinal cord, 866
Blue lunula, in Wilson's disease, 491
Blue sclera, 390
B-lymphocytes, chronic lymphocytic leukaemia, 227

BODE index, 25–26
Body mass index (BMI), 347
Boeck, Caesar PM, 482
Bone marrow, 223
Bone marrow aspirate, 229, 230f
Bone marrow transplant, for osteogenesis imperfecta, 391
Bone matrix, reduction in, 391
Bone protection, assessment for, 344–345
Bone, thyrotoxicosis affecting, 308
Bosentan, for Eisenmenger's syndrome, 126
Boston's sign, 314
Bouchard, C. J., 264f, 265
Bouchard's nodes, 242, 263, 263f
Bouillaud, Jean Baptiste, 799
Bourneville, D. M., 543
Bourneville's disease. See Tuberous sclerosis
Boutonnière deformity, 242, 269, 270f
BPPV. See Benign paroxysmal positional vertigo
Brachial neuritis, 738
Bradyarrhythmias
  indications for permanent pacing, 856–857
  indications for temporary pacing, 856
Bradycardia
  causes, 855–856
  investigations, 856
  nocturnal, 855
  sinus, acute myocardial infarction, 858
Bradykinesia, 679, 681
Bradyphrenia, 682
Brain
  arteriovenous malformations, hereditary haemorrhagic telangiectasia and, 460
  imaging, role of, 878
Brainstem vascular disease, 752
Branch retinal vein occlusion, 399, 400f
  prognosis of, 401
Branham, H. H., 424
Braunwald, Nina, 92
Breast cancer, obesity and, 346
Breathing, patterns of, 3f
Breathlessness management in COPD, 25
Breslow thickness, melanoma and, 487–488
Bright, Richard, 333
Brisk jerk, 621
Brissaud's reflex, 570
British Thoracic Society, step care regimen for chronic asthma, 8
Broadbent sign, 136, 138
Broadbent, W., 138
Broad complex tachycardia, 889
Broca, Pierre Paul, 626
Broca's aphasia, 624
Broca's area, 623–624
Brockenbrough–Braunwald–Morrow sign, 130
Brock, Russell, 42, 82, 131
Brock syndrome, 42
Bronchial cartilage deficiency, 11
Bronchial haemorrhage, control of, 13
Bronchial lavage, 30

Bronchiectasis, 10, 11*f*
  abnormalities associated with, 13
  causes of, 10–11
  in cystic fibrosis, 16*f*
  definition of, 10
  diagnosis of, 10
  examination of, 10
  focal airway obstruction in, 14
  history of, 10
  investigations for, 11
  obstructive pattern, spirometry, 5
  Reid's classification of, 13–14
  respiratory pathogens in, 12
  sicca, 13
  sites for localized disease, 13
  surgery in, indications for, 13
  treatment for, 12–13
Bronchitis, obstructive pattern, spirometry, 5
Bronchoalveolar lavage (BAL), 30, 481
Bronchodilators
  for bronchiectasis, 13
  long-acting, for COPD, 24
  short-acting, for COPD, 23–24
Bronchogenic carcinoma, 46
  chest radiography in, 47, 48*f*
  clubbing in, 46
  contraindications for surgery in, 49
  cutaneous manifestations of, 47
  endocrine manifestations of, 47
  genetic change associated with, 49
  haematologic manifestations of, 47
  investigation of, 47–48
  pleural effusion, 828
  presentation of, 47
  prognosis of, 49
  radiotherapy for, 49
  staging of, 48
  surgery of, 48
Bronchopulmonary sequestration, 842
Bronchoscopy, in bronchogenic carcinoma, 47
Brown-Séquard, Charles-Edouar, 598
Brown-Séquard syndrome, 597, 598*f*
Brucellosis, 38, 177
Bruch, KWL, 516
Brugada ECG patterns, 877*f*
Brugada syndrome, 875, 877*f*
Bruising, 215. *See also Ecchymoses*
  inspection of, 215
  investigations for, 216
Bruits
  in hereditary haemorrhagic telangiectasia, 458
  thyroid, 303
Brunt, Peter, 747
Budd–Chiari syndrome, 163–164, 166
  serum ascites albumin gradient and, 163
Budesonide, inhaled, 7
Bulbar palsy, pseudobulbar palsy and, 693
Bulbospinal muscular atrophy, 342
Bulkeley's membrane, 518
Bullae (blisters), 429
Bullectomy, for COPD, 26

Büller, H. R., 795
Bullous diseases, autoimmune, 430–431
Bullous eruption, 428, 429*f*
Bullous pemphigoid, 429–430
Burkholderia cepacia, 17
Butterfly rash, 284, 285*f*
Bywaters, Eric, 767

C

CADASIL. *See* Cerebral autosomal dominant arteriopathy with subcortical infarcts and leukoencephalopathy
Caeruloplasmin, serum, 184
Café-au-lait spots, 496
Caffeine, in Parkinson's disease, 683
CAG expansion, and Huntington disease, 619
Calcaneocavovarus deformities, 725*f*
Calcification
  aortic valve, 66, 67*f*
  of familial basal ganglia, 685
  intracranial, 535, 537*f*
  subcutaneous, 279
Calcipotriol, 520
Calcium, albumin-corrected total, 326
Calcium pyrophosphate crystal deposition, osteoarthritis with, 893
Calliper shoes, 621
Calmette–Guérin (BCG) vaccine, 51
Camptocormia, 667
Cancer risk
  in cystic fibrosis, 17
  obesity, 346
Candida albicans, in nail infections, 449
Candidal endocarditis, 143
Candida parapsilosis, in nail infections, 449
Capillary permeability, increase in, 382
Caplan, L. R., 733
CAPN3, 650
Carbamazepine, 813, 850*t*
Carbidopa, 683
Carbimazole, for thyrotoxicosis, 307
Carbon monoxide (KCO), 5
Carcinoid syndrome, 338, 339*f*
Carcinoid tumours, 338*b*
  diagnosis of, 339
  gastric, 339
  liver, metastatic, 338–339
  treatment of, 339–340
Carcinoma
  caecum, 159
  colon, 160
  pancreas, 159
  stomach, 159, 411
Cardiac arrhythmias, in unsteadiness, 752
Cardiac catheterization
  for aortic regurgitation, 60
  for aortic stenosis, 66
  for atrial septal defects, 103
  for constrictive pericarditis, 138
  for Ebstein's anomaly, 114

INDEX

for Eisenmenger's syndrome, 125
for hypertrophic cardiomyopathy, 73
for mitral regurgitation, 73
for mitral stenosis, 80
for mixed aortic valve disease, 71
for pulmonary stenosis, 98
for ventricular septal defects, 108
Cardiac failure. *See* Heart failure
Cardiac lesions, initial shunt for, 118
Cardiac pacemakers
  hypertrophic cardiomyopathy, 130
  indications, 856
Cardiac resynchronization therapy, 134
Cardiac rhabdomyomas, tuberous sclerosis, 539
Cardiac silhouette, 98
Cardiac syncope, 873
Cardiac tamponade, 137, 826, 826*f*
Cardiomegaly, 5
Cardiomyopathy, in pregnancy, 881–882
Cardiopulmonary exercise testing, in congestive cardiac failure, 133
Cardiovascular manifestations
  of bronchogenic carcinoma, 47
  of Ehlers–Danlos syndrome, 255
  of hypothyroidism, 322
  of polycystic kidney disease, 194
  of pseudoxanthoma elasticum, 194
Cardiovascular system, 54
  examination of, 54–56
  history of, 54
Carney complex, 299
Carotenaemia, 171
Carotid angioplasties, for carotid transient ischaemic attack, 640
Carotid artery pulsation
  bifid, 847, 847*f*
  jugular venous pulse *vs.*, 847
Carotid artery stenosis, 638
Carotid Doppler, in stroke, during hyperacute phase, 636
Carotid endarterectomy, for carotid transient ischaemic attack, 639–640
Carotid sinus massage, 874
Carotid sinus syndrome, 874
Carotid transient ischaemic attack, 639
Carpal tunnel syndrome, 599, 600*f*
Carpentier's classification, of mitral regurgitation, 74–75
Carpopedal spasm, 325
Carrell, Alexis, 202
Castleman disease, 218, 802–803
Castle, William B., 867
Cataracts, 371, 372*f*
  central, 378*f*
  diabetes mellitus, 371
  in dystrophia myotonica, 674, 677
  treatment of, 372
Catheter-directed thrombolysis, 845
Cauda equina syndrome, 782
  cause of, 783
  conus medullaris syndrome *vs.*, 783

investigation of, 783
types of, 783
vertebral level of lesion in, 783
Caveolin-1, 31
Cavernous sinus, 708
Cazenave, Pierre L. A., 289
CEAP classification, venous disease, 551
Celecoxib, 506–507
Cellulitis, 784, 785*f*
  diagnosis, 786
  hospital admission, 786
  management of, 784–785
  treatment options, 786
Central line insertion, 883
  clinical indications, 885
  complications of, 883
  equipment for, 883–884
  positioning in, 885
  steps for, 884
Central nervous system, alcohol on, 689
Central optic chiasm, lesions of, 643*t*
Central retinal artery occlusion, 374*f*, 604
Central retinal vein occlusion, 399, 400*f*
  clinical course in, 401
  complications of, 401
Central scotoma, 603, 603*f*
  in optic atrophy, 387
Cerebellar degeneration
  alcoholic, 606
  paraneoplastic, 609
Cerebellar dysarthria, 608
Cerebellar signs, 606–607
Cerebellar syndrome, 605
  anti-Yo antibodies with, 609
  causes of, 606–607
  coordination of gait, lack of, 606
  gait abnormalities, 583
  multiple system atrophy and, 666
  tremors in, 606, 723
Cerebellar tumours, role of chaperones in, 609
Cerebellopontine angle, 610
  tumours, 610, 752
Cerebral aneurysms
  inherited conditions, 869
  risk factors, 869
Cerebral arteriovenous malformations, 458
Cerebral autosomal dominant arteriopathy with subcortical infarcts and leukoencephalopathy (CADASIL), 693
Cerebral infarction. *See* Stroke
Cerebral oedema, 393
Cerebral salt wasting syndrome (CSW), 813–814
Cerebrospinal fluid (CSF)
  interpretation of, 896
  in motor neuron disease, 654
  pressure, 896
Cerebrovascular accidents, Eisenmenger's syndrome and, 124
Cervical lymphadenopathy, 236
Cervical myelopathy, 734
Cervical spine, ankylosing spondylitis and, 247

Chaddock reflex, 571
Chagas' disease, 11
Chaperones, role in cerebellar tumours, 609
Charcot foot, 252–253, 253f
Charcot, Jean Martin, 253f, 615–616
Charcot–Marie–Tooth disease, 613
  forme fruste for, 615
  gene mutations in, 615
  inheritance of, 614–615
  types of, 613–614
Charcot's arthropathy, 251. *See also* Neuropathic foot
  causes of, 712
  Rogers and Bevilacqua classification, 252, 252f
Charcot's fever, 171
Chemotherapy
  for carcinoid syndrome, 340
  for small cell lung cancer, 48
Cherry-red spot, at fovea, 373, 374f
Chest
  examination of
    cirrhosis of liver and, 816
    in COPD, 20
  expansion, ankylosing spondylitis and, 247
Chest drain insertion, 886
  contraindications s to, 888
  for pneumothorax, 862
  procedure for, 886–888
  for spontaneous (non-traumatic) pneumothorax, 886
    complications of, 888
Chest pain, 777. *See also* Angina pectoris; Myocardial infarction, acute
  hypertrophic cardiomyopathy, 127
  respiratory diseases associated with, 2
Chest radiography
  of aortic coarctation, 788, 790f
  of aortic regurgitation, 60
  of aortic stenosis, 66, 67f
  of asthma, 5, 7
  of atrial septal defects, 103
  of bacterial pneumonia, 839f
  of bronchogenic carcinoma, 47, 48f
  for central line insertion, 885
  of collapsed lung, 41, 42f
  of congestive cardiac failure, 133
  of constrictive pericarditis, 138
  of cystic fibrosis, 16f
  of dextrocardia, 121, 122f
  of Ebstein's anomaly, 114, 114f, 115f
  of Eisenmenger's syndrome, 125, 125f
  of emphysema, 21f
  of Fallot's tetralogy, 118, 119f
  of hypertrophic cardiomyopathy, 129
  of interstitial pneumonia, 30
  of mitral regurgitation, 73
  of mitral stenosis, 78–79, 79f
  of patent ductus arteriosus, 111
  of pleural effusion, 828, 828f
  of pulmonary stenosis, 98, 98f
  of sarcoidosis, 480
  of spontaneous pneumothorax, 860, 860f
  of stroke, during hyperacute phase, 636
  for swallowing difficulties, 150
  of tricuspid regurgitation, 95
  of tuberculosis, 827
  of ventricular septal defects, 107, 108f
Cheyne–Stoke breathing, 3f
Chiari, H., 713
Chlamydia pneumoniae, 840
Chlorambucil, 227
Chloride channels, in cystic fibrosis, 17
Cholangitis, autoimmune, 746
Cholestasis, pruritus in, 746
Cholesterol. *See also* Hypercholesterolaemia
  crystals, 374f, 375
  embolus, in fundus, 373, 374f
    retinal arterial occlusion, 373, 374f
  pleural fluid, 831
Cholesterolosis, 408
Cholinergic crisis, in myasthenia gravis, 671
Cholinesterase inhibitors, for delirium, 763
Chorda tympani, 704
Chorea, 617
Choroidal haemangioma, 535, 536f
Choroidal neovascularization, in age-related macular degeneration, 368
Chowne, W. D., 282
Christian, Henry A., 447
Christmas disease, 246
Chromosome, in Friedreich's ataxia, 631
Chronically swollen leg, causes of, 785–786
Chronic bronchitis. *See also* Chronic obstructive pulmonary disease
  definition of, 22
Chronic eosinophilic pneumonia, 842
Chronic hypertension, management of, in pregnancy, 881
Chronic inflammatory demyelinating polyradiculoneuropathy, 802
Chronic kidney disease, foods to be avoided, 805
Chronic liver disease
  ascites and, 162–163
  gynaecomastia and, 341
  hepatomegaly and, 173
Chronic lymphocytic leukaemia, 225
  anaemia in, 225–226
  pathogenesis of, 227
  presentation of, 226
  prognosis in, 226
  staging of, 227
  treatment of, 227
Chronic myelocytic leukaemia, 177
Chronic myeloid disorders, 177–178
Chronic myeloid leukaemia (CML)
  accelerated phase, 229
  blast phase, 229
  blood film, 229, 229f
  chronic phase, 229
  examination of, 228
  features of, 228
  haematological malignancies, 229
  history of, 228
  pathophysiology of, 228

prognosis of, 228
prognostic factors, 229
treatment options, 230
Chronic obstructive pulmonary disease (COPD), 20.
    See also Chronic bronchitis; Emphysema
  acute exacerbation of, 24
  BODE index for, 25–26
  cause of death and disability in, 23
  definition of, 22
  differential diagnosis of, 23
  expiratory capacity reduction in, 22
  inflammatory mechanisms in, 22–23
  inhaled steroids for, 24
  left ventricular function and, 34
  long-term domiciliary oxygen therapy
      for, 25
  molecular genetics of, 26
  newer treatments for, 27
  nutrition in, 27
  organisms associated with, 25
  outpatient treatment for, 23–24
  patients' symptoms of, 23
  proteolysis in, 23
  role of surgery for, 26–27
Chronic reflux, lifestyle advice for, 151
Chronic renal failure, polycystic kidney disease
    and, 192
Chronic urticaria, 544
  investigation of, 545
  management of, 545–546
Chronic venous insufficiency, 551
Chronotropic incompetence, 857
Chrysotherapy, 430
Churg, J., 689
Churg–Strauss disease, 292
Churg–Strauss syndrome, 842
Chvostek, Frantisek, 327
Chvostek's sign, 325
Chylothorax, 831
Ciclosporin, 546
Cirrhosis, of liver, 165
  ascites formation in, 162
  causes of, 166
  haemochromatosis and, 179*b*
  hepatic encephalopathy in, 167
  investigation for, 166
  laboratory changes in, 167–168
  management of, 168
  palpable liver and, 174
  poor prognostic factors in, 167
  primary biliary. *See* Primary biliary cirrhosis
  secondary biliary, 747
  sequelae of, 166
  variceal bleeding in, management of, 168
Citalopram, 740
Cladribine, 662
Clasp-knife spasticity, 565
Clasp-knife type, of spasticity, 682–683
Claude, Henri, 719
Claude syndrome, 719
Claudication, neural, 782

Claw hand
  causes of, 730
  ulnar, 728, 729*f*, 730
Click–murmur syndrome. *See* Mitral valve prolapse
Clinical activity score (CAS), 312
Closed spina bifida, 724, 727
Clostridia spp., 784
Clubbing
  in bronchogenic carcinoma, 46
  crackles with, 29, 29*f*
Cluster headache, 575
Clustertic syndrome, 576
CNTNAP2 gene, 624
Coagulopathy, in therapeutic abdominal paracentesis,
    898
Coal tar-based treatments, 520
Coarctation of aorta, 787
  associated conditions, 788
  commoner in men or women, 788
  complications of, 790
  fundal findings in, 790
  intervention for, different types of, 791
  investigations in, 788
  postoperative complications of, 791
  survival improved by surgery, 791
  treatment of, 790–791
  types of, 791
Cocaine, 697*t*
Coeliac disease, 437
Cognitive behavioural therapy (CBT), for anxiety, 740
Cog-wheel rigidity, 565, 679, 681
COL1A1, defects in, 390–391
COL1A2, defects in, 390–391
Colchicine, 259, 825
Cold-related skin conditions, 442
Cold sore, 462–464, 463*f*
Collagen
  metabolism, defect in, 257
  type I mutations, 390–391
Collagen vascular disorder, erythema multiforme from,
    444
Collapse
  brain imaging in, 878
  hypoglycaemia and, 874
  risk stratification scores for, 874
Collapsed lung, 41
Collapsing pulse. *See* Corrigan's pulse
Colonic polyps, 505
Colorectal cancer surveillance, for Crohn's disease, 157
Comedones, 413
Common peroneal nerve entrapment, 601
Communication
  aids, for speech disturbance, 750
  on ward/clinic, 750
Community-acquired pneumonia, antibiotics for, 841
Compression fracture, 742
Computed tomography (CT)
  of aortic coarctation, 788
  of bilateral spastic paralysis, 594
  of bronchiectasis, 11–12
  of bronchogenic carcinoma, 47

Computed tomography (CT) *(Continued)*
    chest, 5
    of congestive cardiac failure, 133
    of constrictive pericarditis, 138
    of facial nerve palsy, 705
    high-resolution
        for bronchiectasis, 11
        in emphysema, 23
        in interstitial pneumonia, 30
        standard *vs.*, 12
    for micturition difficulties, 582
    of multinodular goitre, 316
    for speech disturbance, 596
    spiral, 12
    of spontaneous pneumothorax, 861
    for stroke, during hyperacute phase, 636
    of Sturge–Weber syndrome, 537*f*
    for swallowing difficulties, 150
Conduction disturbances, in infective endocarditis, 143
Confusion, 761
Confusion Assessment Method, 763
Congenital heart disease
    common, 118
    embryology of heart development and, 117–118
    maternal risk in, 881
    mitral regurgitation, 74–75
Congestive cardiac failure, 132
    aetiology of, 132
    devices in, 134–135
    drugs to be avoided in, 134
    fluid retention in, 132
    impaired perfusion in, 132
    in infective endocarditis, 143
    investigation for, 132–133
    with preserved ejection fraction, 134
    symptomatic, with reduced rejection fraction, pharmacologic treatment of, 133–134
    types of, 133
    ventricular dysfunction in, 132
Conjugated bilirubin, renal excretion of, 170, 172
Conjugate gaze, mechanisms to, 645–646
Connective tissue disorders, pyrexia of unknown origin and, 38–40
Consecutive optic atrophy, 388
Consensual light reflex, in optic atrophy, 387
Consolidation, 838
    in bronchogenic carcinoma, 47
    pulmonary, 829
Constipation, in Parkinson's disease, 685
Constrictive pericarditis, 136, 825
    causes of, 136–137
    investigations of, 138
    vs. restrictive cardiomyopathy, 137–138
    treatment of, 138
Constructional apraxia, 626
Continuous nasal positive airway pressure (CPAP), 45
Contralateral subthalamic nucleus, hemiballismus in, 633
Contralateral thalamotomy, for hemiballismus, 634
Contrast aortography, in aortic coarctation, 788
Conus medullaris, 783
    syndrome, 783

Coombs, RRA, 289
Coordination testing, 568, 570
COPD. *See* Chronic obstructive pulmonary disease
COPD Assessment Test, 23
Copper
    -chelating agents, 184
    deposition of, 183
Cor bovinum, 61
Corneal sensation, testing, 564
Corneal ulcerations, 467
Coronary angiography, mitral stenosis, 80
Coronary artery bypass grafting (CABG), for stable angina, 779
Coronary artery disease. *See also* Angina pectoris; Myocardial infarction, acute
    hypertriglyceridaemia and, 439
    obesity patterns and, 348
    pseudoxanthoma elasticum, 516
    resting 12-lead ECG in, 778
Cor pulmonale, 33, 34*f*
Corrigan, Sir Dominic J., 112
Corrigan's pulse (collapsing pulse), 58, 110–112
Corrigan's sign, 58–59
Cortical cataracts, 378*f*
Cortical tubers, tuberous sclerosis, 539
Corticosteroids
    for chronic urticaria, 546
    for COPD, 24
    for Crohn's disease, 157
    for erythema multiforme, 444
    for herpes gestationis, 431
Corticotrophin-releasing hormone (CRH), 336
Cortisol, urinary free, 336
Cor triatriatum, 82
Cottonwool spots, 376, 378*f*
    causes of, 385–386
Cough, 35
    chronic persistent, 36
    persistent purulent, 17
Cough hypersensitivity syndrome, 36
Cough reflex arc, 36
Courvoisier's law, 171
COVID-19
    in adults, 39–40
    clinical features of, 39
    complications of, 39–40
    multiple sclerosis, 662
    pharmacological treatment options, 40
    with pneumonia, 842
Cowden's disease, 507
Cowen's sign, 314
Crackles
    during auscultation, 4
    clubbing with, 29
Cradle cap, 533
Cranial nerves
    examination, 563
    in Guillain–Barré syndrome, 800
Craniopharyngioma, 596
Creatine kinase, serum, 276, 650
Crepitant cellulitis, 784

Crepitus, 784
CREST syndrome, 281
Crocodile tears, 705
Crohn, Burrill Bernard, 158
Crohn's disease, 155, 159, 246
    associated diseases, 156
    complications of, 156
    investigation for, 156–157
    macroautophagy in, 158
    ocular features of, 156
    severity assessment systems in, 157
Cronkhite–Canada syndrome, 507
Crowe's sign, 498
Cruveilhier–Baumgarten murmur, 168
Cryotherapy, for molluscum contagiosum, 490
Crystal deposition, calcium pyrophosphate, osteoarthritis with, 893
CT. *See* Computed tomography
CT pulmonary angiography (CTPA), for non-massive pulmonary embolism, 880–881
CT severity index, 770–771
Cubital tunnel syndrome, 601, 731
CUG-binding protein 1 (CUG-BP1), 675–676
Cullen's sign, 509
Cullen, T. S., 509
Curacao criteria, for hereditary haemorrhagic telangiectasia, 460
CURB65 severity score, for bacterial pneumonia, 839–840
Curettage, for molluscum contagiosum, 490
Cushing, Harvey William, 337
Cushing's disease, 336
    investigations of, 336–337
    management of, 337
Cushing syndrome, 334
    in bronchogenic carcinoma, 47
    causes of, 336
    clinical features of, 334–335, 335f
    investigations of, 336–337
    management of, 337
    in proximal myopathy, 690
    pseudo-, 337
Cutaneous T-cell lymphoma, 432, 433f, 434f
Cutaneous telangiectasia, hereditary haemorrhagic telangiectasia and, 460
Cutler, Elliott, 82
Cyanosis
    differential, 111
    in Ebstein's anomaly, 113
    obstructive sleep apnoea and, 44
Cyanotic heart diseases of infancy, 124
Cyclic citrullinated peptide (CCP) antibodies, 272
Cyclophosphamide, 227, 813
Cylindrical bronchiectasis, 13
Cystic bronchiectasis, 14
Cystic fibrosis, 12, 15
    airway defects in, 17
    bronchiectasis in, 16f
    cancer risk in, 17
    cause of death in, 18
    chest complications of, treatment of, 16–17
    clinical manifestations of, 16
    definition of, 15b
    diagnosis in infancy, 17
    forme fruste of, 19
    inheritance pattern for, 17
    lifespan of patient with, 18
    methods of treatment for, 16–17
    physiotherapy for, 17
    pregnancy in, 19
    transplantation management in, 18
Cystic fibrosis transmembrane conductance regulator (CFTR), 11, 15b
    modulator therapies, 18
Cystoscopy, for micturition difficulties, 582

D

Dalrymple, J., 314
Dalrymple's sign, 310, 311f
Dana, Charles Loomis, 866
Danlos, H. A., 257
Dapagliflozin, 134
Dapsone
    for autoimmune bullous diseases, 430
    for dermatitis herpetiformis, 436
Darier, F. J., 548
Darier's sign, 548
Darwin, Charles, 693
Dawson's fingers, 659f
Day time sleepiness, in Parkinson's disease, 685
DCCV. *See* Direct current cardioversion
D-dimers, 793, 844–845
Deafness. *See* Hearing loss
Deep-brain stimulation, drug-resistant tremor, 723
Deep sulcus sign, 860, 860f
Deep tendon reflexes, 617
Deep vein thrombosis, 792
    causes of, 795–796
    clinical probability estimation, 792–793
    complications of, 794–795
    diagnosis of, 792, 794
    examination, 792
    features of, 792
    history of, 792
    investigation, 793–794
    long-term anticoagulation, 794
    predisposing factors for, 793
    pulmonary embolism, risk of, 795
    recurrent, causes of, 795–796
    standard treatment, 794
    superficial thrombophlebitis and, 508
Degenerative discs/facets, 742
Degenerative spine disease, in Brown-Séquard syndrome, 597
Déjérine, Joseph Jules, 629
Déjérine-Klumpke, Augusta, 731
Delirium, 762
    computed tomography/magnetic resonance imaging, 762
    dementia and, 579, 763–764
    investigations for, 762

Delirium *(Continued)*
  management of, 762–763
  pathophysiology of, 763
  presentation of, 762
  recognition of, importance of, 763
Delphian node, 236
Dementia
  causes of, 578
  delirium and, 579, 763–764
  screening for, 580
de Musset, Alfred, 62
de Musset's sign, 59
Demyelinating disorders, 661
Demyelinating neuropathy, in Guillain–Barré syndrome, 801
Dengue fever, 38
Dentatorubral pallidoluysian atrophy, with spinocerebellar degeneration, 632
Depression
  dementia and, 579
  in Parkinson's disease, 682, 685
  pseudo-Cushing syndrome and, 337
Dermatitis herpetiformis, 435, 436*f*
  conditions associated with, 435
  investigations of, 435–436
  treatment of, 430, 436
Dermatitis, stasis, 549
Dermatographism, 545
Dermatomyositis, 275, 276*f*, 412
  skin manifestations, 276*f*
Dermatophytes, in nail infections, 449
Desferrioxamine, for haemochromatosis, 182
Desmogleins, 430
Detemir, for diabetes mellitus, 357
Devic's disease, 661
Dextrocardia, 121
  associated abnormalities, 121
Dextroversion, 122
Diabetes
  gestational, 882
  type 1. *See* Type 1 diabetes
  type 2. *See* Type 2 diabetes
Diabetes Control and Complications Trial, 381
Diabetes insipidus (DI), 808
Diabetes mellitus
  acanthosis nigricans, 411
  annual review, 360–361
  Bell's palsy and, 705
  HbA1c measurement and monitoring in, 357
  hypopituitarism in, 319
  necrobiosis lipoidica, 494
  neuropathy in, 688, 689*f*
  pancreas–kidney transplantation and, 202
  retinopathy and, duration of, 381
  sixth nerve palsy and, 707
  skin lesions, 495
  third cranial nerve palsy and, 717
  type 2, 354
    control of, 357
    complications of, 354
    diagnostic criteria for, 355
    drug treatment recommendations for, 356–357
    obesity and, 347, 349
    self-monitoring for, 356–357
  in vitreous opacities, 408
Diabetic amyotrophy, 690–691
Diabetic autonomic dysfunction (DAN), 353
Diabetic blindness, 381
Diabetic foot, 358. *See also* Lower extremity ulcers
  Charcot's joint, 253
  cutaneous pressure perception, 361
  diagnosis, 359–361
  ischaemic, 358–359, 360*f*
  management, 359–360
  neuropathic, 359, 360*f*
  neuropathic/ischaemic combined, 358–359
  Neuropathy Disability Score, 361
  types, 359
Diabetic ketoacidosis, 814
Diabetic maculopathy, 379
Diabetic neuropathy, 252, 688
  types of, 689*f*
Diabetic retinopathy, 355, 376, 378*f*
  classification of, 380
  earliest sign of, 382
  management of, 376–378, 380
  screening for, 381–382
  symptoms of, 376, 379–380
  systemic conditions worsen, 381
Dialysis. *See also* Haemodialysis
  acute myocardial infarction and, 202
  carpal tunnel syndrome, 600
  in infants and children, 201
  for polycystic kidney disease, 193
  renal transplantation and, 201
Diarrhoea, 152
  in carcinoid syndrome, 338
  dermatitis herpetiformis and, 435
  investigation for, 153
  mechanisms of, 153
Diastolic dysfunction, 130
Diastolic heart failure, 134
Diastolic murmurs
  in aortic regurgitation, 58, 61
  differential diagnosis of, 137
  effects of inspiration, 56
  in mitral regurgitation, 87
Dickens, Charles, 45
Dicke, W. K., 437
Differentiation syndrome, 234
Diffuse proliferative glomerulonephritis, 143
Digital ulceration, scleroderma, 280, 280*f*
Diplopia (double vision), 610
  monocular, 408
  sixth nerve palsy, 707
  third cranial nerve palsy and, 717
Dipstick, for urinary tract infection, 766–767
Direct current cardioversion, emergency synchronised, 889
  complications of, 889
  delivering the shock during, 890
  indications for, 889

INDEX

Direct light reflex, in optic atrophy, 387
Direct ophthalmoscopy, cataract detection using, 372
Direct oral anticoagulants (DOACs), 890
'Dirty elbows and knees' sign, 319
Disease–improving global outcomes, 766
Dissociated nystagmus, 648
Distal muscular dystrophy, 589f
Diuresis, 814–815
Diuretics
　for patient with cirrhosis and ascites, 163
　for symptomatic heart failure, 134
Diverticular abscess, 160
Dix–Hallpike test, in benign paroxysmal positional vertigo, 753
DMPK gene, 675
DNA chips, 654
Doll's head manoeuvre, 645–646
Dominant hemisphere functions, 625
'Donald Duck' speech, 749
Donnall, Thomas E., 202
Dopamine receptors, 684
Dopaminergic agents, 683
Doppler leg ultrasound, for non-massive pulmonary embolism, 880
Double apical impulse, 127
Double vision. *See* Diplopia
Downbeat nystagmus, 648
Downward-sloping clavicles, 628f
Drainage, closed-tube, for pleural effusion, 831
Dressing apraxia, 626
Dressler syndrome, 826
Dressler, W., 826
Driving, ankylosing spondylitis and, 249
Drooling, in Parkinson's disease, 685
Drug eruptions, 484f
　bullous, 428, 429f
Drug holidays, in levodopa therapy, 683
Drug hypersensitivity, erythema multiforme from, 443
Drug-induced pyrexia, 38
Drug reaction with eosinophilia and systemic symptoms (DRESS) syndrome, 39
Drüsen, 368f, 369f
Dual antibiotic therapy, for community-acquired pneumonia, 841
Duane syndrome, 708
Dubin–Johnson syndrome, 172
Duchenne, Guillaume-Benjamin-Amand, 590, 691
Duchenne muscular dystrophy, 588, 589f
Duhring, L. A., 437
Duke's criteria, for bacterial endocarditis, 141–142
Duodenal metal transporter-1 (DMT-1), 180–181
Duodenitis, 817
Dupuytren's contracture, 242, 816, 817f
Durkan's test, 601
Duroziez, P. I., 62
Duroziez's sign or murmur, 601
Dynamic hyperinflation, 22
Dysarthria, 608, 625
　cerebellar, 608
　communication in, 750

921

　scanning, 606
　types of, 749
Dysdiadochokinesia, 606
Dysferlin, 649
Dyskeratosis congenita, 31
Dyskinesia
　tardive, 685
　upper body, 681
Dyslexia, 626
Dysmetria, 606
Dysmyelopoiesis, of systemic mastocytosis, 547
Dysphasia, 624–625
　description of, 624–625
　expressive, 623–624
　with lateral medullary syndrome, 732
　sensory or receptive, 624
　types of, 749
Dysphonia, 625
Dyspnoea, 54
　aortic regurgitation and, 58
　aortic stenosis and, 63
　degree of, 2
　in Guillain–Barré syndrome, 800
　hypertrophic cardiomyopathy and, 127
　mitral stenosis and, 76
　onset of, 2
　pulmonary stenosis and, 96
Dyspraxia
　orofacial, 624
　verbal, 624
Dyssynergia, 606
Dystrophia myotonica, 674, 675f
　features of, 676
　inheritance in, 675–676
　management of, 678
　prenatal diagnosis of, 678
　surgery for, 677
　tests in, 677–678
　therapeutic modalities in, 676
Dystrophin, 589

E
Early Treatment of Diabetic Retinopathy Study, 378
Eaton–Lambert syndrome, 670–671
Eaton, L. M., 671
Ebstein's anomaly, 113
　indications for surgery, 114–115
　investigations of, 114
　outcome predictors, 114
　pathology in, 113
　treatment of, 115
Ebstein, Wilhelm, 115
Ecchymoses (bruising)
　causes, 522
　purpura, 522, 522f
ECG. *See* Electrocardiography
Echocardiography
　of aortic coarctation, 788
　of aortic regurgitation, 60
　of aortic stenosis, 66

Echocardiography *(Continued)*
  of atrial septal defects, 103
  of constrictive pericarditis, 138
  of Ebstein's anomaly, 114
  of Eisenmenger's syndrome, 125
  of hypertrophic cardiomyopathy, 127–129, 128*f*
  of mitral regurgitation, 73
  of mitral stenosis, 79–80
  of mitral valve prolapse, 84
  of mixed aortic valve disease, 71
  of patent ductus arteriosus, 111
  of pericardial rub, 824–825, 826*f*
  of prosthetic heart valves, 91
  of pulmonary stenosis, 98
  transthoracic, of congestive cardiac failure, 133
  of tricuspid regurgitation, 95
  of ventricular septal defects, 107
Edrophonium (Tensilon) test, in myasthenia gravis, 645
Effective osmolality, 814
Effusive-constrictive pericarditis, 138
Ehlers–Danlos syndrome, 254
  cardiovascular manifestations of, 255
  gastrointestinal manifestations of, 254–255
  management of skin wounds, 255
  types of, 256–257
Ehlers, Edvard, 257
Eighth cranial nerve, testing, 565
Eisenmenger complex, 124
Eisenmenger's syndrome, 123
  age of onset of, 124
  complications of, 124–125
  investigation for, 125
  pregnancy in, 125–126
  prognosis in, 125
  pulmonary hypertension in, 124
  treatment of, 126
Eisenmenger, Victor, 126
Ejection click, 798
  in aortic coarctation, 788
  in aortic regurgitation, 58
  in aortic stenosis, 63, 64*f*
  in pulmonary stenosis, 96
Ejection systolic murmur
  in aortic regurgitation, 58
  in aortic stenosis, 63, 64*f*, 65
  in hypertrophic cardiomyopathy, 127
  other causes of, 65
  in pulmonary stenosis, 96
Elbows, examination of, 244
Elbow tunnel syndrome, 601
Elderly
  aortic stenosis prevalence in, 65
  presentation of hyperthyroidism, 512
  systemic lupus erythematosus, 287
  thyroxine replacement therapy, 322
Electrocardiography (ECG)
  of acute infarction, 780, 781*f*
  of aortic coarctation, 788, 789*f*
  of aortic regurgitation, 59*f*, 60
  of aortic stenosis, 66
  of atrial septal defects, 102–103, 102*f*

  of bradycardia, 856, 856*f*
  of congestive cardiac failure, 133
  of constrictive pericarditis, 138
  of dextrocardia, 121, 122*f*
  of dystrophia myotonica, 676, 676*f*
  of Ebstein's anomaly, 114, 114*f*, 115*f*
  of Eisenmenger's syndrome, 125
  of Fallot's tetralogy, 118–120, 119*f*
  of hypertrophic cardiomyopathy, 129, 129*f*
  of mitral regurgitation, 73
  of mitral stenosis, 78, 78*f*
  of patent ductus arteriosus, 111
  of pericardial rub, 824–825, 825*f*
  of pulmonary stenosis, 97, 97*f*
  regular narrow complex tachycardia on, 890
  rhythms of, 890
  ST-elevation myocardial infarction localization and, 779
  for stroke, during hyperacute phase, 636
  of tricuspid regurgitation, 94
  of ventricular septal defects, 107
Electroencephalogram (EEG), in seizures, 850
Electromyography (EMG)
  of dermatomyositis, 276
  of dystrophia myotonica, 677–678
  of myasthenia gravis, 669
  of primary orthostatic tremor, 722
Elephant man, 500
El Escorial criteria, for amyotrophic lateral sclerosis, 654
Eleventh cranial nerve (accessory nerve), testing, 565
Elicit Branham's sign, 422
Elschnig's spots, 386
Embolization, systemic
  in aortic stenosis, 67
  infective endocarditis, 142
Emergency synchronised direct current cardioversion, 889
  complications of, 889
  delivering the shock during, 890
  indications for, 889
Emergency Synchronized Direct Current Cardioversion
  appropriate energy, 889
  type of, 889
Emery–Dreifuss muscular dystrophy, 589*f*, 590
Emollients, for pruritus, 746
Emotional lability, 652, 692
Empagliflozin, 134
Emphysema. *See also* Chronic obstructive pulmonary disease
  chest radiography in, 23
  definition of, 22
  high-resolution computed tomography in, 23
  molecular genetics of, 26
  obstructive pattern, spirometry, 5
  pleural, 829
Encephalotrigeminal angiomatosis. *See* Sturge–Weber syndrome
Endarterectomy, carotid, for carotid transient ischaemic attack, 639–640

Endarteritis
  aortic coarctation and, 790
  patent ductus arteriosus, 790
Enders, John F., 727
Endobronchial ultrasound (EBUS)-guided transbronchial needle aspirate (TBNA), in bronchogenic carcinoma, 48
Endocarditis
  infective. *See* Infective endocarditis
  from prosthetic valve prosthesis, 91
Endocrine syndromes, of bronchogenic carcinoma, 46
Endocrinology, 302
Endometrial cancer, 346
Endomyocardial biopsy, 129
Endoscopy, upper gastrointestinal, in swallowing difficulties, 150
Enophthalmos, 694
Enroth's sign, 314
Enterococcal endocarditis, treatment of, 142
Entrapment neuropathies, 601–602
Eosinophilia
  in asthmatics, 841
  pleural fluid, 831
  tropical, 842
Epidermal growth factor receptor (EGFR) for diabetes mellitus, 356
Epidermolysis bullosa acquisita, 430
Epidermolytic hyperkeratosis, 469
Epidural metastasis, from spinal cord compression, 595
Epigastric mass, 159
Epilepsy. *See also* Seizures
  tuberous sclerosis, 542
Epinephrine (adrenaline), pupillary responses, 697*t*
Epistaxis, hereditary haemorrhagic telangiectasia and, 460
Epitope spreading, 352
Epitrochlear lymphadenopathy, 236
Epley manoeuvre, 753
Epstein–Barr virus, hairy leukoplakia from, 452
Erasmus GBS Outcome Scale (EGOS), 456
Erb's point, 99
Eruptive xanthomata, 438, 439*f*, 558, 559*f*
  conditions of, 438
Erythema ab igne, 440, 441*f*, 442*f*
Erythema induratum, 447
Erythema multiforme, 443
Erythema nodosum, 446, 447*f*
Erythroderma, 533
Escherichia coli, causing urinary tract infection, 153, 164
Essential thrombocythaemia, 229
Etanercept, 249, 271–272
Ethanol injection, multinodular goitre, 317
Evan syndrome, 212
Exercise
  haemodynamics, mitral stenosis, 80
  in multiple sclerosis, 660
  for osteoarthrosis, 264–265
  response in COPD, 22, 24*b*, 26
Exercise testing
  in aortic regurgitation, 60
  in aortic stenosis, 66
  hypertrophic cardiomyopathy, 129
Exertional syncope, 873
Exophthalmos (proptosis), 310, 311*f*
  investigations, 312
  quantification, 312
  unilateral, management, 312
Expressive dysphasia, 623, 749
External compression, 150
Extramedullary haematopoiesis, 177
Extraocular muscles, 719
Exudates
  causes for, 719
  pleural, causes for, 830
  retinal haemorrhages and, clinicopathologic correlations of, 364–365
  transudate and, 162, 830
Exudative maculopathy, 378*f*
Eye
  examination of, 364, 365*f*, 816
  lesions, Crohn's disease and, 156
  manifestations
    Graves' disease, 305
    of rheumatoid arthritis, 271
    Sturge–Weber syndrome, 536*f*, 537
    thyroid disease. *See* Graves' ophthalmopathy
  movements, testing, 564

F

Fabry's disease, 615
Face, examination of
  acromegaly, 296
  cirrhosis of liver and, 816
  lupus pernio and, 479
  myxoedema, 320*f*
  Parkinson's disease, 679, 680*f*
  red, causes in adults, 531
  for respiratory disease, 3
Facial nerve, 610–611. *See also* Seventh cranial nerve
Facial sensation, testing, 564
Facial synkinesis, 705
Facial weakness
  in facioscapulohumeral dystrophy, 627
  in seventh nerve palsy, 702, 703*f*
Facioscapulohumeral dystrophy, 589*f*, 627, 628*f*
  atypical phenotypes, 629
  genetics of, 629
Factitial panniculitis, 447
Faecal calprotectin, for Crohn's disease, 157
Faecal mass, 160
Fahr's disease, 685
Fallot's pentalogy, 118
Fallot's tetralogy, 116
  anomalies in, 117
  arrhythmias detected with Holter monitoring, 120
  chest radiography for, 118–120, 119*f*
  complications of, 117
  constituents, 116–117
  embryological development of, 117
  investigations for, 118–120

Fallot's tetralogy *(Continued)*
  repaired, long-term complications in, 120
  treatment for, 118
  uncorrected, 116
    survival of, 117
  ventricular septal defect and, 108
Fallot's triology, 118
Falls, 343
  clinic, role of, 345
  frequent, 682
  incidence of, 345
  investigation for, 344
  recurrent, treatment for, 344
  vitamin D deficiency and, 344
Familial adenomatous polyposis (FAP), 506, 612
Familial basal ganglia calcification, 685
Familial juvenile polyposis, 506
Familiar hypercholesterolaemia, 558–559
  treatment of, 559
Fantonetti, G. B., 282
Fasciculation, 654
Fatigue, in Parkinson's disease, 685
Febuxostat, 260
Felty, Augustus R., 188
Felty syndrome, 186, 245, 270
  peripheral blood smear in, 187*f*
Feminizing state, causes, 342
Femoral arteries
  compression, Duroziez's sign, 787
  pistol-shot, 58
  pulses, in aortic coarctation, 787
Ferguson, Anne, 158
Fever, 37
  diagnosis of, 37
  investigations for, 38
  medication inducing, 38–39
Fibrates, 557
Fifth cranial nerve, testing, 564
Finasteride, 418
Finger-nose-finger test, 568
Finger reflexes, 567–568
Fingolimod, 662
First cranial nerve, examination, 563
Fisher scale, 870
'Fisher's one and a half syndrome, 646
Fitz–Hugh–Curtis syndrome, hepatic friction rub, 175
Fleischer, Bruno, 185
Flexor carpi ulnaris, 730
Flick sign, 599
Flint, Austin, 62
Floppy mitral valve. *See* Mitral valve prolapse
Fludarabine, 227
18-Fluorodeoxyglucose positron emission tomography, in speech disturbance, 749
Flushing
  causes of, 338
  facial, 338
Focal monomelic upper limb atrophy, 629
Focal-onset seizures, 850
Follicle-stimulating hormone (FSH), deficiency, 301
Food ingestion, effects in tetraplegia, 715

Food protein enterocolitis syndrome (FPIES), 775
Foot
  Charcot's. *See* Charcot's arthropathy
  cutaneous pressure perception, 361
  diabetic. *See* Diabetic foot
  joint disease, examination, 244–245
Foot deformities. *See also* Pes cavus, in Charcot–Marie–Tooth disease
  Charcot–Marie–Tooth disease, 613, 614*f*
Foot drop
  causes of, 622
  in common peroneal nerve palsy, 621
  high steppage gait, 583–584
Foramen magnum, classical syndrome of, 716
Foramen ovale, patent, 101
Forced expiratory time (FET), 4
Forced expiratory volume in 1s (FEV1), 4*f*
  in COPD, 21*b*
  in cystic fibrosis, 18
  progressive reduction of, 23
Forced vital capacity (FVC), 4*f*, 21*b*
Forme fruste, 615
Foster Kennedy syndrome, 394
Fourth cranial nerve
  examination, 564
  lesion, 717
Foville, Achille LF, 708, 733
Foville syndrome, 708, 733
FOXP2 gene mutations, 624
Frankel, Hans Ludwig, 716
Frankel's classification, of neurological deficit, 716
Frank leukaemia, of systemic mastocytosis, 547
Freckling, in axilla or inguinal region, 498
Fredrickson classification, of hyperlipidaemia, 503–504
Friction rub, hepatic, 175
Friedreich, Nikolaus, 632
Friedreich's ataxia, 403, 630
  foot deformity in, 631*f*
  Harding's criteria for, 631
  mode of inheritance, 630
  pathological changes in, 632
  prognosis of, 631–632
Froment, Jules, 731
Froment's sign, 729*f*, 730
Frontotemporal dementia, 579
Functional residual capacity, 3*f*
Fundal examination
  central scotoma, 604
  cerebellar syndrome, 606
  pseudoxanthoma elasticum, 514, 514*f*
  Sturge–Weber syndrome, 535, 536*f*
Fungal infections
  cure in, 451
  vitiligo *vs.*, 554
Fungal nail disease, 448, 449*f*
Furosemide, for nephrotic syndrome, 34, 752
Fusarium, in nail infections, 449

G
Gag reflex, 565

INDEX

Gait
  abnormal, 583
  apraxia, 626
  cerebellar, 583
  in cerebellar syndrome, 606
  festinating, 583, 680–681
  hemiplegic, 583
  high stepping, 583–584, 621
  parkinsonian, 583
  phases, 584f
  scissor, 584
  sensory ataxic, 583
Gallavardin phenomenon, 69, 88
Gallop rhythm, 797
Gallstones, 346
Gammaglobulin, for Guillain–Barré syndrome, 802
Gamma-interferon, 831
Ganciclovir, for hairy leukoplakia, 453
Gardner's hydrodynamic theory, of syringomyelia, 712
Gardner syndrome, 506
Garrod, Archibald E., 265
Gastric antral vascular ectasia, 817
Gastric carcinoma
  pernicious anaemia and, 866
  phlebitis migrans, 508
Gastric erosions, 817
Gastric neuroendocrine tumours, types of, 339
Gastric ulcer, 817
Gastric veins, 167
Gastritis, 817
Gastrointestinal (GI) bleeding
  aortic stenosis and, 68–69
  pseudoxanthoma elasticum, 516
  upper, 817–818
    risk assessment tools for, 819–820
Gastrointestinal (GI) manifestations
  of cystic fibrosis, 16
  of Ehlers–Danlos syndrome, 254–255
  of polycystic kidney disease, 195
  of pseudoxanthoma elasticum, 516
  of scleroderma, 282
Gastroparesis, 150
Gaucher, P. C. E., 178
Gaucher's disease, 178
Gaze, conjugate, mechanisms to, 645–646
Gee, Samuel J., 437
Gefapixant, 36
Gegenhalten, 682–683
Gemfibrozil, 439
General anaesthesia
  for dystrophia myotonica, 677
  for rheumatoid arthritis, 271
Generalised anxiety disorder (GAD), 739
Generalised-onset seizures, 850
Generalized Anxiety Disorder seven-item scale, 740
Generalized lymphadenopathy, 236
Gene therapy, for cystic fibrosis, 18
Genital infection, herpes simplex virus type 2, 462
Gerbode defect, 108
Gerhardt syndrome, 708
Gestational diabetes mellitus (GDM), 882

Gibb, H. P., 678
Gibson murmur, 110
Gifford's sign, 313
Gilbert syndrome, 171–172
'Gin and tonic,' in myasthenia gravis, 670
Gingival hyperplasia, causes of, 232–233
Gintrac, E., 282
Gitelman, Hillel, 811
Gitelman syndrome, 811
Glabellar tap, 680
Glandular fever, maculopapular rash and, 483
Glargine, for diabetes mellitus, 357
Glasgow coma scale, 870
Glasgow outcome scale, 870
  for acute stroke, 637
Glatiramer acetate, 662
Glaucoma, 399
Glaucomatous optic atrophy, 388
Glenn operation, 118
Gliadin, 436–437
Glial myelinopathy, 613
Glomerulonephritis, 143, 745
GLP-1 mimetic therapy, for diabetes mellitus, 356
Glucosamine, 265
Glucose, 148
  pleural fluid, 830, 832
Glucose-6-phosphate dehydrogenase (G6PD) deficiency, 211–212
Gluten, 436–437
  foods containing, 436
  intolerance, 435
Gluten-free diet, 437
Goeckerman treatment, 520
Goitre
  causes, 320–321
  multinodular, 315
    investigations, 316
    natural history, 316
    non-toxic, 317
    thyroid status, 316
    treatment, 317
  simple, investigations, 321–322
  toxic multinodular, 308, 316–317
    Graves' disease vs., 318
    treatment, 317–318
  WHO grading of, 303
Gonda reflex, 571
Gonococcal perihepatitis, hepatic friction rub, 175
Goodpasture's syndrome, 2
Gordon reflex, 571
Gorlin's sign, 257
Gottron's sign, 275, 276f
Gout, 258, 853
  acute
    diagnostic criteria for, 260
    treatment of, 259
  basic pathophysiology of, 258
  chronic tophaceous, 259, 259f
  clinical differences, 261

Gout *(Continued)*
    different clinical manifestations of, 259
    pseudogout *vs.*, 261
    treatment of hyperuricaemia, 259
Gouty arthritis, 259
Gouty tophi, 259*f*
Gowers' sign, 690
Gowers, Sir W. R., 691
Gradenigo, C., 708
Gradenigo syndrome, 708
Graham Steell murmur, 33
'Granny's tartan,', 440
Granulomatosis with polyangiitis (GPA), 292
Grasp reflex, 570
Graves' disease, 305
    components of, 306
    euthyroid, 310
    examination of, 310
    histopathology, 309
    laboratory test, 306
    monitoring thyroid-stimulating antibodies, 308
    pretibial myxoedema, 306, 510, 512*f*
    radioactive iodine uptake, 306
    toxic multinodular goitre *vs.*, 318
    urticaria with, 545
Graves' ophthalmopathy, 312
    Clinical Activity Score (CAS), 312
    eponyms related to, 313–314
    euthyroid, 312
    management, 312–313
    pathogenesis, 309
    pretibial myxoedema with, 510
    signs, 308, 311*f*, 312–313
Grey Turner, G., 509
Grey Turner's sign, 509
Groenblad, E. E., 516
Groenblad–Strandberg syndrome, 516
Gross, J., 304
Grossman, Werner, 781
Gross, R. E., 112
Grover's disease, 323
Grove's sign, 314
Growth factors, in proliferative retinopathy, 382
Growth hormone
    deficiency, 301
    excess secretion, causes of, 299
Gruentzig, Andreas, 781
Gubler, Adolphe Marie, 708, 733
Guillain–Barré syndrome, 800
    diagnosis of, 800
    differential diagnosis of, 802
    features of, 801
    other variants of, 802
    pathology of, 801
    prognosis of, 802
    treatment of, 802
Guillain, C., 803
Gull, W. W., 323
Gunn, Marcus, 389

Guttman, Sir Ludwig, 716
Guyon's canal, 730
Gynaecomastia, 341

H
Haemangiomas, Sturge–Weber syndrome, 535
Haemarthrosis, spontaneous, 216
Haematological disorders, chorea and, 618
Haematological malignancies (AML), 223
Haematopoiesis, extramedullary, 177
Haemochromatosis, 179, 180*f*, 509
    cause of death in, 182
    early identification of, benefit of, 181
    hereditary, 179
    increased iron uptake, mechanism of, 180–181
    joint pain in, 179
    magnetic resonance imaging of, 181, 181*f*
    management of, 181–182
    screening for, 182
Haemodialysis. *See also* Dialysis
    alternatives to, 423
    arteriovenous fistulae and, 192
    artificial arteriovenous fistula and, 422
    carpal tunnel syndrome, 599
    prosthetic arteriovenous access grafts, 423–424
    renal transplantation and, 200–201
    vascular access options, 422
Haemofiltration, 766
Haemolytic anaemia, 211
    aortic stenosis with, 67
Haemophilia A, 216–217
Haemophilus influenzae, 17, 25
Haemoptysis, 2
    medical causes, 293
    patient's management, 293
Haemorrhage
    Eisenmenger's syndrome and, 124
    gastrointestinal, hereditary haemorrhagic telangiectasia and, 460
    splinter, 456*f*
    subarachnoid, 868
Haemothorax, 832
Hair follicles, growth of, 418
Hair loss. *See also* Alopecia
    associated with scarring, 417
    hypothyroidism, 319
    normal, 417
Hairs, exclamation-point, 416
Hairy leukoplakia, 452, 453*f*
Hallervorden–Spatz disease, 685
Hallucinations, in Parkinson's disease, 684*b*
Haloperidol
    for delirium, 762–763
    for hemiballismus, 634
HALT PKD study, 196
Hamartin, tuberous sclerosis and, 543
Hamman, L. V., 32
Hamman–Rich syndrome, 31
Hammer toes, 614*f*
Hampton's sign, 844

INDEX

Hands
  acromegaly, 296, 297f
  bilateral, 734–736
  Dupuytren's contracture, 242–244
  examination of
    cirrhosis of liver and, 816
    for respiratory disease, 2–3
  joint disease, examination of, 242–244, 243f
  osteoarthritis in, 262
  psoriatic arthritis in, 266
  rheumatoid, 269, 270f
    ulnar deviation of, 273
  scleroderma, 279, 280f
  in syringomyelia, 709
  ulnar nerve palsy, 728
  unilateral, 735–736, 735f
  wasting of small muscles, 735–736, 735f
Handwriting, examination of, 721f
Harding's criteria, for Friedreich's ataxia, 631
Harken, Dwight, 82, 92
Harrington, C. R., 303
Harrington, William, 522
Hasenclever index, 239
Hashimoto, H., 324
Hashimoto's disease
  associated conditions, 323
  thyroid status, 320–321
  urticaria with, 545
Hashimoto thyroiditis, 321
HbA1c, 355
  type 2 diabetes and, 355
Headache, 573
  clinical characteristics of, 575
  diagnosis of, 575
  examination for, 574–575
  history for, 573–574
  medication overuse, 576
  primary, 575
  red flag symptoms of, 575
  types of, 575
Head nodding, with heart beat, 59
Hearing loss
  in cerebellopontine angle tumour, 610
  in facioscapulohumeral dystrophy, 627
  multinodular goitre with, 315
Hearing tests, 565
Heart
  development of, congenital heart disease and embryology of, 117–118
  size, in Addison disease, 331
Heart disease. *See also* Congenital heart disease; Coronary artery disease
  carcinoid syndrome and, 339
  in infective endocarditis, 141
  Marfan syndrome and, 59, 83
Heart failure
  aortic coarctation and, 788
  classifying severity of, 56
  in gallop rhythm, 798
  in hereditary haemorrhagic telangiectasia, 458
  jugular venous pulse, 848

  mechanism of anaemia, 848
  mitral regurgitation, 72, 75
  mitral stenosis, 76
  palpable liver and, 174
  patent ductus arteriosus, 112
  ventricular septal defects, 109
Heart–lung transplantation
  indications for, 18
  pregnancy for, 19
Heart sounds, 54, 55f
  in aortic regurgitation, 58, 59f
  in aortic stenosis, 63, 64f
  in Ebstein's anomaly, 113
  fourth
    abnormal, gallop rhythm, 797, 798f
    causes of, 798–799
    mechanism of production of, 798
    split first heart sound and ejection click, 798
  in mitral regurgitation, 72
  in mitral stenosis, 76
  in mixed aortic valve disease, 88
  in mixed mitral valve disease, 86
  in patent ductus arteriosus, 110, 111f
  in prosthetic heart valves, 90
  in pulmonary stenosis, 96
  second
    in aortic stenosis, 65
    split, 100, 101f
  third
    abnormal, gallop rhythm, 797
    in aortic regurgitation, 58
    in aortic stenosis, 64
    causes of, 798
    implications of, in valvular heart disease, 798
    mechanism of production of, 797
    in mitral regurgitation, 72, 75
    in mixed mitral valve disease, 86
    ventricular, gallop rhythm, 797
Heart transplantation, indications for, 135
Heat exposure, erythema Ab Igne and, 440, 441f, 442f
Heat-related skin conditions, 442
Heberden's nodes, 242, 263, 263f
Heberden, William, 265
Heel–shin test, 570
Heerfordt's disease, 703
Helicobacter pylori, 817
Hemianopia
  bitemporal, 596
  homonymous, 642, 643f
Hemiballismus, 633
Hemiparkinsonism, 682
Hemiplegia, 635. *See also* Stroke
  crossed, 733
  gait, 583
Hemisection, of spinal cord, 597–598
Hemithyroidectomy, multinodular goitre, 317
HEMORR$_2$HAGES score, 795, 795t
Hench, Philip S., 854
Henoch, Eduard Heinrich, 457

Henoch–Schönlein purpura, 454, 455f
  clinical features, 521
  differential diagnosis of, 661–662
  IgA nephropathy vs., 456
  investigations for, 455
  treatment of, 455–456
Hepatic arterial bruit, over liver, 174
Hepatic encephalopathy, cirrhosis of liver and, 167
Hepatic friction rub, 175
Hepatitis A, 170
Hepatitis C infection
  cirrhosis, 166
  lichen planus, 471
Hepatocellular carcinoma, 745
  haemochromatosis and, 179b, 182
Hepatojugular reflux, 847
Hepatomegaly, 173
  carcinoid syndrome and, 338
  causes of, 174
  haemochromatosis and, 179
  investigation of, 174
Hereditary haemorrhagic telangiectasia, 458, 459f
  clinical criteria for, 460
  complications of, 460
  genetics of, 459
Hereditary spastic paraplegia, 594
Heredo-degenerative parkinsonian disorders, 685
Hermansky–Pudlak syndrome, 31
Herniated nucleus pulposus, 742
Herpes gestationis, 431
Herpes gladiatorum, 463
Herpes keratitis, 463
Herpes simplex virus (HSV), 462
  encephalitis, 463
  infection
    complications of, 463
    pathogenesis of, 464
    treatment of, 464
  mucocutaneous infections, 464
  type 2, 462
Herpes zoster syndrome, 465
  complications of, 467
  diagnosis of, 467
  HIV and, 467
  management of, 467
  ophthalmic, 465, 466f
  presentation of, 465
  by sensory fibres, of the nerve, 466f
  transmission of, 466
  vaccination for, 467
Herpetic whitlow, 463, 463f
Hertoghe's sign, 319
HFE gene, mutations in, 181–182
Hib vaccine, Felty syndrome and, 188
Hilal, S. K., 871
Hill's sign, 61
Hip, osteoarthritis in, 262
Hirsutism, Cushing syndrome and, 335b
Histamine, urinary, 548

HIV infection/AIDS
  herpes zoster and, 467
  lipodystrophy and, 478
  molluscum contagiosum, 489
  seborrhoeic dermatitis, 533
  tuberculosis and, 52
HLA
  matching, renal transplantation, 201
  sensitization, before transplantation, 201
HLA-B27-positive patients, with ankylosing spondylitis, 249
Hodgkin's lymphoma, 237–240
  localised, risk factors in, 238–239
  presentation of, 237
  prognostic factors of, 239
  staging system, 237–238
  treatment of, 238
Hodgkin, Thomas, 333
Hoehn–Yahr staging, in Parkinson's disease, 683
Hoffmann, Johann, 324
Hoffmann syndrome, 322
Hoffman's sign, 567
Hollenhorst plaques, 373
Holmes' rebound phenomenon, 606
Holmes, Sir Gordon M., 607
Holter monitoring, hypertrophic cardiomyopathy, 129
Holt, Mary, 105
Holt–Oram syndrome, 102
Homans, J., 796
Homonymous hemianopia, 642, 643f
Hope, James, 75
Hope murmur, 72
Hoppe, H. H., 671
Horizontal nystagmus, 647, 753
Hormonal therapy, for hereditary haemorrhagic telangiectasia, 461
Horner, J. F., 698
Horner syndrome, 694
  causes of, 695
    with unilateral headache, 698
  congenital, 695
  features of, 695, 696f
  intermittent, 697
  lesion localization in, 697
Hospital-acquired pneumonia, 842
Hospital Anxiety and Depression Scale, 740
'Hot-cross bun sign,', 665, 666f
'Hot potato' speech, 749
House–Brackmann grades, of seventh nerve palsy, 702–703
Houssay, Bernado Alberto, 301
Houssay phenomenon, 301
Howell–Jolly body, 187, 187f
Hughes, G. R. V., 796
β-Human chorionic gonadotrophin, plasma, 342
Human herpes virus, 481
Human immunodeficiency virus (HIV). *See* HIV infection/AIDS
Hungerford, David, 230
Hunt & Hessle scale, 870
Huntingtin protein, 618–619

INDEX

Huntington disease, 193, 618–619
Hunt, W. E., 708
Hydrodynamic component, venous pressure and, 551
Hydromyelia, 711
Hydrostatic component, venous pressure and, 551
5-Hydroxyindoleacetic acid (5-HIAA), 339, 339f
Hydroxymethylglutaryl co-enzyme A reductase inhibitors, 557
5-Hydroxytryptamine (5-HT; serotonin), 339, 339f
Hyoid, 45
Hyperacute phase, stroke during, management of, 636
Hypercalcaemia
  causes of, 329–330
  hypocalciuric, 330
  sarcoidosis and, 480
  treatment, 330
Hypercholesterolaemia, 504
Hyperinflation
  in COPD, 21f
  dynamic, 22
Hyperkalaemia, 804
  causes of, 805
  electrocardiographic changes, 805
  emergency treatment, 805
  examination, 804
  features of, 804
  foods to be avoided, 805
  initial step, 804
  nonemergency options, 805
Hyperkeratosis, subungual, 448
Hyperlipidaemia
  causes of, 556
  eruptive xanthomata and, 438
  management of, 556–557
  palmar xanthomata and, 503–504, 504f
Hyperlipidaemia, nephrotic syndrome, 199
Hypermagnesaemia, 326b
Hypernatraemia, 806
  blood volume, 807–808
  diagnosis of, 806
  in elder patients, 807
  examination, 806–807
  features of, 806
  history of, 806–807
  initial step, 806–807
  sodium concentration, 807–808
Hyperparathyroidism. See Primary hyperparathyroidism
Hyperpigmentation, 456f
  Addison disease and, 331
  causes of, 332
  haemochromatosis and, 179
Hypersplenism, 187
  criteria for, 187
Hypertension, 203
  in aortic coarctation, 790
  causes of, 205
  complications of, in pregnancy, 881
  follow-up for, 205–206
  idiopathic intracranial, 395
  in Scheie classification, 384
  malignant, 207

obesity, 346
outpatients, investigations for, 204
polycystic kidney disease and, 194
pulmonary, 34
resistant, 207
screening, 204
stages of, 204
third cranial nerve palsy and, 718
treatment, 205–206
Hypertensive agents, guidelines for initiating, 205–206
Hypertensive retinopathy, 383, 384f, 385f
  grading of, 383–385
  morbidity and, 386
Hyperthyroidism
  amiodarone-induced, 309
  apathetic, 512
  atrial fibrillation, 315, 512
  causes, 307
  iodine uptake, 306
  laboratory tests, 306
  multinodular goitre, 316–317
  presentation in elderly, 512
  prevalence, 308
  tremor and, 721
Hypertonic hyponatraemia, 814
Hypertonic saline, inhaled, for cystic fibrosis, 18
Hypertriglyceridaemia, 438
  causes of, 438–439
  coronary artery disease and, 439
  eruptive xanthomata and, 438
  management of, 439
Hypertrophic cardiomyopathy, 127
  complications, 130
  epidemiology, 130–131
  genetics, 130
  investigations, 127–130
  management, 130
  sudden death predictors, 131
Hypertrophic obstructive cardiomyopathy, 65
Hypertrophic pulmonary osteoarthropathy, 745
Hyperuricaemia
  drug for, 260
  treatment of, 259
Hyperviscosity syndrome, 220
Hypocalcaemia, mechanism of, 326
Hypocalciuric hypercalcaemia, 330
Hypocaloric diets, obesity and, 348
Hypogammaglobulinaemia, chronic lymphocytic leukaemia and, 225
Hypogammaglobulinaemia-related disease, 12
Hypoglycaemia, collapse and, 874
Hypogonadism, bitemporal hemianopia, 596
Hypokalaemia, 809
  acid–base balance, 811
  blood pressure, 811
  causes of, 810
  diagnosis of, 809
  digoxin administration, 810
  electrocardiogram findings, 809–810, 810f
  examination, 809
  features of, 809

Hypokalaemia *(Continued)*
  history of, 809
  intravenous administration, potassium, 811
  life-threatening complications, 810
  periodic paralysis, 810
  potassium replacement, 811
  treatment, 811
Hypokalaemic periodic paralysis, 308
Hypomagnesaemia, 326*b*
Hyponatraemia, 812
  classification, 813
  dehydrated patients, 813
  diagnosis of, 812
  euvolaemic patients, 813
  examination, 812
  features of, 812
  history of, 812
  oedematous patients, 813
  symptoms of, 813
  treatment, after urological operations, 815
Hyponychium, disorders of, 493
Hypoparathyroidism, 325
  acute tetany, management, 326
  biochemical features of, 326
  causes, 326
  causes of, 326
  corrected calcium, 326
  diagnosis of, 325
  examination, 325
  features of, 325
  history of, 325
  post-thyroidectomy, 325
Hypoparathyroid tetany, 326
Hypopigmentation, causes, 555
Hypopigmented macules, tuberous sclerosis, 540, 540*f*
Hypopigmented patches, in vitiligo, 553, 554*f*
Hypopituitarism, 300
  affecting life expectancy, 301
  assessment of, 301
  bitemporal hemianopia, 596
  causes of, 300–301
  treatment of, 301
Hypopnoeas, 44
Hypothyroidism, 319
  cardiovascular manifestations, 319–320
  delayed relaxation, 322
  laboratory indicator for, 321
  management, 322
  neurological manifestations, 322
  prevalence, 323
  salient features of, 319–320, 320*f*
  subclinical, 322
Hypotonic hyponatraemia, 814
  treatment, 814–815
Hypoxia, long-term oxygen therapy, 44
Hysteria, 615

I

Ibrutinib, 227
Ibuprofen, for cystic fibrosis, 18

Ice pack test, in myasthenia gravis, 669
Ichthyosis, 468, 469*f*
  inherited, 468, 469*f*
  lamellar, 469
  malignancy and, 412
  X-linked, 468, 469*f*
Ichthyosis vulgaris, 468, 469*f*
Ideational apraxias, 626
Idebenone, in Friedreich's ataxia, 632
Idelalisib, 227
Ideomotor apraxia, 626
Idiopathic interstitial pneumonias, 29
Idiopathic intracranial hypertension, 395
Idiopathic pulmonary fibrosis, 28
  causes of death in, 31
  investigation of, 30
  management of, 31
  mortality in, 30–31
  pathology of, 29
  prognosis of, 31
IL12B, 519
Ileocaecal abscess, 160
Ileostomy site, pyoderma gangrenosum at, 523, 524*f*
Iliac fossa
  left, mass in, 160
  right, mass in, 160
Immune complex-mediated vasculitis, 456*f*, 457
Immunoglobulin A (IgA)-mediated diseases, 429
Immunoglobulin A (IgA) nephropathy, 456
Immunomodulation, in myasthenia gravis, 671
Immunoreactive trypsinogen (IRT) assay, 17
Immunosuppressive therapy
  for autoimmune bullous diseases, 430–431
  for Crohn's disease, 157
  for erythema multiforme, 444
Implantable cardioverter defibrillators (ICD)
  for heart failure, 134
  hypertrophic cardiomyopathy, 130
Impotence, in Parkinson's disease, 685
Inclusion body myositis, 277
Indolent form, of systemic mastocytosis, 547
Infancy
  cyanotic heart diseases of, 124
  myotonia congenita in, 672
Infant Hercules, 322
Infections
  genital, herpes simplex virus, 463
  nail, non-fungal, 450
  pyoderma gangrenosum *vs.*, 525
  pyrexia of unknown origin and, 38
Infective endocarditis
  aortic coarctation and, 790
  in aortic stenosis, 67
  bacteria in, 141
  complications of, 143
  distal infection in, 142
  patent ductus arteriosus, 112
  pathogenesis of, 141
  prognostic factors for, 142
  prophylaxis against, 104
  prophylaxis in, 143

prosthetic valve, 91
pulmonary stenosis, 98
risk factors for, 141
surgery for, 143
Inferior petrosal sinus sampling, 337
Infertility, male, in cystic fibrosis, 16
Inflammatory arthropathy, 742
Inflammatory bowel disease. *See* Crohn's disease
Inflammatory mechanisms, in COPD, 22–23
Infliximab, 271–272
Inguinal lymphadenopathy, 236
Inherited ichthyosis, 468–470, 469*f*
Inhibitors, 217
Inoue, Kanji, 82
Insomnia, in Parkinson's disease, 685
Insulin
  for diabetes mellitus, 356–357
  hypoglycaemia test, 301
  injection, lipodystrophy and, 476
  resistance, 349, 412
Insulin-like growth factor (IGF-1), plasma, 297
Interferon, 813
  in multiple sclerosis, 662
Interferon-α, lupus pernio, 479
Interleukin-12β (IL12B) gene, 519
Interleukin-23 receptor (IL23R) gene, 519
Intermittent positive pressure ventilation, for asthma, 9
Internuclear ophthalmoplegia, 644, 645*f*
Interstitial lung disease
  dermatomyositis, 275
  restrictive pattern, spirometry, 5
Interstitial pneumonia. *See also* Idiopathic pulmonary fibrosis
  idiopathic, 30
  usual, 29
Intertrigo, 347
Intracranial aneurysms
  heritable connective tissue disorders, 406
  polycystic kidney disease and, 193
Intracranial haemorrhage, aortic coarctation and, 790
Intracranial hypertension, idiopathic, 395
Intracranial pressure, raised, 392
Intramedullary pulse pressure theory, of syringomyelia, 712
Intravenous drug use, 816
Intravenous gammaglobulin, for Guillain–Barré syndrome, 802
Intravenous immunoglobulin, in myasthenia gravis, 671
Intravenous methylprednisolone, in multiple sclerosis, 662
Intrinsic factor antibodies, 866
Invasive coronary angiography, in congestive cardiac failure, 133
'Inverted champagne bottle' legs, 613
Involuntary movements, 722
Iodine
  effect on thyroid status, 308
  radioactive. *See* Radioactive iodine
Ion exchange resin, 557
Iron, increased uptake, 180–181
Irritable bowel syndrome, 153–154

Ischaemic tubular necrosis, 767
Itching. *See also* Pruritus
  classification of, 474–475
  spinal tracts and, 475
Ivabradine, for symptomatic heart failure, 134

J

Janeway, E. G., 144
Janeway lesions, 140
Jaundice, 170
  acutely to secondary care, 171
  bilirubin metabolism, 172
  carotenaemia *vs.*, 171
  investigations of, 171
  postoperative, 172
  postoperative, causes of, 172
Jaw jerk, 564
Jaw-winking, 705
'Jack-in-the box' tongue, 617
Jejunal biopsy, 435
Jellinek's sign, 314
Jendrassik manoeuvre, 570
Jerky nystagmus, 647
Jod–Basedow phenomenon, 308
Joffroy's sign, 313
Johnson, F. C., 445
Joint(s)
  aspiration, 892
  examination, 242–245
  hypermobile, 254, 255*f*, 256*f*, 257
  pain, haemochromatosis and, 179
  position sense, testing, 568, 570–571
Joint disease. *See also* Arthritis
  examination of, 242–244
  in unsteadiness, 752
Jugular venous pressure (JVP), 846
  carotid artery pulsations *vs.*, 847
  causes of raised, 846–847
  in constrictive pericarditis, 136, 137*f*
  in cor pulmonale, 33
  examination of, 54
  hypertrophic cardiomyopathy, 127
  prognostic value in heart failure, 848
  tricuspid regurgitation, 94*f*
  waveforms, 846, 847*f*
Juxtaphrenic peak sign, 42*f*

K

Kalischer, Otto, 538
Kaposi's sarcoma, 232, 421
Kartagener, M., 122
Kartagener syndrome, 11, 13, 121
Kayser, Bernard, 185
Kayser–Fleischer rings, 183
Kearns–Sayre syndrome, 403
Kendall, Edward C., 303, 324
Kennedy disease, 656
Kennedy, Foster, 395
Kennedy, John F., 333
Kennedy syndrome, 342

Keratitis, herpes, 463
Kerley, P. J., 82
Ketones, 148
Khan., F., 795
Kidneys
　bimanual examination of, 148f
　changes after unilateral nephrectomy, 190–191
　palpable, 190, 192
　polycystic kidney, 192
　short-term risks of donation, 191
　transplanted, 160. See also Renal transplantation
　unilateral/bilateral, 193
　　palpable, 190
　warm ischaemic time and, 201
Kimpton, M., 795
Klebsiella species, 25
Klinefelter syndrome, gynaecomastia and, 341
Knee arthrocentesis, 892
Knee aspiration
　complications of, 893
　equipment for, 892
Knee jerks
　absent, conditions with, 631
　examination of, 570
Knee joint
　examination of, 244
　osteoarthrosis in, 262
　painful, 853
Knie's sign, 314
Kocher–Debré–Sémélaigne syndrome, 322
Kocher, Emil Theodor, 324
Kocher's sign, 314
Koch, Robert, 52
Koebner, H., 473
Koebner's phenomenon, 471, 553b
Koenen's subungual angiofibromas, 493
Koilonychia, 491
Kolff, Willem, 767
Kornzweig, A. L., 404
Korsakoff's psychosis, 689
Korsakoff, S. S., 689
Krypton red photocoagulator, 370
Kussmaul, Adolf, 136
Kussmaul breathing, 3f
Kussmaul's sign, 136, 848
Kyphoscoliosis
　ankylosing spondylitis and, 247
　congenital, 13

L
Lactate dehydrogenase, pleural fluid, 830
Lactose-free diet, for Crohn's disease, 157
Lacunar infarcts, 640
Lacunar syndromes, 641
La main succulente, 710
Lambert, E. H., 671
Lamotrigine, 813, 850t
Landmark technique, procedure using, 892–893
Landouzy–Déjérine syndrome, 627, 628f
Landouzy, Louis TJ, 629

Langerhans, P., 453
Language
　disorders, 624–625
　dysphasia, 625
　neurological basis of, 623
　therapy, 150
Language therapists, for speech disturbance, 749–750
Latent tuberculosis, 51
Lateral cauda equina syndrome, 783
Lateral chest wall scars, 90
Lateral medullary syndrome, 732
Lateral optic chiasm, lesions of, 732
Lateral popliteal nerve palsy, 621
Laurence, J. Z., 404
Laurence-Moon-Biedl-Bardet syndrome, 403
Leaching, 805
12-Lead electrocardiography, in syncope, 873
Lead-pipe rigidity, 565
Learning disabilities, in neurofibromatosis, 496, 499
Left iliac fossa, mass in, 160
Left-to-right shunting, patent ductus arteriosus and, 112
Left ventricular assist device, 760
Left ventricular dysfunction
　COPD and, 798
　diastolic, 847
Left ventricular hypertrophy (LVH)
　aortic coarctation and, 788, 789f
　aortic regurgitation, 58–59, 59f
Legius syndrome, 498
Legs
　examination of, cirrhosis of liver and, 165
　lower motor neuron signs in, 724–725
　swollen
　　acutely, 785
　　bilateral, 785
　　chronically, 785–786
Leg ulcers. See Lower extremity ulcers
Leiner's disease, 533
Leishmaniasis, 236
Lenalidomide, 227
Lens extraction, 372
Leonardo da Vinci, 105
Leopard skin spotting, pseudoxanthoma elasticum, 515
Leptin, 347
Lesar–Trelat sign, 412
Lesions, in cauda equina syndrome, 783
Leucocytes, 148
Leukaemia
　acute, 231
　ankylosing spondylitis and, 250
　chronic lymphocytic, 225
　chronic myelocytic, 177
　lymphomas converted to, 227
　in neurofibromatosis, 496
Leukoderma, 555
Leukonychia, 491, 492f
Leukoplakia, hairy, 471, 472f
Leukostasis, 234
Leukotriene antagonists, 546
Levetiracetam, for hemiballismus, 634

INDEX

Levine, Samuel A., 75
Levine's sign, 779
Levodopa, 683
Levoversion, 122
Lewy bodies, 681
Lewy body dementia, Parkinson's disease dementia *vs.*, 579
Lhermitte, J. L., 646, 663
Lhermitte's sign, 660
Libman, E., 144
Lichen planus, 471, 472*f*
    diagnosis of, 471
    examination of, 471
    management of, 473
    prognosis of, 473
Lichen simplex, 474, 475*f*
Lichtheim, Ludwig, 866
Lid lag, 310
Lidocaine, 36
Lid retraction, 311, 311*f*
Life expectancy, in myotonia congenita, 672
Lifestyle modifications, for age-related macular degeneration, 370
Light-headedness, 751
Light's criteria, 829
Limb-girdle muscular dystrophy (LGMD), 589*f*, 590, 629, 649
    mode of inheritance in, 649–650
Limbic encephalitis, 764
Limb spasticity, in multiple sclerosis, 662
Lindsay's half-and-half nail, 491, 492*f*
Linezolid, 813
Lipid-lowering agents
    for familiar hypercholesterolaemia, 559
    for xanthelasma, 557
Lipid profiles, serum
    obesity, 347
    primary biliary cirrhosis, 746
Lipoatrophy, 477*f*
Lipodystrophy, 476, 477*f*
    conditions associated with, 476
    familial, 478
    human immunodeficiency virus and, 478
Liposome, 18
Lisch nodules, 496, 497*f*, 498
Lithium succinate/lithium gluconate, topical, 534
Livedo reticularis, 442, 442*f*
Liver
    biopsy, 746
    cysts, in polycystic kidney disease, 193–194
    enlarged, hepatomegaly and, 173
    hepatic arterial bruit over, 174
    metastatic carcinoid tumours from, 338–339
    palpable, causes of, 174
    percussion of, 173
    pulsatile, 174
    tender, 174
Liver disease
    Dupuytren's contracture, 816, 817*f*
    haemochromatosis and, 179

Liver failure
    acute, serum ammonia level and, 167
    ascites, 162
Liver function tests, 745
Liver transplantation
    for ascites, 163
    for primary biliary cirrhosis, 747
LMWH. *See* Low-molecular-weight heparin
Lobar pneumonia, recurrent or persistent, 14
Local anaesthesia, in chest drain insertion, 886–887
Lock, James F., 82
Loculated ascites, in therapeutic abdominal paracentesis, 899
Loewi's sign, 314
Loeys–Dietz syndrome, 256
Löffler syndrome, 841
Löfgren syndrome, 481
Long-acting antimuscarinic antagonist (LAMA), for COPD, 24
Long-acting beta2-agonist (LABA)
    for asthma, 8–9
    for COPD, 24
Long-acting bronchodilators, for COPD, 24
Long thoracic nerve of Bell, 737
    palsy of, 737
Long thoracic neuropathy, 737
Lorazepam, 851
Low-back pain
    of ankylosing spondylitis, 248
    seronegative arthritic disorders, 248
Lower extremity ulcers
    arterial, 551
    causes of, 420–421, 551
    investigation of, 420
    venous, 420, 549
Lower limbs
    bilateral pyramidal lesions affecting, 658–659
    causes of lower motor neuron signs, 724–725
    deformity of, 724
    factors affecting venous pressure, 551
    limb girdle dystrophy in, 649, 650*f*
    neurological examination, 569*f*
    phlebitis migrans, 508
Lower motor neuron lesions
    inverted supinator reflex, 567
    in legs, 724
    of seventh cranial nerve palsy, 703–706, 703*f*
Lower urinary tract symptoms, 581
    acute urinary retention, 582
    chronic urinary retention, 582
    differential diagnosis, 581–582
    examination, 581
    features of, 581
    history of, 581
    investigations, 582
    obstructive symptoms, 582
Low-molecular-weight heparin (LMWH)
    antenatal period, 880
    for venous thromboembolic disease, in pregnancy, 880

Luftsichel sign, 42f
Lumbar puncture, 895
    complications of, 895
    contraindications s for, 896
    course of action in, 890
    procedure for, 895
    sitting up, 895
Lumbar sprain/strain, 742
Lumbricals, 567
Lung
    abnormal, 5
    base of, dullness at, 829
    cancer. See Bronchogenic carcinoma
    consolidation, 829, 838
    pseudotumour, 831
Lung biopsy
    in interstitial lung diseases, 31
    in interstitial pneumonia, 30
Lung collapse, 41, 42f
    cause of, 41–42
    degree of, 861
    differential diagnosis, 829
Lung disease
    ankylosing spondylitis and, 247
    dermatomyositis, 275
    scleroderma, 280
Lung fibrosis, 745
Lung transplantation
    complications of, 18
    for cystic fibrosis, 18–19
    in idiopathic pulmonary fibrosis, 31
    indications for, 27
    single, for COPD, 27
Lung-volume reduction surgery, for COPD, 26
Lupus erythematosus
    drug-induced, 287
    systemic. See Systemic lupus erythematosus
Lupus nephritis, 287
Lupus pernio, 479, 480f
Luteinizing hormone (LH), deficiency, 301
Lutembacher, R., 82
Lutembacher syndrome, 77
Luthy's sign, 601
LV assist devices, 134–135
Lyme disease, 854
Lymphadenopathy, 235
    ALL AGES mnemonic, 235–236
    CHICAGO, 236
    generalized, causes, 236
    maculopapular rash with, 101
    regional, causes, 236
Lymph nodes
    enlarged, 159
    supraclavicular, 235
Lymphocytosis
    causes of, 233–234
    chronic lymphocytic leukaemia and, 225
    peripheral blood smear demonstrating, 226f
    pleural fluid, 831

Lymphoma
    converted to leukaemias, 227
    cutaneous T-cell, 432, 433f, 434f
Lymphomatoid papulosis, 412

M

Machado–Joseph disease, with spinocerebellar degeneration, 632
Mackenzie, James, 848
Macleod, John JR, 478
Macroautophagy, in Crohn's disease, 158
Macroglossia
    acromegaly and, 296
    causes of, 297
Macula, 364, 365f
Macular degeneration, 367f, 368–369
    age-related. See Age-related macular degeneration
Macular oedema
    central retinal vein occlusion and, 400
    signs of, 380
Maculopapular rash, 483, 484f
Maculopathy, drugs causing, 370
Madras motor neuron disease, 653
Magnetic resonance imaging (MRI)
    of acoustic neurofibroma, 611, 611f
    of aortic coarctation, 788
    of atrial septal defects, 103
    of bilateral spastic paralysis, 594
    of Broca's aphasia, 623
    of congestive cardiac failure, 133
    of constrictive pericarditis, 138
    of Cushing syndrome, 336
    of dermatomyositis, 276
    of facial nerve palsy, 705
    of haemochromatosis, 181, 181f
    of hypertrophic cardiomyopathy, 129
    of hypopituitarism, 301
    of multinodular goitre, 316
    of multiple sclerosis, 660
    of multiple system atrophy, 666f
    of seizures, 850
    of speech disturbance, 749
    of subacute combined degeneration of spinal cord, 865, 865f
    for swallowing difficulties, 669
    of syringomyelia, 710, 711f
    of tricuspid regurgitation, 95
Magnetic resonance spectroscopy, dermatomyositis, 276
Malar flush, 76
Malaria, 38
Malassezia folliculitis, 533
Male pattern baldness, 418
Malignant disease. See also Cancer risk
    ascites, in therapeutic abdominal paracentesis, 899
    cutaneous manifestations of visceral, 412
    dermatomyositis, 412
    erythema multiforme from, 444
    ichthyosis, 412

INDEX

Peutz–Jeghers syndrome, 506
phlebitis migrans, 508
pyrexia of unknown origin and, 38
Malignant retinopathy, 384
Mallory–Weiss tear, 817
Mammalian target of rapamycin (mTOR) pathway, tuberous sclerosis, 543
Mantoux, C., 482
Mantoux test, 480
Marantic endocarditis, 143
Marche à petits pas, 584
Marchiafava–Bignami disease, 689
Marcus Gunn pupil, 394
Marfan syndrome, 11
  heart disease and, 59, 83
  pneumothorax secondary to, 859
Marie, Pierre, 250, 299, 616
Masseters, testing, 564
Mastocytosis, systemic, 547–548
Maternal death, causes of, 880
Mayer sign, 568
McCune–Albright syndrome, 299
McDonald's criteria, in multiple sclerosis, 660
McDonald, William Ian, 663
McLeod syndrome, 590
Mechanical heart valves, 90–92
Mechanical ventilation, for asthma, 9
Medial medullary syndrome, 733
Median nerve, 566f, 567
  innervated by, 730
Mediastinal spread, of bronchogenic carcinoma, 46
Mediastinum, abnormal, 5
Medical pleurodesis, 862
Medication-overuse headaches, 576
Medulloblastoma, 609
Mees' lines, 491, 493f
Meig's syndrome, 832
Melaena, 816
Melanocytes, in vitiligo, 554
Melanoma, malignant, 485
  associated genes, 488
  commonest type of, 107
  different types of, 487
  examination of, 485, 486f
  levodopa for, 683
  patterns of growth of, 487
  prognostic factors in, 488
  risk factors for, 487
  treatment of, 487
Melkersson–Rosenthal syndrome, 703
Memory loss, 577
  investigations for, 578
  neuroimaging for, 578
Ménière, P., 648
Meniere's disease, 752
Meningioma, parasagittal falx, 593
Meningococcus groups A and C vaccine, Felty syndrome and, 188
Meningoencephalitis, 467

Mental status, altered
  in cirrhotic patient, 167
  measuring serum ammonia level in, 167
Meralgia paraesthetica, 601
Merlin, 499
Merrick, John, 500
Meryon, Edward, 590
Mesothelioma, 833
Metabolic acidosis, 329, 811
Metachromatic leukodystrophy, 615
Metamorphosia, 366
Metastases, of bronchogenic carcinoma, 46
Metformin, for diabetes mellitus, 356
Methimazole, 309
Methotrexate, 249, 430, 813
1-Methyl-4-phenyl-1,2,3,6-tetrahydropyridine (MPTP), 679
Microangiopathic haemocytic anaemia, thrombocytopenias associated with, 216
Microarrays, 654
Micro-aspiration, in hospital-acquired pneumonia, 842
Micrographia, 679
Microscopic polyangiitis, 292
Microsomal epoxide hydrolase, in COPD, 26
Microvascular brainstem ischaemia, in internuclear ophthalmoplegia, 644
Micturition difficulties, 581
Mid axillary line, chest drain insertion in, 886
Midline cauda equina syndrome, 783
Midsternal vertical thoracotomy, 90
Midsystolic click, 83
Migraine, 575
Mild retinopathy, 384
Milkmaid's grip, 617
Millard, Auguste LJ, 708, 733
Millard–Gubler syndrome, 708, 733
Miller–Fisher syndrome, 801
Milroy, W. F., 785
Minkowski, O., 299
Minot, George, 866–867
Miosis
  in Horner syndrome, 695, 696f
  senile, causing Argyll Robertson pupil, 587
Mitchell, John Kearsley, 253
Mitochondrial impairment, 619
Mitral leaflet, billowing, 85
Mitral regurgitation, 72
  aortic regurgitation with, 89
  aortic stenosis with, 89
  Carpentier's classification of, 74–75
  causes, 73
  congenital cardiac conditions with, 74
  determination of severity, 75
  diastolic rumble, 87
  flail leaflet, 73
  indications for surgery, 75
  investigations, 73–74
  management, 75
  mechanisms, 74–75
  mild, 75
  moderate, 75

Mitral regurgitation *(Continued)*
  natural history, 75
  severe, 75
  third heart sound in, 72, 75, 798
  tricuspid regurgitation *vs.*, 74
Mitral stenosis, 76
  aortic regurgitation with, 89
  aortic stenosis with, 88–89
  causes, 77, 81
  complications, 78
  determination of severity, 78
  haemodynamic changes, 82
  indications for surgery, 81
  investigations, 78
  management, 80–81
  mitral regurgitation *vs.*, 86
  moderate, 81
  natural history, 77
  pathology, 77
  severe (tight), 81
  surgical procedures, 81
Mitral valve
  Carpentier's nomenclature, 84
  cross-sectional area, 80
  prostheses, 90
  repair, 75
Mitral valve disease
  aortic valve disease with, 88
  mixed, 86
Mitral valve prolapse, 83
  associated conditions with, 84
  click mechanism in, 84
  complications of, 84
  management of, 84
  prevalence of, 83
  segments, 84–85
Mitral valve replacement
  atrial fibrillation, 92
  mitral stenosis, 81
Mobitz type I heart block, 856*f*
Mobitz type II heart block, 856*f*
Möbius, P. J., 706
Möbius' sign, 313
Möbius syndrome, 708
Model for End-Stage Liver Disease, 168
Moderate retinopathy, 384
Modified British Medical Research Council questionnaire, 23
Modified Rankin scale, 870
Modified Rankin Scale, for acute stroke, 637
Moles, 485, 486*f*
  ABCDE description of, 485
  atypical, 485, 486*f*
Molluscum contagiosum, 489, 490*f*
Monoclonal antibodies, 813
Monoclonal gammopathy of undetermined significance (MGUS), 220
Monocular diplopia, 408
Mononeuritis multiplex, causes of, 688
Moon, R. C., 404
Moraxella catarrhalis, 25

Morning stiffness, 250, 262
Morton, Newton, 591
Morton's metatarsalgia, 601
Morton, T. G., 602
Morvan syndrome, 712
Moschcowitz, E., 522
Moschcowitz syndrome, 522
Motor neuron disease (MND), 652. *See also* Amyotrophic lateral sclerosis
  characteristic features of, 653
  clinical patterns of, 653
  diagnosis of, 652
  palliative care in, 655
  Parkinsonism and, 665
  pathology of, 654
  symptoms of, 652–653
  treatment of, 655
  types of, 653–654
  wasting of small muscles of hand, 735*f*
Motor neuropathy, causes of, 688
Moulds, in nail infections, 449
Mouniere-Kuhn syndrome, 12
Mouth
  lichen planus in, 471, 472*f*
  Peutz–Jeghers syndrome in, 505, 506*f*
  ulcers in, 473
  white lesions, 473
Mouth ulcers
  erythema multiforme and, 443
  systemic lupus erythematosus, 284, 285*f*
Movements
  involuntary, 722
  poverty of, in Parkinson's disease, 679, 681
MRI. *See* Magnetic resonance imaging
MSCRAMMs, 143
Mucormycosis, rhinocerebral, 718
Muehrcke's nail, 491
Muller's sign, 59
Multifocal intraocular lens implants, 372
Multiple endocrine neoplasia (MEN) type 1, 298
Multiple myeloma, 220*f*
  anaemia of, 219
  bone marrow patients, 220
  complications of, 219
  diagnostic criteria, 220
  erythema multiforme from, 444
  examination, 218
  features of, 218
  IgM, 219
  kidney disease, 219
  light chain deposition disease, 220–221
  treatment, 220
Multiple sclerosis, 657
  in Brown-Séquard syndrome, 597
  clinical categories of, 660
  during coronavirus pandemic, 662
  diagnosis of, 660–662
  exercise in, 660
  Friedreich's ataxia and, 631
  in internuclear ophthalmoplegia, 644
  investigations of, 658

INDEX 937

in jerky nystagmus, 647
medications for, 661
modifiable risk factors for, 661
MRI in, 659f, 660–661
natural history of, 660
pathogenesis of, two-hit model in, 662–663
in pregnancy, 660
presentation of, 659–660
prevalence of, 659
prognostic markers for, 661
risk factors for, 661
treatment for, 662
Multiple system atrophy (MSA), 664
  diagnosis of, 665–666
  diagnostic criteria for, 666–667
  pathogenesis of, 667
  pure autonomic failure vs., 665
  radiological signs of, 665
  types of, 664–665
Murmurs, 56
  in aortic coarctation, 787
  in aortic regurgitation, 58, 61
  in carcinoid syndrome, 338
  continuous, 111
  diastolic
    in aortic regurgitation, 58, 61
    differential diagnosis of, 137
    effects of inspiration, 56
    in mitral regurgitation, 87
  in Ebstein's anomaly, 113
  hypertrophic cardiomyopathy, 127
  mitral regurgitation, 72, 74
    radiation to neck, 74
  mitral stenosis, 76, 78
  mitral valve prolapse, 83
  mixed aortic valve disease, 70, 71f
  pansystolic, 55
    causes, 74
    hypertrophic cardiomyopathy, 127
    mitral regurgitation, 127
  patent ductus arteriosus, 110, 111f
  severity of aortic stenosis, 65
  systolic
    in aortic regurgitation, 58
    effects of inspiration, 56
    Levine's grading, 74
    mitral regurgitation, 72
    short, at apex, 72
  ventricular septal defects, 107, 108f
Murphy's sign, 170
Murphy, William P., 866–867
Murray, Joseph E., 202
Muscle
  atrophy, mechanism of, 727
  biopsy, 276
  delayed relaxation, 322
  hypertrophy, in myotonia congenita, 672
  wasting, in dystrophia myotonica, 675f
Muscleblind-like 1 (MBNL1), 675–676
Muscle fibres, type 1 vs. type 2, 691

Muscle power
  grading, 567
  testing, 568
Muscle tone, assessing, 565–566, 568–569
Musicians, hypermobile joints advantages to, 257
Mutant huntingtin, 619
Myasthenia gravis, 668, 669f, 745
  age and, 668
  associated disorders in, 671
  differential diagnosis of, 724
  drugs causing, 670
  'gin and tonic' exacerbate, 670
  grading of, 670
  groups of muscles in, 669
  immunomodulation in, 671
  investigations in, 669
  treatment modalities for, 670
Myasthenic crisis, 671
Mycobacterium avium, 12
Mycoplasma pneumoniae, 840
Mycosis fungoides, 432, 433f, 434f
Myelodysplastic syndrome (MDS)
  blood film show, 222–224
  classification, 223
  diagnosis of, 222–223
  examination, 222
  feature of, 222
  prognosis of, 224
Myelodysplastic syndromes, 178
Myelofibrosis, 178, 178f, 229
Myeloid metaplasia, 177
Myeloma, osteosclerotic, 802–803
Myeloproliferative disorders, 176
Myerson's sign, 680
Myocardial infarction
  acute
    in dialysis patients, 202
    risk factors for, 779
    sinus bradycardia, 858
  complications of, 779–780
  ST-elevation, localization of, 779
Myogenic stem cell transplant, 590
Myopathies
  dermatomyositis, 277
  distal weakness, 677
  history and examination of, 571–572
  proximal, 690
    causes of, 691
  in unsteadiness, 752
  X-linked, 590
Myositis
  disorders associated with, 277
  inclusion body, 277
Myotonia, 672, 676
Myotonia congenita, 672
Myotonic dystrophy, 677f
Myxoedema. *See also* Hypothyroidism
  facies, 320f
  history, 323
  origin of term, 323
  pretibial, 306, 510, 512f

N

N-acetylcysteine (NAC) infusion
  acute paracetamol overdose, 822
  antidote, paracetamol overdose, 822
  common infusion regime, 823
  side effects of, 823
  staggered paracetamol overdose, 822
Nail(s)
  examination of, 242
    for alopecia areata, 416, 417f
  pitting, 518f
  scrapings, 450
  splinter haemorrhages in, 140, 140f
Nail changes, 491
  disorder of hyponychium, 493
  disorders of lunula, 491
  pitting, 491
  psoriasis and, 266, 501, 517, 518f
  scleroderma, 279
Nail disease, fungal, 448, 449f
Nailfold
  adhesion of, lichen planus and, 472f
  disorders of, 491–493
  telangiectasia, 491
Nail-plate
  disorders of, 491
  thickening, 448–449
Natalizumab, 662
National Institute for Health, in multiple sclerosis, 661
National Institute of Health Stroke Scale, for acute stroke, 637
Natriuretic peptide, serum B-type, in congestive cardiac failure, 132
Naxos disease, 876
Neck
  circumference, obstructive sleep apnoea and, 45
  examination of, 302, 303f
    for COPD, 20
    for respiratory disease, 3–4
  radiation of murmurs to, 74
  stiffness, causes of, 406
  thyroid disease, 305
  visible carotid pulsation in, 58
Necrobiosis lipoidica, 494, 495f
Necrolytic migratory erythema, 509
Necrotizing fasciitis, 786
Nelson syndrome, 331, 337
Nephropathy, immunoglobulin A (IgA), 456
Nephrotic syndrome, 197
  cause of, 198–199
  complications of, 198
  defined, 197
  diagnosis of, 197
  examination of, 197
  history of, 197
  hyperlipidaemia, 199
  oedema, 198
  renal causes of, 198–199
  treatment of, 198
Nerve conduction studies, 601, 622
Nerve injury, 622

Nerves, thickened, causes of, 687
Nervus intermedius (of Wrisberg), 704
Neural canal defects, 727
Neural claudication, 782
Neuralgic amyotrophy, 738
Neurally mediated syncopal syndromes
  description, 873
  pathophysiology of, 873–874
Neural tube defects, 727
Neurapraxia, 622
Neuritis, brachial, 738
Neuroendocrine tumours, 338b
Neurofibromas, 498
  associated abnormalities of, 499
  biopsy of, 498
  plexiform, 498
  type 2 signs, in cerebellopontine angle tumour, 610
Neurofibromatosis, 496
  annual screening, 499
  in child, 499
  inheritance, 499
  type 1, 497f, 498
  type 2, 498
Neurofibromin, 499
Neurogenic itch, 475
Neuroimaging
  for memory loss, 578
  for seizures, 850
Neuroleptic malignant syndrome, 39
Neurological examination, 565–568
  cranial nerves, 563–565
  history, 563
  lower limbs, 568–571, 569f
  for micturition difficulties, 581
  upper limbs, 565–568, 566f
Neurological manifestations
  bronchogenic carcinoma, 47
  hypothyroidism, 322
  of polycystic kidney disease, 194
  of rheumatoid arthritis, 272
  Sturge–Weber syndrome, 537, 537f
  of Wilson's disease, 184
Neurology case, 563
Neuronal axonopathy, 613
Neuropathic foot (ulcers). See also Charcot's arthropathy
  causes, 359
  diabetic, 358, 360f
Neuropathic itch, 474
Neuropathy Disability Score, 361
Neurosyphilis, 586
Neurotmesis, 622
Neutropenic sepsis, 836
Newsom–Davies clinical grading, for myasthenia, 670
Niacin, 439
Nicotinic acid derivatives, 557
Night blindness, in retinitis pigmentosa, 403
Nikolsky, P. V., 431
Nikolsky's sign, 429
Ninth cranial nerve, testing, 565
Nitrites, 148
Node of Cloquet, 236

INDEX 939

Nodular sarcoidosis, 480f
Non-atopic dermatitis, 426
Nondominant hemisphere functions, 625
Non-dominant hemisphere functions, 625
Non-fungal nail infections, 450
Non-Hodgkin's lymphoma, 238
 classification of, 238
 investigations, 239–240
 symptoms of, 238
Non-invasive stress tests, in congestive cardiac failure, 133
Non-invasive ventilation, for COPD, 25
Non-massive pulmonary embolism, in pregnancy, 880–881
Non-proliferative retinopathy, 380
 clinical presentation of, 381
 visual loss in, 380–381
Non-resolving vitreous haemorrhage, surgical technique for, 382
Non-small cell lung cancer (NSCLC)
 drugs used in, 48
 prognosis of, 49
 surgery for, 49
Non-steroidal anti-inflammatory drugs (NSAIDs)
 for ankylosing spondylitis, 249
 for rheumatoid arthritis, 271
Non-traumatic pneumothorax, chest drain insertion for, 886
Noonan syndrome, 98–99
Normal flow–volume loop, 5, 5f
NO SPECS mnemonic, 311–312
Nothnagel, Carl Wilhelm, 719
Nothnagel syndrome, 719
Nowell, Peter, 230
NSAIDs. See Non-steroidal anti-inflammatory drugs
Nucleus pulposus, herniated, 742
Number needed to treat (NNT), 780
Number 3 sign, 788, 790f
Nutrition, in COPD, 27
Nystagmus, 564, 753
 in cerebellar syndrome, 605
 definition of, 647
 dissociated, 648
 downbeat, 648
 horizontal, 647
 in internuclear ophthalmoplegia, 644
 jerky, 647
 pendular, 647
 types of, 647
 upbeat, 648
 vertical, 647
 vestibular, 648

O

Obesity, 346
 acanthosis nigricans in, 412
 adverse health consequences of, 347, 348f
 central, 348
 diet types, 350
 genetic origin, 347
 management, 348–349, 348f
 mechanisms of, 349
 morbid, 347
Obesity hypoventilation syndrome, 44
Ob gene, 347
Obstructive sleep apnoea, 43
Ochsner, A. J., 731
Ochsner's clasping test, 731
Octreotide
 for acromegaly, 299
 for carcinoid syndrome, 340
Oculomotor nerve. *See* Third cranial nerve
Oculopharyngeal dystrophy, 589f
Oedema, non-pitting, pretibial myxoedema, 511
Oesophageal cancer, 150–151
Oesophageal candidiasis, 150
Oesophageal manometry, 151
Oesophageal rupture, pleural effusions and, 830
Oesophageal stricture, 150
Oesophageal submucosal veins, 166
Oesophageal varices, 817
Oesophagitis, 817
Oesophagogastric tumours, 818
Ofatumumab, 227
Oldfield's theory, of syringomyelia, 712
Oligodendroglial α-synucleinopathy, transgenic mouse models of, 667
Olivopontocerebellar atrophy, 665
Olivopontocerebellar degeneration, 685
 with spinocerebellar degeneration, 632
Omega-3 fatty acids, 438
Onychogryphosis, 491
Onycholysis, 491, 501, 502f
 fungal infections and, 448
 management of, 501–502
 psoriasis, 501
Onychomycosis, 448, 449f, 491
Open lung biopsy, for interstitial lung diseases, 31
Ophthalmoplegia, internuclear, 644, 645f
Oppenheim's disease, 676–677
Oppenheim sign, 571
Optic atrophy, 387, 388f
 consecutive, 388
 differential diagnosis of, 387–388
 glaucomatous, 388
 in jerky nystagmus, 647
 in multiple sclerosis, 657
 primary *vs.* secondary, 388
Optic discs, 364
 examination, 604
Optic nerve (cranial nerve II)
 examination of, 563
 lesions of, 643t
Optic neuritis, 659
Optic neuropathy
 compressive, 603, 603f
 investigation of, 388–389
Optic tract, lesions of, 643, 643f
Optokinetic system, 645
Oral appliances, for obstructive sleep apnoea, 45
Oral contraceptives, 446

Oram, Samuel, 105
Orbitopathy. *See* Graves' ophthalmopathy
Orchitis, viral, gynaecomastia and, 341
Ord, W. M., 323
Orlistat, 349
Orthostatic hypotension, in Parkinson's disease, 685
Orthostatic proteinuria, 148
Ortner, N., 82
Ortner syndrome, 82
Osler's nodes, 140, 140*f*
Osler–Weber–Rendu Syndrome, 458, 459*f*
  clinical criteria for, 460
  complications of, 460
Osler, William, 144, 461
Osserman grading, for myasthenia, 670
Osteoarthritis, 262
Osteoarthrosis
  nodal, 263
  types and causes of, 263
Osteogenesis imperfecta, 390, 391*f*
Osteolytic lesions, 219
Osteomalacia, 185
Osteoporosis, 343
  Cushing syndrome and, 334
  management, 345
Ototoxic medication, in vertigo, 752
Ovarian tumours, 160
Overlap syndrome, 277
Oxygen therapy
  for cor pulmonale, 34
  long-term domiciliary, 24

P

Pacemakers. *See* Cardiac pacemakers
Pacemaker syndrome, 857–858
Paganini, Niccolò, 257
Pain
  in cauda equina syndrome, 782
  in Parkinson's disease, 685
  sensation loss of, 709
  spinal tracts and, 475
Pallidectomy, for hemiballismus, 634
Pallidotomy, unilateral posteroventral medial, 684
Palmar hyperkeratosis, 412
Palmar xanthomata, 503, 504*f*, 556, 557*f*
Palms, examination of, 242–244
Palpations
  of abdomen, 147
  of chest, 4
  of thyroid gland, 302
Pancoast, Henry K., 697
Pancoast's tumour, 697
Pancreas–kidney transplantation, 202
Pancreatic carcinoma, 612
Pancreatic disease, associated dermatoses, 509
Pancreatitis, acute. *See* Acute pancreatitis
Panniculitis, 447
Pansystolic murmurs, 55
Panton–Valentine leukocidin-producing *Staphylococcus aureus*, 841

Papillitis, 394
Papilloedema, 392, 393*f*
  causes of, 393–394
  in cerebellopontine angle tumour, 610
  differential diagnosis of, 394
  field defect in, 393
  first manifestation of, 392
  papillitis *vs.*, 394
  simulate, conditions, 394
  stages of, 395
Papulopustular rosacea, 531*f*
Paracentesis, for ascites, 163
Paracetamol overdose
  acute, 822
  antidote, 822
  diagnosis of, 821
  examination, 821
  features of, 821
  history, 821
  King's College Criteria, liver transplant, 823
  maximum oral recommendation, 821
  staggered, 822
  toxicity dose, 822
  treatment nomogram, 822*f*
Paralytic poliomyelitis, 726
Paramembranous defect, 108
Paranasal sinusitis, 13
Paraneoplastic syndrome. *See also* Malignant disease
  in bronchogenic carcinoma, 46
Paraplegia-in-extension, 593
Paraplegia-in-flexion, 593
Paraplegin, 594
Parapneumonic effusion, 831
Parathyroid hormone (PTH), 327
Paraumbilical veins, 167
Parietal anterior circulation syndrome, 640–641
Parietal lobe sign, 625
Parkinsonian gait, 583
Parkinsonism, 682
  heredo-degenerative, 685
  lower half, 683
  motor neuron disease and, 664
  multiple system atrophy and, 666
Parkinson plus syndromes, 685
Parkinson's disease, 679, 680*f*
  causes of, 682
  dementia, 578
  gait, 679
  management of, 683
  mental status in, 682
  pathological changes in, 681–682
  protein diets in, 683
  seborrhoeic dermatitis, 532
  severity of, grading of, 683
  tremors in, 720, 721*f*
Parks–Bielschowsky three-step test, 564
Paronychia, 491
Parry, Caleb Hillard, 314
Parsonage–Turner syndrome, 738
Pars plana vitrectomy, 382, 401
Past-pointing, 606

INDEX **941**

Patellar clonus, 568
Patellar tap (ballottement), 244, 245f
Patent ductus arteriosus, 110
  complications of, 112
  congenital cardiac lesions dependent on, 112
  continuous murmur of, in pulmonary hypertension, 111
  indications for closure of, 112
  lesions associated with, 111
Patent foramen ovale, 101b
Pauling, Linus, 214
Pautrier's microabscesses, 432
PCSK9 inhibitors, for familiar hypercholesterolaemia, 559
Pegaptanib, for age-related macular degeneration, 369
Pegvisomant, 299
Pelger–Huet neutrophils, 229
Pemberton, H. S., 304
Pemberton's sign, 302
Pemphigoid
  bullous, 429–430
  cicatricial, 430
Pemphigus, 429
  pathogenesis of, 430
Pemphigus erythematosus, 429
Pemphigus foliaceus, 429
Pemphigus vegetans, 429
Pemphigus vulgaris, 429
  management of, 429
Pendred syndrome, 315, 322
Pendular nystagmus, 647
Penicillamine
  for myasthenia gravis, 668, 670
  for Wilson's disease, 184
Penicillin, erythema multiforme from, 443
Pentostatin, 813
Percussion
  chest, 4
  in COPD, 21
Percutaneous coronary intervention (PCI)
  for stable angina, 779
  for ST-elevation myocardial infarction, 780
Pericardial effusion, 825
Pericardial knock, 137, 137f
Pericardial rub, 824
  admission indications, 825
  characteristic features of, 824
  examination of, 824, 825f, 826f
  in pericarditis, 824, 825f, 826f
Pericardiocentesis, 825
Pericarditis
  acute, 824–825
  constrictive, 136, 824–825
  effusive-constrictive, 138
  pericardial rub in, 824, 825f, 826f
  tuberculous, 138
Pericardium, function, 826
Periodic paralysis, hypokalaemic, 308
Peri-partum cardiomyopathy, 881–882

Peripheral blood smear
  following splenectomy, 187, 188f
  with large granular lymphocytes, 188f
Peripheral neuropathy, 687
  of diabetes, drugs for, 688
  hereditary, 615
  pyramidal weakness with, 630
  in unsteadiness, 752
Peripheral nystagmus, 753
Peritoneovenous shunting, for ascites, 163
Peritonitis, spontaneous bacterial, ascites and, 164
Pernicious anaemia, 866
Peroneal muscular atrophy. *See* Charcot–Marie–Tooth disease
Peroxisome proliferator-activated receptor-γ coactivator 1α (PGC-1α), 619
PERRLA mnemonic, 563
Persistent purulent cough, 17
Pes cavus, in Charcot–Marie–Tooth disease, 613, 615
Petechiae, 140
Peutz–Jeghers syndrome, 505, 506f
p53 gene, 177
Phacoemulsifacation, 372
Phaeochromocytoma, in neurofibromatosis, 499
Phalen's test, 599, 600f
Pharyngeal phase, of swallowing, 150
Phasic nystagmus, 648
Philadelphia chromosome, 177, 230
Phlebitis
  catheter-associated, 508, 509f
  migrans, 508
  treatment, 509
Phlebotomy, for haemochromatosis, 181
Phlegmasia cerulea dolens, 794
Phonation, 625
Phonation, dysphonia, 625
Phosphodiesterase-4 inhibitors, for COPD, 24
Phosphodiesterase 5 inhibitors, for Eisenmenger's syndrome, 126
Photocoagulation
  for diabetic retinopathy, 370
  for retinal vein occlusion, 401
Photodynamic therapy, for age-related macular degeneration, 369
Phototherapy
  for pruritus, 747
  psoriasis, 520
  in vitiligo, 555
Photothermolysis, port-wine stains, 537
pH, pleural fluid, 830
Phrenic nerve palsy, 467
Physiotherapy, for cystic fibrosis, 17
Phytanic acid storage disease, 403
Pickwick, Mr., 45
Piebaldism, 555
Pigmentation
  generalized, 182
  increased. *See* Hyperpigmentation
  venous ulcers, 549
Pill-rolling movement, 679, 720
Pinprick testing, 568

942 INDEX

Pitt-Rivers, R., 304
Pituitary necrosis, postpartum, 300
Pituitary tumours
  bitemporal hemianopia, 299
  causing acromegaly, 297
  Nelson syndrome and, 337
Pityriasis amiantacea, 533
Pityriasis versicolor, 554
Pityrosporum folliculitis, 533
PKD1 gene, 195
PKD2 gene, 195
Plantar response, 569*f*, 570
Plasma exchange/plasmapheresis
  for autoimmune bullous disease, 430
  for Guillain–Barré syndrome, 802
Platelets, in therapeutic abdominal paracentesis, 898
Pleural biopsy, 829
Pleural effusion, 827
  closed-tube drainage for, 830–831
  differential diagnosis, 829–830
  drug-induced, 832
  exudate *vs.* transudate, 829–830
  investigation in, 850
  malignant, 830
  tuberculous, 832
  ultrasonography for, 831
Pleural fluid
  abnormal accumulation of, mechanisms for, 833
  bloody, 832
  cytology of, 831
  earliest radiological signs of, 832
  investigations in, 850
Pleural tap. *See* Thoracocentesis
Pleural thickening, 829
Pleurodesis, medical, 862
Plexiform neurofibroma, 498
Plummer's nails, 502
Pneumococcal vaccine, Felty syndrome and, 188
Pneumonia
  atypical, 840
  bacterial
    aetiology of, 839
    chest radiography of, 839*f*
    CURB65 severity score for, 839–840
    poorly resolving or recurrent, 840
    suspected, investigation of, 839
  chronic eosinophilic, 841
  community-acquired, 841
  complications of, 840–841
  healthcare-associated, 842
  hospital-acquired, 842
  lobar, recurrent or persistent, 14
  mycoplasma, 840
  survival benefit, 842
  ventilator-acquired, 842
Pneumothorax
  causes of, 861
  investigation of, 860–861
  management of, 861–862
  size of, estimation of, 861
  spontaneous, 859

chest drain insertion for, 886
classification of, 860
tension, 862
POEMS syndrome, 218–219, 802–803
Poliomyelitis
  lower limb deformity in, 726, 802
  provocation, 726
  vaccine-associated paralytic, 726
Polio vaccines, 726
Polycystic kidney disease, 192
  abdominal pain in, causes of, 194
  causes of death, 195
  complications of, 194–195
  diagnostic criteria of, 193
  genetic transmission of, 195
  hypertension in pregnancy, 196
  management of, 193
  pathology of, 194
  prevalence of, 193
  prognostic factor in, 195
  renal manifestations of, 194
  screening in, 195
  treatment for, 196
Polycystins, 194
Polycythaemia rubra vera, 229
Polycythaemia vera, 177, 178*f*
Polydactyly, 402
Polyglandular syndromes, 332
Polymerase chain reaction (PCR) test, 39
Polyneuropathies, classification of, 687–688
Popper, Hans, 175
Portal hypertension, ascites and, 161, 163, 897
Portal hypertensive gastropathy, 817
Portosystemic collaterals, cirrhosis of liver and, 166–167
Port-wine stain
  histology, 537
  Sturge–Weber syndrome, 535
  trigeminal nerve distribution, 537
Positron emission tomography (PET)-CT, in bronchogenic carcinoma, 47
Postcardiotomy syndrome, 826
Posterior circulation syndrome, 641
Posterior parietal lobe, lesions of, 643
Postherpetic neuralgia, 467
Post-partum cardiomyopathy, 881–882
Postpoliomyelitis muscular atrophy, 725
Post-thyroidectomy hypoparathyroidism, 325
Post-transplant immunosuppression, drugs for, 201
Postural hypotension, 664
Potain, Pierre Carl Édouard, 799, 848
Potassium adaptation, 804
Potts shunt, 118
Power
  grading, 567
  testing, 569–570
Predominantly sensory neuropathy, causes of, 688
Preeclampsia, 199
Pre-eclampsia, in hypertension, 881
Pregabalin, for anxiety, 740

INDEX

Pregnancy, 879
  atrial septal defects and, 104
  cardiomyopathy in, 881–882
  chronic hypertension in, 881
  in cystic fibrosis, 19
  diabetic retinopathy and, 381
  Eisenmenger's syndrome and, 125–126
  hypertension in, 881
  maternal death, causes of, 880
  medical problem in, 881
  multiple sclerosis in, 660
  non-massive pulmonary embolism in, 880–881
  polycystic kidney disease and, 196
  propylthiouracil and, 308
  seizures and, 850
  thyroxine replacement therapy, 322
  venous thromboembolic disease in, 880
  ventricular septal defects, 109
Pre-procedure analgesia, in chest drain insertion, 886
Preproliferative retinopathy, 378f
Pressure hydrocephalus, 579–580
Pressure perception, feet, 361
Pressure test, carpal tunnel syndrome, 601
Pretibial myxoedema, 510, 512f
  histology of, 511
  pathogenesis of, 511
  treatment of, 511
  types of, 511
Primary adrenal insufficiency, 332
Primary biliary cirrhosis, 744
  associated diseases to, 745
  association with cancer, 745
  cancer risk to, 745
  corticosteroids, 747
  cure for, 747
  decompensate, 745
  diagnosis of, 745
  examination, 744–745
  features of, 744–745
  history of, 744
  investigations of, 745–746
  liver biopsy, 746
  liver transplantation, 747
    indications, 747
    survival after, 747
  patient investigation, 745–746
  phases of, 745
  presentation of, 745
  stages of, 746
  symptoms, 744
  treatment of, 746
  ursodeoxycholic acid, 747
  in women, 745
Primary ciliary dyskinesia, 11
Primary hypercholesterolaemia, 504
Primary hyperparathyroidism
  biochemical consequences of, 329
  diagnosis of, 328
  examination, 328
  features of, 328
  history of, 328

  multiple endocrine neoplasia 1 (MEN1), 329
  multiple endocrine neoplasia 2 (MEN2), 329
  serum calcium, 329
Primary lateral sclerosis, 653
Primary progressive aphasia, 749
Pringle, J. J., 543
Pringle's disease. *See* Tuberous sclerosis
Prins, M. H., 795
Probiotics, for Crohn's disease, 157
Procainamide, in myotonia congenita, 673
Prognathism, acromegaly and, 296
Progressive muscular atrophy, 653
Progressive supranuclear palsy, 680f
Proliferative retinopathy, 376, 377f, 380
  complications of, 380
Propionibacterium acnes, 413
Proprotein convertase subtilisin/kexin type 9 protease (PCSK9), 559
Proptosis. *See* Exophthalmos
Propylthiouracil, 307
Prosopagnosia, 626
Prostate-specific antigen (PSA), for micturition difficulties, 582
Prosthetic arteriovenous haemodialysis-access graft, 423–424, 423f
Prosthetic heart valves, 90
  aortic, 90
  causes of anaemia, 91
  complications, 91
  heart sounds, 90
  indications for, 91
  mitral, 91
  types, 90–91
Prosthetic valve endocarditis, 91, 142–143
Protein, 148
Protein diets, in sudden and substantial loss of mobility, 683
Proteinuria, with rheumatoid arthritis, 272
Proteolysis, in COPD, 23
Prothrombin time (PT), prolonged, normal APTT and, 216
Proton pump inhibitors (PPIs), 813
  for gastrointestinal bleeding, 816
Proximal muscle weakness, 275
Proximal myopathy, 690
Pruritoceptive itch, 474
Pruritus (itching), 744. *See also* Primary biliary cirrhosis (PBC)
  atopic dermatitis, 425
  in cholestasis, 746
  control, 746
  jaundice and, 170
  pathogenesis of, 746
  phototherapy for, 747
  primary biliary cirrhosis and, 746
  treatment of, 746
Pseudobulbar palsy, 692
  bulbar palsy and, 693
Pseudo-Cushing syndrome, 337
Pseudogout, 259f, 260
Pseudogout attack, 261

Pseudohypoparathyroidism, 326
  description, 326
  physiological effects of, 327
Pseudomonas aeruginosa, 17, 25, 450
Pseudopseudohypoparathyroidism, 326
Pseudotumour cerebri, 395
Pseudoxanthoma elasticum, 513, 514*f*, 515*f*
Psoriasis, 517, 518*f*
  clinical features of, 517
  erythrodermic, 519
  estimating severity of, 518
  exacerbating factors of, 519
  genetics of, 519
  guttate, 519
  inverse, 519
  management of, 519–520
  nail changes in, 266, 501, 517, 518*f*
  nose, ears, fingers and toes, 520
  pathogenesis and therapy of, 268
  patterns of joint involvement, 266–267
  plaque, 519
  prevalence of, 517
  pustular, 519
  types of, 518–519
Psoriatic arthritis, 248, 266, 267*f*, 517
  pathogenesis and therapy of, 268
  patterns of joint involvement, 266
  prognosis of, 267
PSORS1 gene, 519
Psychogenic itch, 475
Psychological symptoms, of Parkinson's disease, 685–686
Psychosis, in Parkinson's disease, 685
Pterygoids, testing, 564
Ptosis, 694
  in Argyll Robertson pupil, 586
  bilateral, causes of, 677
  causes of, 697
  in dystrophia myotonica, 674
  third cranial nerve palsy and, 717
Pulfrich effect, 663
Pulmonary arteriovenous malformations, 458
Pulmonary artery, unilateral absence of, 13
Pulmonary balloon valvuloplasty, 118
Pulmonary embolism
  anticoagulation recommendation, 845
  chest X-ray, 844
  defined, 844
  diagnosis of, 844
  electrocardiogram findings, 844, 845*f*
  examination, 843
  features of, 843–844
  gold standard investigation, 844
  history of, 843
  non-massive, in pregnancy, 880–881
  pulmonale and, 34*f*
  risk of, in below-knee thrombi, 795
Pulmonary eosinophilic disorders, 841–842

Pulmonary fibrosis. *See also* Interstitial pneumonia
  caveolin in, 31
  genetic disorders with, 31
  idiopathic, 28
Pulmonary function tests, in interstitial pneumonia, 30
Pulmonary haemorrhages, restrictive pattern, spirometry, 5
Pulmonary hypertension, 34
  in atrial septal defects, 101, 104
  in mitral stenosis, 81
  in patent ductus arteriosus, 111
  in ventricular septal defects, 106, 109
Pulmonary oedema, restrictive pattern, spirometry, 5
Pulmonary regurgitation, ventricular septal defects, 106
Pulmonary rehabilitation, for bronchiectasis, 13
Pulmonary stenosis, 96
  associated syndromes, 98–99
  balloon valvotomy in, 99
  cause of, 96–97
  complications of, 98
  grading of severity, 98
  types, 97
Pulmonary tuberculosis, 50
  antituberculous treatment, 52
  contacts screening, 51
  diagnosis of, 50
  early diagnosis of, 51
  examination of, 50
  features of, 50
  history of, 50
  risk factors, 50–51
  sputum-positive, 51
  treatment, 51
Pulmonary valve area, 97
Pulse(s)
  aortic regurgitation, 59, 59*f*
  aortic stenosis, 63, 64*f*
  arterial leg ulcers, 420
  bradycardia, 855
  collapsing, 110, 422, 760
  examination of, for respiratory disease, 3
  jerky, mitral regurgitation, 72, 74
  mixed aortic valve disease, 70
  pseudoxanthoma elasticum, 513
Pulse pressure
  in aortic coarctation, 787
  in aortic regurgitation, 59
  in aortic stenosis, 64
Pulse rate, slow, 855
Pulsus paradoxus, acute severe asthma and, 8
Pulsus parvus et tardus, 63
Pupillary light reflex, nerve pathways of, 587
Pupils
  eccentric, 587
  examination, 563
  grossly unequal. *See* Anisocoria
  small, 587. *See also* Miosis
Pure sensory stroke, 641
Purpura, 521, 522*f*
  palpable, 454*b*
Pursuit movements, testing, 564

Pursuit system, 645
Pustules, 456f
Putnam–Dana syndrome. *See* Subacute combined degeneration, of spinal cord
Putnam, James Jackson, 866
Pyoderma gangrenosum, 523, 524f
  associated conditions, 525
  differential diagnosis, 523
  ileostomy site, 523, 524f
  variants, 523
Pyogenic bacterial infection, 784
Pyostomatitis vegetans, 524
Pyramidal lesions, bilateral, in lower limbs, 658–659
Pyramidal weakness, with peripheral neuropathy, 631
Pyrexia of unknown origin, differential diagnoses of, 38

Q

Queen Anne's sign, 319
Quick sequential organ failure assessment (qSOFA), 836
Quincke, H. I., 62
Quincke's sign, 58
Quinidine, in myotonia congenita, 673
Quinton, Paul M., 19

R

Radial nerve
  cutaneous supply of, 701
  entrapment, 602
  in forearm, branches of, 701
  muscles supplied by, 701
  origin of, 701
  testing, 731
Radial nerve palsy, 699, 700f
  high, 700–701
  low, 701
  management of, 701
  sensory impairment in, 699, 700f
Radial pulse, absent, 757
Radicular pain, in tetraplegia, 714
Radioactive iodine
  therapy
    advantages and disadvantages, 307
    advice to patients, 308
    contraindications to, 307–308
    hyperthyroidism, 307
    hypothyroidism after, 319
    multinodular goitre, 317
    thyroid eye disease, 313
    uptake in Graves' disease, 306
Radiography. *See also* Chest radiography
  for cellulitis, 785
  of Charcot's foot, 253f
  of osteoarthrosis, 263f, 264
  of psoriatic arthritis, 267
  for pyogenic bacterial infection, 785
Radiotherapy. *See also* Radioactive iodine, therapy
  for acromegaly, 318
  for bronchogenic carcinoma, 49

Rai staging, chronic lymphocytic leukaemia, 226–227
Raja, O. G., 863
Ramsay Hunt, James, 706
Ranibizumab, for age-related macular degeneration, 369
Ranson criteria, 770–771
Rapid eye movement behaviour disorders, in Parkinson's disease, 685
Rashes
  dermatomyositis, 275
  erythema Ab Igne and, 441f, 442, 442f
  erythema multiforme and, 443
  in herpes zoster, 465
  maculopapular, 483, 484f
  purpuric, 454
  reticulated, 442
  in systemic lupus erythematosus, 284, 285f
Raymond–Cestan syndrome, 716
Raymond syndrome, 708
Raynaud, Auguste-Maurice, 283
Raynaud's phenomenon, 527, 528f
  causes of, 528–529
  investigations for, 529
  primary Raynaud's *vs.*, 527–528
  scleroderma, 279, 527, 528f
  treatment of, 529
Raynaud syndrome, 745
Reactive arthritis, 854
Reading difficulty, 626, 642
Rebound phenomenon, 606
Receptive dysphasia, 749
Rectal bleeding, aortic stenosis with, 68
Rectal submucosal veins, 167
Recurrent venous thrombosis, 795–796
Reddish-brown macules, 547
Red reflex, 364
Refsum's disease, 403, 613
Refsum, Sigvald, 404
Regional lymphadenopathy, 236
Rehabilitation, after stroke, 638
Reid's classification, of bronchiectasis, 13–14
Reiter, H. C., 250
Reiter syndrome, 246
Rejection of transplanted kidneys, 202
Relaxation techniques, for anxiety, 740
Rembrandt, 531
Renal calculi, in polycystic kidney disease, 195
Renal cysts
  bilateral, 193
  in polycystic kidney disease, 193
  tuberous sclerosis, 541
Renal disease
  chronic. *See* Chronic renal failure
  end-stage, 200
  scleroderma, 280b
  systemic lupus erythematosus, 286
Renal replacement therapy, indications for, 766
Renal transplantation
  blood transfusion before, 201
  complications of, 201
  contraindications to, 201

Renal transplantation *(Continued)*
  dialysis, in age group, 201
  HLA-matching, 201
  indications for, 200
  rejection of, 202
  survival rate of, 202
  timing of referral, 200
  warm ischaemic time and, 201
Renal tubular acidosis type 1 (RTA 1), 810
Rendu, HJLM, 461
Rendu–Osler–Weber disease. *See* Hereditary haemorrhagic telangiectasia
Resistant hypertension, 207
Resistin, 349
Respiratory case, 2
Respiratory failure, acute, treatment for, 25
Respiratory manifestations, of cystic fibrosis, 16
Respiratory system
  examination of, 2
  history of, 2
Restless legs, in Parkinson's disease, 685
'Rest pain' syndrome, 419
Retinal arteriolar narrowing, 385
Retinal artery occlusion, 373, 374*f*
  central, 604
Retinal detachment, 396, 397*f*
  pathology of, 396
  surgical procedures for, 398
  surgical technique for, 382
  types of, 396–398
Retinal haemorrhages, exudates and, clinicopathologic correlations of, 364–365
Retinal pigment, loss, age-related macular degeneration, 369*f*
Retinal vein occlusion, 398
  branch, 399, 400*f*
    prognosis of, 401
  central, 399, 400*f*
    clinical course in, 401
    complications of, 401
    management of, 401
    vascular responses to, 401
Retinal vein thrombosis, 393, 400*f*
  branched, 400*f*
    occlusion sites of, 400–401
  central, 400*f*
Retinal vessels, 364
Retina, telangiectasias, 627
Retinitis pigmentosa, 102, 403*f*
  genetics of, 403–404
  inverse, 404
  management of, 404
  ocular conditions are associated with, 404
  present, 403
  prognosis in, 402
  secondary, 404
  sine pigmento, 404
  systemic disorders associated, 403

Retinopathy
  diabetic, 380
  hypertensive, 383, 384*f*, 385*f*
    grading of, 383–385
    morbidity and, 386
Retinopexy, pneumatic, 398
Retroperitoneal lymphadenopathy, 159
Reversible ischaemic neurological disease, 640
Rhegmatogenous retinal detachment, 396–397
Rheumatic heart disease, 86
Rheumatoid arthritis, 29
  anaemia in, 270–271
  anti-cyclic citrullinated peptide antibodies of, 272–273
  cadherins in, 273
  causes of proteinuria, 272
  cutaneous manifestations of, 272
  Felty syndrome and, 186
  hands, 269, 270*f*
  joints affected in, 271
  neurological manifestations of, 272
  palindromic, 271, 854
  phosphatidylinositol 3′-kinase-γ in the Rheumatoid arthritis
    pathogenesis of, 273
  pleural effusions and, 830
  poor prognostic factors of, 273
  pulmonary manifestations of, 271
  skin lesions, 270
  treatment of, 271–272
Rheumatoid factor, pleural fluid, 831
Rheumatoid nodules, 269, 270*f*
Rheumatology, 242
  case studies on, 242
Rhinophyma, 530, 531*f*
Rib notching, 788–789
Riboflavin, for migraine, 575
Rich, A. R., 32
Richet, Charles, 776
Richter's syndrome, 227
Rickets, Wilson's disease and, 185
Rifampicin, for bacterial endocarditis, 142
Right heart catheterization, 133
Right iliac fossa, mass in, 159
Right internal jugular catheter, insertion of, steps for, 884–885
Right ventricular failure, pulmonary stenosis, 96
Rigidity, 682–683
  examination, 565
  in Parkinson's disease, 679, 681
Riley–Day syndrome, 11
Riluzole, for motor neuron disease, 655
Rimonabant, 349
RIND. *See* Reversible ischaemic neurological disease
Ringworm, 449
Rinne, H. A., 572
Rinne's test, 565
Risperidone, for delirium, 762–763
Rituximab, 227, 271–272, 430
  Graves' ophthalmopathy, 312–313
  systemic lupus erythematosus, 287–288

INDEX

Robbins, Frederick C., 727
Rockall score, 819
Rockall, Tim, 820
Roflumilast, for COPD, 24
Roger, Henri, 109
Romberg, M. H., 727
Romberg's test, 571
Roosevelt, Franklin Delano, 727
Rosacea, 530
Rosenbach's sign, 313
Rosenberg, E. F., 854
Rosenmüller node, 236
Roth, M., 144
Roussy–Lévy disease, with spinocerebellar degeneration, 632
Roussy–Lévy syndrome, 615
Roux-en-Y gastric bypass, 349

S

Saccadic movements, testing, 564
Saccadic system, 645
Saccular bronchiectasis, 14
Sachs, B. P., 389
Sacks, B., 144
Sacroiliitis
    ankylosing spondylitis and, 248
    psoriatic arthritis and, 266
Saddle anaesthesia, 782
Salicylates, erythema multiforme from, 443
Saliva, drooling of, 679
Salt-wasting nephropathies, 811
Salt wasting syndrome, 813–814
San Francisco Syncope Rule (SFSR), 874
Sarcoglycan complex of proteins, 649
Sarcoidosis
    cardiac, 482
    cutaneous, 479–480
    investigation for, 480–481
    nodular, 480*f*
    ocular manifestations of, 481
    presentation of, 480
    prognosis of, 481
    treatment of, 481
    viral infections and, 481
Sarcopenia, in unsteadiness, 752
SARS-CoV-2, 37, 39
Saturday night palsy, 699
Savitz, S. I., 733
Scapula, winging of, 738*f*
Scapulohumeral dystrophy, 629
Schaefer reflex, 571
Scheie Classification, of hypertensive retinopathy, 384, 385*f*
Schilder's disease, 661
Schirmer filter paper test, 272
Schmidt syndrome, 332
Schober's test, 247
Schönlein, Johannes Lucas, 457
Schwannomas, 498
Schwannomin, 499

Schwartz, William, 815
Scissor gait, 584
Scleral buckling, 398
Sclerodactyly, 279, 745
Scleroderma
    diffuse cutaneous, 281
    limited cutaneous, 281
    Raynaud's phenomenon, 279, 523, 524*f*
    sine scleroderma, 281
Scopulariopsis brevicaulis, in nail infections, 449
Scotoma
    caecocentral, 603
    central, 603, 603*f*
    definition, 604
Scrapings, nail, 450
Seborrhoeic dermatitis, 532, 533*f*
Secondary biliary cirrhosis, 747
Secondary hypercholesterolaemia, 504
Secondary retinal detachment, 397–398
Second cranial nerve. *See* Optic nerve
Seizures, 849. *See also* Epilepsy
    causes of, 850
    classification of, 849–850
    investigation of, 850
Seldinger technique, in right internal jugular catheter insertion, 884–885
Selective serotonin reuptake inhibitors (SSRIs), 740, 813
Semmes–Weinstein monofilaments, 361
Senile macular degeneration. *See* Age-related macular degeneration
Sensation
    loss of, in common peroneal nerve palsy, 621
    testing, 568, 570
Sensorimotor stroke, 641
Sensory ataxia, 583, 607
Sensory loss
    in Brown-Séquard syndrome, 598*f*
    in common peroneal nerve palsy, 621
    dissociated, 710
        causes of, 710
        onion-skin pattern, of face, 709, 711
    in radial nerve palsy, 699*b*, 700*f*
    in tetraplegia, 714
Sepsis
    diagnosis of, 835
    examination, 834–835
    features of, 834–835
    history of, 834
    neutropenic sepsis, 836
    prognosis of, 836–837
    risk group, 835
    shock, 835
Sepsis shock, 835
Septic arthritis, 853
    causative agent of, 854
    risk factors, 854
Septic emboli, to vasa vasorum, 143
Serotonin (5-HT), 339, 339*f*
Serotonin noradrenaline reuptake inhibitors (SNRIs), for anxiety, 740

Serratus anterior, 738
  action of, 738
Seventh cranial nerve (facial nerve)
  branches of, 704–705
  reflexes involving, 705
  sensory component of, 704
  testing, 564–565
Seventh cranial nerve palsy (facial nerve palsy), 702
  bilateral, 703
  House–Brackmann grades, 702–703
  imaging studies of, 705–706
  localization of lesion, 705
  lower motor neuron type, 703, 703f
  Lyme disease, 854
  unilateral, 703–704
  upper motor neuron type, 703, 703f
Sexual dysfunction
  in multiple sclerosis, 662
  SSRI medication and, 740
Sézary–Lautner cells, 432
Sézary syndrome, 434
Shagreen patches, 539
Shawl sign, 275
Sheehan syndrome (postpartum pituitary necrosis), 300
Sherlock, Sheila, 175
Sherrington, Sir Charles, 626
Shh pathway, 609
Shifting granuloma sign, 42f
Shingles. *See* Herpes zoster syndrome
Shins, skin lesions, 495
Shipbuilder, 833
Short-acting bronchodilators, for COPD, 23–24
SHOVE mnemonic, 563
Shovlin, Claire, 461
Shy–Drager syndrome, 664–665
Sibutramine, 349
Sicca syndrome, 745
Sick euthyroid syndrome, 323
Sickle cell disease, 214
Sillence classification, of osteogenesis imperfecta, 391
Single-nucleotide polymorphisms (SNPs), 49, 654
Sinopulmonary infection, chronic, 13
Sister Joseph's nodule, 237, 237f
Sitostanol-ester margarine, 557
Situational syncope, 872
Situs inversus, 13, 121
Situs solitus, 121
Sixth cranial nerve
  examination, 768
  nucleus of, 708
  palsy, 707
Sjögren's syndrome, 28, 271, 745
  in urticaria, 544b
Skeletal defects, restrictive pattern, spirometry, 5
Skeleton
  abnormalities in, 390
  lesions, in neurofibromas, 498
Skin
  bleeding, aortic stenosis with, 68–69

  temperature, of Charcot's foot, 252
  tumours, histology of, 498
  wounds, Ehlers–Danlos syndrome, 254
Skin biopsy
  for dermatitis herpetiformis, 435
  for Henoch–Schönlein purpura, 455
  for mycosis fungoides, 432
  for pseudoxanthoma elasticum, 516
  for pyoderma gangrenosum, 525
Skin lesions
  in dermatomyositis, 275, 276f
  in diabetes, 495
  in Ehlers–Danlos syndrome, 254, 255f
  heat or cold-related, 442
  in malignant disease, 412
  in pancreatic disease, 508
  in rheumatoid arthritis, 270
  in shins, 495
Skin moisturisers, for pruritus, 746
Skin rashes. *See* Rashes
Skin tags
  in acanthosis nigricans, 411
Skull radiography
  bitemporal hemianopia, 596
  Sturge–Weber syndrome, 537f
SLE. *See* Systemic lupus erythematosus
Sleep apnoea, obstructive, 43
Sleep-disordered breathing, patterns of, 44f
'Slit-like void sign,', 665, 666f
Small cell lung cancer (SCLC)
  prognosis of, 49
  single-nucleotide polymorphisms in, 49
  surgery of, 48
Small-vessel ANCA-associated vasculitis, 291f
  Churg–Strauss disease, 292
  classification, 291–292
  diagnosis of, 291
  examination, 290–291
  features of, 290–291
  history of, 290
  microscopic polyangiitis, 292
  patient investigation, 293
  respiratory complications, 293
  Wegener's granulomatosis, 292
Smell, assessing sense of, 563
Smith antigen, 286b
Smith, Robert W., 499
Smithy, Horace, 82
Smoking
  cataracts and, 371
  communicating spirometry results and, 27
  in emphysema, 26
  Graves' ophthalmopathy and, 310, 313
  in Parkinson's disease, 679
Snout reflex, 705
Sodium, restriction of, for patient with cirrhosis and ascites, 163
Sodium valproate, 722, 813
Solomon, D. H., 314
Sonic hedgehog (Shh) pathway, 609
Sore throat, 39

Souttar, Henry, 82
Spasticity, 682–683
  Ashworth scale and, 658
  in tetraplegia, 714
Spastic paralysis/paraparesis
  bilateral. *See* Spastic paraplegia
  in Brown-Séquard syndrome, 598*f*
  multiple sclerosis and, 657
  one leg, 594
  scissor gait, 584
Spastic paraplegia (bilateral spastic paralysis), 592
  causes, 593
  hereditary, 594
  intracranial causes, 593
  investigations, 594
  lesion localization, 594–595
  tropical, 594
Speech
  components of, 625
  genetics of, 624
  scanning, 606
Speech disturbance, 748. *See also* Dysarthria; Dysphasia
  management of, 693
Spender, J. K., 265
Spina bifida, 710, 724, 726
  closed, 724, 727
  prenatal screening tests for, 727
Spinal bulbar muscular atrophy, 656
Spinal cord
  arteriovenous malformations, hereditary haemorrhagic telangiectasia and, 460
  hemisection of, 597–598
  relationship to vertebrae, 782–783
  subacute combined degeneration of, 864
Spinal cord compression
  epidural metastasis, 595
  incomplete, 593
Spinal cord lesions
  Frankel's classification of neurological deficit, 716
  hemisection. *See* Brown-Séquard syndrome
  localization, 594
  non-traumatic causes for, 715
  partial transection, 593
  total transection, 593*t*
Spinal injuries, acute high, air transport, 716
Spinal muscular atrophy, 342, 653
Spinal stenosis, 742
Spine, osteoarthritis in, 263
Spinocerebellar degeneration, 632
Spinothalamic sensation, loss of, 597
Spirometry, 4*f*
  communicating results to patients, 27
Spironolactone, gynaecomastia caused by, 341
Spleen
  enlarged, 176
  palpable, 177
Splenectomy
  indications for, 187
  peripheral blood smear following, 187, 187*f*

Splenomegaly, 176
  causes of, 176
  diagnosis of, 176
  differential diagnosis of, 177
  Felty syndrome and, 186
  lymphadenopathy with, 235
Splenorenal shunts, 167
Splinter haemorrhages, 140, 140*f*, 456*f*
Splints, 701
Spondylarthropathies, classification models, 248
Spondylolisthesis, 742
Spontaneous (non-traumatic) pneumothorax, chest drain insertion for, 886
Sputum cytology, in bronchogenic carcinoma, 47
Sputum-positive pulmonary tuberculosis, 51
Squint, 717
Stable angina, 778–779
Staphylococcal superinfection, atopic dermatitis and, 426
Staphylococcus aureus
  causing persistent purulent cough, 17
  in nail infection, 450
  Panton–Valentine leukocidin-producing, 841
STarT Back Tool, 743
Stasis dermatitis, 549
Statins
  for familiar hypercholesterolaemia, 559
  for xanthelasma, 557
Status epilepticus
  description, 851
  treatment procedures, 852
Steatorrhoea, treatment of, 16
Steele–Richardson–Olszewski disease, 685
Steinberg's triad, 658
ST-elevation myocardial infarction (STEMI)
  localization of, 779
  therapy for, 780
Stellwag's sign, 313
Stem cells, for Parkinson's disease, 684
Stereotactic radiosurgery, 612
Sternomastoid muscles, testing, 565
Steroids
  cataracts and, 372
  for chronic asthma, 7
  continuous use of, 8
  in multiple sclerosis, 660
  for sarcoidosis, 481
Stevens, A. M., 445
Stevens–Johnson syndrome, 444
Still disease, 245
Stokes–Adams syndrome, 858
Stokes, W., 858
Strandberg, J., 516
Strauss, L., 689
Streptococcus pneumoniae, 12
Striatonigral degeneration, 664
Stridor, multinodular goitre with, 315
Stroke
  acute
    imaging in, 636
    ischaemic, blood pressure reduction in, 636–637

Stroke *(Continued)*
    thrombolysis in, 637
    tools for, 637
  annual risk of, 890
  causes of, 636
  causing expressive dysphasia, 623
  classification of, 640–641
  discharge of, 638
  in hemiballismus, 633
  during hyperacute phase, management of, 636
  lateral medullary syndrome caused by, 732
  obstructive sleep apnoea and, 43
  polycystic kidney disease and, 192
  rehabilitation after, 638
  risk factors for, 639
  understanding, 640
Strümpell, Adolf, 250
Sturge–Weber syndrome, 535, 536f
  inheritance, 535
  treatment, 537
Sturge, William A., 538
Stuttering, 624
Subacute combined degeneration, of spinal cord, 864
  investigation of, 865–866
  pathology of, 865
Subarachnoid haemorrhage
  cause of, 406–407
  complications of, 870
  deterioration in, 407
  diagnosis of, 868
  examination, 868
  features of, 868
  heritable connective tissue disorders, 516
  history of, 868
  management of, 407
  non aneurysmal, 871
  noninvasive method, 869
  patient investigation, 869
  pharmacological agent, 870
  in polycystic kidney disease, 194
  scoring systems, 870–871
Subhyaloid haemorrhage, 405, 406f
  cause of, 406–407
  investigations of, 407
Subthalamic nucleus, contralateral, hemiballismus in, 633
Subungual angiofibromas, 493, 541f
Subungual hyperkeratosis, 448, 450
Sudden death
  in aortic stenosis, 66
  hypertrophic cardiomyopathy, 131
Suker's sign, 314
Sulfapyridine, for dermatitis herpetiformis, 556
Sulfasalazine, for ankylosing spondylitis, 249
Sulindac, 522
Sulphonamides, erythema multiforme from, 443
Summation gallop, 797
Superoxide dismutase (SOD), in amyotrophic lateral sclerosis, 654
Supinator reflex, 567
  inversion, 567

Supraclavicular lymph nodes, 235
Suprascapular nerve entrapment, 602
Surviving Sepsis Campaign, 835–836
Swab, throat, Henoch–Schönlein purpura and, 455
Swallowing
  difficulties, 149
    causes of, 149
    differential diagnosis of, 150
    investigation in, 150
    management of, 150
  oesophageal phase of, 150–151
  oral phase of, 150
  stages of, 150
Swan-neck deformity, 242, 269, 270f
Sweating
  in Horner syndrome, 697
  in Parkinson's disease, 685
Sweat testing, in cystic fibrosis, 17
Sweet, R. D., 224
Sweet syndrome, 223, 223f
Sydenham's chorea, 617–618
Synacthen test, 301
Synchysis scintillans, 408
Syncope, 872
  in aortic stenosis, 63, 66
  cardiac, 127
  causes of, 873
  circumstances in, 872
  diagnosis of, 873
  electrocardiogram findings, 875–876
  episodes of, duration and frequency of, 872
  hypertrophic cardiomyopathy and, 127
  medical history in, 872
  medication history in, 872
  neurally mediated, 873–874
  preceding symptoms of, 872
  tilt table test in, 874–875
  triggers of, 872
Syndrome X, 778
Synovial fluid, 893
  in osteoarthrosis, 264
  uric acid crystals and, 258
Syphilis, 374, 388. *See also* Neurosyphilis
Syringobulbia, 586
Syringomyelia, 709
  associated abnormalities, 710
  of Charcot's joint, 712
  clinical features of, 710
  formation of, theories of, 712
  investigations of, 710
  la main succulente, 710
  management of, 712–713
  treatment of, 711–712
Syrinx, cavity of, 711
Systemic disease, 661
Systemic inflammatory response syndrome (SIRS)
    scoring, 770–771, 836
Systemic lupus erythematosus (SLE), 275, 284, 745
  causes of death, 288
  clinical features of, 284–285, 285f
  diagnostic criteria of, 286–287

drug-induced, 287
management of, 287–288
in older patients, 287
pathogenesis of, 288–289
pleural effusions and, 830
skin manifestations of, 286
in urticaria, 544*b*
Systemic mastocytosis, 547
Systemic sclerosis. *See* Scleroderma

T

T3. *See* Triiodothyronine
T4. *See* Thyroxine
Tachyarrhythmia, in emergency synchronised direct current cardioversion, 889
Tachypnoea, 3*f*
Tactile agnosia, 625–626
Taft, William Howard, 45
Takayasu's arteritis, 758–759
Tamoxifen, gynaecomastia, 342
Tandem walking test, 571, 607
Tardive dyskinesia, 685
Target-shaped lesions, erythema multiforme and, 443
Tarsal tunnel syndrome, 601
Taussig–Bing syndrome, 120
Teare, Donald, 131
Teeth, abnormalities in, 390
Telangiectasia
　hereditary haemorrhagic, 458, 459*f*
　　clinical criteria for, 460
　　complications of, 460
　lupus pernio, 479, 480*f*
　nailfold, 491
Telogen effluvium, 418
Temporal lobe, lesions of, 643*t*
Temporary external pacing
　complications of, 901
　indications, 900
　steps of, 900
Tendon reflexes, deep
　grading, 570
　lower limb, 569*f*, 583
　tetraplegia in, 714
　upper limb, 566*f*, 567
Tendon xanthoma, 558
Tension, 575
Tension pneumothorax, 862
Tension-type headache, 575
Tenth cranial nerve, testing, 565
Terry's nail, 491, 492*f*
Terry, T. L., 516
Terson syndrome, 405, 406*f*, 407
Testicular atrophy, haemochromatosis and, 179
Tetany, hypoparathyroid, acute attack of, management, 326
Tetrabenazine haloperidol, for hemiballismus, 634
Tetracycline, rosacea, 531
Tetralogy of Fallot. *See* Fallot's tetralogy
Tetraplegia, 714
　lesion localization of

　　to eighth cervical root level, 716
　　to fifth cervical root level, 715
　　to first thoracic root level, 716
　　to seventh cervical root level, 716
　　to sixth cervical root level, 715–716
Tetrathiomolybdate, 184
Thalamic stimulation, drug-resistant tremor, 723
Thalamotomy
　contralateral, for hemiballismus, 634
　drug-resistant tremor, 723
Thalidomide, 36
Therapeutic abdominal paracentesis, 897
　complications of, 898
　contraindications to, 898–899
　procedure for, 898–899
Thiazides, hypertension, 206
Thionamide, 307
Thiopurine methyltransferase, for rheumatoid arthritis, 272
Third cranial nerve
　anatomy of, 719
　examination, 564
Third cranial nerve palsy, 717
　causes of, 718
　investigation of, 718
Thompson, Richard, 158
Thomsen, AJT, 673
Thomsen's disease, 672
Thoracic outlet syndrome, 735*f*
Thoracocentesis
　complications of, 832
　for pleural effusions, 827
Thoracotomy, for pneumothorax, 862
Throat swab, Henoch–Schönlein purpura and, 455
Thrombectomy, 845
Thromboangiitis obliterans, 508
Thrombocytopenia
　bruising, 522
　microangiopathic haemocytic anaemia and, 216
Thrombocytopenic purpura, 745
　idiopathic, 522
　thrombotic, 522
Thrombolysis
　in acute stroke, 637
　indications of, 845
　in stroke, during hyperacute phase, 636
Thrombophlebitis. *See also* Phlebitis
　septic, 509
　superficial, 509
Thrombosis, Eisenmenger's syndrome and, 124–125
Thrombotic thrombocytopenic purpura (TTP), 216, 522
Thunderclap headache, 869–870
Thymectomy, in myasthenia gravis, 671
Thymoma, 671
Thyroid acropachy, 305
Thyroid bruit, 303
Thyroid dermopathy, 511, 512*f*
Thyroid examination, 302, 303*f*
Thyroid eye disease. *See* Graves' ophthalmopathy

952   INDEX

Thyroid function
    clinical signs of, 302
    screening recommendations, 511–512
Thyroid function tests
    acute non-thyroidal illness, 323
    for chronic urticaria, 545
    hypothyroidism, 322
    multinodular goitre, 316
Thyroid-stimulating antibody, 308
Thyroid-stimulating hormone (TSH)
    deficiency, 301
    isolated elevation, 321
    isolated suppression of, 306–307, 321
    pretibial myxoedema, 511
    serum, 306, 321
Thyrotoxicosis. *See also* Hyperthyroidism
    affecting bone, 308
    gynaecomastia and, 341
    pregnancy and, management of, 308
    treatment of, 307
Thyroxine (T4)
    replacement therapy, 322
    serum free, 307, 321
    therapy for multinodular goitre, 317
Tilt table test, in syncope, 874–875
Tinea pedis, 448*b*
Tinea unguium, 449
Tinel, Jules, 602
Tinel's sign, 599, 600*f*
Tissue plasminogen activator, in stroke, 637
Tizanidine, 662
Tolosa, E., 708
Tolosa–Hunt syndrome, 708
Tone. *See* Muscle tone
Tongue
    enlarged. *See* Macroglossia
    hairy leukoplakia and, 452, 453*f*
    involuntary movements, 617
Top of the basilar syndrome, 608–609
Total anterior circulation syndrome, 640
Tourniquet test, carpal tunnel syndrome, 601
Tracheal compression, multinodular goitre, 316
Tracheobronchomegaly, 12
Traction retinal detachment, 380
Transbronchial biopsy, for interstitial lung diseases, 31
Transcriptional dysregulation, 619
Transgenic mouse models, of oligodendroglial α-synucleinopathy, 667
Transient global amnesia, 764
Transient ischaemic attack, 639
Transjugular intrahepatic portosystemic stent shunt (TIPS), for ascites, 163
Transoesophageal echocardiography
    mitral regurgitation, 73
    mitral stenosis, 80
Transplanted kidney, 200. *See also* Renal transplantation
Transthoracic echocardiography
    of congestive cardiac failure, 133
    for weight loss, 141

Transudate
    exudate and, 162, 829–830
    pleural, causes for, 829–830
Transverse myelitic syndrome, 593
Trapezius muscle
    paralysis of, 738
    testing, 565
Traube, L., 62
Traube's sign, 58
Trauma
    in cauda equina syndrome, 782
    osteoarthritis, 263
    painful knee joint, 853
    to spine, in Brown-Séquard syndrome, 597
Tremors, 720
    cerebellar, 723
    classification of, 722
    drug-associated, 722
    essential, 721*f*, 723
    intention, 721–722
    neuropathic, 723
    palatal, 723
    in Parkinson's disease, 679, 681, 720, 721*f*
    pathophysiology of, 723
    physiological, 720, 723
    postural (action, kinetic), 722
    primary orthostatic, 722
    psychogenic, 723
    resting, 720
    treatment of, 723
Trichophyton interdigitale, in nail infections, 449
Trichophyton rubrum, in nail infections, 449
Trichorrhexis nodosa, 418
Trichotillomania, 418
Tricuspid annuloplasty, 115
Tricuspid regurgitation, 93
    carcinoid syndrome and, 338
    causes of, 93–94
    in Ebstein's anomaly, 113
    indications for intervention in, 94
    investigation of, 94–95
    jugular venous pulse, 94*f*
    mitral regurgitation *vs.*, 74
    pulsatile liver in, 174
Tricuspid valve replacement, 115
Trientine dihydrochloride, 184
Trigeminal neuralgia, 576
Triglycerides, serum. *See also* Hypertriglyceridaemia
    coronary artery disease and, 439
Triiodothyronine (T$_3$)
    pretibial myxoedema, 312
    serum free, 307, 321
Tripe palms, 411
Triplet repeat, diseases associated to, 619
Triptan, for migraine, 575
Tritschler, T., 795
Tropical eosinophilia, 842
Tropical spastic paraplegia, 594
Trotter syndrome, 322
Trousseau, Armand, 327, 333, 509
Trousseau's sign, 325, 508

Tryptase, serum, 548
Tschernogobow, A., 257
TSH. *See* Thyroid-stimulating hormone
Tuberculin test, 669
Tuberculous meningitis, 50
Tuberculous pericarditis, 138
Tuberin, 543
Tuberous sclerosis, 539, 540*f*, 661
  benign metastasis hypothesis, 542
  diagnostic criteria, 541–542
  genetics, 542
  management, 542
  pathogenesis, 543
  prevalence, 541
  subungual angiofibromas, 493
  subungual fibromas, 539
Tubular myopathy, X-linked, 590
Tumour necrosis factor-alpha (TNF-α), in COPD, 26
Tumour necrosis factor (TNF) antagonists, 249
Turcot, J., 507
Turcot syndrome, 506
Turner syndrome, aortic coarctation and, 787
Turner-Warwick, Dame Margaret, 32
Tylosis, 412
Type 1 diabetes
  in adults, 353
  autoimmune thyroid disease, 353
  coeliac disease, 353
  diabetic autonomic dysfunction, 353
  diagnosis of, 352
  epitope spreading, 352
  examination, 351–352
  feature of, 351–352
  genetic markers, 352
  history of, 351
  immune markers, 352
  latent autoimmune diabetes, adults, 352
  pathology, 352
Type 2 diabetes
  flash glucose monitoring, 357
  oral diabetes medications, 356
Tzanck smear, 467

U

Uhthoff's symptom, 660
Ulcerations, superficial, 456*f*
Ulcerative colitis, prognostic factors in, 153
Ulcers, mouth, 473
Ulnar claw hand, 728, 729*f*, 730
  tardy, 731
Ulnar nerve, 566*f*, 567
  affected wrist, 730
  muscles supplied by, 728–730
Ulnar nerve palsy, 728
  elbow lesions, 730
Ulnar paradox, 730
Ultrasonography
  in bilateral renal cysts, 193
  multinodular goitre, 315
  for pleural effusion, 832
  in polycystic kidney disease, 193
Ultraviolet B phototherapy, psoriasis, 520
Unsteadiness, 751
Upbeat nystagmus, 648
Upper limbs. *See also* Hands
  limb girdle dystrophy in, 649, 650*f*
  neurological examination, 566*f*
Upper motor neuron lesions
  jaw jerk, 564
  lower limb examination, 568–571
  upper limb examination, 565–568
Upper motor neuron, of seventh cranial nerve, 703, 703*f*
Uric acid crystals, 261
Urinalysis, for micturition difficulties, 582
Urinary pH, 148
Urinary tract symptom, lower, 581
Urinary urgency, in Parkinson's disease, 685
Urine dipstick, 148
Urine, Henoch–Schönlein purpura and, 454
Urticaria, 456*f*, 544, 545*f*
  chronic, 544
Urticaria pigmentosa, 547, 548*f*
Urticaria, wheal, 773*f*
Usher's disease, 403
Usual interstitial pneumonia (UIP), 28
Uveitis, anterior
  ankylosing spondylitis and, 247
  sarcoidosis and, 481
Uveoparotid fever, 703
Uvula, systolic pulsations of, 59

V

Vaccination
  Felty syndrome and, 188
  for herpes zoster, 467
Vaccine-associated paralytic poliomyelitis, 726
Valsalva, Antonio Maria, 62
Valsalva retinopathy, 604
Valve destruction, in infective endocarditis, 143
Vancomycin, for bacterial endocarditis, 142
Variceal bleeding, in cirrhosis, 168*t*
Varicose bronchiectasis, 13
Varicose veins, 550*f*
  in absence of skin changes, 551
  treatment, 550
Vascular endothelial growth factor (VEGF), 48
  inhibitors, for age-related macular degeneration, 369
Vasculitis, 455
  immune complex-mediated, 456*f*, 457
  pyoderma gangrenosum *vs*., 525
  in urticaria, 544
Vasodilators, in aortic regurgitation, 61–62
Vasopressin analogues, 813
Vasospastic conditions, 529
Vegan diet, 214
VEGF. *See* Vascular endothelial growth factor
Venetoclax, 227
Venlafaxine, 813

Venous hum, abdominal, portal venous hypertension and, 174
Venous insufficiency, chronic, 550
Venous pressure, legs, factors affecting, 551
Venous thromboembolism
 in pregnancy, 880
 superficial thrombophlebitis and, 508
Venous ulcers, 420, 549
Venous valve component, venous pressure and, 551
Ventilation perfusion scan, 844
Ventilator-acquired pneumonia, 842
Ventricular arrhythmias, Fallot's tetralogy and, 120
Ventricular biopsy, in congestive cardiac failure, 133
Ventricular infarction, 780
Ventricular septal defects (VSD), 106, 107f
 associated lesions, 108–109
 causes, 107
 complications of, 107
 diagnosis of, 106
 effect of pregnancy, 109
 investigations, 107–108
 management, 109
 surgery for, 109
 types, 108
Ventricular tachycardia (VT), hypertrophic cardiomyopathy, 129
Verapamil, for migraine, 575
Vertebral arteries, 609
Vertebrobasilar artery, 609
Verteporfin, for age-related macular degeneration, 369
Vertical nystagmus, 647, 753
Vertigo
 causes of, 751–752
 treatment of, 753
Vesicles, 456f
Vestibular neuronitis, 751–752
 clinical examination, 752
 clinical signs, 752
Vestibular nystagmus, 648
Vestibular schwannomas
 in acoustic neurofibroma, 610, 611f
 in neurofibromatosis, 498
Vestibuloocular system, 645–646
Vibration sense testing, 568
Viral exanthems, maculopapular rash and, 483
Viral hepatitis, 174
Virchow node, 236
Virchow, Rudolph, 796
Virchow triad, 794
Visual acuity testing, 563
Visual agnosia, 626
Visual evoked potentials, in multiple sclerosis, 658
Visual field defects
 bitemporal hemianopia, 596
 central scotoma, 603, 603f
 homonymous hemianopia in, 642
 papilloedema, 393
 unsteadiness and, 752
Visual fields, testing, 563

Visual loss
 in age-related macular degeneration, 366, 369–370
 in non-proliferative retinopathy, 380
 pseudoxanthoma elasticum, 516
Vital capacity, in myasthenia gravis, 669
Vitamin B$_{12}$, 658
 deficiency, 865, 865f
 treatment with, neurological lesions to, 866
Vitamin D deficiency, falls and, 344
Vitiligo, 553, 554f, 745
 associated conditions with, 553–554
 diagnosis of, 553
 histology of, 555
 management of, 555
 types of, 554
Vitiligo Area Scoring Index, 555
Vitiligo European Task Force system, 555
Vitrectomy, pars plana, 380
Vitreous haemorrhage. *See* Terson syndrome
Vitreous humour, haemorrhage and, 405
Vitreous opacities, 408
 causes of, 408
Vocal fremitus, 4, 20
Vocal resonance, 21
von Bechterew, Vladimir, 250
von Economo disease, 682
von Graefe's sign, 310
von Hebra, Ferdinand, 289, 437
von Hippel–Lindau disease, 609
von Leber, T., 38
von Recklinghausen, Friedreich Daniel, 182, 499
von Recklinghausen's disease, 498
von Volkmann, R., 731
von Willebrand disease, 216
von Willebrand factor defects, in aortic stenosis, 68–69
von Willebrand's disease, 216, 522
V/Q scanning, for non-massive pulmonary embolism, 880–881
Vulvovaginitis, 462

W
Waddling gait, 584
Wallace, Angus, 500
Wallenberg's syndrome, 732
 vessel, 733
Wallenburg, Adolf, 733
Walton, John, 651
Warfarin, HEMORR$_2$HAGES score, 795
Warm-up phenomenon, in myotonia, 672
Wartenberg's sign, 568, 729f
Watermelon stomach, 917
Waterston shunt, 118
Watson syndrome, 99
Weber–Christian disease, 447
Weber, F Parkes, 461, 538
Weber-Liel, F. E., 572
Weber, Sir HD, 447
Weber's syndrome, 733
Weber's test, 565
Wedge biopsy, of erythema nodosum, 446

Wegener's granulomatosis, 292
Weight loss, 139
  investigation for, 141–144
  obesity and, 348–349
Weil's disease, presentation of, 170
Weiss, Nathan, 327
Welander's distal myopathy, 677
Weller, Thomas H., 727
Werdnig–Hoffman's disease, 653
Wernicke, K., 648, 689
Wernicke's area, 623–624, 749
Wernicke's encephalopathy, 165, 167
Wheezing, 2
  asthma and, 2
Whiplash, neck pain and, 249
Whipple, George, 866–867
White atrophy, venous ulcers, 549
White cell count, in CSF, 738
Whitlow, herpetic, 463, 463f
Wickham, L. F., 473
Wickham's striae, 471
Wiggers, Carl, 848
Wilks, Sir Samuel, 671
Willan–Plumbe syndrome. *See* Psoriasis
Williams–Campbell syndrome, 11, 13
Williamson, O. K., 863
Williamson sign, 863
Williams, Roger, 747
Williams syndrome, 68–69, 99
William's theory, of syringomyelia, 712
Willis, Thomas, 671
Wilson, Samuel A. K., 185
Wilson's disease, 183, 371, 682
  biochemical changes in, 184
  clinical stages of, 185
  diagnosis of, 183
  inheritance of, 184
  pathophysiology of, 184
  radiographic features of, 185
  treatment of, 184

Withering, William, 811
Wolff–Chaikoff effect, 308
Wolff–Parkinson–White syndrome, 114
  Ebstein's anomaly and, 113, 114f
Woltman's sign, 322
Wood, Paul, 126, 848
Wood's lamp examination, 554–555
World Federation of neurological surgeons grading, 870
Woronoff's ring, 517
Wrist extension test, 601
Wrist splints, carpal tunnel syndrome, 601

X

Xanthelasma, 556, 557f, 744
Xanthochromia, 869, 896
Xanthomata
  conditions of, 438
  eruptive, 438, 439f, 495, 558, 559f
  histology of, 504
  palmar, 503, 504f, 558, 559f
  planar, 559f
  tendon, 558, 559f
  tuberoeruptive, 559f
  types of, 558
X-linked ichthyosis, 468–469, 469f
X-linked spinal muscular atrophy, 653
X-rays, diagnostic. *See* Radiography

Y

Yacoub, Sir Magdi, 19, 135
Yeasts, in nail infections, 449
Yellow nail syndrome, 13
Young syndrome, 11, 13

Z

Zinc, 369
Zollinger–Ellison syndrome, 328, 339

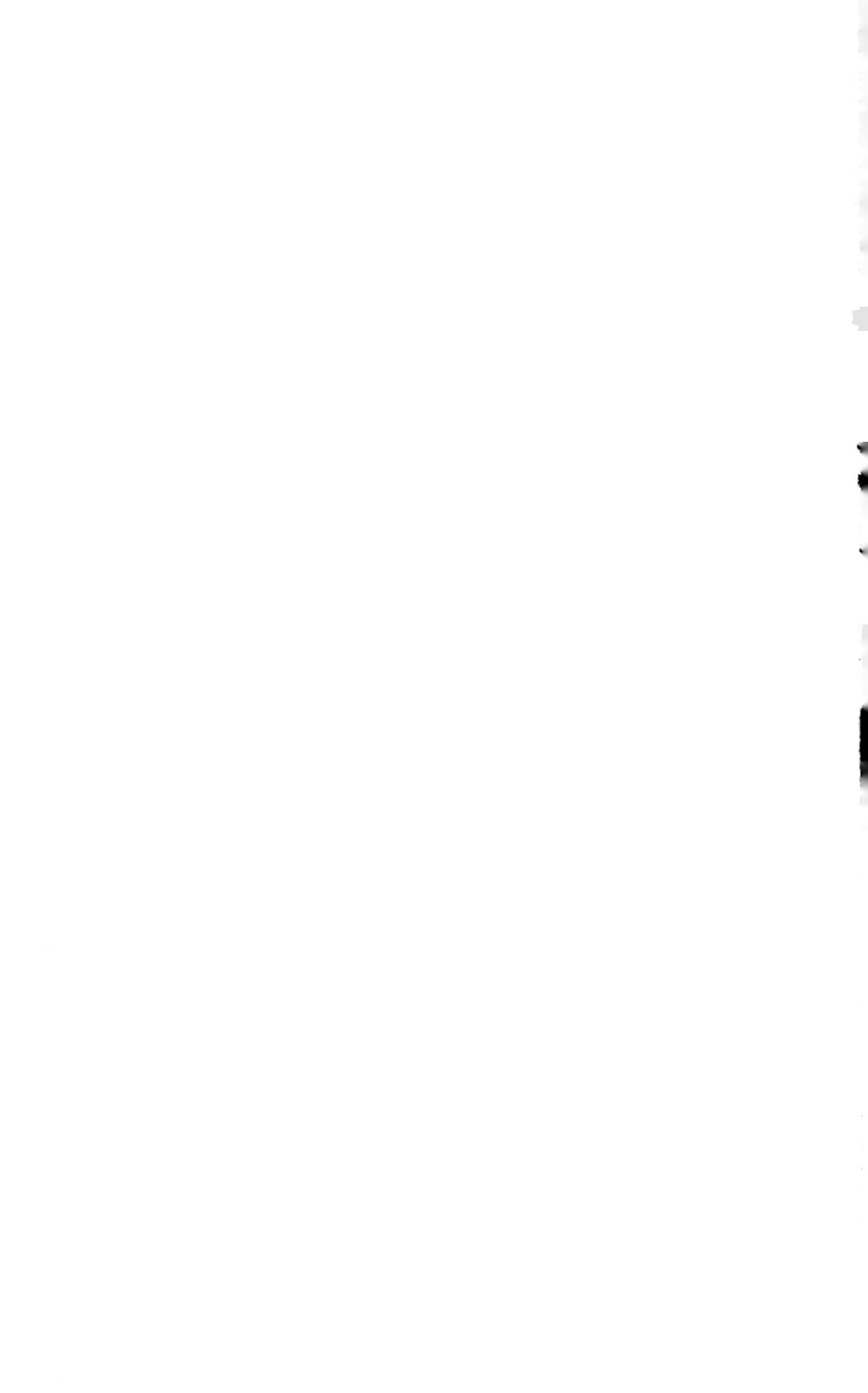